CRITICAL CARE MEDICINE

John M. Luce, M.D.

Associate Professor of Medicine and Anesthesia,
University of California, San Francisco;
Associate Director, Medical-Surgical Intensive Care Unit,
San Francisco General Hospital,
San Francisco, California

David J. Pierson, M.D.

Professor of Medicine,
University of Washington;
Medical Director, Respiratory Care Department,
Harborview Medical Center,
Seattle, Washington

with

Contributors from the
University of California, San Francisco, and the
University of Washington, Seattle

Illustrations by Phyllis Wood

1988

W. B. SAUNDERS COMPANY
Harcourt Brace Jovanovich, Inc.

Philadelphia   London   Toronto   Montreal   Sydney   Tokyo

W. B. SAUNDERS COMPANY
Harcourt Brace Jovanovich, Inc.

The Curtis Center
Independence Square West
Philadelphia, PA 19106

Library of Congress Cataloging-in-Publication Data

Luce, John M.

Critical care medicine.

1. Critical care medicine.   I. Pierson, David J.
   II. Title.   [DNLM: 1. Critical Care.   WX 218 L935c]

RC86.7.L83   1988   616'.028   87–26589

ISBN 0–7216–1711–5

Editor: John Dyson
Designer: W. B. Saunders Staff
Production Manager: Carolyn Naylor
Manuscript Editor: W. B. Saunders Staff
Indexer: Ellen Murray

Critical Care Medicine   ISBN 0–7216–1711–5

Last digit is the print number: 9 8 7 6 5 4 3 2 1

Contributors

Wendell P. Fleet, M.D.
Associate Professor of Medicine,
University of Washington;
Attending Physician, Nephrology Section,
Harborview Medical Center,
Seattle, Washington

Nora F. Goldschlager, M.D.
Clinical Professor of Medicine,
University of California, San Francisco;
Director, Coronary Care Unit, and
Director, Electrocardiographic Laboratory,
San Francisco General Hospital,
San Francisco, California

James H. Grendell, M.D.
Associate Professor of Medicine and Physiology,
University of California, San Francisco;
Director, Gastroenterology Research Laboratory
San Francisco General Hospital,
San Francisco, California

Michael S. Hickey, M.D.
Assistant Clinical Professor of Surgery,
University of California, San Francisco;
Surgical Director, Nutritional Support Service,
San Francisco General Hospital,
San Francisco, California

Judith A. Luce, M.D.
Assistant Clinical Professor of Medicine,
University of California, San Francisco;
Director, Inpatient Oncology Service,
San Francisco General Hospital,
San Francisco, California

Susan M. Ott, M.D.
Assistant Professor of Medicine,
University of Washington;
Attending Physician, Nephrology Section,
Harborview Medical Center,
Seattle, Washington

Kristin Weaver, R.N., M.S.
Head Nurse, Nutritional Support Service,
San Francisco General Hospital,
San Francisco, California

D. Scott Weigle, M.D.
Assistant Professor of Medicine,
University of Washington;
Attending Physician, Section of Metabolism,
Endocrinology and Nutrition,
Harborview Medical Center,
Seattle, Washington

Richard A. Zager, M.D.
Professor of Medicine,
University of Washington;
Head, Nephrology Section,
Harborview Medical Center,
Seattle, Washington

Preface

Critical Care Medicine is no more—and no less—than medicine practiced in intensive or critical care units. Such units were first created in the 1950s to group hospitalized patients with imminently life-threatening problems, especially those related to single or multiple organ system dysfunction or failure. Intensive care units (ICUs) can now be found in almost all large and medium-sized American hospitals. In general, the units offer a high nurse-to-patient ratio, ready access to physicians, and the services of respiratory therapists and other skilled health professionals. The units also provide a variety of diagnostic and therapeutic techniques ranging from electrocardiographic and hemodynamic monitoring to mechanical ventilation and acute hemodialysis.

As ICUs have proliferated in the United States and other developed countries, the kind of medicine practiced in them has evolved almost into a separate speciality. Critical care medicine necessarily embraces physicians from many parent disciplines, including medicine, surgery, anesthesia, and pediatrics, who spend much, if not most, of their time in the ICU. In addition, as noted earlier, nurses, respiratory therapists, and other health professionals are vital constituents of the critical care team. All these clinicians must have special training, experience, and competence in managing the complex problems of their patients. They must develop mechanical skills such as endotracheal intubation and the placement of intravascular catheters. They must interpret the data obtained by many kinds of monitoring devices, and they must integrate this information with their knowledge of the pathophysiology of disease.

This book has been written to help physicians, nurses, and respiratory therapists manage critically ill patients. Although our concern is for the "whole patient," the book is divided into sections on organ systems to facilitate its use. Each section contains chapters that are devoted to the diseases commonly encountered in ICUs. Whenever possible, each disease is discussed in terms of its definition, pathophysiology, diagnosis, management, and outcome. Certain chapters within the organ system sections cover specific monitoring techniques and therapies; these are generally discussed in terms of their indications, contraindications, techniques, discontinuation, and possible complications. Each chapter concludes with a list of recommended readings. We and the other contributors hope that this organized approach will make the book a ready reference to the growing field of critical care.

John M. Luce, M.D.
David J. Pierson, M.D.

Contents

SECTION III
Pulmonary Disorders

SECTION IV
Renal and Fluid and Electrolyte Disorders 256

x Contents

Physiologic Principles of Critical Care

1. Overview of Respiratory Failure*

John M. Luce

David J. Pierson

DISORDERS OF TISSUE OXYGENATION

Critically ill patients usually manifest failure or dysfunction of one or more major organ systems. Although the degree of failure differs from patient to patient, as does the number of organ systems involved, the most common underlying abnormality is inadequacy of tissue oxygenation. This inadequacy is due to cardiovascular, pulmonary, hematologic, or other problems alone or in combination. It results in neurologic disturbance, diminished renal function, inadequate liver metabolism, or other abnormalities. It yields significant changes in systemic arterial blood gases, regional blood flow, urine output, or other variables. It is treated with transfusions, supplemental oxygen, inotropic drugs, or other agents. Whatever its cause and possible correction, impaired tissue oxygenation is the most important and time-consuming part of critical care.

Disorders of tissue oxygenation may be lumped together physiologically as abnormalities of respiration. In its totality, the term respiration refers to the exchange of oxygen (O_2) and carbon dioxide (CO_2) between an animal, such as man, and the environment. This process is also called extracellular respiration because it includes the entire body. Within individual cells, respiration involves the chemical combustion of O_2 and foodstuffs—carbohydrate, protein, and fat—to generate the energy necessary to run the complex cellular machinery. Carbon dioxide and water are byproducts of this vital reaction.

Human respiration may be divided arbitrarily into four sequential steps. These include: (1) ventilation, the exchange of respiratory gases between the atmosphere and the lungs; (2) pulmonary gas exchange, in which O_2 and CO_2 cross the alveolar-capillary membrane in opposite directions, and mixed venous blood returning from the peripheral tissues

---

*Portions of this chapter appeared, in different form, as Pierson DJ, Luce JM: Cardiopulmonary components of respiratory failure. In Fallat RJ, Luce JM (eds): Cardiopulmonary Critical Care Management. New York, Churchill Livingstone, Inc., 1987.

becomes oxygenated as it traverses the lungs; (3) gas transport, the conveying of arterial blood from the lungs to the peripheral tissues via the systemic circulation and of mixed venous blood with a high CO_2 tension back to the pulmonary circulation; and (4) tissue gas exchange, in which O_2 is extracted from arterial blood by the tissues, which release CO_2 for transport back to the lungs.

In theory, impairment in any or all of these steps could result in respiratory failure. However, that term has traditionally been used to describe an abnormally high systemic arterial CO_2 tension ($PaCO_2$) or an abnormally low O_2 tension (PaO_2) or both. Specific levels of $PaCO_2$ and PaO_2 differ among investigators and depend in part on the altitude at which these variables are analyzed. Nevertheless, most would agree that respiratory failure is present at any altitude if the PaO_2 is 50 mm Hg or less or if the $PaCO_2$ is 50 mm Hg or more or both.

This traditional definition of respiratory failure evolved at a time when systemic arterial blood gas analysis was introduced to clinical practice. By focusing on blood gas abnormalities, the definition reminded clinicians of the importance of pulmonary function in many diseases. However, it did not grant equal status to the cardiovascular, hematologic, and other systems, and it did not stress the utility of laboratory tests other than systemic arterial blood gas analysis. Such tests include analysis of pulmonary arterial blood, determination of hemoglobin concentration, and measurement of cardiac output, among others. They are commonly employed in critical care units, where patients have complicated problems involving many organ systems.

Because of these limitations of the traditional definition of respiratory failure, this condition can best be regarded as a disturbance in any or all of the steps of respiration that is sufficiently severe to threaten life. At the same time, clinicians should focus on tissue oxygenation and the four forms of respiratory failure that can disturb it: (1) failure of ventilation, (2) failure of arterial oxygenation, (3) failure of O_2 transport to the tissues, and (4) failure of the tissues to use the O_2 available to them (Table 1–1).

DETERMINANTS OF TISSUE OXYGENATION

Tissue O_2 utilization is the same as the body's consumption of O_2 ($\dot{V}O_2$). This variable is defined physiologically by the Fick equation, which states that $\dot{V}O_2$ is equal to the amount of O_2 transported to the tissues, the systemic O_2 transport ($\dot{D}O_2$), minus the amount of O_2 returned to the lungs. Systemic oxygen transport is the product of the O_2 content of systemic arterial blood (CaO_2) and the cardiac output ($\dot{Q}_T$); thus, $\dot{D}O_2 = CaO_2 \times \dot{Q}_T$. The CaO_2 is equal to the normally large amount of O_2 carried by hemoglobin (1.34 ml O_2/g hemoglobin $\times$ g hemoglobin/100 ml blood

TABLE 1–1. DISORDERS OF TISSUE OXYGENATION

CONDITION	DEFINITION	CLINICAL EXAMPLES	LABORATORY ABNORMALITIES
Ventilatory failure	Abnormal CO_2 elimination by the lungs	Sedative drug overdosage, chronic obstructive pulmonary disease	High $PaCO_2$
Failure of arterial oxygenation	Abnormal O_2 uptake by the lungs	Pneumonia	Low PaO_2
Failure of O_2 transport	Limited O_2 delivery to peripheral tissues so that aerobic metabolism cannot be maintained	Cardiogenic shock, anemia, carbon monoxide poisoning	Low $P\bar{v}O_2$, $S\bar{v}O_2$, $C\bar{v}O_2$, lactic acidosis
Failure of O_2 uptake	Inability of tissue to extract O_2 from blood and use it for aerobic metabolism	Cyanide poisoning, septic shock	High $P\bar{v}O_2$, $S\bar{v}O_2$, $C\bar{v}O_2$, lactic acidosis

$PaCO_2$ = systemic arterial carbon dioxide tension; PaO_2 = systemic arterial oxygen tension; $P\bar{v}O_2$ = mixed venous oxygen tension; $S\bar{v}O_2$ = mixed venous oxygen saturation; $C\bar{v}O_2$ = mixed venous oxygen content.

$\times$ arterial O_2 saturation [SaO_2]) plus the normally small amount of O_2 dissolved in blood (0.003 ml O_2/100 ml blood $\times$ PaO_2). The amount of O_2 returned to the lung is the product of the O_2 content of mixed venous blood ($C\bar{v}O_2$) and $\dot{Q}_T$. Thus, $\dot{V}O_2 = \dot{Q}_T \times (CaO_2 - C\bar{v}O_2)$ or $C(a - \bar{v})O_2$.

Implicit in the Fick equation are two assumptions: (1) O_2 demand by the tissues ($\dot{V}O_2$) determines O_2 supply to them ($\dot{D}O_2$), and (2) an increase in $\dot{V}O_2$ will normally be met by an increase in $\dot{Q}_T$, $C(a - \bar{v})O_2$, or both, as supply meets demand. In keeping with the latter assumption, the $C(a - \bar{v})O_2$ and the $C\bar{v}O_2$ have been used as indicators of the adequacy of tissue oxygenation. Thus, oxygenation is considered adequate if the $C(a - \bar{v})O_2$ is near the normal level of 5 ml O_2/dl of blood and the $C\bar{v}O_2$ is appropriately 15 ml O_2/dl. Even more popular indicators are the PO_2 of mixed venous blood ($P\bar{v}O_2$) and the mixed venous O_2 saturation ($S\bar{v}O_2$) obtained by pulmonary artery catheterization. It is generally accepted that a marked decline in $P\bar{v}O_2$ from the normal level of 40 mm Hg or a $S\bar{v}O_2$ much below 75 percent signifies inadequate tissue oxygenation because it is believed that the peripheral tissues are extracting more O_2 from their diminished supply of oxygenated blood. Assuming that CaO_2 remains normal, the inadequacy of tissue oxygenation is attributed to the $\dot{Q}_T$ in most instances. As a result, the $P\bar{v}O_2$ and $S\bar{v}O_2$ are frequently used to estimate the $\dot{Q}_T$, especially when other techniques are not available.

Although using mixed venous blood gas values to approximate $\dot{Q}_T$

may be appropriate in many patients, this approach cannot be employed in everyone. Indeed, recent studies have shown that $\dot{V}O_2$ is determined by $\dot{D}O_2$ rather than vice versa at critically low levels of $\dot{D}O_2$ in certain patients with sepsis and the adult respiratory distress syndrome (ARDS). As a result, the $C(a - \bar{v})O_2$ may not vary with changes in $\dot{Q}_T$ to the degree expected if $\dot{V}O_2$ remains constant. The mechanisms accounting for these findings are not clear, although alterations in regular blood flow or O_2 extraction may be responsible, as will be discussed. The important point for clinicians to remember is that the $C\bar{v}O_2$, $P\bar{v}O_2$, and $S\bar{v}O_2$ values cannot be used to assure the adequacy of tissue oxygenation in all individuals.

Ventilatory Failure

Ventilation, the first step of respiration, involves the exchange of O_2 and CO_2 between the environment and the lungs. Although respiratory gases are inspired for this purpose, not all the gas that enters the lungs crosses the alveolar-capillary membrane and participates in respiration. Total minute ventilation ($\dot{V}E$) can be divided into that portion of gas actually exposed to the membrane, the alveolar ventilation ($\dot{V}A$), and that portion not available for gas exchange, the dead space ventilation ($\dot{V}D$). The CO_2 produced by the body ($\dot{V}CO_2$) during respiration is removed almost entirely by $\dot{V}A$ and is directly dependent upon it for excretion. This is expressed by the alveolar ventilation equation: $\dot{V}CO_2 = PACO_2/\dot{V}A = PACO_2/(\dot{V}E - \dot{V}D)$, in which $PACO_2$ refers to the tension of CO_2 in the alveoli.

Because equilibration of CO_2 is normally complete across the alveolar-capillary membrane, the tension of CO_2 in the alveoli and in systemic arterial blood is the same, that is, $PACO_2$ is equal to $PaCO_2$. Thus, $PaCO_2 = \dot{V}CO_2/\dot{V}A$, and changes in $PaCO_2$ reflect the adequacy of $\dot{V}A$ to meet the body's metabolic needs. Although $\dot{V}A$ cannot be predicted by physical examination or measured easily, $PaCO_2$ can be determined by systemic arterial blood gas analysis. An elevation of $PaCO_2$ above the normal level of 40 mm Hg (at sea level) is called hypoventilation. An elevation of $PaCO_2$ to 50 mm Hg or more constitutes ventilatory failure.

Although chronic ventilatory failure is associated with certain physiologic abnormalities, this condition is tolerated by many patients. This is not true of acute increases in $PaCO_2$, which are potentially life-threatening for three reasons: (1) the CO_2 not excreted by the lungs is converted into carbonic acid, which depresses the pH below its normal level of 7.40, causing respiratory acidosis, and may precipitate fatal dysrhythmias and organ dysfunction; (2) an increase in $PaCO_2$ is accompanied by a decrease in PaO_2, as predicted by the alveolar gas equation discussed later; and (3) acute elevations of $PaCO_2$ cause an increase in cerebral blood flow (and thereby intracranial pressure) through cerebral vasodilatation.

The alveolar ventilation equation predicts that three mechanisms can lead, individually or in combination, to ventilatory failure: (1) increased $\dot{V}CO_2$, (2) increased $\dot{V}D$, and (3) decreased $\dot{V}A$ (or $\dot{V}E$). Increased $\dot{V}CO_2$ from fever or other hypermetabolic states rarely causes ventilatory failure by itself but may contribute to such failure in patients who cannot increase $\dot{V}E$. The same is true of increased $\dot{V}D$, which may represent more than half of $\dot{V}E$ in some patients with pulmonary embolism (PE) and other forms of pulmonary vascular disease. Decreased $\dot{V}A$, the most common cause of ventilatory failure, may result from disorders of any part or parts of the ventilatory pump: the ventilatory control center in the brainstem, the nerves that supply the respiratory muscles, the muscles themselves, the chest wall, the airways, or the lung parenchyma. The purest form of ventilatory failure is narcotic or sedative drug overdose, which reduces $\dot{V}A$ by depressing the brainstem ventilatory control center. Alveolar ventilation is decreased primarily by airflow obstruction in patients with chronic obstructive pulmonary disease (COPD).

Monitoring patients with ventilatory failure usually requires only the analysis of systemic arterial blood gases at appropriate intervals. The treatment of ventilatory failure involves normalizing $\dot{V}CO_2$ or $\dot{V}D$ if these variables are elevated and, most often, normalizing $\dot{V}A$. Patients whose $\dot{V}CO_2$ is increased by fever should receive antipyretics, for example. Although $\dot{V}D$ can rarely be reduced to normal in such patients, its further increase may be prevented by, say, anticoagulation in patients with PE. Normalization of $\dot{V}A$ can be accomplished by pharmacologic reversal of narcotic or sedative drugs in patients with ventilatory control center depression. Other measures such as the administration of bronchodilators or ventilatory stimulants may be necessary in COPD patients. If these measures fail, mechanical ventilation may be required to normalize $\dot{V}A$.

Failure of Arterial Oxygenation

The alveolar PO_2 (PaO_2) is determined by (1) the PO_2 in inspired gas (PiO_2), corrected for water vapor; (2) the alveolar PCO_2 ($PaCO_2$), for which the $PaCO_2$ can be substituted; and (3) the respiratory quotient (R), which is the ratio of $\dot{V}CO_2$ and $\dot{V}O_2$ and depends upon the foodstuff being metabolized. This relationship is spelled out in the alveolar gas equation: $PaO_2 = PiO_2$ corrected for water vapor $- PaCO_2/R$. Assuming a normal corrected PiO_2 of 150 mm Hg at sea level, a normal $PaCO_2$ of 40 mm Hg, and an R of 0.8, the normal PaO_2 at sea level is 100 mm Hg.

During its passage through the pulmonary circulation, mixed venous blood with a low PO_2 is exposed to alveolar gas with a high PO_2.

Pulmonary capillary blood exposed to alveolar gas with a given PO_2 equilibrates with that PO_2; for example, the PO_2 of capillary blood exposed to a normal P_{AO_2} of 100 mm Hg is, itself, 100 mm Hg. Before the capillary blood leaves the left atrium, however, it mixes with a small amount of blood, including that from the bronchial veins, that has bypassed the pulmonary circulation. The addition of this unoxygenated mixed venous blood causes the PaO_2 to be lower than the P_{AO_2}; this difference, the $P(A - a)O_2$, should be less than 20 mm Hg in normal adults. When combined with the alveolar gas equation, this information yields the following equation: $PaO_2 = P_{AO_2} - 20$ mm Hg $= P_{IO_2}$ (corrected for water vapor) $- PaCO_2/R$.

From this equation, it follows that the PaO_2 can fall below the normal adult minimum of 80 mm Hg at sea level if (1) P_{IO_2} decreases, (2) $PaCO_2$ increases, or (3) $P(A - a)O_2$ increases. A decrease in P_{IO_2} might occur during a fire, when O_2 is consumed. An increase in $PaCO_2$ (hypoventilation) occurs during ventilatory failure. Increases in $P(A - a)O_2$ are due either to (1) diffusion limitation, which is seen during extreme exercise at high altitude, (2) ventilation-perfusion mismatching, as occurs with COPD, and (3) intrapulmonary shunt, as happens in diseases like pneumonia or ARDS in which the alveoli are filled with fluid and mixed venous blood cannot be oxygenated. A decrease in PaO_2 to 50 mm Hg or less by any of these mechanisms is called failure of arterial oxygenation.

As is true of ventilatory failure, failure of arterial oxygenation is both diagnosed and monitored by systemic arterial blood gas analysis. Treatment likewise involves normalization of the physiologic variables involved: P_{IO_2}, $PaCO_2$, or $P(A - a)O_2$. Supplemental O_2 can correct the P_{IO_2}. Correction of $PaCO_2$ was discussed earlier under the subject of Ventilatory Failure. Normalization of $P(A - a)O_2$ can only be accomplished by reversing underlying disease processes such as pneumonia and ARDS. Pending such reversal, administering O_2 at a high P_{IO_2} or reducing atelectasis and redistributing lung water with positive end-expiratory pressure (PEEP) are generally required.

Failure of Oxygen Transport

Although the PaO_2 is used to assess the adequacy of systemic arterial oxygenation, clinicians should remember that it primarily reflects the concentration and kinetic energy of O_2 molecules and hence their tendency to travel by diffusion and enter into chemical reactions. As noted earlier, the actual amount of O_2 in systemic arterial blood, the O_2 content (CaO_2), is equal to the amount of O_2 carried by hemoglobin (1.34 ml O_2/g hemoglobin $\times$ g hemoglobin/100 ml blood $\times$ SaO_2) plus the amount of O_2 dissolved in blood (0.003 ml O_2/100 ml blood $\times$ PaO_2). Assuming a normal hemoglobin concentration of 15 g/dl, a PaO_2 of nearly 100 mm Hg and an SaO_2 of 97 percent, the CaO_2 is approximately 20 ml O_2/dl blood.

The relationship between SaO_2 and PaO_2 depends on the shape of the oxyhemoglobin dissociation curve, illustrated in Figure 1–1. Although the position of the curve is affected by the functional status of hemoglobin and its affinity for O_2, these conditions are not always considered during systemic arterial blood gas analysis. Indeed, the SaO_2 is often derived mathematically from the PaO_2 in such circumstances under the assumption that the oxyhemoglobin curve has a normal configuration. Yet its configuration is not normal in many critically ill patients. Alkalemia and hypothermia will shift the curve to the left for example, increasing the SaO_2 for a given PaO_2 but inhibiting O_2 release to the tissues. On the other hand, acidemia and hyperthermia will shift the curve to the right, decreasing the SaO_2 for a given PaO_2 but making more O_2 available for intracellular metabolism.

In addition, clinicians should recall that although the CaO_2 indicates the amount of O_2 carried in blood, it does not necessarily reflect the amount of O_2 transported to the tissues. This is because, as noted earlier, tissue O_2 transport ($\dot{D}O_2$) depends not only on the CaO_2 but also on the cardiac output ($\dot{Q}_T$): $\dot{D}O_2 = CaO_2 \times \dot{Q}_T$. Because $\dot{Q}_T$ equals approximately

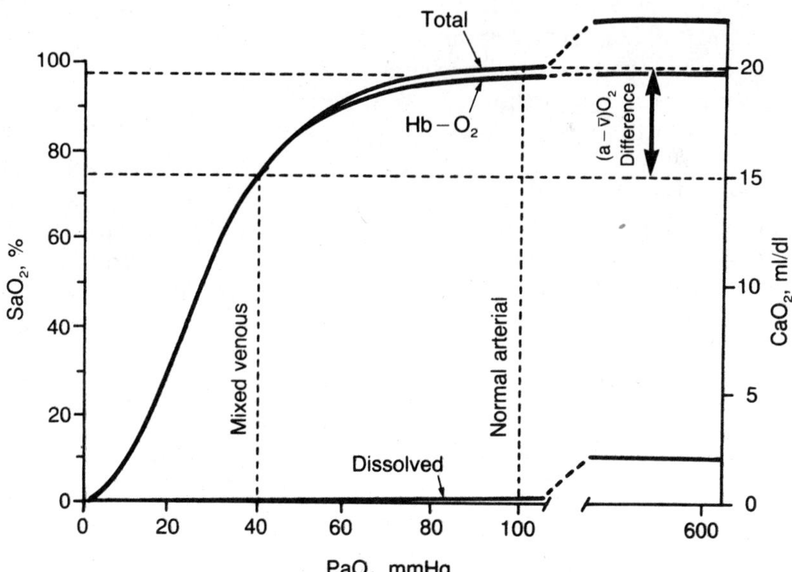

FIGURE 1–1. Oxyhemoglobin dissociation curve. See text for explanation. (Reproduced, with permission, from Luce JM, Tyler ML, Pierson DJ: Intensive Respiratory Care. Philadelphia, W. B. Saunders Co., 1984, p. 26.)

5 L/min in health, $\dot{D}O_2$ is approximately 20 ml O_2/dl blood $\times$ 5 L/min, or 1 L O_2/min. The actual $\dot{D}O_2$ in a given patient can be calculated by multiplying the CaO_2 by the $\dot{Q}_T$, which can be determined by the thermodilution technique during pulmonary artery catheterization.

Cardiac output is the product of heart rate (HR) and stroke volume (SV). Normally SV is the dominant variable, with HR changing little unless required to by stress or exercise. However, HR may become an important factor in disease states. In such circumstances it also is helpful to analyze SV into the three components that govern it: (1) preload, the length of ventricular muscle fibers at end-diastole, which is equated with end-diastolic volume and approximated by end-diastolic pressure; (2) afterload, the wall tension developed by the ventricle to eject blood, which is approximated by the vascular resistance of the circulation into which the ventricle is emptying; and (3) contractility, the inotropic state of the ventricular muscle fibers, which is inferred by the velocity of circumferential muscle fiber shortening and by other means.

Failure of O_2 transport may be caused by any process that reduces CaO_2 or $\dot{Q}T$, or both. Among the most common causes of a reduction in CaO_2 is failure of arterial oxygenation, which is manifested by low PaO_2. Profound anemia also reduces the CaO_2 by depressing the hemoglobin concentration rather than the PaO_2. Carbon monoxide (CO) poisoning, which also does not alter the PaO_2, reduces the CaO_2 by two mechanisms: (1) Because of its greater affinity for CO than O_2, circulating hemoglobin is unable to carry O_2, creating a situation similar to severe anemia. (2) In the presence of CO, the oxyhemoglobin dissociation curve is left-shifted, making less O_2 available to the tissues.

Depression of $\dot{Q}_T$ is the most common cause of failure of O_2 transportation. Such depression results from alterations either in HR, as may occur with brady- or tachydysrhythmias, or in SV. Hypovolemic shock is an example of failure of O_2 transport due to deficiency of preload (in addition to deficiency of CaO_2 due to anemia if red blood cells have been lost). In massive PE, obstruction of the main pulmonary arteries by clot increases right ventricular afterload and prevents blood from flowing through the lungs. Cardiogenic shock is characterized by an increase in preload, a decrease in contractility, and a compensatory increase in left ventricular afterload that imposes an additional burden on the failing left ventricle.

Although systemic arterial blood gas values are helpful in diagnosing and monitoring failure of arterial oxygenation in patients with failure of O_2 transport, they provide little information about CaO_2 and none about $\dot{Q}_T$. However, pulmonary arterial catheterization may provide key data regarding $\dot{Q}_T$ and $C\bar{v}O_2$. Normally, the $C\bar{v}O_2$ is 15 ml O_2/dl, the $P\bar{v}O_2$ is 40 mm hg, and the $S\bar{v}O_2$ is 75 percent, as noted earlier. In general, failure of O_2 transport is said to be present when the $C\bar{v}O_2$ is less than 10 ml O_2/

dl, the $P\bar{v}O_2$ less than 30 mm Hg, and the $S\bar{v}O_2$ less than 60 percent. The absolute values are less important than the downward trend in the variables. This trend is paralleled by an elevation of serum lactate that reflects anaerobic metabolism. It often correlates with decreased mentation, reduced urine output, and other signs of inadequate tissue perfusion.

Failure of arterial oxygenation is treated by normalizing CaO_2 and $\dot{Q}_T$. In anemic patients, this involves red blood cell transfusions or, as a stopgap measure, increasing the PIO_2 so that more O_2 is dissolved in plasma. Carbon monoxide poisoning is also treated with O_2, which drives CO off hemoglobin molecules so that they can transport O_2. Depression of $\dot{Q}_T$ can be reversed by reestablishing an adequate HR and SV. This means treating dysrhythmias, providing preload in the form of intravenous fluids or red blood cells when necessary for hypovolemia, reducing right ventricular afterload in patients with PE, and reducing left ventricular preload and afterload and improving contractility in patients with cardiogenic shock.

Failure of Oxygen Uptake

As noted earlier, the Fick equation implies that $\dot{D}O_2$ is established by tissue needs. Similarly, it is correctly assumed in most clinical settings that tissue O_2 extraction and utilization will progress normally once sufficient O_2 is delivered to the tissues. The tissues appear to insure adequate O_2 delivery by the release of vasoactive substances that regulate regional blood flow. Although shifts in the oxyhemoglobin dissociation curve also affect O_2 extraction, they are outweighed by regional blood flow alterations in most persons.

Despite normal assumptions, situations exist in which the peripheral uptake of O_2 is impaired and $\dot{V}O_2$ markedly decreases. Among these situations is cyanide (CN) poisoning, a condition characterized by disruption of intracellular respiration through the reaction of cyanide with the iron in cytochrome oxidase. Patients with CN poisoning have a normal PaO_2, SaO_2, CaO_2, and $\dot{D}O_2$ but cannot use O_2 for aerobic metabolism. Blood returning to the heart from the tissues thus has an abnormally high $P\bar{v}O_2$, $S\bar{v}O_2$, and $C\bar{v}O_2$ in the face of lactic acidosis. In general, failure of O_2 uptake is present when such acidosis is present and the $C\bar{v}O_2$ is greater than 18 ml O_2/dl, the $P\bar{v}O_2$ greater than 60 mm Hg, and the $S\bar{v}O_2$ greater than 80 percent. Again, the absolute values are less important than the upward trend in the variables.

The most clinically important cause of failure of O_2 uptake is septic shock associated with ARDS, as noted earlier. The latter condition is characterized by increased pulmonary microvascular permeability that leads to the formation of pulmonary edema at low intravascular pressures.

In combination with diffuse atelectasis, the edema produces severe hypoxemia that is usually treated with mechanical ventilation and PEEP. Bacterial sepsis, with or without lung involvement, causes renal and other organ system dysfunction that is complicated by poor tissue perfusion. Yet patients in septic shock usually manifest a high $\dot{Q}_T$ and increases in $P\bar{v}O_2$, $S\bar{v}O_2$, and $C\bar{v}O_2$. These findings suggest either that the O_2 in systemic arterial blood is shunted by the tissues or that they cannot extract it, owing to some circulating toxin. Because a disturbance in regional blood flow is the more likely mechanism, septic shock is considered a form of distributive shock.

As noted earlier, the low $\dot{V}O_2$ in patients with sepsis and ARDS seems to result from a reduced $\dot{D}O_2$ and not vice versa. The exact level of $\dot{D}O_2$ at which $\dot{V}O_2$ falls varies from patient to patient, but in general it is around 9 ml O_2/kg/min. Below this level, mixed venous blood values may not accurately reflect the adequacy of tissue oxygenation in patients with sepsis and ARDS, as noted earlier. If the $C\bar{v}O_2$, $P\bar{v}O_2$, and $S\bar{v}O_2$ begin to fall rather than remaining elevated in patients with septic shock, another insult such as left ventricular failure may have been superimposed.

Implications for Monitoring

Given the limitations of following the $P\bar{v}O_2$, $S\bar{v}O_2$, and $C\bar{v}O_2$ in certain patients, what is the optimal indicator of tissue oxygenation? Some day clinicians may be able to monitor the intracellular PO_2 and other metabolic variables with miniature electrodes. Alternatively, they may determine tissue activity or performance through measurements of lactate levels from key tissue beds as reflections of aerobic metabolism or with sophisticated tests of brain, heart, and other organ function. As yet, these tests are not generally available, even in a research setting. Until they are, clinicians must assess all physiologic variables and clinical data that they can now obtain with catheters and other devices in concert with simple bedside observation, including skin temperature and neurologic examination.

RECOMMENDED READING

Comroe JH, Batelho S: The unreliability of cyanosis in the recognition of arterial anoxemia. Am J Med Sci 214:1, 1947.

Danek SJ, Lynch JP, Weg JG, et al: The dependence of oxygen uptake on oxygen delivery in the adult respiratory distress syndrome. Am Rev Respir Dis 122:387, 1980.

Luce JM: The cardiovascular effects of mechanical ventilation and positive end-expiratory pressure. JAMA 252:807, 1984.

Mithoefer JD, Bossman OG, Thibeault DW, et al: The clinical estimation of alveolar ventilation. Am Rev Respir Dis 98:868, 1968.

Mohsenifer Z, Goldbach P, Tashkin DP, et al: Relationship between O_2 delivery and O_2 consumption in the adult respiratory distress syndrome. Chest 84:267, 1983.

Pierson DJ: Acute respiratory failure. In Sahn SA (ed): Pulmonary emergencies. New York, Churchill Livingstone, Inc., 1982, p. 75.

Pierson DJ, Hudson LD: Monitoring hemodynamics in the critically ill. Med Clin North Am 7:1347, 1983.

Weil MH, Henning RJ: New concepts in the diagnosis and fluid treatment of circulatory shock. Anesth Analg 58:124, 1979.

Winter PM, Miller JN: Carbon monoxide poisoning. JAMA 236:1502, 1976.

Cardiovascular Disorders

2. Cardiopulmonary Arrest and Resuscitation

Nora F. Goldschlager

INTRODUCTION

Cardiac arrest is present when effective cardiac pump function ceases. It is due either to ventricular fibrillation (VF), which is usually preceded by ventricular tachycardia, or, more rarely, to ventricular asystole. The success of cardiopulmonary resuscitation (CPR) depends directly on the elapsed time between the cardiac arrest and the institution of resuscitative efforts.

INDICATIONS

The indication for the institution of CPR in the intensive care unit (ICU) is the occurrence of cardiovascular collapse or respiratory arrest without cardiac arrest. If the patient's cardiac rhythm is not being monitored at the time of the arrest, cardiovascular collapse is assumed to be present if a pulse cannot be felt and the blood pressure cannot be obtained. In a monitored patient, VF or ventricular asystole will be seen on the cardiac monitor. Patients arresting with electromechanical dissociation (EMD) can have any cardiac rhythm but no effective mechanical systole, and blood pressure will be unobtainable. The significance of EMD relates to the underlying clinical picture: EMD occurring as a consequence of cardiac tamponade or tension pneumothorax is treatable and thus potentially reversible, whereas end-stage heart disease is usually not treatable, and thus the EMD has an extremely poor prognosis.

TECHNIQUE

An effective airway must be established. If respiratory arrest has occurred, the possibility of foreign body obstruction should be considered and measures taken to relieve it manually, by delivery of a series of sharp blows to the interscapular area, or by performing the Heimlich maneuver, which consists of a series of sharp upward thrusts in the epigastric area. Oral and esophageal obturator airways, while of some use in the field, are not effective substitutes for endotracheal intubation, which should be performed without delay. While awaiting intubation, ventilation of the patient, using an Ambu bag with supplemental oxygen, is recommended. If CPR has already begun, interruption during endotracheal intubation should not exceed 15–20 seconds in order to avoid anoxic brain damage.

If the cardiac rhythm is observed to be VF, a series of sharp blows to the precordium ("thumpversion") may be tried, provided that only seconds have elapsed. Defibrillation should then be performed immediately, using 200–400 joules (see Chapter 19). Defibrillation should also be carried out in patients in whom the rhythm is not being monitored at the time of the arrest, since valuable time will be lost in attempting to document the rhythm by an electrocardiogram (ECG); VF can be assumed, since it is the most common rhythm during cardiac arrest; if the rhythm turns out to be severe bradycardia or asystole, defibrillation will have done no harm. "Fine" VF is less responsive to defibrillation than is "coarse" VF and can sometimes be converted to coarse VF by 0.1–1.0 ml epinephrine 1:1000 solution diluted to 10 ml. If the epinephrine is administered early enough in the CPR procedure, the intravenous route may suffice; if not, the intracardiac route should be used. Defibrillation is also less likely to be achieved if hypoxia and acidosis are present, and these must be corrected early by adequate ventilation, supplemental oxygen, and, rarely, sodium bicarbonate (50 mEq intravenously [IV] initially with frequency of administration determined by arterial pH determinations). Sodium bicarbonate should not be given once an effective cardiac rhythm has been restored unless warranted by specific arterial pH determinations.

Drugs that may be useful in treating refractory ventricular tachycardia/fibrillation unresponsive to defibrillation attempts are lidocaine (50–150 mg as an IV bolus), bretylium (300–500 mg IV over 5–10 minutes), procainamide (500–1000 mg IV over 10–20 minutes), and propranolol (1.5 mg IV as a bolus). Continuous infusion of the appropriate antidysrhythmic agent(s) should be begun when the cardiac rhythm has stabilized.

If the cardiac rhythm is asystole, precordial thumps may be tried and CPR begun immediately thereafter. Atropine (0.6–1.2 mg IV) or isoproterenol (1–20 µg/ml) may be used in patients with bradycardia but are ineffective in asystole. Transvenous endocardial pacing should be instituted if a rhythm is not obtained. Transthoracic pacing is usually ineffective and its use is obsolete. An external transthoracic demand pacemaker, in which two large electrodes are positioned on the anterior and posterior thorax and connected to a portable pacemaker generator, can be used to pace the patient through the chest wall at energy levels sufficiently high to produce myocardial stimulation (as well as chest wall muscle stimulation) but not so high as to be painful to the patient. External demand pacing is a temporary measure only and should be replaced with a transvenous endocardial pacing system as soon as it is feasible.

Hyperkalemia, often associated with cardiac arrest, is recognized by loss of P-wave voltage with eventual loss of P waves, atrioventricular (AV) block (rare), and intraventricular conduction disturbances, producing markedly broad and bizzare QRS complexes having a sine-wave pattern. Since the P waves are often not discerned because of their low voltage, the wide QRS rhythm is mistaken for ventricular tachycardia. Hyperkalemia is treated with 10–30 ml (1–3 g) of 10 percent calcium chloride, given IV over 1–5 minutes, repeated as needed, since its effect is transitory, and with glucose, insulin, and sodium bicarbonate. Owing to EMD, cardiac pacing will be ineffective until the hyperkalemia is corrected.

EMD is of ominous prognostic import unless it is the result of potentially reversible conditions such as severe acidosis, electrolyte imbalance (especially hyperkalemia), Type I antidysrhythmic drug toxicity (procainamide, quinidine, disopyramide), or cardiac tamponade (see Chapter 13). If these associated complications are effectively treated and EMD persists, primary myocardial failure is probably present. Cardiac pacing is obviously not indicated in EMD, since the problem is not one of rhythm but of ineffective mechanical systole in response to the rhythm.

COMPLICATIONS

Vigorous CPR can result in fracture of the sternum, hemothorax, pneumothorax, and laceration of abdominal viscera, especially the liver. Cardiac complications include rupture of either ventricle, and of the atria, aorta, and tricuspid valve apparatus; the apparent incidence is about 7 percent. If the patient survives CPR, these potential complications should be borne in mind, as they may cause problems in the resuscitated patient.

RECOMMENDED READING

Ad Hoc Committee on Cardiopulmonary Resuscitation of the Division of Medical Sciences, National Academy of Sciences—National Research Council: Cardiopulmonary resuscitation. JAMA 198:245, 1966.

American Heart Association: Advanced Cardiac Life Support. Dallas, American Heart Association, 1975.

American Heart Association: Standards for CPR and ECC. JAMA 255:2841, 1987.

Goldberg AH: Cardiopulmonary arrest. N Engl J Med 290:3811, 1974.

Heissenbuttel RH, Bigger JT Jr: Bretylium tosylate, a newly available drug for ventricular arrhythmias. Ann Intern Med 91:229, 1979.

Lie KI, Wellens HJ, Van Capella FJ, et al: Lidocaine in the prevention of primary ventricular fibrillation. A double-blind randomized study of 212 consecutive patients. N Engl J Med 291:1324, 1974.

Morgan JP, Sanders FH, Raizes GS, et al: High-energy versus low-energy defibrillation:

Experience in patients (excluding those in the intensive care unit) at Mayo Clinic–affiliated hospitals. Mayo Clin Proc 59:829, 1984.

Pantridge JF, Adgey AAJ, Geddes JS: The Acute Coronary Attack. New York, Grune & Stratton, Inc., 1975, pp. 66–78.

Pennington JE, Taylor J, Lown B: Chest thump for reverting ventricular tachycardia. N Engl J Med 283:1192, 1970.

Wolff GA, Veith F, Lown B: A vulnerable period for ventricular tachycardia following myocardial infarction. Cardiovasc Res 2:111, 1968.

3. Dysrhythmias

Nora F. Goldschlager

DEFINITION

A dysrhythmia is defined as any cardiac rhythm other than sinus rhythm at a normal rate. Cardiac dysrhythmias comprise tachydysrhythmias and bradydysrhythmias. Tachydysrhythmias can originate in virtually any portion of the heart: they are generally classified as supraventricular (originating in the sinus node, atrium, coronary sinus, atrioventricular [AV] node, and His bundle) and ventricular (originating in the Purkinje system or ventricular myocardium). Bradydysrhythmias are similarly categorized as atrial or ventricular bradycardias.

PATHOPHYSIOLOGY

There are three mechanisms of dysrhythmia production: (1) disorders of impulse formation, (2) disorders of impulse conduction, and (3) triggering. Cardiac tissue that has the capability of undergoing diastolic depolarization to reach threshold and discharge is called automatic tissue. Under certain circumstances, abnormal impulse formation occurs in automatic tissue, leading to enhancement of intrinsic firing rate and to tachycardia.

Delay in, or failure of, impulse conduction can result in either bradycardia or tachycardia. Failure of impulse transmission is followed by an (atrial or ventricular) asystolic period, which is terminated by an impulse generated in an *escape focus*; the ectopic focus then generates an *escape rhythm*, which persists until the dominant pacemaker resumes its activity.

If an impulse (usually premature) is blocked in one pathway of conduction but travels slowly in another, it can reexcite the previously blocked pathway, provided that sufficient time has elapsed for the pathway to recover (Fig. 3–1). This *reentry* of the slowly conducted impulse into the previously refractory pathway can lead to reentry tachycardias. Reentry can occur in the sinus and AV nodes, atrium, bundle branches, and ventricular myocardium; accessory (extra-AV nodal) pathways (such as the Kent bundle in WPW syndrome) can also be involved.

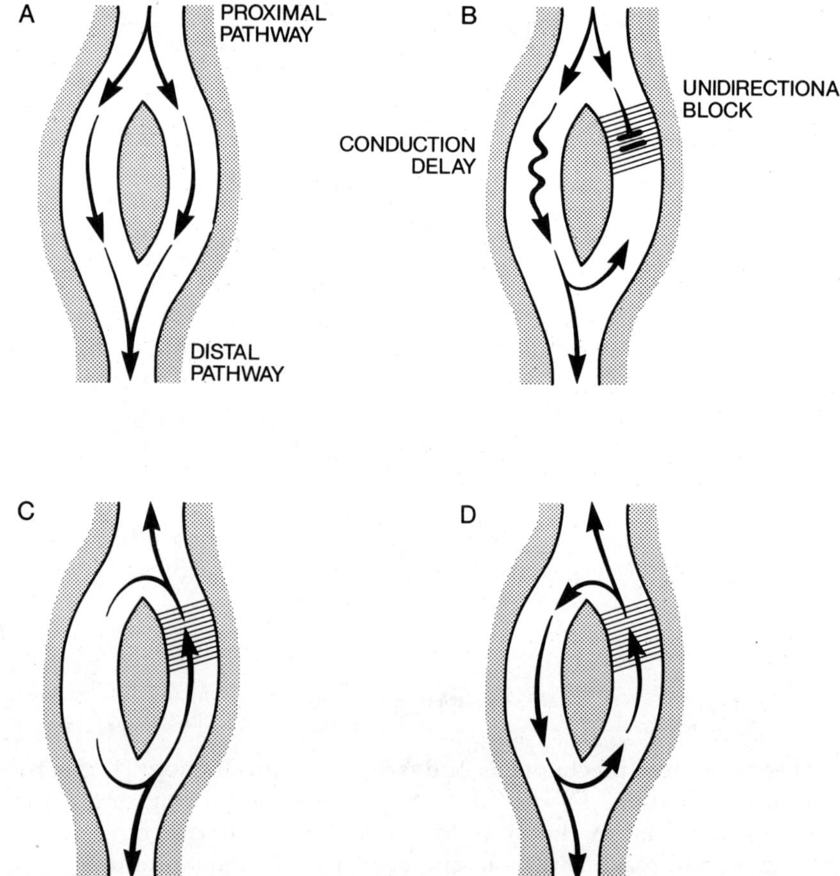

FIGURE 3–1. Mechanism of reentry dysrhythmia. Instead of homogeneous conduction (A), the presence of a conduction delay and a unidirectional block (B) can lead to retrograde as well as antegrade conduction (C) and a sustained tachycardia (D).

Triggered rhythms are generated in fibers in which an afterdepolarization occurs during or following full repolarization. If the afterdepolarization reaches threshold, another action potential and another afterdepolarization can result, perpetuating the rhythm for variable periods of time. These fibers are not themselves automatic but must be driven (discharged) by others. Abnormal triggering has been demonstrated in Purkinje fibers and in atrial and ventricular muscle fibers; it has been related to excess catecholamines and to digitalis: exercise-induced tachycardias and the rhythms of digitalis toxicity may be triggered in origin.

Tachydysrhythmias can cause hemodynamic embarrassment, including ischemic cardiac pain due both to rapid rate and to loss of AV synchrony. If, for example, the atria contract against closed AV valves (owing to short PR or RP intervals), ventricular filling is impaired and stroke volume falls; in addition, the atrial stretch that results from the increased atrial volume causes reflex hypotension. If, on the other hand, atrial contraction is dissociated from ventricular contraction, the ventricles can at times receive the atrial volume, leading to variable, but not necessarily low, stroke volumes. Rate alone should never be used as a criterion of rhythm diagnosis, nor should the diagnosis of a specific rhythm be altered merely because the patient is or is not tolerating it. (This applies most importantly to ventricular tachycardia, which is often well tolerated.) Cardioversion should be employed in all tachydysrhythmias that cause hemodynamic deterioration unless they result from digitalis toxicity (see Chapter 18).

Bradydysrhythmias can cause syncope, near syncope, dizziness, and confusion, owing to cerebral hypoperfusion; they can also cause weakness, lassitude, and signs of low cardiac output. Symptomatic bradycardias or those resulting in hemodynamic impairment require temporary or permanent cardiac pacing (see Chapter 16).

DIAGNOSIS AND MANAGEMENT
OF TACHYDYSRHYTHMIAS

Supraventricular Tachydysrhythmias

Sinus Tachycardia. The sinus rate in sinus tachycardia usually does not exceed 150/min unless circulating levels of catecholamines are extremely high (acute myocardial infarction with shock and/or pulmonary edema, pheochromocytoma, alcohol withdrawal, cocaine or amphetamine overdose), in which case sinus rates of 180/min or more can occur. The P waves are normal in contour and have a normal axis. If the rate is very rapid they will be buried in the preceding T waves and may be difficult to discern, leading to mistaken diagnoses; this is especially dangerous if the QRS complexes are wide. Carotid sinus massage (CSM) can transiently slow the rate, allowing identification of P waves; however, CSM is usually without effect if the patient is significantly sympathetically stimulated. Correction of accompanying conditions leads to slowing of the rate without specific therapy. Intravenous or oral β-blockers should be used only in those clinical circumstances in which the tachycardia *per se* is detrimental, such as in patients with myocardial ischemia or infarction.

Paroxysmal Supraventricular Tachycardia (PSVT). PSVT is due to a reentry mechanism, most often involving the AV node alone, or the AV node and an extra-AV nodal bypass tract. Infrequently, the sinoatrial node is involved. The QRS complexes are narrow unless preexistent or rate-

Text continued on page 28

TABLE 3–1. PROPERTIES OF ANTIDYSRHYTHMIC AGENTS USED IN
ACUTE CLINICAL SETTINGS

Drug	Intravenous Dose	Oral Dose	Metabolism	Time to Peak Effect
Lidocaine	LOADING 1. 1–2 mg/kg at 50–100 mg/min; may repeat 1 mg/kg bolus after 5 min if no response; a third 1 mg/kg bolus may be tried after 10 min 2. 50–75 mg IV every 5 min to maximum of 2 mg/kg MAINTENANCE 30–35 µg/kg/min continuous infusion	—	Exclusively hepatic	20 min
Procainamide	LOADING 20–50 mg/min up to total of 1 g, dysrhythmia is controlled, or hypotension or QT interval prolongation greater than 50 per cent occur MAINTENANCE 2–6 mg/min continuous infusion	LOADING 500–1000 mg (IM loading is same) MAINTENANCE 350–1000 mg q 3–6 hr depending on preparation	Predominantly renal	*IV* 20 min *Oral* 60 min
Quinidine	6–10 mg/kg at 0.3–0.5 mg/kg/min	LOADING 600–1000 mg MAINTENANCE 200–600 mg QID	Predominantly hepatic	*IV* sulfate 90 min, gluconate 3.5 hr
Tocainide	500–750 mg over 15 min immediately followed by 800 mg orally	LOADING 400–600 mg MAINTENANCE 400–800 mg q 8–12 hr	Predominantly hepatic but renal significant	*Oral* 1 hr

TABLE 3–1. PROPERTIES OF ANTIDYSRHYTHMIC AGENTS USED IN
ACUTE CLINICAL SETTINGS *Continued*

HALF-LIFE	THERAPEUTIC SERUM LEVEL	ACUTE ADVERSE EFFECTS	CAUTIONS AND COMMENTS
1.5 hr	1.5 μg/ml	*CNS*— Dose-related confusion, paresthesis, delirium, seizures, stupor, coma *Cardiac*—Occasional sinus node and His-Purkinje exit block	Low serum levels 20–40 minutes after single bolus followed by continuous infusion; may require second bolus of 1 mg/kg to restore therapeutic levels Reduce maintenance dose in elderly and in patients with reduced hepatic flow, hepatic disease, or CHF Use caution in patients with high degree AV block
3–5 hr (NAPA—8 hr or longer)	4–10 μg/ml (PA + NAPA—15–25 μg/ml)	*GI*—nausea, vomiting, diarrhea *Cardiac*—sinus node depression, orthostatic hypotension, polymorphic ventricular tachycardia	Active metabolite NAPA may have prolonged half-life at larger procainamide doses (>10 hrs); dosage should be decreased in patients with decreased renal function Sustained-release oral preparations preferred in view of relatively short half-life
6 hr	3–6 μg/ml	*GI*—diarrhea, nausea, vomiting, abdominal pain *Cardiac*—significant hypotension common with IV infusion; this route is not advised Prolongation of QRS duration, QT interval, polymorphic ventricular tachycardia *CNS*—tinnitus, hearing loss, confusion, delirium *Hematologic*— thrombocytopenia	Anticoagulant drugs may shorten half-life and reduce serum concentration Lower doses may be required in patients with decreased hepatic function and CHF May increase serum digoxin level, thus requiring digoxin dosage reduction
12–16 hr	6–10 μg/ml	*CNS*—same as for lidocaine	Narrow therapeutic-to-toxic ratio Elimination impaired in patients with renal insufficiency, and 50 per cent dose reduction is recommended; no evidence of impaired hepatic elimination in mild CHF

Table continued on following page

TABLE 3–1. PROPERTIES OF ANTIDYSRHYTHMIC AGENTS USED IN
ACUTE CLINICAL SETTINGS *Continued*

DRUG	INTRAVENOUS DOSE	ORAL DOSE	METABOLISM	TIME TO PEAK EFFECT
Flecainide	1.5–2 mg/kg	100–300 mg q 12 hr	Predominantly hepatic	*Oral* 1–6 hr
Encainide	0.6–0.9 mg/kg over 5 min	25–75 mg q 6–8 hr	Predominantly hepatic	*Oral* 1–2 hr
Propranolol	0.1–0.5 mg every 5 min to total of 0.20 mg/kg	10–200 mg q 6–8 hr	Hepatic	*IV* 1–5 min *Oral* 1–3 hr
Esmolol	LOADING 500 µg/kg bolus MAINTENANCE 50–250 µg/kg	—	Blood, liver	5 min
Bretylium	LOADING 500 µg/kg bolus over 1 min followed by 50–250 µg/kg continuous infusion	—	Renal	*IV* 5–30 min
Bethanidine	5–20 mg/kg	LOADING 20–30 mg MAINTENANCE 5–10 mg/kg q 8 hr	Renal	*Oral* 30–60 min

TABLE 3–1. PROPERTIES OF ANTIDYSRHYTHMIC AGENTS USED IN
ACUTE CLINICAL SETTINGS *Continued*

HALF-LIFE	THERAPEUTIC SERUM LEVEL	ACUTE ADVERSE EFFECTS	CAUTIONS AND COMMENTS
20 hr	0.2–1.0 µg/ml	*Cardiac*—negative inotropic effect common; AV and His-Purkinje conduction block *CNS*—metallic taste, blurred vision, dizziness, headache, nausea	Initial dose should not exceed 100 mg q 12 hr Avoid doses >400 mg/day in CHF, renal failure, elderly, <50 kg weight Contraindicated in cardiogenic shock Cimetidine reduces both renal and nonrenal clearance; dosage reduction is required
3–4 hr	0.5–1.0 µg/ml	*Cardiac*—Prolongs PR, HV, and QRS intervals, polymorphic ventricular tachycardia in absence of prolonged QT interval *CNS*—dizziness, diplopia, ataxia	Two highly active metabolites (ODE and MODE) Plasma concentrations vary as much as 50-fold; therefore, adjust dosage based on response of dysrhythmia, QRS widening, or tolerance
3–6 hr	0.04–0.90 µg/ml	*Cardiac*—negative inotrophy, bradycardia (sinus bradycardia, AV block), hypotension after IV administration *CNS*—depression *GI*—nausea, vomiting *Other*— bronchospasm, impaired glucose tolerance, masking of response to hypoglycemia	If used to treat intractable VT or VF, must be used with extreme caution
10 min	—	Hypotension	Cardioselective Ultrashort-acting β-adrenergic blocking agent. No effect seen 30 min after discontinuation of infusion
8–14 hr	0.5–1.5 µg/ml	Nausea with rapid IV administration; hypertension followed by hypotension, anxiety, flushing, substernal pressure, nasal stuffiness	Initial hypertension can be blocked by pretreatment with β-adrenergic blocking agent May prove useful in refractory VT or VF Hypotension may require dopamine Contraindicated in digitalis toxicity May be less effective at low serum potassium levels
14 hr	0.18–1.5 µg/ml	Orthostatic hypotension common unless pretreatment with tricyclic antidepressant	Chemical structure and pharmacologic properties similar to bretylium tosylate but oral absorption is better May be less effective at low serum potassium levels

Table continued on following page

TABLE 3–1. PROPERTIES OF ANTIDYSRHYTHMIC AGENTS USED IN
ACUTE CLINICAL SETTINGS *Continued*

DRUG	INTRAVENOUS DOSE	ORAL DOSE	METABOLISM	TIME TO PEAK EFFECT
Amiodarone	2.5–10 mg/kg over 30 min	LOADING 800–1200 mg QID for 1–4 weeks MAINTENANCE 200–800 mg QID	Hepatic	*IV* 10 min *Oral* 4 hr
Verapamil	LOADING 0.075–0.15 mg/kg, or 10 mg IV over 1–2 min MAINTENANCE 0.005 mg/kg/min continuous infusion	80–160 mg every 6–8 hr	Hepatic	*IV* 3–5 min *Oral* 60–120 min
Digoxin	LOADING 0.75–1.0 mg in 24 hrs (or less in atrial fibrillation)	LOADING 1–2 mg in 24 hr MAINTENANCE 0.25–0.75 mg depending upon ventricular response to atrial fibrillation	Hepatic	*IV* 1–5 hr *Oral* 2–6 hr
Mexilitine	LOADING 250 mg in 5 min to total of 750 mg in 3 hr MAINTENANCE 0.5–1.0 mg/min	LOADING 400–600 mg MAINTENANCE 200–300 mg TID	Liver	*IV* 15–30 min

AV = atrioventricular; SA = sinoatrial; CHF = congestive heart failure.

dependent bundle branch block is present or antegrade conduction to the ventricles occurs over an extra-AV nodal pathway (such as a Kent bundle in WPW syndrome). Atrial depolarization is retrograde, resulting in inverted P waves in ECG leads 2, 3, and aV_F. The P waves may occur just before, during, or after the QRS complexes; they are not discerned if they occur during the QRS complexes.

Termination of the rhythm is accomplished by blocking impulse conduction in either the antegrade or retrograde direction. Vigorous CSM

TABLE 3–1. PROPERTIES OF ANTIDYSRHYTHMIC AGENTS USED IN
ACUTE CLINICAL SETTINGS *Continued*

HALF-LIFE	THERAPEUTIC SERUM LEVEL	ACUTE ADVERSE EFFECTS	CAUTIONS AND COMMENTS
30–50 days	0.15–5 μg/ml	Hypotension; worsened conduction system disease, depressed cardiac index, polymorphic ventricular tachycardia Constipation, tremor, ataxia, thyroid dysfunction, pulmonary fibrosis	Oral absorption slow and erratic Hypotension common at 5 mg/kg IV administration rate If concomitant digoxin therapy, decrease digoxin dose
3–7 hr	0.1–0.15 μg/ml	Negative inotropic effect, hypotension, bradycardia, AV block	Use caution when giving to patients with depressed myocardial function Avoid if patient is receiving β-blocking agents Contraindicated in advanced heart failure, and in 2° or 3° AV block without pacemaker in place Can increase serum digoxin level
40 hr	0.5–2.5 μg/ml	Peripheral vasoconstriction with hypertension (uncommon)	Serum levels increased by quinidine, verapamil, amiodarone, some antibiotics May increase myocardial oxygen demand Cardioversion not contraindicated if serum level is in the therapeutic range, or low energy used In atrial fibrillation, dose should be titrated against ventricular rate
10 hr	0.5–2.0 μg/ml	Hypotension, bradycardia, QRS widening, nausea, tremors, nystagmus	Not useful in supraventricular dysrhythmia; low toxic:therapeutic ratio. Use IV route with caution.

should be attempted first; the maneuver will either terminate the tachycardia or have no effect; a Valsalva maneuver can also be tried. Intravenous verapamil is the drug of choice (5–10 mg over 10–20 min). Intravenous (IV) propranolol or esmolol may also be used; they are contraindicated in patients receiving calcium entry blocking agents. Edrophonium (Tensilon), metaraminol (Aramine), and digoxin (0.25–0.50 mg) are less useful. Pressor agents should not be used in patients with chest pain or preexisting hypertension. Rapid atrial pacing can terminate the rhythm, but catheter placement requires fluoroscopic guidance for optimum positioning. If the

QRS complexes are broad and ventricular tachycardia cannot be ruled out, IV lidocaine (Table 3–1) can be used without harm. Cardioversion is required if hemodynamic decompensation (including chest pain) is present, regardless of the rate of the tachycardia.

Atrial Flutter. Atrial flutter may be sustained or paroxysmal. The atrial rate is 280–320/min. Rapid atrial rates are associated with sympathetic stimulation or digitalis therapy; slower atrial rates are associated with antidysrhythmic drug therapy, large and hypertrophied atria, or intraatrial conduction delay. The AV conduction ratio is usually 2:1 in untreated flutter; AV nodal Wenckebach periodicity with changing AV conduction ratios is common. CSM may produce AV block and illustrate the flutter waves and their rate; termination of the dysrhythmia does not occur by this maneuver.

Therapy of choice in sustained atrial flutter is DC cardioversion, using low energy levels (25–50 joules; see Chapter 18); pace termination by overdrive techniques is also effective in selected patients. Pharmacologic conversion is accomplished by first digitalizing the patient (1.0–1.5 mg IV over 12 hr) then treating with intramuscular or oral quinidine sulfate (400 mg initially, followed by 200 mg q 6 h for 24 hr, 300 mg q 6 h for 24 hr if the first regimen fails, and 400 mg q 6 h if the second regimen fails [Table 3–1]). Procainamide may also be used (500–1000 mg sustained-release preparation initially, followed by 250–500 mg q 6 h). Digoxin alone is not expected to slow the ventricular rate; pushing digitalis to achieve this end is contraindicated, since toxic rhythms will occur. Quinidine and procainamide slow the atrial rate, allowing the possibility of 1:1 AV conduction if a full digitalizing dose has not been given. The vagolytic effect of quinidine resulting in enhancement of AV conduction is rarely encountered in clinical practice; if 1:1 AV conduction of flutter impulses occurs, it is usually the result of slowing of the atrial rate. When sinus rhythm is restored, antidysrhythmic therapy is continued for variable periods of time, depending on the clinical situation.

Atrial Fibrillation. Atrial fibrillation (AF) may be either sustained or paroxysmal. It is characterized by a varyingly irregular ventricular rate. The faster the ventricular rate, the more regular it may appear. CSM may be used to slow AV conduction and to illustrate the atrial mechanism. Initial management consists of IV digoxin to slow the ventricular rate (0.25–0.50 mg q 4–6 h until the desired rate is achieved); the dosage and frequency of administration are titrated against the ventricular rate. Serum levels of digoxin in patients with AF are almost always high and are of little use in management. If digitalis alone is insufficient to slow the ventricular rate, IV verapamil (0.5 mg/kg loading dose followed by 0.005 mg/kg/min continuous infusion) or IV diltiazem (0.25 mg/kg loading dose followed by 0.001–0.002 mg/kg/min continuous infusion) may be added. Since the effect of digoxin on the AV node is primarily vagal, enhanced sympathetic tone may result in difficulty in achieving the desired ventricular rate; verapamil and diltiazem slow AV conduction by direct effect on AV nodal cells, thus synergizing with digitalis. Caution is required in patients with depressed myocardial function whenever calcium entry blocking agents are used. Verapamil may cause an increase in the serum digoxin level.

Conversion of the rhythm to sinus is accomplished using quinidine or procainamide (Table 3–1); DC cardioversion is also successful, provided that the associated clinical condition is optimized. Urgent cardioversion is required if hypotension or severe chest pain due to rapid ventricular rate are present (see Chapter 18). If the patient is hyperthyroid, cardioversion should be delayed for 1–2 months after euthyroidism is achieved.

In patients with known WPW syndrome, or in patients with AF and broad, bizarre QRS complexes that could signify antegrade conduction over an accessory pathway, digitalis and verapamil are contraindicated, since an increase in ventricular rate, sometimes leading to ventricular fibrillation, can result. (Any agent that causes hypotension can accelerate the ventricular rate.) IV procainamide (100 mg q 5 min to 1000 mg), lidocaine, or DC cardioversion are preferred. Propranolol has little effect on accessory pathway conduction and should not be used.

Recognition of digitalis toxicity in patients with AF consists of identifying the presence of high-grade or complete AV block and an ectopic pacemaker that stimulates the QRS rhythm. Because the ectopic pacemaker discharges at regular intervals, the ventricular rate will be regular. Type I (Wenckebach) or Type II exit block from the focus of origin of the rhythm may occur, resulting in the expected changes in RR cycle lengths. Treatment consists of withdrawal of digitalis and any other AV nodal blocking agent the patient may be taking; temporary cardiac pacing (see Chapter 16) is indicated if the ventricular rate is unacceptably slow.

As with atrial flutter, antidysrhythmic agents are often required for variable periods of time, depending upon the clinical situation, once conversion to sinus rhythm has occurred. If the AF is paroxysmal, antidysrhythmic therapy is given preventively.

Ectopic (Automatic) Atrial Tachycardia. In automatic atrial tachycardia, the atrial rate is 150–200/min; the AV conduction ratio is usually 1:1, but Type I (Wenckebach) and Type II AV block can occur. Atrial tachycardia with block is usually a rhythm of digitalis toxicity. The P waves have a normal frontal plane axis, a short duration, and a peaked morphology. CSM produces AV block, allowing the P waves to be seen; there is no change in atrial rate, and the tachycardia does not terminate.

Management consists of discontinuing digitalis and correcting underlying disease processes, most commonly severe congestive heart failure and chronic lung disease. Administration of potassium, an older therapy, is virtually never required. Cardioversion is usually unsuccessful, as the conditions that gave rise to the rhythm remain unchanged; if the rhythm is due to digitalis toxicity, cardioversion is contraindicated. Antidysrhythmic agents are also generally not useful.

Multifocal Atrial Tachycardia. Multifocal atrial tachycardia (MAT) is an automatic rhythm characterized by P waves of varying morphologies and by varying PR intervals. Although the AV conduction ratio is usually 1:1, AV block can occur. It is usually seen in patients with chronic obstructive pulmonary disease or severe metabolic disorders and is usually unassociated with symptoms or signs of hemodynamic deterioration. Therapy is directed at the underlying clinical condition, since the rhythm is affected very little or not at all by antidysrhythmic agents, digitalis, and DC cardioversion. A transient and occasionally long lasting response to IV verapamil may occur. The major differential diagnosis is AF; it is important to distinguish the two in order to avoid pushing digoxin (which is not indicated in MAT) to toxicity in an attempt to slow the ventricular rate.

Accelerated Junctional Rhythm and Junctional Tachycardia. The rate of an accelerated junctional rhythm is 60–120/min; the rhythm usually results from enhanced automaticity of the AV junction and is *not* caused by AV block. Since the ventricles are depolarized by the junctional focus and the atria by the sinus node (or other mechanism), AV dissociation is present. No specific treatment is indicated.

The rate of junctional tachycardia is 120–200/min. It occurs in patients with severe congestive heart failure, after open heart surgery, and as a result of digitalis toxicity. It may not be distinguishable electrocardiographically from PSVT, but the response to vagal maneuvers or AV nodal blocking drugs clarifies the issue. Treatment is similar to that for automatic atrial tachycardia.

Ventricular Tachydysrhythmias

Isolated premature ventricular beats of uniform morphology, even if occurring in bigeminal fashion, usually require no therapy, except perhaps in the setting of acute myocardial infarction. General principles of management include insuring adequate oxygenation, correction of fluid and electrolyte abnormalities, and control of pain. Frequent premature beats of multiform contour and in doublets and triplets usually require suppression, as they may presage a sustained dysrhythmia.

Monomorphic Ventricular Tachycardia. Monomorphic ventricular tachycardia (VT) refers to a VT of uniform morphology, which is often, but not always, sustained. The tachycardia frequently has a superior mean frontal plane QRS axis, and concordance (similarity) of QRS complex morphology across the precordium. Lead VI often shows a QR, RR', or pure R wave, and Lead V6 shows QS or RS configuration (Table 3–2). A 12–lead ECG

TABLE 3–2. INTRAVENTRICULAR ABERRATION VS VENTRICULAR ECTOPY

ABERRATION	ECTOPY
• Preceded by premature P wave	• Not preceded by premature P wave
• rSR′ in V_1; Rs with wide S in V_6	• R, RR′, QR in V_1; QR or rS in V_6
• Fixed coupling absent	• Fixed coupling present
• QRS duration usually less than 0.14 sec	• QRS duration often greater than 0.14 sec
• Resembles a defined bundle branch block pattern	• Frontal plane QRS axis often markedly superior

should be performed in all patients with a wide QRS complex tachycardia in order to fully assess the QRS morphology. Monomorphic VT may be reasonably well tolerated, in which case it can be managed medically, using IV lidocaine (50–100 mg bolus followed by 1–4 mg/min continuous infusion) or IV procainamide (100 mg q 5 min to 1000 mg, followed by 1–6 mg/min continuous infusion) (Table 3–1). If urgent rhythm conversion is required for hemodynamic deterioration, cardioversion is the method of choice (see Chapter 18). If the VT is refractory to initial pharmacologic or electrical management or both, IV bretylium (300–500 mg loading dose followed by 1–3 mg/min continuous infusion) may be tried. Amiodarone may be useful in refractory cases, as may small doses of IV propranolol (Table 3–1). Selected patients with VT that continues to be refractory to medical management should be referred for cardiac catheterization or electrophysiologic study or both.

Polymorphic VT. This is a nonsustained VT that has an irregular rate. The QRS complexes are of varying morphology; sometimes they appear to undulate around an isoelectric baseline (*les torsades de pointes*). Polymorphic VT occurs during acute myocardial ischemia, Type I antidysrhythmic drug toxicity (quinidine, procainamide, disopyramide), hypokalemia, hypomagnesemia, and congenital long QT interval syndrome. It may also occur in patients taking amiodarone and the experimental agent sotalol. Since polymorphic VT can degenerate to ventricular fibrillation, suppression is required. Many patients with polymorphic VT have a long QT interval; thus, antidysrhythmic agents that act to increase this interval (Type I agents) are generally not used (their appropriate use in this condition should be documented in the electrophysiologic laboratory). Isoproterenol (1–6 μg/min) is useful if the VT is bradycardia-dependent (that is, has its onset after a relatively long RR interval); however, use of this β-agonist is contraindicated in many acutely ill patients for other reasons. Cardiac pacing is the treatment of choice; it is best performed from the atrium, but ventricular pacing is also successful. Some normomagnesemic patients respond to IV magnesium sulfate (2–3 g over 1 min followed by 10 g in 5–6 hr). Some hypokalemic patients will respond to potassium replacement only after IV magnesium has been administered.

Bidirectional VT. This rhythm is almost always due to digitalis toxicity and is characterized by QRS complexes that have an alternating configuration. Withdrawal of digitalis is required, and if the tachycardia causes hemodynamic embarrassment, digoxin-specific antibodies should be used if available, since the rhythm is usually unresponsive to other therapies.

Accelerated Ventricular Rhythm (AVR). AVR is a benign rhythm in which the intrinsic firing rate of the ventricles is enhanced above its normal 30–40/min. It emerges upon slowing of the sinus rate (and is thus an escape rhythm), and disappears as the sinus rate accelerates; its onset and offset are often characterized by fusion complexes. Since the rate of the rhythm is not rapid, hemodynamic embarrassment does not occur, and no specific therapy is indicated. Increasing the sinus rate by any means will abolish the rhythm. AVR should be distinguished from slow VT, which has its onset by a premature ventricular beat; slow VT usually requires suppression by pharmacologic means.

Diagnosis and Management of Bradydysrhythmias

Bradydysrhythmias may result from sinus bradycardia, sinoatrial exit block, or sinus pauses, or from second degree or complete AV block. Treatment will vary depending on the cause of the bradycardia, so correct recognition is essential.

Sinus Bradycardia. The sinus rate is below 60/min. In the ICU setting, sinus bradycardia is usually the result of hypervagotonia and can be seen in patients with inferior wall or right ventricular myocardial infarction or both, increased intracranial pressure, and visceral distention. It is common during endotracheal suction, intubation, and vagal maneuvers such as vomiting; despite its transient nature, asystole of several seconds' duration can result. Use of β-blocker therapy is a common cause, and sinus rate can be depressed for up to 48 hours after discontinuing these medications. Usually no treatment is required. If the slow rate causes hemodynamic embarrassment or symptoms of cerebral hypoperfusion, atropine (0.8–1.0 mg q 2 min to total dose of 2.0 mg) should be given. Occasionally, atropine produces sinus tachycardia that, if AV conduction is impaired, may cause varying degrees of AV block. If atropine has no effect, temporary cardiac pacing is required. Isoproterenol, although useful in enhancing sinus rate and AV conduction, is usually not indicated in critically ill patients because of its dysrhythmogenic potential and the associated increase in myocardial oxygen demand.

Ventricular Bradycardia. Ventricular bradycardia results from high degree or complete AV block or from a slow junctional or ventricular escape rhythm. Slow escape rhythms usually originate distal to the His bundle and do not respond to treatment with atropine or isoproterenol; cardiac pacing is required. If the bradycardia results from AV nodal block, treatment is similar to that for sinus bradycardia. Temporary cardiac pacing may be necessary if the AV block is distal to the AV node. (Intra-AV nodal and intraHis block are characterized by narrow QRS complexes with long PR intervals of conducted P waves; block distal to the His bundle is characterized by normal PR interval of conducted P waves and QRS complexes having a bundle branch block pattern.) If atropine is used to facilitate AV conduction in patients with AV block, an increase in sinus rate can cause an exacerbation of the AV block, resulting in an even slower ventricular rate. Increases in heart rate due to atropine can produce myocardial ischemia and ventricular dysrhythmias, especially in patients with acute myocardial infarction.

RECOMMENDED READING

Ferrer MI: The sick sinus syndrome. Circulation 47:635, 1973.

Friedberg CK, Donoso E: Arrhythmias and conduction disturbances due to digitalis. Prog Cardiovasc Dis 2:408, 1959.

Giardina EGV, Heissenbuttel RH, Bigger JT Jr: Intravenous procainamide to treat ventricular arrhythmias. Ann Intern Med 78:183, 1973.

Harrison DC, Meffin PJ, Winkle RA: Clinical pharmacokinetics of antiarrhythmic drugs. Prog Cardiovasc Dis 20:217, 1977.

Hindman MC, Wagner GS, JaRo M, et al: The clinical significance of bundle branch block complicating acute myocardial infarction. 2. Indications for temporary and permanent pacemaker insertion. Circulation 58:689, 1978.

Josephson ME, Kastor JA: Supraventricular tachycardia: mechanisms and management. Ann Intern Med 87:346, 1977.

Lown B, Wyatt NF, Levine HD: Paroxysmal atrial tachycardia with block. Circulation 21:129, 1960.

Phillips J, Spano J, Burch G: Chaotic atrial mechanism. Am Heart J 78:171, 1969.

Rosen M, Reder R: Does triggered activity have a role in the genesis of cardiac arrhythmias? Ann Intern Med 94:794, 1981.

Sanna G, Arcidiancon R: Chemical ventricular defibrillation of the human heart with bretylium tosylate. Am J Cardiol 32:982, 1973.

Shine KI, Kastor J, Yurchak PM: Multifocal atrial tachycardia. N Engl J Med 279:344, 1968.

Singh BN, Ellrodt G, Peter CT: Verapamil: A review of its pharmacological properties and therapeutic use. Drugs 15:169, 1978.

Smith TW, Haber E, Yeatman L, et al: Reversal of advanced digoxin intoxication with Fab fragments of digoxin-specific antibodies. N Engl J Med 294:797, 1976.

Smith WM, Gallagher JJ: "Les torsades de pointes:" an unusual ventricular arrhythmia. Ann Intern Med 93:578, 1980.

Von Cappeler D, Copeland GD, Stern TN, et al: Digitalis intoxication. A clinical report of 148 cases. Ann Intern Med 50:869, 1959.

Waxman MB, Wald RW, Sharma AD, et al: Vagal techniques for termination of supraventricular tachycardia. Am J Cardiol 46:655, 1980.

Wellens HJJ, Bar FW, Bassen WR, et al: Effects of drugs in the Wolff-Parkinson-White syndrome. Am J Cardiol 46:665, 1980.

Wellens HJJ, Bar FW, Lie KI: The value of the electrocardiogram in the differential diagnosis of tachycardia with a widened QRS complex. Am J Med 6:27, 1978.

4. Acute Myocardial Infarction

Nora F. Goldschlager

DEFINITION

Acute myocardial infarction (MI) describes the condition involving death of myocardial tissue. More than 1,000,000 people suffer an MI each year, and 500,000 people die of coronary artery disease (CAD) each year, many suddenly. The major mortality occurs within the first several hours, before hospitalization. Despite this, MI and "rule out" MI diagnoses constitute the highest percentage of intensive care unit (ICU) admissions. The major contributions of the ICU setting to patients with MI are the recognition and treatment of atrial and ventricular dysrhythmias and the aggressive management of ischemic pain.

PATHOPHYSIOLOGY

Acute MI is usually caused by atherosclerotic CAD, in which an abrupt decrease in coronary artery flow produces ischemic necrosis. Hemorrhage under or rupture into an atherosclerotic plaque may be the proximate cause; thrombus is often superimposed upon an obstruction in patients with transmural MI. MI may also be caused by prolonged vasospasm, coronary artery embolism, and vasculitis. Generalized myocardial necrosis not due to disease of the coronary arteries can be caused by excessive catecholamine stimulation (in which a marked increase in myocardial oxygen demand is not met by the available supply), penetrating and nonpenetrating chest trauma, and severe acute hypertension. The location and extent of MI depend on the severity of the underlying CAD, the adequacy of the collateral circulation to the infarct area, and the presence of prior MI. MI causes ischemic dysfunction of the ventricles, in which both systolic and diastolic function are impaired, resulting in increased ventricular pressures and volumes and reduced stroke volumes.

DIAGNOSIS

Chest pain is usually substernal, often with radiation to the jaw, neck, shoulders, and arms. Radiation to the back should suggest the possibility of aortic rupture or dissection (see Chapter 10). The chest pain is described as pressing, crushing, or burning; epigastric symptoms may predominate. Associated symptoms can include shortness of breath, diaphoresis, nausea and vomiting, syncope or near-syncope, and profound weakness; these symptoms may dominate the clinical picture, chest pain being a minor complaint or even being absent. More rarely, the patient can present with a cerebrovascular accident, pulmonary edema, shock, or ventricular tachycardia, with chest pain not being a major symptom. A prodromal syndrome, usually consisting of crescendo angina (worsening chest pain) or unstable angina (worsening chest pain including rest pain), can be elicited in up to 50 percent of patients; a minority seek medical attention. This chapter will deal only with the phase of MI treated in the hospital.

Physical examination reveals an acutely ill and anxious patient with pain severe enough to require opiates. The physical findings in acute ischemic heart disease are often transient and are neither sensitive nor specific for the diagnosis. They include an S4 gallop, murmur of mitral regurgitation, and paradoxically split S2. If significant left ventricular (LV) dysfunction is present, an enlarged rocking PMI, S3 gallop, and pulmonary rales may be present. If right ventricular (RV) MI has occurred, central venous pressure will be elevated, provided the patient is not hypovolemic.

The admission electrocardiogram (ECG) is generally very helpful in establishing the diagnosis of MI but may fail to show the classical findings in up to 50 percent of cases, especially if prior MI has occurred. The recorded ST segment changes, whether depression or elevation, may normalize without further evolution, thus representing unstable angina rather than MI. Patients with abnormalities in ECG leads 2, 3 and aV_F should always have RV precordial leads recorded to diagnose or exclude an RVMI: RVMI is common in patients with inferior wall MI; it occurs in 15–45 percent of such patients, and ST elevation in $V_{2-4}R$ is both sensitive and specific for this diagnosis. Abnormal left ventricular depolarization (e.g., left bundle branch block and WPW conduction) is associated with left ventricular repolarization abnormalities; thus, recognizing MI with certainty in the presence of these patterns is not possible. Left anterior fascicular block (LAFB) will mask the pattern of inferior MI, and left posterior fascicular block (LPFB) will mask the pattern of lateral MI. LAFB and LPFB patterns can also mimic MI by inscribing Q waves in the lateral and inferior leads, respectively; however, they are usually neither sufficiently deep (25 percent of the height of the R wave) nor wide enough (0.04 seconds) to constitute infarction Q waves. Evolution of an infarction pattern is required for the diagnosis of MI, whether it is "transmural" (Q wave) or "nontransmural" (non-Q wave). Rapid development of Q waves (2–4 hours) can occur (and is the rule if intravenous or intracoronary thrombolytic therapy is used), but the time course of their development is usually 24–36 hours. (Q waves can develop in the absence of MI in patients with vasospastic angina, pulmonary embolism, chronic lung disease, pancreatitis, and fascicular blocks; they are usually transient, and the differential diagnosis is clear.) Persistence of ST elevation beyond 2 weeks is unexpected and indicates significant left ventricular akinesis or dyskinesis; it is usually permanent.

Creatine kinase (CK) levels are elevated to at least twice normal in MI; elevations less than this are common in patients with unstable angina. Since CK elevation *per se* is seen in cardiac disorders other than MI (inflammatory myocarditis, contusion, penetrating trauma) and in many noncardiac disorders, the myocardial fraction (MB) is the more specific test for myocardial necrosis. Normal levels of CK and CK-MB vary with the individual laboratory. CK-MB is detectable by 8 hours after the onset of symptoms and reaches a peak at 24 hours; both appearance time and time to peak level are significantly shorter if thrombolytic therapy is used and reperfusion successful (if reperfusion has not occurred, the time course of CK-MB elevation resembles that in patients who have not had an intervention). If the MI is suspected of having occurred 2–3 days before admission, the CK may be normal and MB absent. Serum LDH, with isoenzyme 1 exceeding isoenzyme 2, helps establish the diagnosis, as these enzyme abnormalities peak at 72 hours.

Neither thallium scintigraphy nor echocardiography is helpful in the diagnosis of *acute* MI. Technetium-labeled pyrophosphate (TcPYP) can be used to identify and localize myocardial necrosis (of any etiology) if administered 3–4 days after the onset of symptoms; since a positive scan can be seen in calcific valve disease and in calcified thrombus, a follow-up scan must be performed after one week to ascertain resolution of the abnormality. TcPYP may be useful in establishing MI in patients with left bundle branch block in whom the history is suggestive but CK-MB determinations nondiagnostic and in patients whose MI is thought to have occurred several days prior to admission and in whom the LDH isoenzymes are nondiagnostic.

MANAGEMENT

General principles of management consist of adequate analgesia, oxygen (2–4L/min by nasal cannulae or 5–6L/min by face mask), and sedation. Intravenous morphine sulfate is the analgesic of choice, since it has no significant myocardial depressant effects; side effects include nausea and vomiting and hypotension. The hypotension is due to reduction in venous tone and is responsive to the Trendelenburg position and fluid therapy. Naloxone (0.4 mg IV) is given PRN if respiratory distress occurs. Sublingual and topical nitrates relieve pain in up to 25 percent of patients; hypotension is treated with fluids. If pain does not resolve within 24 hours, pericarditis or continuing ischemia may be present; ECGs during and after pain should always be obtained to exclude the presence of transient and reversible ST segment changes that could reflect vasospasm.

Dysrhythmia monitoring is done throughout the intensive care unit stay. Bradycardias occur in up to one third of patients, usually with inferior wall MI (see Chapter 3). Atrial dysrhythmias occur in 10–15 percent of patients; the rhythm is usually atrial fibrillation, which is seen in the setting of pericarditis but is usually due to significant left ventricular dysfunction. Ventricular dysrhythmias of some type occur in almost 100 percent of patients with MI. Lidocaine prophylaxis against ventricular fibrillation is not required in the acute care setting; "warning dysrhythmias," including the R-on-T phenomenon, are not predictive for the occurrence or nonoccurrence of ventricular fibrillation. Lidocaine, if administered to treat ventricular dysrhythmias, should be discontinued after 24 hours; tapering of the dose is not required prior to discontinuation.

Intravenous or intracoronary thrombolytic therapy using streptokinase should probably be reserved for patients having their first MI that is anterior in location. Patients receiving this therapy are subsequently anticoagulated with heparin. Prior to discharge, cardiac catheterization should be performed, and if reperfusion has occurred and ventricular function is thereby preserved, definitive revascularization procedures should be strongly considered. Aspirin therapy is often continued indefinitely.

The complications of acute MI include post–MI angina, congestive heart failure (see Chapter 11), shock (see Chapter 8), acute mitral regurgitation due to papillary muscle dysfunction or ruptured papillary muscle tip (see Chapter 6), and ventricular septal rupture. Invasive hemodynamic monitoring is often required to clarify the cause of the complication (see Chapter 15) and to expedite appropriate management. Post-MI angina should be aggressively treated with intravenous, topical, and oral nitrates, calcium channel and β-blockers (Tables 4–1 and 4–2), and intraaortic balloon counterpulsation if necessary (see Chapter 17). Ventricular septal rupture and rupture of the mitral valve supporting apparatus require urgent hemodynamic stabilization and early cardiac surgery; aortocoronary bypass procedures often have to be performed concomitantly.

Pericardial effusion occurs in 25–30 percent of patients with MI, especially those with anterior MI and congestive heart failure. Pericarditis is not always associated with the effusion; thus, the effusion is not specific for the diagnosis of pericarditis. Anticoagulation has not been documented to cause hemorrhagic effusion with cardiac tamponade in these patients, and if it is being used for other reasons it need not be discontinued.

TABLE 4–1. ANTIANGINAL AGENTS USED IN THE ICU SETTING

PHARMACO-DYNAMIC EFFECTS	ACUTE THERAPY	LONG-TERM MANAGEMENT				
	Sublingual Nitroglycerin	Nifedipine	Long-Acting Nitrates	β-Blockers	Diltiazem	Verapamil
Vasodilatory effect						
Coronary arteries (conductance vessels)	+ + +	+ + +	0/ +	0	+ +	+ +
Coronary arterioles (resistance vessels)	− /?	+ + +	0/ +	—	?	?
Peripheral vessels	+ +	+ + +	0/ +	0/ −	+	+ +
Preload (venous capacitance)	↓ ↓ ↓	0/ ↓	↓ ↓	·0	0	0
Afterload	↓ ↓	↓ ↓ ↓	↓	0	↓	↓ ↓
LV function	↑	↑	0	↓ ↓	0/ ↓	↓
Heart rate	↑ ↑	↑ /0	↑ /0	↓ ↓ ↓	↓ ↓	↓
AV conduction	0	0	0	↓ ↓	↓ ↓	↓ ↓ ↓

Post-ICU Management

The patient should be transferred to a facility with telemetry capability and should remain there for 1–2 days. Ventricular dysrhythmias identified by telemetry should be treated (see Chapter 3). Inpatient rehabilitation should commence. Antianginal medications should not be used routinely in the absence of pain. Prior to discharge, low-dose β-block therapy (e.g., timolol 20 mg BID) is indicated in patients at moderate and high risk for recurrent MI; it is probably not necessary to treat low-risk patients.

TABLE 4–2. CALCIUM ENTRY BLOCKING AGENTS USED IN ISCHEMIC HEART DISEASE

AGENT	DOSE	COMMENTS
Verapamil	75–150 µg/kg IV 80–160 mg PO q 6–8 h	With β-blocker, may lead to asystole, AV block, hypotension, CHF
Nifedipine	10–40 mg PO q 6–8 h	May be used safely with β-blocker Side effects: hypotension, dizziness, flushing, nausea
Diltiazem	75–150 µg/kg IV 30–90 mg PO q 6–8 h	With β-blocker, may cause AV block Side effects: hypotension, dizziness, flushing, bradycardia

Outcome

The outcome depends on the extent of MI, severity and extent of underlying CAD, whether the MI is a Q-wave or a non–Q-wave one, and the category of risk, assessed at the time of hospital discharge, into which the patient falls. Pump failure is associated with MI involving over 40 percent of the myocardium; most patients with cardiogenic shock fall into this category. Patients with non–Q-wave MI have a relatively uncomplicated hospital course but have a higher incidence of post–MI angina, reinfarction, congestive heart failure, and death. Early cardiac catheterization, and myocardial revascularization in selected cases, is an appropriate course of action. Calcium channel blocking agents may have some role in prevention of post–MI complications in patients with non–Q-wave MI.

Risk stratification after MI can be made according to the results of 24-hour ambulatory ECG monitoring, resting LV ejection fraction, and low level exercise test in those who qualify. Patients without evidence of ongoing ischemia, an ejection fraction greater than 40 percent, and no complex ventricular ectopy have a 2–4 percent one-year mortality. No specific intervention is required. Those with ongoing ischemia and/or significant ventricular dysrhythmias and/or ejection fraction less than 40 percent have a 10–15 percent one-year mortality. Medical management, including revascularization in patients with continued ischemia, should be considered in this group. Patients with LV ejection fraction less than 40 percent and complex ventricular dysrhythmias who cannot undergo exercise testing because of ventricular dysfunction have a 35–50 percent one-year mortality; treatment is aimed at suppressing ventricular dysrhythmias and optimizing hemodynamic function.

In patients with diffuse myocardial necrosis not due to CAD, prognosis depends on the extent of myocardial damage that has occurred.

RECOMMENDED READING

Alonzo A, Simon AB, Feinlieb M: Prodromata of myocardial infarction and sudden death. Circulation 52:1056, 1975.

Blomberg DJ, Kimber WD, Burke MD: Creatine kinase isoenzymes: Predictive value in the early diagnosis of acute myocardial infarction. Am J Med 59:464, 1975.

Bruno FP, Cobb FR, Rivas F, et al: Evaluation of 99m technetium stannous pyrophosphate as an imaging agent in acute myocardial infarction. Circulation 54:71, 1976.

Buckley MJ, Mundth ED, Daggett WH, et al: Surgical management of ventricular septal defects and mitral regurgitation complicating acute myocardial infarction. Ann Thorac Surg 16:598, 1971.

Candell-Riera J, Figueras J, Valle V, et al: Right ventricular infarction: relationships between ST segment elevation in V_4R and hemodynamic, scintigraphic, and echocardiographic findings in patients with acute inferior myocardial infarction. Am Heart J 101:281, 1981.

Cohn JN, Guiha NH, Broder MI, et al: Right ventricular infarction: clinical and hemodynamic features. Am J Cardiol 33:209, 1974.

DeWood MA, Spores J, Notske R, et al: Prevalence of total coronary occlusion during the early hours of transmural myocardial infarction. N Engl J Med 303:897, 1980.

Engel TR, Meister SG, Frankl WS: The "R-on-T" phenomenon: an update and critical review. Ann Intern Med 88:221, 1978.

Forrester J, Chatterjee K, Parmley WW, et al: Hemodynamic profiles in acute myocardial infarction and their therapeutic implications. Circulation 48 (Suppl IV):59, 1973.

Forrester JS, Diamond G, Chatterjee K, et al: Medical therapy of acute myocardial infarction by application of hemodynamic subsets. N Engl J Med 295:1356, 1404, 1976.

Forrester JS, Diamond GA, Swan HJC: Correlative classification of clinical and hemodynamic function after acute myocardial infarction. Am J Cardiol 39:137, 1977.

Hassett MA, Williams RR, Wagner GS: Transient QRS changes simulating acute myocardial infarction. Circulation 62:975, 1980.

Hutter AM, Sidel VW, Shine KI, et al: Early hospital discharge after myocardial infarction. N Engl J Med 288:1141, 1973.

Kim YI, Williams JF: Large-dose sublingual nitroglycerin in acute myocardial infarction: relief of chest pain and reduction of Q wave evolution. Am J Cardiol 49:842, 1982.

Lie KI, Wellens HJ, VanCapelle FJ, et al: Lidocaine in the prevention of primary ventricular fibrillation. A double-blind randomized study of 212 consecutive patients. N Engl J Med 291:1324, 1974.

Meltzer LE, Kitchell JB: The incidence of dysrhythmias associated with acute myocardial infarction. Prog Cardiovasc Dis 9:50, 1966.

5. Unstable Angina

Nora F. Goldschlager

Nora F. Goldschlager

DEFINITION

Unstable angina is characterized by (1) anginal pain that occurs at rest and is of sufficient severity to warrant hospitalization to "rule out myocardial infarction (MI)"; (2) ST-T wave abnormalities that are transient and reversible, occurring with pain and returning toward or to baseline when pain has resolved; and (3) lack of rise of creatine kinase (CK) and myocardial fraction (MB) characteristic of an MI. Unstable angina occurs in patients with normal coronary arteries and in those with fixed atherosclerotic coronary artery disease (CAD); it may also occur during or shortly after acute MI.

PATHOPHYSIOLOGY

In contrast to effort angina, which occurs as a result of a primary increase in myocardial oxygen (O_2) demand (such as from an increase in heart rate and/or blood pressure) not being met by the available blood supply, unstable angina occurs as a result of a primary decrease in myocardial O_2 supply in the absence of an increase in O_2 demand. A decrease in O_2 supply can result from focal vasospasm occurring in normal or diseased coronary arteries, a generalized increase in coronary vasomotor tone, thrombus formation, or hemorrhage into or rupture of an atherosclerotic plaque. One or more of these variables may be operative alone or in combination. The arterial occlusion that results can obstruct coronary flow to varying degrees. The process is often transient, owing to relief of the underlying vasospasm, reduction in vasomotor tone, and lysis of the thrombus. Interaction at the endothelial surface of the coronary artery among platelets and vasoactive peptides as well as loss of endothelial integrity are currently areas of intense research activity.

DIAGNOSIS

The patient has severe chest pain at rest. A pre-admission crescendo (worsening) pain pattern may be elicited. The chest pain is often described by the patient as resembling his or her usual anginal pain but more severe in nature. If the unstable angina occurs in a patient without underlying CAD, a history of prior angina or MI is absent; however, the patient may complain of nocturnal angina that may awaken him from sleep. Associated symptoms (radiation of pain, shortness of breath, diaphoresis) resembling those of acute MI may be present. If the patient has been taking antianginal medications, including sublingual nitroglycerin, there is often a lack of response to these agents, and several sublingual nitroglycerin tablets may be required for any reduction in pain.

Physical examination is usually unremarkable, although a transient S3 gallop, murmur of mitral regurgitation, paradoxically split S2, and pulmonary rales are occasionally appreciated during the pain. The chest roentgenogram is normal or unchanged from prior examinations.

The electrocardiogram (ECG) reveals ST-T wave abnormalities during pain that resolve after the pain is relieved. The ST-T abnormalities may consist of ST-segment depression or isolated T-wave inversion (nontransmural or subendocardial ischemia), elevation (transmural ischemia), or "pseudonormalization," in which the ST-T waves appear more normal during pain than during the patient's baseline ECG. Any or all of these may be present in a given patient at different times, and up to 65 percent of episodes may be clinically silent, unaccompanied by symptoms. Total CK and MB fraction may be slightly elevated, but not above twice normal. Significant rises in CK-MB indicate acute MI, rather than unstable angina.

MANAGEMENT

The patient should be admitted to an intensive care unit with continuous ECG monitoring. The monitoring lead should reflect the abnormal ST-segment deviation as disclosed on the 12-lead ECG; lead II or modified V_{2-4} leads provide the greatest diagnostic yield.

Pain should be aggressively treated with sedation, analgesics, O_2, antianginal agents (see Tables 4–1 and 4–2), and antiplatelet agents. Calcium entry blocking agents should be employed to protect against vasospasm; sublingual, topical, and oral nitrate preparations are used to reduce preload and to dilate the epicardial coronary vessels; β-blocking agents may be useful in treating hypertension and/or tachycardia, including the tachycardia that may occur with use of some of the calcium entry blocking medications. Aspirin should be used as an antiplatelet agent.

Patients who continue to have pain despite aggressive medical therapy and normal or low blood pressure and heart rate should have a pulmonary artery catheter placed to guide further therapy. Intravenous thrombolytic therapy using heparin or streptokinase should be considered in these patients. If ischemic pain continues, intraaortic balloon counterpulsation should be initiated (see Chapter 17), and cardiac catheterization performed; myocardial revascularization should be undertaken in appropriate patients.

Patients who become asymptomatic with medical therapy should be transferred to a ward with telemetric capability and should undergo gradual increase in activity much like the patient recovering from an acute MI. A low-level exercise test prior to hospital discharge should be performed in order to identify continuing ischemia; if myocardial ischemia is demonstrated, cardiac catheterization should be carried out, preferably prior to discharge.

OUTCOME

Up to 10 percent of patients with unstable angina have normal coronary arteries on cardiac catheterization, and prognosis is good. Spasmolytic agents and nitrates may, however, be required for variable lengths of time.

Ten to 15 percent of patients have left main CAD and should undergo aortocoronary bypass surgery. The remainder have single vessel (about 35 percent) or multivessel CAD (about 50–60 percent); surgical treatment is generally recommended in the latter, angioplasty in the former.

Overall outcome depends on the extent and severity of the underlying CAD, the degree of preexisting left ventricular dysfunction, and the presence and severity of ongoing ischemia, as in the case of the patient with acute MI. Myocardial revascularization should be performed if continuing ischemia can be documented and should be strongly considered in patients with multivessel CAD and impaired ventricular function who are relatively asymptomatic.

RECOMMENDED READING

Ambrose JA, Winters SL, Arora RR, et al: Coronary angiographic morphology in myocardial infarction: a link between the pathogenesis of unstable angina and myocardial infarction. J Am Coll Cardiol 6:1233, 1985.

Ambrose JA, Winters SJ, Stern A, et al: Angiographic morphology and the pathogenesis of unstable angina pectoris. J Am Coll Cardiol 5:609, 1985.

Cairns JA, Gent M, Singer J, et al: Aspirin, sulfinpyrazone, or both in unstable angina. N Eng J Med 313:1369, 1985.

Figueras J, Singh BN, Ganz W, et al: Mechanism of rest and nocturnal angina: observations during continuous hemodynamic and electrocardiographic monitoring. Circulation 59:955, 1979.

Golding LAR, Loop FD, Sheldon WC, et al: Emergency revascularization for unstable angina. Circulation 58:1163, 1978.

Haines DE, Raabe DS, Gundel WD, et al: Anatomic and prognostic significance of new T-wave inversion in unstable angina. Am J Cardiol 52:14, 1983.

Johnson SM, Mauritson DR, Winniford MD, et al: Continuous electrocardiographic monitoring in patients with unstable angina pectoris: identification of high-risk subgroup with severe coronary disease, variant angina, and/or impaired early prognosis. Am Heart J 103:4, 1982.

Mandelkorn JB, Wolf NM, Singh S, et al: Intracoronary thrombus in nontransmural myocardial infarction and in unstable angina pectoris. Am J Cardiol 52:1, 1983.

National Cooperative Study Group: Unstable angina pectoris: National Cooperative study group to compare surgical and medical therapy. Am J Cardiol 42:839, 1978.

Oliva PB: Unstable rest angina with ST-segment depression. Ann Intern Med 100:424, 1984.

Rahimtoola SH: Unstable angina: current status. Mod Concepts Cardiovasc Dis 54:116, 1985.

Singh BN, Nademanee K: Beta-adrenergic blockade in unstable angina pectoris. Am J Cardiol 57:992, 1986.

6. Valvular Disruption

Nora F. Goldschlager

Nora F. Goldschlager

DEFINITION

Valve disruption refers to the loss of integrity or separation of any portion of a cardiac valve and can involve the leaflet, annular attachment, chordae tendineae, or muscular support. Valve disruption is a potentially life-threatening occurrence if the aortic or mitral valves are involved. The resulting valvular insufficiency is often refractory to medical management, necessitating urgent surgical intervention. Disruption of the tricuspid valve is less emergent and can often be managed medically.

ACUTE TRICUSPID REGURGITATION

Pathophysiology

Rupture of the papillary muscle support to the tricuspid valve is rare and is due to trauma or to myocardial infarction (MI). Chordal rupture may be due to trauma or to infective endocarditis (IE) or may occur spontaneously in patients without structural heart disease and in those with tricuspid valve prolapse due to myxomatous degeneration. Fenestration of the valve leaflets may be due to trauma but most often results from endocarditis.

Insufficiency of the tricuspid valve produces a volume overload to the right atrium and right ventricle, which then dilate as a compensatory mechanism. Central venous pressures rise, causing right-sided "congestive failure." If the tricuspid regurgitation (TR) is massive, underfilling of the left heart can result, leading to a low output syndrome.

Diagnosis

The physical examination will vary with the cause. Pure TR is initially unaccompanied by central venous pressure elevation, and is manifested by a prominent systolic regurgitant wave in the neck. If the right atrium is normal in size and volume and has normal compliance, inspiratory increase in intensity of the murmur is expected to be present; however, if the right atrium is dilated and very compliant, alterations in intensity of the murmur with changes in pressure and flow may not occur.

A parasternal lift will be present in right ventricular volume overload. P2 is normal unless pulmonary hypertension is present; a right ventricular S3 gallop that increases with inspiration is heard. The murmur of TR is usually not holosystolic and is often crescendo-decrescendo in contour; its quality varies from blowing to harsh, depending on the etiology and the flow pattern across the valve. A thrill may be present. If the regurgitant volume is very large, a diastolic flow murmur following the S3 gallop will be present; it is distinguished from organic tricuspid stenosis by the clinical setting and the absence of associated findings. Long-standing TR is accompanied by an increase in central venous pressure, hepatomegaly (sometimes painful), peripheral edema, and ascites. Jaundice may be present, and marked abnormalities of liver function may be found.

The electrocardiogram (ECG) is usually within normal limits in isolated TR, although tall P waves suggesting right atrial abnormality may be seen. If TR accompanies right ventricular MI, evidence of inferoposterior and right ventricular infarction will be present. The chest roentgenogram may disclose right atrial and right ventricular enlargement, depending on the chronicity of the disease. The echocardiogram may reveal a large right atrium and ventricle and paradoxical motion of the interventricular septum, which contributes to right ventricular ejection in right ventricular volume overload. The etiology of the TR may also be seen (for example, regional wall motion disorder of ischemic heart disease, vegetations in IE, tricuspid and mitral valve prolapse).

Management

Management is medical unless the TR is due to trauma requiring surgery for other reasons or to IE with recurrent septic pulmonary emboli. Care must be taken not to overdiurese the patient, as left ventricular underfilling with low cardiac output can occur. Afterload-reducing agents to lower pulmonary vascular resistance may be tried, but their use is usually limited by systemic hypotension due to decreased systemic vascular resistance. Tricuspid valve repair or replacement may be performed in selected patients; long-term anticoagulation is required in the latter.

Outcome

Prognosis depends on the cause of the tricuspid regurgitation and is often benign, even if the etiology is IE.

ACUTE MITRAL REGURGITATION

Pathophysiology

Rupture of the mitral valve or its supporting apparatus is a potentially fatal occurrence. Rupture of the base of a papillary muscle is usually due to ischemic necrosis. Because a papillary muscle supplies chordal support to both anterior and posterior leaflets, rupture at its base results in a flail valve, a situation that is incompatible with life. Rupture of a papillary muscle tip is also invariably due to MI. However, it is compatible with survival, since fewer chordae, often supplying only one leaflet, arise from a papillary muscle tip; thus, although incompetent, the mitral valve is not a flail valve. The posteromedial papillary muscle ruptures more frequently than the anterolateral papillary muscle, and this rupture is seen during acute inferoposterior wall MI. Chordal rupture is due to IE or to myxomatous degeneration such as is seen in Marfan's syndrome or in valve prolapse; it may be spontaneous, occurring in normal individuals, and can occur after nonpenetrating chest trauma. Fenestration is usually the result of IE.

Acute mitral regurgitation (MR) may not be severe, especially if it is due to rupture of a few chordae tendineae, and thus may be compatible with long-term survival. Acute severe MR, in contrast, produces pulmonary edema that is often refractory to medical management, left ventricular volume overload, and passive pulmonary hypertension. The pulmonary edema and pulmonary hypertension (which sometimes causes right-sided failure) result from sudden left atrial hypertension caused by acute volume overload in a chamber of normal size and compliance.

Diagnosis

The primary symptom is dyspnea. Physical examination discloses a dynamic, nondisplaced cardiac apical impulse. A parasternal lift may be present and is due either to right ventricular enlargement resulting from pulmonary hypertension or to "paradoxical" systolic expansion of the more posteriorly located left atrium. Both S3 and S4 gallop sounds are heard; the presence of an S4 gallop distinguishes acute MR from chronic MR, the latter usually being associated with atrial fibrillation and thus absence of S4. P2 may be increased if pulmonary hypertension is present. The MR murmur is of variable intensity, depending on its degree and on the cardiac output; it is sometimes not holosystolic and may be crescendo-decrescendo in contour. If chordal rupture to the posterior leaflet is present, the murmur radiates to the base and can be confused with that of aortic stenosis; however, there are no associated findings such as slowly rising pulses, sustained apical impulse that is displaced downward and to the left, and diminished to absent A2. If chordal rupture to the anterior leaflet has occurred, the murmur radiates to the axilla, to the back, and up the spine. Both leaflets are often involved, and the murmur is very loud and widespread. In patients with acute MI who develop hemodynamic decompensation and a systolic murmur, the differential diagnosis of acute MR, ruptured interventricular septum, or severe papillary muscle dysfunction cannot always be made on clinical grounds alone (although the presence of a thrill suggests a ventricular septal defect [VSD]), and bedside catheterization of the right heart is required.

The ECG may be normal or may show evidence of MI. Patterns compatible with left atrial abnormality or left ventricular hypertrophy occur in patients in whom the MR is more chronic. Sinus rhythm is usually present; atrial fibrillation is suggestive of chronic MR. The chest roentgenogram may reveal pulmonary edema. The left atrial size is normal. In chronic MR, left atrial, left ventricular, and right ventricular enlargement will be present on the chest roentgenogram.

The echocardiogram is very helpful in evaluating the etiology of the MR, as well as in confirming the presence of left ventricular volume overload by showing hyperdynamic motion of the interventricular septum and posterior walls. Exaggerated left ventricular wall motion may not be seen in patients with MI who have regional wall thinning and reduced movement. Mitral valve prolapse may be seen, as may flail chordae or papillary muscle tip and valvular vegetations. Chamber size and regional wall motion can be evaluated and severity of the MR estimated from Doppler flow studies.

Bedside flow-directed balloon catheterization of the right heart discloses a prominent systolic regurgitant wave in the pulmonary artery wedge pressure tracing; mean wedge pressure may be normal. If the MR is severe, the regurgitant wave can be superimposed on the pulmonary artery pressure tracing itself as a second wave occurring in systole, prior to the dicrotic notch. The regurgitant wave amplitude may approach left ventricular systolic pressure. Right heart catheterization can exclude the diagnosis of ruptured interventricular septum in patients in whom the diagnosis is in doubt, since an oxygen step-up at the level of the right ventricle (or the right atrium if significant streaming occurs) signifying left-to-right shunt will not be present.

Management

Medical management is used to stabilize the patient hemodynamically prior to surgical treatment. Diuretics are used to treat the pulmonary edema; digitalis may be helpful, but caution is warranted in patients with acute MI, since the drug lowers the threshold for ventricular fibrillation. Afterload-reducing agents are given intravenously to lower systemic vascular resistance and enhance stroke volume, thereby reducing the regurgitant volume to the left atrium. Nitroprusside is the agent of choice and is administered in doses sufficient to reduce the regurgitant wave to a reasonable value (15–25 mm Hg; mean pulmonary artery wedge pressure 12–18 mm Hg). Hypotension is treated with dopamine if it is not improved by reduction in the regurgitant volume. Intraaortic balloon counterpulsation (see Chapter 17) may be required for hemodynamic stability. Cardiac catheterization with coronary angiography should be carried out in patients with papillary muscle tip rupture secondary to acute infarction, since myocardial revascularization is undertaken at the same time as valve replacement. Catheterization may have to be performed with the patient receiving balloon counterpulsation. Cardiac catheterization is not absolutely required in other cases of mitral valve disruption, and surgery should not be delayed in order to perform this procedure. Despite the high surgical risk, surgery is preferable to medical therapy in patients with valve disruption causing severe MR.

Outcome

Patients who have rupture of a few chordae tendineae may be able to tolerate acute MR by virtue of left atrial and ventricular dilatation and hypertrophy; they then have a clinical course resembling chronic MR. Patients who have undergone mitral valve replacement follow the course of those with valve replacement for any reason. Anticoagulation is required. Patients who have mitral valve replacement associated with myocardial revascularization have a higher surgical risk (10–25 percent) and a poorer early and late result than those who have valve replacement alone, owing primarily to the extent and severity of ischemic left ventricular dysfunction. Patients with rupture of chordal support to the posterior leaflet of the mitral valve are candidates for mitral valvuloplasty, in which redundant leaflet tissue is plicated; anticoagulation is not required in these cases, and the surgical results are generally excellent.

ACUTE AORTIC REGURGITATION

Pathophysiology

Acute aortic regurgitation (AR) imposes a large volume overload at high (aortic diastolic) pressure to the left ventricle, which, if the ventricle is of normal size and compliance, cannot adapt acutely by dilating. Because of the marked increase in left ventricular diastolic pressure in the face of a near-normal diastolic volume, there is an early impairment in ejection, which results in low forward stroke output, left atrial hypertension, and pulmonary edema.

The usual etiologies are IE, aortic dissection, and nonpenetrating chest or upper abdominal trauma. Aortic dissection (see Chapter 10) produces AR by causing aortic root dilatation with separation of the aortic cusps, by displacement of a cusp due to the pressure of a hematoma, and by shearing off a cusp from its annular support structure. IE causes AR by fenestration of a cusp or by leaflet destruction.

Diagnosis

The patient appears acutely ill, with tachycardia, peripheral hypoperfusion, and congestive heart failure. Fever and positive blood cultures are present in patients with IE, and anterior chest and back pain are present in those with aortic dissection. Physical examination discloses a somewhat widened pulse pressure but not so wide as in chronic AR. The widened pulse pressure may be the earliest sign of acute AR. The left ventricular impulse is dynamic and nondisplaced. A2 is normal. S1 is diminished, owing to premature closure of the mitral valve by the regurgitant jet, and there is no S4. The diastolic murmur may be of variable intensity, depending upon the direction of the regurgitant jet as well as its volume; often the tachycardia precludes accurate auscultation. A holodiastolic murmur indicates only that there is regurgitation throughout diastole; a murmur that ends in early or mid diastole indicates only that the regurgitation ceases partway through diastole. The differential diagnosis of this finding is insignificant AR or life-threatening AR in which the AR is so severe that the left ventricular end-diastolic pressure equals aortic diastolic pressure early in diastole. The clinical picture clarifies the issue. For similar reasons, bounding, bisferiens, and water-hammer pulses are not felt, and Quincke's pulses are not seen if the acute AR is severe.

The ECG may be normal or, if aortic dissection is present, may reveal left ventricular hypertrophy due to preexisting hypertension, pericarditis, or inferior wall MI due to right coronary artery dissection or shearing off of the artery from the aorta. The chest roentgenogram shows normal chamber size unless preexisting left ventricular hypertrophy is present; abnormalities of the aortic shadow, such as widening of the mediastinal shadow, may suggest dissection. Caution should be used in interpreting anteroposterior chest roentgenograms, however, since significant anatomic distortion can be present. Pulmonary congestion is present.

The echocardiogram shows diastolic fluttering and premature closure of the mitral valve (before the onset of the QRS complex). The dynamic ventricular wall motion and dilatation seen in chronic AR are not present. In patients with aortic dissection, the dissection itself, an intimal tear, and pericardial fluid may be visualized. Vegetations or a flail leaflet that prolapses into the left ventricular outflow tract in diastole may be demonstrated in patients with IE. Doppler flow studies allow estimation of the severity of the regurgitation.

Management

Medical management is usually employed only temporarily until surgery can be performed. Pulmonary edema should be treated with diuretics. Afterload-reducing agents are used to lower systemic vascular resistance, thereby increasing forward stroke volume and reducing regurgitant volume. Intraaortic balloon counterpulsation is contraindicated, owing to its effect of augmenting aortic diastolic pressure, thus increasing the AR. Cardiac catheterization may be performed to identify aortic dissection or to evaluate the possibility of other diagnoses such as ruptured sinus of Valsalva with fistula formation. However, surgery should not be delayed, especially when the diagnosis seems clear. Similarly, surgery should never be delayed in patients with IE in order to attempt to complete a full course of antibiotic therapy, since surgery can be performed safely even in patients with positive blood cultures.

Outcome

When aortic valve replacement is accomplished, the patient's course resembles that of any patient with a prosthetic aortic valve. Anticoagulation is required. Prosthetic valve dehiscence is more common in patients with aortic prostheses than in those with mitral valve prostheses and should be considered if symptoms and signs recur.

PROSTHETIC VALVE DEHISCENCE

Dehiscence of a prosthetic valve may result from technical problems or from undermining of the suture lines, owing to infection or necrosis in surrounding tissue. Prosthetic valve dehiscence imposes the same deleterious conditions upon the heart as do acute severe regurgitant lesions in native valves. Dehiscence of the aortic valve is the most common and the most serious. Fluoroscopy may demonstrate excessive motion of the prosthesis. Treatment is surgical (except in tricuspid valve dehiscence, which does not constitute an emergency) and should be performed without undue delay.

RECOMMENDED READING

Cheng TO, Bashour T, Adkins PC: Acute severe mitral regurgitation from papillary muscle dysfunction in acute myocardial infarction. Circulation 46:491, 1972.

Goodman D, Kimbiris D, Linhart JW: Chordae tendineae rupture complicating the systolic click–late systolic murmur syndrome. Am J Cardiol 33:681, 1974.

Griffin FM, Jr, Jones G, Cobbs CG: Aortic insufficiency in bacterial endocarditis. Ann Intern Med 76:23, 1972.

Howe JP, Alpert JS: Acute mitral regurgitation. In Dalen JE (ed): Valvular Heart Disease. Boston, Little, Brown & Co., Inc., 1981, p. 135.

Morganroth J, Perloff JK, Zeldis SM, et al: Acute severe aortic regurgitation. Ann Intern Med 87:223, 1977.

Selzer A, Kelly JJ, Jr, Vannitamby M, et al: The syndrome of mitral insufficiency due to isolated rupture of the chordae tendineae. Am J Med 43:822, 1967.

Simpson P, Bristow JD: Acute diseases of native and prosthetic cardiac valves. In Scheinman MM (ed): Cardiac Emergencies. Philadelphia, W. B. Saunders Co., 1984, p. 213.

White AF, Dinsmore RE, Buckley MJ: Cineradiographic evaluation of prosthetic cardiac valves. Circulation 48:882, 1973.

7. Myocardial Contusion

Nora F. Goldschlager

DEFINITION AND PATHOPHYSIOLOGY

Myocardial contusion describes a condition in which petechiae and ecchymoses are present in one or more layers of myocardium. They are usually the result of non-penetrating injury to the chest. Nonpenetrating chest trauma can result in a spectrum of myocardial pathology, ranging from contusion to cardiac rupture; the clinical presentation can therefore vary from an asymptomatic state to a life-threatening emergency. Myocardial contusion is usually unrecognized clinically, since it does not produce significant symptoms; accompanying chest trauma usually predominates the clinical picture. The diagnosis of myocardial contusion is most often made by specific laboratory investigations.

DIAGNOSIS

The most common symptom is precordial pain. The pain may resemble that of acute myocardial infarction but often has a pleuritic or pericarditic component or both. The pain is unresponsive to nitroglycerin and coronary artery spasmolytic agents but may respond to antiinflammatory drugs.

The electrocardiogram (ECG) usually shows nondiagnostic ST-T wave abnormalities but may disclose features typical of pericarditis. Q waves signifying myocardial necrosis are not usually seen unless myocardial injury is severe or a coronary artery is lacerated or thrombosed. The patient with suspected myocardial contusion should have an ECG performed upon admission and serially thereafter for several days, in order to assess the occurrence of an evolutionary pattern of myocardial necrosis. If the ECG is normal on admission, contusion is unlikely.

Serial determinations of creatine kinase-myocardial fraction (CK-MB) activity should be performed to assess the extent of myocardial necrosis. The recognized causes of false-positive CK-MB assays (hypothermia, bowel infarction, pancreatitis, hypothyroidism, and intracerebral infarction) are relevant in the trauma patient and should be excluded when evaluating the significance of an elevated enzyme level.

Echocardiography may be helpful in establishing the diagnosis of contusion. The findings might include demonstration of a regional wall motion disorder (which usually involves the right ventricle) and will show pericardial fluid if this is present. The echocardiographic findings will reflect the extent of myocardial injury and thus may be absent in patients with mild trauma. Specificity of the findings in patients with past myocardial infarction due to coronary artery disease is substantially reduced.

Radionuclide imaging is a sensitive and relatively specific means of evaluating myocardial contusion. Technetium-labeled pyrophosphate (TcPYP) will be concentrated in areas of myocardial necrosis ("hot spots"); scans should be performed one week apart to assess resolution of the necrotic process. Positive pyrophosphate scans may also be seen in patients with remote myocardial infarction in which calcium is present (as in a calcified thrombus) and in patients with calcific valvular disease. Radionuclide ventriculography may reveal a hypokinetic or akinetic segment of ventricular muscle (usually the right ventricle); extravasation of the isotope into the pericardial space indicates myocardial rupture. The right ventricular ejection fraction may be transiently depressed; a depressed left ventricular ejection fraction should prompt a search for other etiologies. Radionuclide ventriculography is a highly sensitive and specific test for myocardial injury.

Although dysrhythmias are common in patients with myocardial contusion, they are neither sensitive nor specific for the diagnosis. Atrial dysrhythmias may reflect pericarditis or high circulating catecholamine levels. Sustained ventricular tachycardia is extremely rare, whereas ventricular extrasystoles and nonsustained bursts of ventricular tachycardia (lasting less than 30 seconds and not requiring intervention) are quite common. Ventricular dysrhythmias can deteriorate into ventricular fibrillation. Evidence of sinus node dysfunction and atrioventricular and intraventricular conduction disturbances can be seen and are usually transient; their occurrence may reflect the presence of patchy, localized areas of hemorrhagic myocardial necrosis.

MANAGEMENT

The management of patients with myocardial contusion suspected on the basis of the clinical picture and an abnormal ECG is similar to that of patients with acute myocardial infarction. They should be admitted to an acute care area with rhythm monitoring capabilities. Ventricular dysrhythmias should be managed with intravenous lidocaine or procainamide if lidocaine is ineffective (Table 3–1). Prophylactic antidysrhythmic therapy is probably not warranted. When the diagnosis of myocardial contusion is established, management proceeds along the lines of the postinfarction patient, with progressive ambulation prior to discharge. For the first two to three days after the acute unit stay, rhythm monitoring by telemetry is necessary. Persistent dysrhythmias may require treatment if they are frequent, sustained, or clinically symptomatic. If the diagnosis of contusion is not established, the patient may be discharged at the discretion of the treating physician.

Outcome

Prognosis is generally excellent in patients with myocardial contusion if no chronic underlying heart disease, such as coronary artery disease, is present and if the area of contusion is not large. Late and unusual complications, such as ventricular aneurysm formation, recurrent systemic embolism, congestive heart failure, and pericardial constriction have been reported but are rare.

RECOMMENDED READING

Allen RP, Liedtke AJ: The role of coronary artery injury and perfusion in the development of cardiac contusion secondary to nonpenetrating chest trauma. J Trauma 19:153, 1979.

Dugani BV, Higginson LAJ, Beanlands DS, et al: Recurrent systemic emboli following myocardial contusion. Am Heart J 108:1354, 1984.

Katz S, Gimmon Z, Appelbaum A: Cardiac contusion in the patient with multiple injuries. Injury 12:180, 1980.

Liedtke AJ, DeMuth WE Jr: Nonpenetrating cardiac injuries: a collective review. Am Heart J 86:687, 1973.

Parmley LF, Manion WC, Mattingly TW: Nonpenetrating trauma of the heart. Circulation 18:371, 1958.

Potkin RT, Werner JA, Trobaugh GB, et al: Evaluation of noninvasive tests of cardiac damage in suspected cardiac contusion. Circulation 66:627, 1982.

Ruder MA, Flaker GC, Alpert MA, et al: Right ventricular myocardial contusion simulating constrictive pericardial disease. Am Heart J 108:1353, 1984.

Stein PD, Sabbah HN, Viano DC, et al: Response of the heart to nonpenetrating cardiac trauma. J Trauma 22:364, 1982.

Sutherland GR, Driedger AA, Holliday RL, et al: Frequency of myocardial injury after blunt chest trauma as evaluated by radionuclide angiography. Am J Cardiol 52:1099, 1983.

Symbas PN: Cardiac trauma. Am Heart J 92:387, 1976.

8. Shock

Nora F. Goldschlager

Shock describes a condition in which severe circulatory impairment is present such that tissue underperfusion, with failure of delivery of substrates and removal of metabolites and eventual organ dysfunction and damage, results unless the process is reversed. The major forms of shock are hypovolemic, anaphylactic, septic, and cardiogenic. Spinal shock, which is less common, is discussed in Chapter 72.

Pathophysiology

A "preshock" state ("compensated hypotension") exists during which systemic vasoconstriction and tachycardia are present. (Tachycardia may not be marked in patients with sinus node dysfunction, autonomic insufficiency, advanced age, and in those taking β-blocking medications.) With progression, the blood pressure declines despite the compensatory tachycardia and peripheral vasoconstriction, and organ hypoperfusion resulting in clinical symptoms occurs. The full-blown picture of shock eventuates and consists of (1) systolic arterial blood pressure less than 90 mm Hg; (2) urine output less than 20 ml/hr; (3) often cool, clammy skin, although the skin may be warm in septic shock; (4) alteration in mental state (impaired consciousness, agitation, stupor, coma, restlessness, confusion); and (5) metabolic acidosis. The acidosis, caused by anaerobic metabolism and lactate production, renal failure with retention of organic acids, and hypoxia, can lead to peripheral vasodilatation and a decreased responsiveness to sympathomimetic amines, as well as to myocardial depression. Hyperglycemia may be present, owing to the effects of excess circulating epinephrine. Respiratory acidosis may compound the metabolic acidosis. Disseminated intravascular coagulation may occur, further aggravating the tissue hypoperfusion. Irreversible shock is present when cellular membrane integrity is violated and organ failure has occurred. All compensatory mechanisms may be decreased with advanced age.

Tissue hypoperfusion is the result of the interaction of two mechanisms: blood flow to an organ (cardiac output) and the arteriolar resistance of that organ. If the vascular resistance is very high owing to vasoconstriction or microcirculatory occlusion, organ damage can occur even though blood flow and pressure are normal. If the vascular resistance is very low, physiologic arteriovenous shunting through the tissue, which precludes normal organ metabolic processes, may occur despite normal or high blood flow.

If the preshock syndrome is not immediately treated, irreversible shock with microcirculatory failure and violation of cellular integrity follows. Cellular membrane damage can release lysosomal enzymes with further cellular destruction and can alter the permeability to electrolytes and water. Specific tissue damage results in renal tubular necrosis and transudation of fluid into the extravascular space; myocardial depression may eventually occur.

DIAGNOSIS

The clinical pictures of "preshock" and full-blown shock were described earlier. The diagnosis of specific kinds of shock are covered later in this chapter.

MANAGEMENT

Principles of management consist of circulatory support and correction of acidosis along with measures to correct the underlying etiology and to prevent complications such as renal failure and acute respiratory distress syndrome. Invasive hemodynamic monitoring to define the hemodynamic picture is essential in cardiogenic and septic shock and expedites management of all shock syndromes, especially if the patient has other underlying diseases. Central venous pressure usually is insufficient to indicate the blood volume; thus, unless central venous pressure is low in patients whose left ventricular function is likely to be normal, pulmonary artery catheterization is required (see Chapter 15). Since cuff and intraarterial blood pressure measurements can be discrepant up to 50 mm Hg, especially if there is severe peripheral vasoconstriction, direct intraarterial monitoring should be performed. Continuous electrocardiographic (ECG) monitoring is mandatory. Urine output must be continuously monitored, and frequent determinations must be made of systemic arterial blood gases, pulmonary function, BUN, creatinine and electrolytes, and clotting factors. An arterial oxygen tension (PaO_2) of 60–70 mm Hg should be maintained; intubation may be required. Pressor agents useful in shock are listed in Table 8–1. Newer inotropic-vasodilating agents are listed in Table 8–2, and the predominant vascular effects of commonly used

TABLE 8–1. CATECHOLAMINES IN CARDIOGENIC SHOCK

DRUG	MAJOR RECEPTOR(S)	USUAL DOSES (μg/kg/min)
Dopamine	B_1†, dopaminergic§	1–30
Dobutamine	B_1†	5–50
Isoproterenol	B_1†, B_2‡	0.02–0.20
Norepinephrine	α*	0.01–0.05
Epinephrine	α* (at larger doses), B_1†	0.05–0.15
Phenylephrine	α*	0.5–1.0
Methoxamine	α*	5–20

*α effects: Vasoconstriction of cutaneous, renal, mucosal, skeletal muscle, and intestinal vascular beds

†B_1 effects: Increased force and rate of cardiac contraction

‡B_2 effects: Vasodilatation of skeletal muscle and mesenteric vascular beds; bronchodilatation

§Dopaminergic: Vasodilatation of renal and mesenteric vascular beds

TABLE 8–2. HEMODYNAMIC EFFECTS OF NEWER INOTROPIC-VASODILATING AGENTS

	HEART RATE	BLOOD PRESSURE	CARDIAC OUTPUT	SYSTEMIC VASCULAR RESISTANCE	PULMONARY ARTERY WEDGE PRESSURE	RIGHT ATRIAL PRESSURE
Amrinone	↑	↑	↑ ↑	↓ ↓	↓ ↓	↓ ↓
Milrinone	↑	↓	↑ ↑	↓ ↓	↓ ↓	↓ ↓
Posicor	↑	↓	↑ ↑	↓ ↓	↓ ↓	↓ ↓
MDL 17043	↑	↓	↑ ↑	↓ ↓	↓ ↓	↓ ↓
MDL 19043	↑	↓	↑ ↑	↓ ↓	↓ ↓	↓ ↓

TABLE 8–3. COMPARISON OF EFFECTS OF VASODILATORS

	PREDOMINANT EFFECT	
DRUG	*Preload* (Venous Dilation)	*Afterload* (Arteriolar Dilation)
Captopril	X	X
Diazoxide		X
Hydralazine		X
Isosorbide Dinitrate	X	
Minoxidil		X
Nitroglycerin	X	
Nitroprusside	X	X
Phentolamine		X
Phenoxybenzamine		X
Prazosin	X	X

vasodilating agents are listed in Table 8–3. Adequate intravascular volume, guided by hemodynamic monitoring, must be maintained.

OUTCOME

The outcome depends upon the etiology of the shock. Cardiogenic shock continues to have a mortality of about 80–90 percent despite the availability of newer drugs and techniques to treat the condition (see Cardiogenic Shock below). The mortality in septic shock is around 60 percent. Early recognition of the preshock state and aggressive management can reduce mortality significantly.

HYPOVOLEMIC SHOCK

Definition

Hypovolemic shock results from intravascular volume depletion most often due to hemorrhage, vomiting, diarrhea, burns, overdiuresis, diabetes mellitus, and pancreatitis. Gastrointestinal and retroperitoneal bleeding or hemorrhage into an aortic aneurysm may be occult.

Pathophysiology

Intravascular volume depletion in hypovolemic shock is responsible for the pathophysiologic events described previously.

Diagnosis

Hypovolemic shock is diagnosed by the demonstration of a decreased intravascular volume in the setting of hypotension and end-organ abnormalities such as abnormal mental status and diminished urine output. From a hemodynamic standpoint, central venous and pulmonary artery wedge pressures are low; cardiac output is low, owing to reduced filling pressures. Systemic vascular resistance is normal or increased as a compensatory mechanism. Sinus tachycardia is present and can reach rates of 150–160/min. The hypotension will be compensated for by tachycardia and peripheral vasoconstriction if blood volume loss does not exceed 20 percent.

Management

Rapid intravenous (IV) infusion of volume load (300 ml normal saline in 10–20 minutes) may be all that is required for hemodynamic stability and should be given before any vasoactive agents are used. The volume load can be repeated once or twice if blood pressure does not rise, provided that central venous pressure remains normal (or low) and pulmonary rales are not present. Crystalloids may be used, but albumin is expensive and has a short half-life, plasma can cause hepatitis, and dextran or hetastarch can interfere with coagulation. If evidence of left ventricular failure is present, pulmonary artery catheterization is required. Early use of vasoactive agents before restoration of intravascular volume can lead to more marked vasoconstriction and further reduction in organ perfusion as well as to increased impedance to left ventricular ejection and to depression of cardiac performance. If shock is due to blood loss, transfusion is necessary; whole blood should be used initially if available unless the patient has underlying cardiac disease, in which case packed cells are preferred in order to avoid pulmonary edema. Inotropic agents are not indicated in hypovolemic shock, since myocardial pump failure is not the problem.

Outcome

Outcome depends on the percentage of intravascular volume lost. If this does not exceed 500 ml, compensation is complete. If 20 percent of the total blood volume is lost, hypotension can be compensated for by tachycardia and vasoconstriction. If more than 45 percent of the blood volume is lost, shock is usually irreversible. If volume can be rapidly restored, prognosis is generally good, depending upon the etiology of the shock. The major complication of therapy is pulmonary edema, which can be avoided if pulmonary artery catheterization is performed and pulmonary artery wedge pressures serially followed; this is particularly important in patients with underlying cardiac disease.

ANAPHYLACTIC SHOCK

Definition

Anaphylaxis is an immediate hypersensitivity reaction to reexposure to an antigen in patients previously sensitized to that antigen. The reaction is mediated by IgE antibody and results from release of substances from mast cells and basophils. The usual causative agents in the intensive care unit (ICU) setting are antibiotics (penicillins, cephalosporins, tetracyclines, aminoglycosides, and amphotericin B), local anesthetics (lidocaine, procaine), animal sera (horse and rabbit sera), and, occasionally, dextran. Anaphylactic reactions to iodinated dyes and nonsteroidal antiinflammatory agents (acetylsalicylic acid, indomethacin) occur more rarely.

Pathophysiology

In sensitive individuals (a positive skin test does not predict the occurrence of anaphylaxis, although the possibility is more likely), the release of certain agents, including histamine, prostaglandins, and kinins, results in constriction of bronchial smooth muscle, an increase in vascular permeability with loss of intravascular volume, induction of platelet aggregation and degranulation, and a decrease in peripheral vascular smooth muscle tone, resulting in vasodilatation and hypotension.

Diagnosis

The patient is agitated, may be wheezing or choking, and may be cyanotic. The cutaneous reactions include erythema, urticaria, and angioedema of the eyes, lips, and tongue. Upper airway obstruction due to laryngeal edema can cause acute respiratory distress and death. Lower airway obstruction due to bronchoconstriction causes hypoxemia and hypercarbia and is not effectively treated by intubation alone. Circulatory collapse can occur with or without pulmonary involvement, and may be associated with ECG abnormalities suggesting myocardial ischemia.

The hemodynamic profile of anaphylactic shock is similar to that of septic shock, which is discussed in the next section. Because of the acute nature of the process, laboratory data are generally not helpful.

Management

If applicable, a tourniquet should be placed on the extremity into which the antigen was introduced, in order to avoid its absorption. Epinephrine, 0.2–0.5 ml of a 1:1000 solution, should be immediately administered subcutaneously. This dose, diluted in 10 ml of sodium chloride, may be given IV every 5 to 15 minutes until a response is observed; care must be taken to avoid extreme blood pressure and heart rate increases, since myocardial ischemia or necrosis can result. IV aminophylline, aerosolized β-adrenergic agonists, and supplemental O_2 are used to treat the bronchospasm. Fluids should be administered rapidly (200–300 ml normal saline to start) to treat the intravascular volume depletion. Antihistamines and steroids are not useful in the management of anaphylactic shock but may be useful to avoid further deterioration once treatment has been initiated.

Outcome

Outcome is either recovery or death, sometimes within minutes. Survivors of anaphylactic shock must be told to identify themselves as having had allergic drug reactions, and medical records should contain this information in a highly visible place. If certain medications such as penicillin must be given, skin testing should first be performed; if the skin test is positive, an allergic reaction may not occur, but if it is negative, the drugs can be used. Desensitization must sometimes be done by knowledgeable personnel. If diagnostic studies using iodine must be performed in allergic patients, premedication with antihistamines (50–100 mg diphenhydramine) and steroids (1 mg/kg methylprednisolone) should be given.

SEPTIC SHOCK

Definition

Shock that accompanies septicemia probably results from endotoxin. Any organism can cause the syndrome, but gram-negative bacteria are more commonly encountered in the ICU setting. The source is usually apparent but may be occult in patients who are found to have abscesses or infective endocarditis.

Pathophysiology

Although incompletely understood, the effects of endotoxin include endothelial damage, enhanced vascular permeability, thrombocytopenia and leukopenia, and microcirculatory stasis with microthrombus formation. Activation of both coagulation and fibrinolytic systems occurs, leading to hyper- and hypocoagulability.

Diagnosis

Fever, chills, rigors, tachypnea, and diaphoresis are usually present. Respiratory alkalosis and metabolic acidosis are present. Mentation may be normal, urine output adequate, and hypotension not profound initially, but rapid deterioration occurs if treatment is not undertaken immediately. The white blood cell count is usually elevated with a left shift.

Unless the shock is advanced or irreversible, patients with septic shock characteristically have a normal or high cardiac output, reduced arteriovenous oxygen difference, and reduced systemic vascular resistance, often to levels of less than 800 dynes-sec cm^{-5} ("warm shock"). The vasodilatation may produce an erythema. With more profound circulatory collapse, the hemodynamic picture changes to one of low cardiac output, profound vasoconstriction with elevated systemic vascular resistance, and severe hypotension.

Management

Documentation of the source of infection is necessary. Previously placed monitoring lines, indwelling catheters, and urinary catheters should be removed and replaced. Surgical debridement or drainage is required if applicable and should not be delayed awaiting stabilization of the patient. Appropriate broad-spectrum antibiotics should be administered as soon as appropriate cultures and baseline laboratory data have been obtained, pending the results of tests of sensitivities of the organism. Generally, an aminoglycoside is used with a semisynthetic penicillin or cephalosporin; antibiotics tailored to culture results may be continued for at least two weeks. Fluids should be administered to maintain a pulmonary artery wedge pressure of 10–15 mm Hg or, in patients with underlying cardiac disease, to maintain an optimum filling pressure as determined by the left ventricular stroke work index. Pressor agents that increase systemic vascular resistance may be needed; dopamine is the agent of choice (Table 8–2); other vasoactive agents may produce excessive vasoconstriction that can further contribute to organ underperfusion. Unless documented myocardial depression is present (fall in left ventricular stroke work index, reduction in ejection fraction as determined by two-dimensional echocardiography or radionuclide angiography), inotropic agents are usually not useful.

The acidosis often responds to fluid therapy, but IV sodium bicarbonate may be required to reverse it, with care taken to avoid pulmonary edema in patients with cardiac disease.

The use of corticosteroids (especially if given more than 24 hours after the diagnosis) and of heparin, if disseminated intravascular coagulation is present, have not been shown to improve outcome, and their use cannot be recommended. In fact, corticosteroids may actually be harmful in patients with septic shock unless adrenal insufficiency is present.

Outcome

The severity of the underlying disease determines prognosis rather than the specific infectious agent or antibiotic regimen. Thus, survival ranges from 85 percent to 10 percent, with an average of about 60 percent. Survival depends upon the integrity of pulmonary, renal, hepatic, and myocardial functions. Serum lactate levels exceeding 8 mmol/L indicate an ominous prognosis.

CARDIOGENIC SHOCK

Definition

Cardiogenic shock may result from pump failure, dysrhythmias, mechanical factors, and obstruction to flow, as occurs with aortic stenosis. The most common etiology of cardiogenic shock in the ICU setting is acute myocardial infarction (MI) due to severe and extensive underlying coronary artery disease (CAD). Patients with shock usually have 40 percent or more of their left ventricular myocardium infarcted. It is important to distinguish between pump failure due to severe left ventricular (LV) dysfunction and underfilling of the left ventricle due to right ventricular (RV) MI, since the latter can be effectively treated, whereas the former is generally not amenable to any therapeutic regimen. The phrase "cardiogenic shock" should probably be reserved for patients with markedly impaired contractile function of the left ventricle due to a large MI.

Pathophysiology

As noted in Chapter 1, left ventricular performance is determined by preload (end-diastolic fiber length, which is proportional to end-diastolic volume and estimated clinically as LV filling pressure or pulmonary artery wedge pressure), afterload (developed pressure or wall stress during ejection, which is estimated clinically as the systemic vascular resistance), and contractility (which cannot be assessed clinically). For a given preload, the lower the afterload, the greater the extent of muscle shortening and, thus, the larger the ejection fraction and stroke volume. As contractility increases, the stroke volume increases at the same loading conditions.

The compensatory mechanisms of tachycardia and vasoconstriction are detrimental to cardiac function in acute MI: Tachycardia, although an inotropic stimulus, increases myocardial O_2 demand; and vasoconstriction, while maintaining perfusion of vital organs, imposes an increased afterload on the heart, which also increases myocardial oxygen demand. The increased O_2 demand cannot be met by the available coronary artery supply, resulting in aggravation of the existing ischemia/infarction.

Diagnosis

Right Ventricular Myocardial Infarction (RMVI). Systemic hypotension and decreased urine output are present. Central venous and right atrial pressures are characteristically elevated; volume infusion will bring this out if not immediately apparent. If tricuspid regurgitation due to papillary muscle dysfunction is present, the right atrial pressure tracing will show a prominent systolic regurgitant wave. The right atrial, RV systolic, and pulmonary artery systolic pressures will be identical if the RV is so dysfunctional as to act as a conduit from the right atrium to the pulmonary artery. Since RV dilatation is limited by the pericardium, a wave form having a dip-plateau contour resembling pericardial constriction may be inscribed; this wave form may be transmitted to the right atrial pressure trace as well. Total pulmonary and pulmonary vascular resistances (see Chapter 15) are normal. RV stroke work index is depressed. Systemic vascular resistance is variable, depending on the degree of systemic hypotension and on the amount of infarcted left ventricular myocardium.

Left Ventricular (LV) Pump Failure. Cardiac output and LV stroke work index are reduced, and pulmonary artery wedge pressure is elevated, reflecting congestive heart failure as well as impaired contractile function. RV stroke work index and right atrial pressure may be low, reflecting the low cardiac output, or elevated if passive pulmonary hypertension resulting from LV failure is present. Total pulmonary and pulmonary vascular resistances will be elevated if passive pulmonary hypertension is present. Systemic vascular resistance is characteristically markedly elevated, often exceeding 2000 dynes-sec cm^{-5}. The arteriovenous difference of O_2 (C(a $- \overline{v})O_2$) is widened, often above 10 ml/dl, reflecting the low cardiac output and maximal tissue O_2 extraction. This is in contrast to septic shock, in which C(a $- \overline{v})O_2$ is narrowed.

Management

RMVI. Fluids should be administered to maintain a pulmonary artery wedge pressure sufficiently high to produce adequate LV stroke volume. Whereas this LV filling pressure is often in the range of 15–18 mm Hg, the diastolic stiffness that accompanies an acute MI might cause higher filling pressures to be required. Optimum filling pressures should be assessed by following serially the LV and RV stroke work indices. The amount of fluids required can be as high as 6 L/day. Central venous pressure elevation, hepatomegaly, and even anasarca may develop as a result; however, as right ventricular function improves, these signs resolve. Inotropic support (Table 8–2) is given as needed to maintain ventricular function; however, pressor agents should be avoided, as the resulting increase in systemic vascular resistance can be detrimental to LV function. Lowering of the impedance to right ventricular ejection (pulmonary resistance) using afterload reducing agents is usually not helpful, since pulmonary resistance is not abnormally elevated; moreover, the concomitant fall in systemic vascular resistance with resulting arterial hypotension aggravates the shock state.

LV Pump Failure. Inotropic agents (dopamine or dobutamine) are used along with diuretics (IV furosemide [Lasix] is the drug of first choice) to improve cardiac output and to relieve pulmonary congestion. Low-dose dopamine (2–5 µg/kg/min) augments renal perfusion and may reduce systemic vascular resistance; inotropic effects are seen at 5–8 µg/kg/min; vasoconstrictor effects are usual at doses exceeding 10 µg/kg/min.

Although intraaortic balloon counterpulsation (Chapter 17) has been used in patients with cardiogenic shock, weaning is difficult, and prognosis is unaltered. Intravenous and intracoronary thrombolytic therapy, early angioplasty, and aortocoronary bypass procedures have not been uniformly successful in altering the dismal prognosis and should be considered only in patients seen within two hours of the onset of chest pain who are young and who are having their first infarction.

Outcome

Cardiogenic shock due to acute MI with pump failure continues to have a mortality of over 80 percent. Prognosis is nil in cardiogenic shock due to congestive cardiomyopathy. Prognosis in patients with RVMI depends upon the amount of infarcted LV myocardium and may be excellent if left ventricular function is reasonably normal. RV function usually normalizes over days to weeks; rarely, the result is a clinical picture of chronic RV failure, frank tricuspid regurgitation, and central venous pressure elevation with hepatomegaly and peripheral edema.

RECOMMENDED READING

Benotti JR, McCue JE, Alpert JS: Comparative vasoactive therapy for heart failure. Am J Cardiol 56:19B, 1985.
Cohn JN, Luria MH, Daddario RC, et al: Studies in clinical shock and hypotension. V. Hemodynamic effects of dextran. Circulation 35:316, 1967.
Francis GS, Sharma B, Hodges M: Comparative hemodynamic effects of dopamine and

dobutamine in patients with acute cardiogenic circulatory collapse. Am Heart J 103:995, 1982.

Holzer J, Karliner JS, O'Rourke RA, et al: Effectiveness of dopamine in patients with cardiogenic shock. Am J Cardiol 32:79, 1973.

Kones RJ: The catecholamines: reappraisal of their use for acute myocardial infarction and the low cardiac output syndromes. Crit Care Med 1:203, 1973.

Kreger BE, Craven DE, McCabe WR: Gram-negative bacteremia. IV. Re-evaluation of clinical features and treatment in 612 patients. Am J Med 68:344, 1980.

Leier CV, Unverferth DV: Dobutamine. Ann Intern Med 99:490, 1983.

Loeb HS, Winslow EBJ, Rahimtoola SH, et al: Acute hemodynamic effects of dopamine in patients with shock. Circulation 44:163, 1971.

Mancini D, LeJemtel T, Sonnenblick E: Intravenous use of amrinone for the treatment of the failing heart. Am J Cardiol 56:8B, 1985.

Massie BM, Chatterjee K: Medical therapy for pump failure complicating acute myocardial infarction. In Schienman MM (ed): Cardiac Emergencies. Philadelphia, W. B. Saunders Co., 1984, p. 29.

Parker MM, Shelhamer JH, Bacharach SL, et al: Profound but reversible myocardial depression in patients with septic shock. Ann Intern Med 100:483, 1984.

Ratshin RA, Rackley CE, Russell RO: Hemodynamic evaluation of left ventricular function in shock complicating myocardial infarction. Circulation 45:127, 1972.

Regnier B, Safran D, Carlet J, et al: Comparative hemodynamic effects of dopamine and dobutamine in septic shock. Intensive Care Med 5:115, 1979.

Shine KI, Kuhn M, Young LS, et al: Aspects of the management of shock. Ann Intern Med 93:723, 1980.

Shoemaker WC, Monson DO: The effect of whole blood and plasma expanders on volume-flow relationships in critically ill patients. Surg Gynecol Obstet 137:453, 1973.

Tarazi RC: Sympathomimetic agents in the treatment of shock. Ann Intern Med 81:364, 1974.

Taylor SH, Verma SP, Hussain M, et al: Intravenous amrinone in left ventricular failure complicated by acute myocardial infarction. Am J Cardiol 56:29B, 1985.

Terradellas JB, Bellot JF, Saris AB, et al: Acute and transient ST segment elevation during bacterial shock in seven patients without apparent heart disease. Chest 81:4, 1982.

Wilson JN: The management of acute circulatory failure. Surg Clin North Am 43:469, 1963.

9. Hypertensive Crises

Nora F. Goldschlager

DEFINITION

A hypertensive crisis is present when there is an accelerated rise in arterial pressure or a pressure sufficiently high to cause potentially irreversible vascular damage to vital organs (brain, heart, kidneys, vascular system). Thus, an excessively high blood pressure *per se* may not constitute hypertensive crisis in one patient, whereas the same level of pressure may do so in another. Patients without prior hypertension may develop crises at blood pressure levels generally well tolerated by those with chronic hypertension. "Malignant" hypertension is characterized by an arterial diastolic pressure exceeding 130 mm Hg and papilledema; hypertensive crisis need not be present in all patients with malignant hypertension.

PATHOPHYSIOLOGY

Hypertensive crisis can result from either primary or secondary hypertension. Secondary hypertension in the intensive care unit (ICU) setting may result from acute volume expansion (especially in patients with renal insufficiency), acute renal failure of any etiology, stimulation of the sympathetic nervous system (use of sympathomimetic agents, including amphetamines and cocaine, rebound after withdrawal of antihypertensive medications, induction of anesthesia, endotracheal intubation, release of stored catecholamines such as might occur with the use of bretylium and in pheochromocytoma), and eclampsia of pregnancy. Other, less frequent, etiologies include renal artery embolism, scleroderma, polyarteritis, and quadriplegia, especially after the acute phase.

The pathophysiology underlying specific target organ damage varies. For example, hypertensive encephalopathy probably results from both cerebral vasoconstriction in response to extremely high systemic blood pressure and from arteriolar dilation, transudation (cerebral edema), and rupture, leading to multiple small hemorrhages. Loss of cerebrovascular autoregulatory processes occurs when vasoconstriction is maximal; vasodilation with increase in cerebral blood flow results. Acute left ventricular

70

failure results from the marked elevation in afterload against which the left ventricle cannot develop sufficient pressure. Myocardial ischemia or infarction results from an increase in myocardial oxygen consumption (determined by heart rate, intraventricular pressure, and inotropic state but clinically estimated from the double product—heart rate multiplied by systolic blood pressure) not met by the available oxygen supply via the coronary arteries. Both left ventricular failure and ischemia/infarction can contribute to the development of pulmonary edema. Necrotizing renal vasculitis can result from renal afferent arteriolar vasoconstriction, leading to increased release of renin and to further hypertension.

Diagnosis

Since hypertensive crisis is defined as a blood pressure high enough to produce potential target organ damage, reversible symptoms are expected to be present. Hypertensive encephalopathy is characterized by headache, nausea and vomiting, confusion, drowsiness, blurred vision, diplopia, agitation, and coma. Physical examination may disclose coma, myoclonus, and seizures, as well as retinal vasospasm, hemorrhages, and exudates. Papilledema is seen in malignant hypertension in which the diastolic pressure often exceeds 120 mm Hg. Focal findings are not present, and the cerebrospinal fluid is usually normal (care should be taken if lumbar puncture is contemplated, as herniation of the brain is a possibility if spinal fluid pressure is extremely high). Microangiopathic hemolytic anemia may be present. Computerized tomography may be required to exclude intracranial mass lesions such as tumor, and an electroencephalogram (EEG) is sometimes useful in excluding a seizure focus in patients who are comatose. The amelioration of the patient's condition with lowering of the blood pressure is itself an excellent and reliable diagnostic feature.

In patients presenting with hypertension and pulmonary edema, it is not always clear whether the hypertension caused the left ventricular failure or the left ventricular failure caused the hypertension by means of excessive sympathetic stimulation. The electrocardiogram (ECG) is often not helpful and may show left ventricular hypertrophy, nondiagnostic ST- and T-wave abnormalities, a bundle branch block pattern, or a myocardial infarction pattern, the age of which may not always be clear. Acute myocardial infarction should be ruled out by serial creatine kinase–myocardial fraction (CK-MB) determinations; serial ECG changes, unless a definite Q-wave infarction pattern evolves, do not establish a diagnosis of myocardial necrosis, since these may occur as a nonspecific finding as the blood pressure normalizes.

If the hypertension is associated with activation of the renin-

TABLE 9–1. DRUGS USED INTRAVENOUSLY IN HYPERTENSIVE EMERGENCIES

Drug	Mechanism of Action	Initial Dosage	Onset of Action	Duration of Action	Maintenance Dosage	Side Effects
Sodium nitroprusside	Arterial and venous vasodilator	0.5–1.5 µg/kg/min; increase rate every 2–3 min to desired response	Immediate	3–5 min	0.1–10.0 µg/kg/min infusion	Thiocyanate toxicity, nausea, vomiting, twitching, psychosis, restlessness
Hydralazine hydrochloride	Arterial vasodilator	10–25 mg IV bolus or in 20 ml NaCl over 10 min or 50–150 µg/min infusion	10–20 min	2–6 hr	Repeat effective dose every 3–6 hr 50–150 µg/min infusion	Nausea, vomiting, tachycardia, headache, flushing, angina
Nifedipine	Arterial vasodilator, calcium channel blocker	10–30 mg PO every 6 hr; 10 mg sublingually	30 min (PO), 5–10 min (sublin-gually)	4–6 hr	10–30 mg every 6–8 hr	Tachycardia, flushing, headache
Trimethaphan camsylate	Sympathetic and parasympathetic ganglionic blocking agent	0.5–4.0 mg/min; increase infusion rate every 5–8 min	1–5 min	2–10 min	1–15 mg/min infusion	Urinary retention, ileus, constipation, orthostatic hypotension, tachyphylaxis, cycloplegia, xerostomia
Furosemide	Diuretic, venous vasodilator	20–80 mg IV over 1–2 min	1–5 min	2–4 hr	40–80 mg every 4–12 hr as needed	Hyponatremia, hypokalemia, dehydration

Propranolol	β-adrenergic receptor blocking agent	1–5 mg IV; repeat after 2 min if needed	2–5 min	2–6 hr	1–3 mg every 4–6 hr	Bradycardia, asthma, heart block, fatigue, lassitude
Methyldopa	Central and peripheral sympathetic blocking agent	250–500 mg in 100 ml IV over 30 min	½–2 hr	2–8 hr	250–500 mg every 6–8 hr	Sedation, somnolence, fever, liver function abnormalities
Reserpine	Central and peripheral sympathetic blocking agent	0.25–5 mg IM	1–4 hr (may be delayed)	6–24 hr	0.25–5 mg every 8–12 hr	Prolonged hypotension, nasal stuffiness, increased gastric acidity and gastrointestinal motility, sedation, somnolence
Diazoxide	Arterial vasodilator	2.5–5 mg/kg or 100–, 200–, 300–mg sequential injections at 10-min intervals or 15–30 mg/min	1–2 min	3–12 hr	Repeat effective dose every 6–12 hr	Hypotension, hyperglycemia, flushing, nausea, vomiting, tachycardia, sodium retention
Labetalol	α- and β-blocking agent (the latter predominates)	20–80 mg at 10–15-min intervals	1–10 min	Up to 12 hr	0.5–2.0 mg/kg/min	Bradycardia, AV block, nausea, vomiting, flushing, asthma

Adapted, with permission, from Perloff D: Hypertensive emergencies. In Scheinman MM (ed): Cardiac Emergencies. Philadelphia, W. B. Saunders Co., 1984, p. 181.

angiotensin-aldosterone system, metabolic alkalosis with hypokalemia and hypochloremia may be present; if renal insufficiency is present (often seen in patients with left ventricular failure and low cardiac output) oliguria, azotemia, and hyperkalemia can occur. As in any acutely ill hypertensive patient, blood pressures in both arms should be periodically checked and examination of the peripheral pulses made so as not to miss the occurrence of aortic dissection.

MANAGEMENT

Monitoring of the cardiac rhythm, intraarterial and cuff blood pressures (since there may be significant discrepancy between the two), and urine output should be instituted and the blood pressure lowered (Table 9–1). A normal blood pressure is neither easily achieved nor necessarily desirable in patients with chronic hypertension who may experience a damaging fall in cerebral perfusion pressure if their blood pressure is lowered too aggressively. Relatively rapid and easily achieved blood pressure reduction can occur, however, in patients who have not had significant hypertension in the past. In patients with congestive heart failure, resolution of the pulmonary edema will not be achieved unless the blood pressure has been adequately controlled; underlying myocardial disease is often a factor, but its presence need not necessarily be assumed.

Nitroprusside, having both arteriolar and capacitance vessel dilating effects, is the agent of choice in reducing blood pressure, since accurate and moment-to-moment titration of dosage against blood pressure response is possible (Table 9–1). Drugs having a long duration of action should not be used initially, in order to avoid unwanted hypotension. Oral or sublingual nifedipine (the sublingual form is given by breaking the capsule and squirting the contents into the mouth) are also useful, especially if ischemic chest pain is present. Intravenous nitroglycerin is an arteriolar dilating agent at high doses only but may be helpful under certain circumstances such as in the patient with myocardial ischemia or infarction. If not contraindicated by bronchospasm, bradycardia, or frank pulmonary edema, β-blocking agents are used. They may be employed in patients with compromised myocardial function to maintain blood pressure, once it is in the optimal range, without causing pulmonary edema and should be considered if the antihypertensive agents produce significant tachycardia; this is especially important in patients with congestive heart failure and myocardial ischemia or infarction. Labetalol, an α- and β-blocking agent, has been used successfully to acutely lower blood pressure without producing reflex tachycardia; since the β-blocking effects of the drug predominate, cautions similar to the use of any β-blocking drugs are advised. Labatalol is particularly helpful in treating the hypertension associated with pheochromocytoma or stimulant drug overdosage (see Chapter 88). If marked vasoconstriction is not present, loop diuretics such as furosemide are useful; they are generally required along with most antihypertensive medications, owing to the effects of the antihypertensives of expansion of intravascular volume via sodium and water retention. Methyldopa should probably be avoided because of the side effect of drowsiness. Thiazide diruetics will be relatively ineffective, especially if renal function is impaired. Diazoxide is generally not indicated in patients with coronary artery disease because of the side effects of angina (which occurs in up to 30 percent of patients) and tachycardia. If aortic dissection is present, agents that produce tachycardia and increase inotropic state (such as hydralazine) should not be used.

If intravascular volume status is unclear or if significant lability of the arterial pressure in response to treatment is encountered, hemodynamic monitoring using a balloon-tipped flow-directed pulmonary artery catheter should be performed. Serial cardiac output determinations by thermodilution technique (with periodic validation by assessment of arteriovenous difference of oxygen, using arterial and pulmonary artery oxygen content) will allow the assessment of changes in systemic vascular resistance during therapy. If antihypertensive treatment results in impairment in renal function, temporary dialysis may be necessary; the presence of renal insufficiency is not a contraindication to aggressive lowering of the blood pressure.

Early transition to an oral antihypertensive regimen should be accomplished. If the patient is postoperative and antihypertensive agents were withdrawn prior to surgery, the preoperative regimen should be reinstituted.

OUTCOME

If the hypertensive emergency is not immediately and aggressively treated, life-threatening complications (myocardial infarction, severe pulmonary edema, intracranial hemorrhage, aortic dissection, and renal failure) may occur. Control of blood pressure is mandatory to prevent recurrences and associated complications. If complications have occurred, outcome will depend upon the degree and type of organ damage sustained. In patients with renal insufficiency, even those requiring dialysis during treatment, long-term blood pressure control has been shown to have a favorable effect in preserving renal function.

RECOMMENDED READING

Ahearn DJ, Grim CE: Treatment of malignant hypertension with sodium nitroprusside. Arch Intern Med 133:187, 1974.

Becker CE, Benowitz NL: Hypertensive emergencies. Med Clin North Am 63:127, 1979.
Beer N, Gallegos I, Cohen A, et al: Efficacy of sublingual nifedipine in the acute treatment of systemic hypertension. Chest 79:571, 1981.
Dinsdale HB, Robertson DM, Haas RA, et al: Cerebral blood flow in acute hypertension. Arch Neurol 31:80, 1974.
Frishman WH, Weinberg P, Peled HB, et al: Calcium entry blockers for the treatment of severe hypertension and hypertensive crisis. Am J Med 104:35, 1984.
Gifford RW, Jr., Westbrook E: Hypertensive encephalopathy: Mechanisms, clinical features, and treatment. Prog Cardiovasc Dis 17:115, 1974.
Houston MC: Treatment of hypertensive urgencies and emergencies with nifedipine. Am Heart J 111:963, 1986.
Mroczek WJ, Davidov M, Gavrilovich L, et al: The value of aggressive therapy in the hypertensive patient with azotemia. Circulation 40:893, 1969.
Perloff D: Hypertensive emergencies. In Scheinman MM (ed): Cardiac Emergencies. Philadelphia, W. B. Saunders Co., 1984, p. 181.
Prys-Roberts C, Meloche R: Management of anesthesia in patients with hypertension or ischemic heart disease. Int Anesthesiol Clin 18:181, 1980.
Vidt DG, Gifford RW Jr: A compendium for the treatment of hypertensive emergencies. Clin Pharmacol Update 51:421, 1984.
Wheat MW, Jr., Palmer RF, Bartley TD, et al: Treatment of dissecting aneurysms of the aorta without surgery. J Thorac Cardiovasc Surg 50:364, 1965.
Whelton PK, Flaherty JT, MacAllister NP, et al: Hypertension following coronary artery bypass surgery: Role of preoperative propranolol therapy. Hypertension 2:291, 1980.

10. Aortic Dissection

Nora F. Goldschlager

DEFINITION

Aortic dissection is caused by an intimal tear in the aorta (not demonstrable in 10 percent of cases), subsequent hematoma formation in its medial layer, and longitudinal separation of the layers of the aorta. Circumferential dissection usually does not occur. Associated conditions include hypertension, Marfan's syndrome, coarctation of the aorta, congenital bicuspid aortic valve, and, possibly, pregnancy (third trimester). Dissection may also result from cardiac catheterization and arterial cannulation for any reason such as placement of an intraaortic balloon catheter or prior to cardiopulmonary bypass. Blunt chest or abdominal trauma may also cause dissection. Two thirds of cases involve the ascending aorta (proximal dissection), and the intimal tear is usually located several centimeters above the aortic valve. A reentry tear, at the point at which the false channel recommunicates with the true lumen, may also be present. One third of cases involve the descending aorta (distal dissection), usually arising just distal to the left subclavian artery. The most common cause of death is aortic rupture.

PATHOPHYSIOLOGY

Hypertension and degenerative diseases of the aorta predispose to dissection, possibly because of weakening of the medial layer: Medial degenerative conditions seem to be essential for dissection to occur. The process of dissection itself also depends upon the rate of change in left ventricular pressure (LV dP/dt); reduction in dP/dt is a goal of therapy in arresting the progression of the dissection.

DIAGNOSIS

Severe pain is almost invariably present unless the patient presents with altered consciousness due to cerebrovascular accident or syncope. The pain is described as ripping, cutting, and tearing and changes its location as the dissection proceeds. If the pain is limited to the anterior precordium, proximal dissection should be suspected; if it is felt both anteriorly and posteriorly, the dissection may involve either the proximal or the distal aorta; and if it is felt posteriorly only (usually in the interscapular area), distal dissection is probably present. If syncope is the presenting symptom, proximal dissection with rupture of the aorta into the pericardial space causing cardiac tamponade should be suspected.

If congestive heart failure of acute onset is described and a murmur of aortic regurgitation is heard, proximal dissection with separation of the aortic cusps due to aortic root dilatation, displacement of an aortic cusp due to pressure of the hematoma, or frank shearing off of a cusp of the aortic valve with consequent loss of leaflet support is likely to be present. Cardiac tamponade due to hemopericardium might complicate this picture. Cerebrovascular accidents, paraplegia, acute renal insufficiency (with increasing hypertension), and cold, pulseless extremities occur (this last might be confused with arterial embolism) and are due to compromise of the true arterial lumens by the dissection, with ischemia/infarction of the organs supplied by those vessels. Occasionally, an intimal flap obstructs arterial flow intermittently, leading to changing pulse amplitude, blood pressures, and organ function.

Physical examination usually reveals a normal or elevated blood pressure with differential blood pressures and pulses, depending upon the location and extent of the dissection. Hypotension should suggest cardiac tamponade or aortic rupture (which occurs in up to 20 percent of cases). New aortic regurgitation establishes the diagnosis of proximal dissection.

The electrocardiogram (ECG) may reveal left ventricular hypertrophy or only nonspecific ST-T wave abnormalities. Acute atrioventricular (AV) conduction disturbances can occur if a proximal dissection extends into the AV node.

The chest roentgenogram may show mediastinal widening. If intimal calcium is separated from the outer aortic shadow by more than 6 mm in the lateral projection, dissection is present. Although specific, the finding is insensitive. This finding is not useful in the frontal plane, owing to imaging of different levels of the aorta. Rupture of the aorta into the lung is characterized by unilateral haziness of the left lung field. Echocardiography and computerized tomography have been used to establish the diagnosis but may be inordinately time-consuming. Contrast angiography is the diagnostic procedure of choice, since the origin and extent of dissection can be best visualized by this technique.

MANAGEMENT

The patient should have continuous ECG and blood pressure monitoring. The pulmonary artery wedge pressure should be monitored by means of a balloon-tipped flow-directed catheter if underlying cardiac disease is present or if intravascular volume status is unclear. Sedation and analgesia are important therapeutic adjuncts. Blood pressure should be aggressively lowered using nitroprusside (up to 3 μg/kg/min) but not to a point at which renal and cerebral circulation are compromised. Cyanide and thiocyanate toxicities resulting from nitroprusside use should be watched for after 36–48 hours of infusion; symptoms are metabolic acidosis, confusion, and seizures. In patients without significant brady-cardia, AV block, congestive heart failure, or bronchospasm, the pulsatility of aortic flow should be reduced by intravenous β-blockers (e.g., propran-olol 0.5–1.0 mg every 5 minutes, up to 10–15 mg for full β-blockade) to abort further dissection. Even if the patient is normotensive, β-blockers may be used. Once the progress of the dissection is arrested, pain becomes easier to manage. If the patient is intolerant of nitroprusside, trimethaphan (beginning with 1 mg/min) can be used; it is essential to watch for ganglionic blockade effects of urinary retention and paralytic ileus. Vaso-dilator agents such as hydralazine may be useful to produce hypotension, but the consequent reflex tachycardia must be avoided or managed with adequate β-blockade.

Medical management is generally indicated in patients with distal dissection and in patients with proximal dissection who are at very high risk for surgery. Surgery is indicated for most patients with proximal dissection (emergently, if required, or after medical stabilization) and in those with distal dissection complicated by rupture of the aorta or compromise of the blood supply to a vital organ.

OUTCOME

Without aggressive therapy, mortality approaches 75 percent in 48 hours. Aortic rupture is associated with early fatality in most cases. If the dissection process can be arrested, patients must remain on antihyperten-sive and β-blocking agents for life, with good control of blood pressure being mandatory.

Late complications of treated dissection include recurrence, aortic aneurysm formation due to the weakening of the aortic wall produced by the dissection, and progressive aortic regurgitation, requiring valve re-placement with or without aortic graft placement and coronary artery bypass. If aortic valve replacement has been required emergently, the usual potential problems associated with valvular prostheses are present.

RECOMMENDED READING

Anagnostopoulos CE, Prabhakar MJS, Kittle CF: Aortic dissection and dissecting aneurysms. Am J Cardiol 30:263, 1972.

Daily PO, Trueblood HW, Stinson EB, et al: Management of acute aortic dissections. Ann Thorac Surg 10:237, 1970.

Hirst AE Jr, Johns VJ Jr, Kime SW Jr: Dissecting aneurysm of the aorta: a review of 505 cases. Medicine 37:217, 1958.

Kolff J, Bates RJ, Balderman SC, et al: Acute aortic arch dissection: re-evaluation of the indications for medical and surgical therapy. Am J Cardiol 39:727, 1977.

Large D, Beloir C, Vasile N, et al: Computed tomography of aortic dissection. Radiology 136:147, 1980.

Matsumoto M, Matsuo H, Ohara T, et al: A two-dimensional echoaortocardiographic approach to dissecting aneurysms to prevent false-positive diagnosis. Radiology 127:491, 1978.

Parker FB Jr, Neville FF Jr, Hanson EL, et al: Management of acute aortic dissection. Ann Thorac Surg 19:436, 1975.

Roberts WC: Aortic dissection: anatomy, consequence and causes. Am Heart J 101:195, 1981.

Slater EE, DeSanctis RW: Clinical recognition of dissecting aortic aneurysm. Am J Med 60:625, 1976.

Wheat MW Jr, Palmer RF, Bartley TD, et al: Treatment of dissecting aneurysms of the aorta without surgery. J Thorac Cardiovasc Surg 50:364, 1965.

11. Congestive Heart Failure

Nora F. Goldschlager

DEFINITION

Congestive heart failure (CHF) describes a condition in which the heart cannot pump sufficient blood to meet the metabolic needs of the body. The phrase "congestive heart failure" should probably be reserved for situations in which the heart failure is due to myocardial disease (such as dilated cardiomyopathy or acute myocardial infarction) rather than to acute mechanical problems (such as disruption of a valve) that occur in the presence of normal myocardial function. Similarly, circulatory congestion, which often results from fluid overload, is not CHF.

PATHOPHYSIOLOGY

Myocardial failure results in a reduction in stroke volume. The compensatory mechanisms that act to restore stroke volume (Fig. 11–1) are sympathetic stimulation, which causes tachycardia and systemic vasoconstriction, and activation of the renin-angiotensin-aldosterone system. The tachycardia is an inotropic stimulus and thus serves to increase myocardial oxygen (O_2) demands. Systemic arteriolar vasoconstriction produces increased afterload, also resulting in an increase in myocardial O_2 requirements. Venous constriction produces increased left ventricular filling pressure and end-diastolic volume (preload) and acts to restore stroke volume through the Frank-Starling mechanism; however, the increase in ventricular volume produces an increase in wall tension, which increases myocardial O_2 demands. Activation of the renin-angiotensin system results in retention of salt and water, which also causes increased preload. Thus, the compensatory mechanisms in CHF are all potentially detrimental to myocardial function.

DIAGNOSIS

The history often reveals the cause of the myocardial failure, such as acute or remote myocardial infarction (MI), hypertension, or alcoholism.

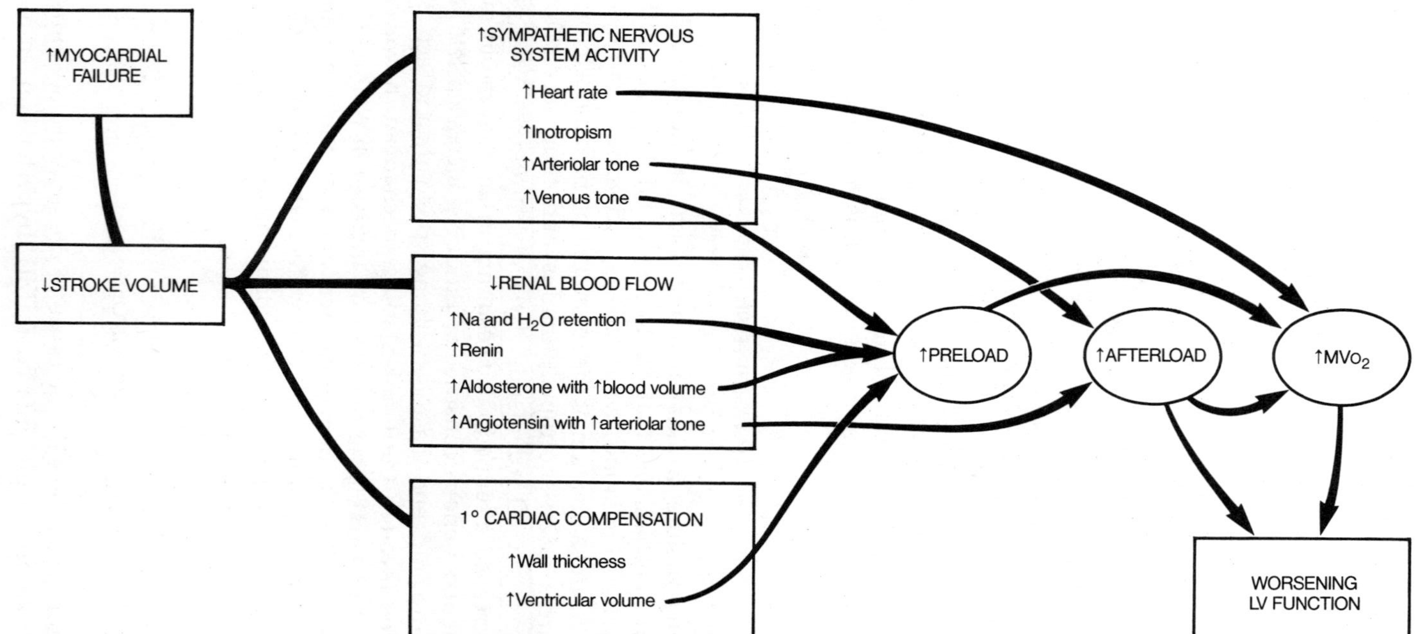

FIGURE 11–1. Compensatory mechanisms in congestive heart failure. See text for further explanation. MVO_2 = myocardial oxygen consumption.

The patient is short of breath, initially on effort and eventually at rest, and often cannot tolerate the supine position; in severe CHF, the patient sits bolt upright or leans over a table in order to breathe. Pulsus alternans or a dicrotic pulse or both indicate severe CHF, usually due to dilated cardiomyopathy or aortic stenosis. Central venous pressure is elevated, and a and v waves are equal unless tricuspid regurgitation (TR) is present. Pulmonary rales can extend to the lung apices.

If right ventricular (RV) failure is present, there is a parasternal lift and an RV S3, the latter often heard best during inspiration or with abdominal compression to increase venous return. P2 is accentuated if pulmonary hypertension is present. A holosystolic murmur of TR, reflecting right ventricular dilatation, may be heard and may increase with inspiration if right atrial chamber size and compliance are normal. Hepatomegaly is felt, and the area is tender if the CHF has occurred rapidly or recently; a pulsatile liver is not expected unless TR is present. Peripheral pitting edema is seen, as well as sacral edema, especially if the patient has been at bed rest.

If left ventricular (LV) failure is present, the apical impulse is usually displaced laterally and downward. An LV lift is felt. S1 is diminished, owing to poor LV contractile function. S2 is often normal; P2 will be accentuated if pulmonary hyptertension is present. A2 is accentuated if systemic hypertension is present and is diminished to absent if significant aortic stenosis is present. S2 is sometimes paradoxically split if LV ejection is delayed relative to RV ejection (common causes of this finding are aortic stenosis, acute ischemia, and a QRS rhythm paced from the RV). An S3 gallop is present (or a summation gallop if the heart rate is rapid). A blowing systolic murmur of mitral regurgitation (MR) due to LV dilatation is often heard. The cause of the heart failure may be apparent from the physical examination; for example, a harsh basal systolic murmur with radiation into the neck, diminished or absent A2, and S4 with a sustained LV impulse suggest the diagnosis of valvular aortic stenosis. If the LV failure is chronic, passive pulmonary hypertension will result: P2 will be accentuated, a parasternal RV lift will be felt, and central venous pressure will be elevated.

The electrocardiogram (ECG) may provide a clue as to the etiologic diagnosis. For example, a pattern of left ventricular hypertrophy suggests past hypertension, valvular aortic stenosis, or hypertrophic subaortic stenosis; acute or remote MI with persistent ST-segment elevation suggests ischemic heart disease with ventricular aneurysm.

Laboratory data are nonspecific. Arterial hypoxemia and metabolic acidosis are common; if tachypnea is marked, respiratory alkalosis can also occur.

The chest roentgenogram shows cardiomegaly and pulmonary congestion or frank pulmonary edema. Vascular redistribution to the

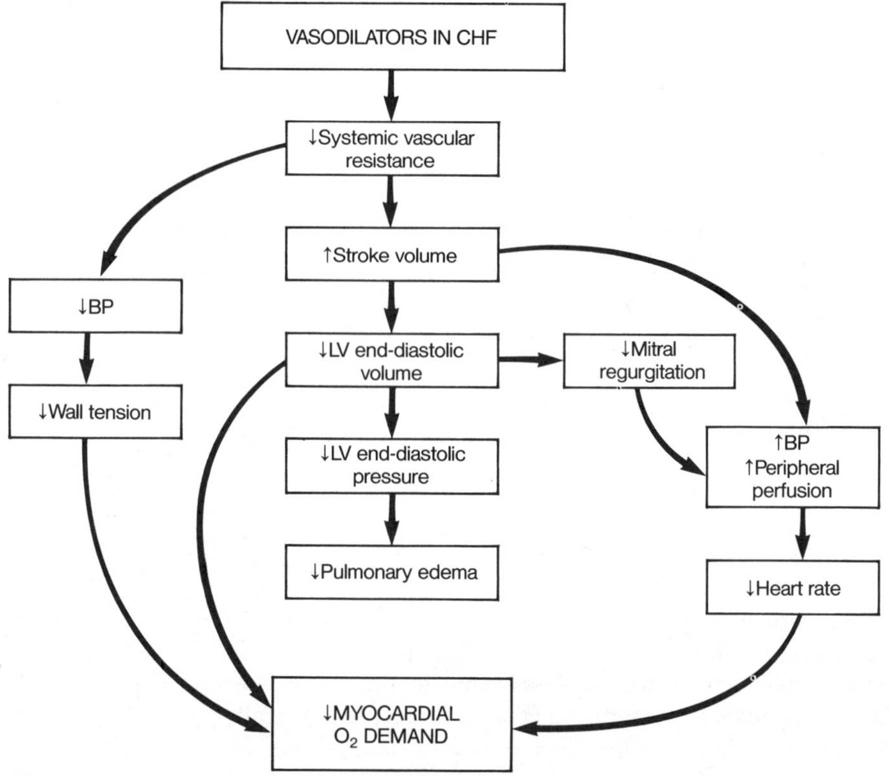

FIGURE 11–2. Action of vasodilators in congestive heart failure (CHF). See text for further explanation.

upper lobes suggests pulmonary congestion. The cause of the CHF may be apparent; for example, a large, tortuous aortic shadow might suggest hypertensive disease.

If invasive monitoring is required, the hemodynamic picture will be characterized by elevated pulmonary artery wedge pressure, low cardiac output, and systemic vasoconstriction with elevated system vascular resistance. If significant passive pulmonary hypertension is present, pulmonary artery pressure is elevated, and total pulmonary resistance is high; pulmonary vascular resistance is normal (see Chapter 15). The arteriovenous difference of O_2 (C ($a - \bar{v}$) O_2) may be widened in association with low cardiac output.

MANAGEMENT

The principles of management of acute CHF are reduction of preload for relief of pulmonary edema, reduction of afterload with vasodilators

(Fig. 11–2) to enhance stroke volume, and enhancement of contractile function. Strict intake and output measurements must be maintained. Continuous ECG monitoring is required, especially since use of diuretics with resulting hypokalemia and hypomagnesemia can produce lethal ventricular dysrhythmias (see Chapter 3). Aggravating factors such as anemia, hyperthyroidism, and infection should be identified and corrected. Mechanical problems such as valvular disruption should be managed with surgical consultation.

Preload reduction is accomplished by intravenous (IV) diuretics and nitrates; the calcium entry blocking agent nifedipine can also be used in selected cases. Although initial diuretic therapy is administered IV, an oral regimen should be substituted as soon as feasible, with IV supplements as needed. Furosemide (with metolazone, or ethacrynic acid in refractory cases) can be used in large doses even in patients with renal insufficiency (Table 11–1); in addition to its diuretic action, it increases venous capacitance, thereby reducing venous return to the heart.

Complications of aggressive diuresis include volume depletion, prerenal azotemia, orthostatic hypotension, hyponatremia, hypokalemia, hypomagnesemia, and contraction metabolic alkalosis due to sodium and chloride depletion. Polymorphic ventricular tachycardia (see Chapter 3) is a potential lethal complication of diuretic therapy. Blood urea nitrogen, creatinine, and electrolytes should be monitored daily and potassium chloride and magnesium supplementation provided as required.

Nitrates can be administered transdermally (nitropaste 1–2 inches q 4 h), orally (isosorbide dinitrate 10–40 mg q 6 h), sublingually (0.4 mg nitroglycerin as often as required), buccally, or intravenously (25–500 μg/min usually suffices). The transdermal route is extremely efficacious in the acute care setting; the paste can be rapidly wiped off if untoward

TABLE 11–1. DIURETICS USEFUL IN CONGESTIVE HEART FAILURE

	IV DOSE	AVERAGE DAILY ORAL DOSE	DURATION OF ACTION (PO)
Loop Diuretics			
Furosemide	20–40 mg; double q 2–4 h until desired effect	40–200 mg	6–8 hours (1–3 hours IV)
Ethacrynic acid	50 mg; may repeat q 3–4 h	50–100 mg	6–8 hours (1–3 hours IV)
Thiazides and Related Drugs			
Hydrochlorthiazide	—	50–100 mg	12 hours
Chlorothiazide	—	500–1000 mg	6–12 hours
Metolazone	—	5–10 mg	24 hours
Potassium-Sparing Agents			
Spironolactone	—	100 mg	3–4 days
Triamterene	—	100–200 mg	12–18 hours

TABLE 11–2. HEMODYNAMIC EFFECTS OF VASODILATORS AND ANGIOTENSIN-CONVERTING ENZYME INHIBITORS IN CHRONIC HEART FAILURE

	HEART RATE	BLOOD PRESSURE	CARDIAC OUTPUT	PULMONARY CAPILLARY WEDGE PRESSURE	RIGHT ATRIAL PRESSURE	SIDE EFFECTS
Nitrates	↔	↔↓	↔↑	↓↓	↓↓	Tolerance Headache Fluid retention
Hydralazine	↔↑	↔↓	↑↑	↔↓	↔↓	Fluid retention Gastrointestinal symptoms Headache Lupus erythematosus Polyneuropathy Angina
Minoxidil	↔↑	↔↓	↑↑	↔↓	↔↓	Fluid retention Headache Hair growth
Prazosin	↔↓	↓↓	↑	↓↓	↓	Fluid retention Hypotension Central nervous system symptoms Tachyphylaxis
Captopril	↔↓	↓↓	↑	↓↓	↓↓	Hypotension Skin rash Proteinuria Leukopenia Nephropathy
Enalapril	↔↓	↓↓	↑	↓↓	↓↓	Attenuation of effects Hypotension

hypotension occurs. Both IV nitroglycerin and nitroprusside (50–500 µg/min) are useful if the pulmonary edema is associated with significant hypertension. Invasive hemodynamic monitoring is recommended if these agents are used. IV hydralazine may also be used (starting dose 10–25 mg); the reduction in systemic vascular resistance with consequent enhancement of stroke volume often counterbalances the reflex tachycardia produced by this agent.

The calcium entry blocker nifedipine has been used with some success as a preload-reducing agent; it also has arteriolar dilating effects, thus reducing impedance to left ventricular ejection, increasing stroke volume, and reducing filling pressure *pari passu*. Nifedipine is particularly useful if ischemic chest pain is present. Since the calcium entry blockers verapamil and diltiazem have the capability of depressing left ventricular contractility, they should be used with caution, if at all, in this setting.

Orally administered afterload-reducing agents and angiotensin-converting enzyme inhibitors are more useful in the chronic than in the acute setting (Table 11–2).

Enhancement of contractility using inotropic agents is costly in the setting of acute pulmonary edema, since they cause an increase in myocardial O_2 demand. Since aggressive preload and afterload reduction therapy is almost always successful, there is little need for inotropic agents unless shock is present (see Chapter 8). Digitalis is a weak inotropic agent and has little place in the management of acute CHF.

OUTCOME

The outcome varies with the etiology of the myocardial failure. Acute CHF in association with severe hypertension can be effectively prevented with vigorous antihypertensive therapy and good blood pressure control. CHF occurring during the course of acute myocardial infarction is an ominous sign, and if it is still present on hospital discharge, it is associated with a 35–50 per cent one-year mortality. Severe CHF due to dilated cardiomyopathy of any etiology has an extremely poor prognosis; pharmacologic agents that normalize cardiac dynamics and produce compensated heart failure do not prolong survival. Myocardial hypertrophy or dilatation or both can develop as compensatory mechanisms, with chronic CHF resulting.

RECOMMENDED READING

Armstrong PW, Walker DC, Burton JR, et al: Vasodilator therapy in acute myocardial infarction. Circulation 52:1118, 1975.

Chatterjee K, Parmley WW, Massie B, et al: Oral hydralazine therapy for chronic refractory heart failure. Circulation 54:879, 1976.

Cohn JN, Franciosa JA: Vasodilator therapy of cardiac failure. N Engl J Med 297:27, 1977.

Cohn JN, Franciosa JA: Selection of vasodilator, inotropic or combined therapy for the management of heart failure. Am J Med 65:181, 1978.

Colucci WS, Wright RF, Braunwald E: Medical progress: new positive inotropic agents in the treatment of congestive heart failure. N Engl J Med 314:290, 349, 1986.

Crandall ED, Staub NC, Goldberg HS, et al: UCLA conference: Recent developments in pulmonary edema. Ann Intern Med 99:808, 1983.

Gavras H, Faxon DP, Berkoben J, et al: Angiotensin-converting enzyme inhibition in patients with congestive heart failure. Circulation 58:763, 1978.

Guiha NH, Cohen JN, Mikulic E, et al: Treatment of refractory heart failure with infusion of nitroprusside. N Engl J Med 291:587, 1974.

Leier CV, Bambach D, Thompson M, et al: Reports on therapy: Central and regional hemodynamic effects of intravenous isosorbide dinitrate, nitroglycerin and nitroprusside in patients with congestive heart failure. Am J Cardiol 48:1115, 1981.

Leier CV, Heban PT, Huss P, et al: Comparative systemic and regional hemodynamic effects of dopamine and dobutamine in patients with cardiomyopathic heart failure. Circulation 58:466, 1978.

Ribner HS, Bresnahan D, Hsieh A-M, et al: Acute hemodynamic responses to vasodilator therapy in congestive heart failure. Prog Cardiovasc Dis 25(1):1, 1982.

Zelis R, Flaim SF: Alterations in vasomotor tone in congestive heart failure. Prog Cardiovasc Dis 26(6):437, 1982.

12. Acute Pericarditis

Nora F. Goldschlager

DEFINITION

Acute pericarditis is an inflammatory process involving the visceral or parietal pericardium, often including the epimyocardium.

PATHOPHYSIOLOGY

Acute pericarditis may be fibrinous or serofibrinous, purulent, or adhesive. Fibrinous and serofibrinous pericarditis are the most common forms and may result from infection, myocardial infarction, collagen-vascular diseases (systemic lupus erythematosus, rheumatoid arthritis), uremia, malignancy (commonly metastatic from lung, melanoma, and breast or from involvement with Hodgkin's disease, leukemia, and lymphoma), and drug therapy (hydralazine, procainamide, and phenytoin). Purulent pericarditis is often related to a cardiac or a mediastinal infectious process such as a stab wound, infective endocarditis with abscess formation, pneumonia, and infected pacing leads. Adhesive pericarditis may follow cardiac surgery and mediastinal radiation therapy (often by months to years).

DIAGNOSIS

Pericardial pain is usually retrosternal in location but may be epigastric. It often radiates to the shoulders (a symptom that may predominate), arms, and back (where it may be mistaken for aortic dissection). The pain may have a pleuritic component, becoming worse with inspiration or coughing, and may be related to position, being aggravated by lying supine; it may also be increased by swallowing. The character of the pain is variable and is described as knifelike, aching, dull, sharp, and squeezing; episodic sharp pain may occur, superimposed upon a duller pain. Fever and leucocytosis may be present. Dyspnea and tachypnea may occur, related primarily to pain but also to accompanying pleuritis.

Physical examination reveals a normal blood pressure without paradox and normal venous pressure without evidence of Kussmaul's sign (note that inspiration often accentuates the pattern of the venous waves; this accentuation should not be confused with elevation of the venous pressure). A pericardial rub may be heard at various times during the patient's course and in varying locations. Auscultation should be performed with the patient supine, semirecumbent, and sitting, during normal breathing and during held inspiration and held expiration. While a three-component rub is classic, only one or two components may be heard; a one-component rub may be mistaken for tricuspid or mitral regurgitation. The rub is often transient, disappearing within a few hours. The presence of a rub does not exclude the presence of a large pericardial effusion or even cardiac tamponade.

The electrocardiogram (ECG) initially shows diffuse J-point elevation with straight or concave upward ST segments. Q waves and coving of the ST segments suggestive of myocardial infarction are not seen. ST segment depression, if present, is confined to leads AVR and V_1. A prominent T wave of atrial repolarization is neither sensitive nor specific for the diagnosis. T-wave inversion is seen after several days, with resolution of the ST elevation (in myocardial infarction T-wave inversion occurs before the ST segments have returned to baseline). Electrical alternans is not seen in pericarditis; its presence should suggest the diagnosis of a large pericardial effusion, which often has a malignant etiology.

Results of the chest roentgenogram and the echocardiogram are often within normal limits but may provide clues to the etiology of the process. The echocardiogram will also reveal small amounts of pericardial fluid that are not clinically detectable. Pericarditis may produce a positive technetium pyrophosphate scan if there is associated myocardial infarction.

MANAGEMENT

Chest pain is managed by analgesics (including opiates) and by antiinflammatory agents: indomethacin 50–75 mg TID-QID or aspirin 10 grains QID should be used. Disappearance of pain often precedes by hours to days disappearance of the pericardial rub. Steroid therapy should be reserved for patients with severe pain unresponsive to the usual measures; consideration should be given to its use if effusion is present. A short course is advised, as discontinuing steroids is often associated with recrudescence of the pericardial inflammation. Occasionally, chronic steroid therapy for chronic relapsing pericarditis must be used; pericardial stripping in these patients is of uncertain benefit.

Atrial premature beats and bursts of atrial tachycardia often accompany acute pericarditis. Unless they lead to sustained atrial tachydysrhythmias, treatment is not warranted. If atrial fibrillation or atrial flutter are present, intravenous digoxin is used to slow the ventricular rate in atrial fibrillation and to maintain a degree of atrioventricular nodal block prior to undertaking pharmacologic conversion of the atrial flutter. DC cardioversion should not be attempted until all evidence of inflammation is resolved, in order to achieve and maintain sinus rhythm. Prophylactic antidysrhythmic therapy may be continued for four to six weeks.

Routine echocardiography to "rule out" pericardial effusion in patients with uncomplicated pericarditis is not warranted, since its predictive accuracy for the subsequent development of effusion is poor in patients in whom fluid is not demonstrated, and its contribution to the management of those patients in whom it is demonstrated is questionable (unless pericardiocentesis for diagnostic purposes is being considered). Pericardiocentesis or pericardial biopsy with or without concomitant drainage procedures for diagnostic purposes is warranted if the etiology is unclear or if purulent pericarditis is suspected. Diagnostic pericardiocentesis is often unproductive, especially if the effusion is small or is posteriorly located. Because of the slight but definite risk of ventricular puncture with consequent tamponade and of cardiac arrest from pericardiocentesis, a surgical approach is preferred, during which both pericardial tissue and fluid can be obtained as well as drainage tubes placed, if required.

Anticoagulant drugs should not be used in patients with pericarditis because of the possibility of developing hemorrhagic cardiac tamponade. If the patient is already receiving anticoagulants that must be continued, heparin should be substituted, since the heparin can be reversed with protamine, if necessary.

Outcome

The clinical course of pericarditis depends upon its etiology, the establishment of which is of prime importance. Viral pericarditis usually has no sequelae but may relapse, as may pericarditis associated with the postcardiotomy syndrome. Occasionally, pericardiectomy is required. Hemodynamically significant pericardial effusion can develop, and cardiac tamponade can occur abruptly. Purulent pericarditis can be fatal if undiagnosed (failure of diagnosis occurs in over 15 per cent of cases), since appropriate antibiotic therapy will not be provided.

All pericarditides may eventuate in pericardial constriction, which often becomes apparent years after the initial insult and can mimic congestive heart failure.

RECOMMENDED READING

Cohen MV, Greenberg MA: Constrictive pericarditis: early and late complication of cardiac surgery. Am J Cardiol 43:657, 1979.

Cohn KE, Stewart JR, Fajardo LF, et al: Heart disease following radiation. Medicine 46:281, 1967.

Comty CM, Cohen SL, Shapiro FL: Pericarditis in chronic uremia and its sequels. Ann Int Med 75:173, 1971.

Fowler NO: Constrictive pericarditis: new aspects. Am J Cardiol 50:1014, 1982.

Franco AE, Levine HD, Hall AP: Rheumatoid pericarditis. Report of 17 cases diagnosed clinically. Ann Int Med 77:837, 1972.

Gore JM, Haffajee CI, Love JC, et al: Isolated right ventricular tamponade after pericarditis from acute myocardial infarction. Am J Cardiol 53:372, 1984.

Hancock EW: Cardiac tamponade. Med Clin North Am 63:223, 1979.

Hirschmann JV: Pericardial constriction. Am Heart J 96:110, 1978.

Horowitz MS, Rossen R, Harrison DC: Echocardiographic diagnosis of pericardial disease. Am Heart J 97:420, 1979.

Isner JM, Carter BL, Bankoff MS, et al: Computed tomography in the diagnosis of pericardial heart disease. Ann Int Med 97:473, 1982.

Klacsmann PG, Bulkley BH, Hutchins GM: The changed spectrum of purulent pericarditis: an 86 year autopsy experience in 200 patients. Am J Med 63:666, 1977.

Kumar S, Lesch M: Pericarditis in renal disease. Prog Cardiovasc Dis 23:357, 1980.

Olson HG, Lyons KP, Aronow WS, et al: Technetium-99m stannous pyrophosphate myocardial scintigrams in pericardial disease. Am Heart J 99:459, 1980.

Rinkenberger RL, Polumbo RA, Bolton MR, et al: Mechanism of electrical alternans in patients with pericardial effusion. Cathet Cardiovasc Diagn 4:63, 1978.

Rooney JJ, Crocco JA, Lyons HA: Tuberculous pericarditis. Ann Int Med 72:73, 1970.

Shabetai R, Fowler NO, Guntheroth WG: The hemodynamics of cardiac tamponade and constrictive pericarditis. Am J Cardiol 25:480, 1970.

Spodick DH: Pericardial rub: prospective. Multiple observer investigation of pericardial friction in 100 patients. Am J Cardiol 35:357, 1975.

Sutton FJ, Whitley NO, Applefeld MM: The role of echocardiography and computed tomography in the evaluation of constrictive pericarditis. Am Heart J 109:350, 1985.

Wong B, Murphy J, Chang CJ, et al: The risk of pericardiocentesis. Am J Cardiol 44:1110, 1979.

13. Pericardial Effusion and Tamponade

Nora F. Goldschlager

DEFINITION

Pericardial effusion refers to the development of fluid within the pericardial space. It may occur in response to any inflammatory and/or mechanical injury to the pericardium. Tamponade occurs when cardiac filling is interfered with to such an extent that cardiac output is significantly compromised.

PATHOPHYSIOLOGY

The pericardium is a relatively stiff structure. The intracardiac volume and the volume of the pericardial sac make up the intrapericardial volume. The intrapericardial pressure is normally the same as the intrapleural pressure. The difference between the intracardiac pressures and the intrapericardial pressure constitutes the transmural distending pressure of the heart. If the intrapericardial pressure is very high and approaches atrial pressures and ventricular diastolic pressures, the transmural cardiac pressure falls, leading to inability of the heart to fill; this results in a reduction in preload (diastolic volume) with consequent reduction in stroke volume.

The normal pericardial space contains 15–50 ml of fluid. If a pericardial effusion develops slowly, up to 2000 ml may accumulate without an increase in intrapericardial pressure and thus without producing clinical symptoms. If, however, fluid accumulation is rapid, 150–250 ml may be sufficient to cause a significant rise in intrapericardial pressure with a resulting fall in transmural cardiac filling pressure, limitation to cardiac filling, and cardiac tamponade. The less distensible the pericardium, the smaller the effusion required to result in clinical symptoms. The pericardium may be rendered relatively nondistensible by fibrosis from any cause, by tumor invasion, or by the accumulation of calcium, as is seen in pericardial constriction. Compensatory mechanisms in tamponade that serve to maintain perfusion to the heart and brain are the following: more complete emptying during systole, leading to an increase in ejection fraction; tachycardia; and peripheral vasoconstriction. The ejection fraction may approach 80 percent in tamponade.

DIAGNOSIS

Mild to moderate pericardial effusion may not produce symptoms. The major symptoms of cardiac tamponade are agitation, dyspnea, tachypnea, and orthopnea.

Physical examination in patients with significant effusion reveals sinus tachycardia, *pulsus paradoxus* (which may not be prominent if severe hypotension, left ventricular failure, or aortic regurgitation are present), elevated central venous pressure with equal a and v waves, and a prominent x descent with obliteration of the y descent; the wave forms may be difficult to ascertain at the bedside, owing to the presence of tachypnea and tachycardia. Kussmaul's sign is not seen in tamponade. The chest may be clear to auscultation or rales may be present. The cardiac apical impulse may be normal, and the heart sounds, although often muffled, may be of normal quality despite hemodynamically significant effusion. A pericardial friction rub may be heard; its presence should not exclude the diagnosis of tamponade. Hypovolemia or hypotension can mask the physical findings of tamponade, which become apparent upon volume loading.

The electrocardiogram (ECG) may be normal or may show nondiagnostic ST-T wave abnormalities, the pattern of pericarditis, low voltage (nondiagnostic *per se*, but helpful if it develops over days and involves the precordial as well as the limb leads), acute myocardial infarction (in which case rupture of the heart should be suspected), and electrical alternans. Electrical alternans usually involves the QRS complexes but can occasionally also involve the P, T, and U waves. Electrical alternans is not necessarily a sign of cardiac tamponade, although it does suggest a large effusion, often malignant in nature, or other pathology such as end-stage congestive cardiomyopathy. It is not the same as, nor does it predict, mechanical alternans.

Dysrhythmias other than sinus tachycardia are not a prominent feature of effusion and tamponade. However, abrupt bradycardia signifies severe tamponade with impending electromechanical dissociation and imminent death.

The chest roentgenogram reveals an enlarged cardiac silhouette if 250 ml or more of fluid is present. Tamponade may be present with a normal roentgenogram. The "water-bottle" configuration of the cardiac shadow is suggestive but not diagnostic of effusion, since it is seen in congestive cardiomyopathy as well. Pulmonary edema is not usually found. Fluoroscopy may show diminished pulsations if the effusion is acute, and right atrial angiography may show a separation between the right cardiac border and the right atrial cavity of 5 mm or more. Computed tomography can also show pericardial effusion and might be especially helpful if localized effusion with local tamponade is suspected. These diagnostic techniques are rarely necessary in the acute care setting, since the echocardiogram provides a rapid diagnosis, having the capability to detect 25 ml or more of pericardial fluid. The echocardiographic findings suggesting (but not proving) tamponade consist of compression of the right ventricle in diastole, reduction in the EF slope of the mitral valve, swinging motion of the heart, pseudoatrioventricular valve prolapse, accentuation of the normal inspiratory increase and expiratory decrease in the right ventricular dimension, and a large anterior and posterior echo-free space. In patients with loculated fluid causing tamponade, such as may occur after cardiac surgery, the echocardiogram may fail to show these typical features.

Cardiac catheterization in tamponade reveals equilibration of diastolic pressures throughout the heart, attenuation or obliteration of the y descent in the atrial pressure tracings (resulting in an "M" or "W" configuration), and reduction in calculated stroke volume. The intraarterial pressure trace is normal in contour but illustrates *pulsus paradoxus*. Kussmaul's sign (an inspiratory increase in venous pressure) is not expected; its presence should prompt consideration of a diagnosis of pericardial constriction (with or without effusion) or other pathologic condition such as right ventricular myocardial infarction, pulmonary embolism, or obstructive pulmonary disease. Invasive monitoring is usually not required to establish a diagnosis of tamponade and should not be undertaken if definitive therapy will thereby by delayed.

MANAGEMENT

Pericardiocentesis should be performed for diagnosis in patients with mild to moderate effusion. Evacuation of the pericardial space should be undertaken emergently in patients with tamponade. Surgical drainage, together with pericardial biopsy, is often preferred in electively performed procedures (fluid cytology may be falsely negative in certain lymphomas) and is the procedure of choice in purulent effusion (in which complete drainage is required) and in hemorrhagic effusion (in which clot formation precludes adequate needle aspiration). If tamponade is present and the effusion is very large, needle aspiration (with concomitant arterial and venous pressure monitoring and echocardiography, if available) is the procedure of choice. If tamponade is present and the effusion is small (normal cardiac size on chest roentgenogram), loculated (as demonstrated on echocardiography), or posteriorly located (indicated by the absence of an anterior echo-free space on echocardiograph), surgical drainage should be carried out emergently. Needle aspiration in these circumstances is often time-consuming and unproductive due to the small volume of fluid and is associated with a significant incidence of complications, including coronary artery laceration, myocardial puncture with further tamponade, and potentially lethal dysrhythmias. Support of the circulation with fluids (despite the elevated central venous pressure) and pressor agents must be maintained until definitive corrective measures are undertaken. Vasodilator therapy is contraindicated, since reduction in cardiac filling pressures is not desired.

OUTCOME

Outcome of treatment of pericardial effusion and tamponade depends upon the underlying etiology. Recurrence is common with malignant and uremic effusions, and surgical drainage with pericardiotomy should be considered. Purulent pericarditis with effusion or tamponade may result in mediastinitis if inadequately treated. Pericardial constriction not infrequently occurs months to years later, and pericardectomy is occasionally required.

RECOMMENDED READING

Guberman BA, Fowler NO, Engel PJ, et al: Cardiac tamponade in medical patients. Circulation 64:633, 1981.

Hancock EW: Subacute effusive-constrictive pericarditis. Circulation 43:183, 1971.

Hancock EW: Cardiac tamponade. In Scheinman MM (ed): Cardiac Emergencies. Philadelphia, W. B. Saunders Co., 1984, p. 252.

Horowitz MS, Schultz CS, Stinson EB, et al: Sensitivity and specificity of echocardiographic diagnosis of pericardial effusion. Circulation 50:239, 1974.

Krikorian JF, Hancock EW: Pericardiocentesis. Am J Med 65:808, 1978.

Kuhn LA: Acute and chronic cardiac tamponade. Cardiovasc Clin 7:177, 1976.

Ofori-Krakye SK, Tyberg TI, Geha AS, et al: Late cardiac tamponade in open heart surgery: incidence, role of anticoagulants in its pathogenesis and its relationship to the postcardiotomy syndrome. Circulation 63:1323, 1981.

Reddy PS, Curtiss EI, O'Toole JD, et al: Cardiac tamponade: hemodynamic observations in man. Circulation 58:265, 1978.

Schiller NB, Botvinick EH: Right ventricular compression as a sign of cardiac tamponade. An analysis of echocardiographic ventricular dimensions and their clinical implications. Circulation 56:774, 1977.

Settle HP, Adolph RJ, Fowler NO, et al: Echocardiographic study of cardiac tamponade. Circulation 56:951, 1977.

Shabetai R: The pathophysiology of cardiac tamponade and constriction. Cardiovasc Clin 7:67, 1976.

Shabetai R, Fowler NO, Guntheroth WG: The hemodynamics of cardiac tamponade and constrictive pericarditis. Am J Cardiol 26:480, 1970.

14. Infectious Endocarditis

Nora F. Goldschlager

DEFINITION

Infectious endocarditis (IE) describes a pathologic process caused by infectious agents that attack cardiac tissue. Generally speaking, the infectious process involves the cardiac valves, although the endocardium (in mural endocarditis) and myopericardium may be exclusively involved. Even with a changing clinical and bacteriologic spectrum, IE continues to have an associated mortality of 10–40 percent despite antibiotic therapy. Morbidity and mortality are almost always the result of cardiac complications. The incidence of IE in patients with rheumatic heart disease has declined recently and has increased in patients with congenital and calcific valvular disease and prosthetic valves. In addition, right-sided endocarditis now accounts for about 15 percent of all cases of IE and for over 50 percent in intravenous drug users.

PATHOPHYSIOLOGY

Structurally normal valves are relatively resistant to infection; nevertheless, in some autopsy series, over 50 percent of cases of IE occurred on anatomically normal valves. Structurally abnormal valves are prone to infection. The etiologies of valvular damage precedent to IE include rheumatic and calcific disease, congenital deformity, and past endocarditis. The valvular damage causes turbulent flow, which contributes further to the structural damage already present. The damaged valve becomes the site of sterile vegetation formation, the lesion consisting of platelets and fibrin; infection occurs via bacteremia from any cause. The infected vegetation has a core of bacteria surrounded by platelets, fibrin, and bacteria. Host defenses cannot penetrate the vegetation to reach the core, in part because of the avascular nature of the valve leaflet or the metal surface of a prosthetic valve; thus, bactericidal antibiotics must be used in treatment.

DIAGNOSIS

Fever and constitutional symptoms are common; absence of fever is often associated with prior antibiotic use in suboptimal dosages. Endocarditis can cause seeding of various organs by bacteria; it can cause an immune complex response with consequent arthritis, glomerulonephritis, and vasculitis; it can also cause systemic or pulmonary embolism (which occurs in up to 50 percent of patients). Cardiac involvement may take the form of myocarditis, myocardial abscess formation with atrioventricular (AV) and intraventricular (mainly left bundle branch block) conduction disturbances, purulent pericarditis, fistula formation, mycotic aneurysm of the aortic root or of a coronary artery, and valvular destruction. Valvular destruction causes valvular insufficiency and can be life-threatening. Valvular stenosis is not produced by endocarditis; rarely, a very large vegetation (such as a fungus ball) can obstruct flow across a valve, producing the hemodynamic picture of stenosis, but the valve itself is not stenotic. The classic signs of endocarditis—splenomegaly, Osler's nodes, Janeway lesions, splinter hemorrhages, and changing murmurs—are now seen in only about 20 percent of cases.

The diagnosis of endocarditis is made by demonstrating cardiac involvement in a patient with bacteremia. In up to 40 percent of patients, the source of infection is not known. Bacteremia is present in over 95 percent of patients with bacterial IE; culture-negative endocarditis is thus distinctly unusual and may signify fungal IE. Cardiac murmurs may be absent initially in 15 percent of patients. The usual murmur present in any patient with bacteremia is a systolic semilunar valve flow murmur that accompanies the fever and tachycardia of systemic infection. A flow murmur is *not* an indication of valvular endocarditis; therefore, bacteremia in a patient with a murmur does not necessarily constitute a diagnosis of infective endocarditis. The murmurs of endocarditis are those that indicate valvular insufficiency and those that are generated by movement of the vegetation itself. The latter murmurs are often harsh or grating, may be inconsistent, and may respond variably to maneuvers such as hand grip, passive leg raising, and respiration. If the murmurs of the vegetation arise from the tricuspid or the mitral valve, they may be confused with regurgitant murmurs; however, the associated findings of AV valve regurgitation are not present. If they arise from the aortic or the pulmonic valves, they may be confused with stenotic murmurs; however, since valve stenosis is not present, the associated findings are absent.

The complete blood count shows leucocytosis, left shift, and often a normochromic, normocytic anemia. Urinalysis can show hematuria, pyuria, and proteinuria; the abnormalities may be due to renal embolism with infarction (present in over 50 percent of autopsied patients) or to bacterial seeding. Azotemia may be present. Clinically important renal dysfunction does not usually occur. A normal erythrocyte sedimentation rate is unexpected and warrants a search to establish another diagnosis.

The electrocardiogram (ECG) may show only sinus tachycardia or may disclose evidence of atrial or ventricular hypertrophy; hypertrophy patterns usually represent precedent heart disease. P-wave abnormalities may be transient, depending on atrial volume and pressure. Patients who develop AV block (4 percent of patients) usually have abscess formation due to *Staphylococcus aureus.* ST-T wave abnormalities may suggest pericarditis, or rarely, myocardial infarction due to septic coronary artery embolism.

The chest roentgenogram may show atrial or ventricular enlargement or both, pulmonary venous congestion, evidence of septic pulmonary emboli, as well as pleural and pericardial effusion. If a prosthetic valve is in place, fluoroscopy can be used to assess its extent of motion, which, if excessive, can suggest dehiscence.

The two-dimensional echocardiogram (2-DE) is useful in confirming the presence of a vegetation in those patients suspected of having it. Failure to demonstrate a vegetation in such patients does not exclude its presence, since the vegetation must of a certain size in order to be detected. Vegetations are frequently large in fungal IE. The yield of 2-DE is poor in patients in whom the physical examination does not suggest vegetations; sensitivity and specificity are largely unknown. Moreover, mural endocarditis without associated valvular involvement is not readily diagnosable. Thus, the routine use of 2-DE to "look for" vegetations in patients with bacteremia is not warranted. When vegetations are demonstrated, 2-DE will allow their measurement, which can then be followed serially during and after treatment. 2-DE can also demonstrate valvular disruption (see Chapter 6) and evaluate chamber size and function; in patients with prosthetic valves, inordinate motion suggesting dehiscence can sometimes be demonstrated.

Computerized tomography may be useful in localizing the source of infection in patients with bacteremia persisting after a full course of antibiotic therapy.

Cardiac catheterization is rarely required in IE and should never delay emergent surgery. Angiography can be helpful in selected patients to demonstrate sinus of Valsalva aneurysms, fistulae, and ventricular septal defects; however, false-negative studies can occur. Dislodgement of vegetations with resulting embolism is a potential serious complication of cardiac catheterization, especially in patients with large mobile vegetations demonstrated echocardiographically and in those in whom recent embolism has occurred.

MANAGEMENT

Prior to beginning antibiotic treatment, two sets of blood cultures should be drawn over a 3–4 hour period. Antibiotic therapy is given as outlined in Tables 14–1 and 14–2. Patients who have bacteremia and a

TABLE 14–1. THERAPEUTIC REGIMENS FOR PATIENTS WITH ENDOCARDITIS BEFORE CULTURE RESULTS ARE KNOWN

CLINICAL SETTING	LIKELY PATHOGEN	THERAPY*
NATIVE VALVE ENDOCARDITIS		
No valvular disease known, acute course usual, severe illness, rapidly progressive	*Staphylococcus aureus* Group A streptococcus *Streptococcus pneumoniae* Enterococcus	Penicillin G 2 mU q 4 h IV and Nafcillin 1.5 gm q 4 h IV or Vancomycin 500 mg q 6 h IV plus Gentamicin 1 mg/kg q 8 h IV or IM
Known past valvular disease, often subacute course	Streptococcus Enterococcus	Penicillin 2 mU q 4 h IV or Ampicillin 1.5 gm q 4 h IV or Vancomycin 500 mg q 6 h IV plus Gentamicin 1 mg/kg q 8 h IV or IM
PROSTHETIC VALVE ENDOCARDITIS		
Early onset	*Staphylococcus epidermidis* *Staphylococcus aureus* Gram-negative rod	Vancomycin 500 mg q 6 h IV plus Gentamicin 1 mg/kg q 8 h IV or IM plus
Late onset	Streptococcus Gram-negative rod	Rifampin 300 mg q 12 h PO
ENDOCARDITIS IN A PARENTERAL DRUG USER†		
	Staphylococcus aureus Streptococcus Enterococcus *Pseudomonas*	Nafcillin 1.5 gm q 4 h IV or Vancomycin 500 mg q 6 h IV plus Gentamicin 1 mg/kg q 8 h IV or IM

*Doses are based on that prescribed for a 70-kg adult with normal renal function.

†Vancomycin and gentamicin are preferred if methicillin-resistant *S. aureus* or *enterococcus* occur regionally. If *Pseudomonas* endocarditis is a possibility, piperacillin or mezlocillin 3 gm q 4 h IV should be added to the regimen.

Adapted, with permission, from Chambers HF, Mills J: Management of infective endocarditis and its complications. In Scheinman MM (ed): Cardiac Emergencies. Philadelphia, W. B. Saunders Co., 1984, p. 234.

flow murmur do not have endocarditis, and appropriate alterations in duration of treatment should be made. Management of septic shock (rare in endocarditis) is outlined in Chapter 8. The minimal inhibitory and bactericidal concentrations of the antibiotic agents used should be evaluated as a test of susceptibility of the organism to the selected antibiotic, and serum concentration of the drugs should be maintained in therapeutic range (1:8 dilution of the patient's serum should kill a standard inoculum of the organism). Persistent bacteremia (bacteremia of 7–10 days' duration despite adequate antimicrobial therapy) should prompt a search for the focus of infection. Extracardiac sites (joints, bones, pleural fluid) should

TABLE 14–2. THERAPEUTIC REGIMENS FOR ENDOCARDITIS OF KNOWN ETIOLOGY

	ANTIBIOTIC REGIMEN*	DURATION (Weeks)
GRAM-POSITIVE ORGANISMS		
Streptococcus viridans	1. Penicillin G 2 mU q 4 h IV	4
	2. Procaine penicillin 1.2 mU q 6 h IM	2–4
	or Penicillin G 2 mU q 4 h IV plus	2–4
	streptomycin 500 mg q 12 h IM	2
	3. Vancomycin 500 mg q 6 h IV	4
	4. Cephalothin 2 gm q 4 h IV	4
Enterococcus†	1. Penicillin G 3 mU q 4 h IV	4–6
	streptomycin 1 gm q 12 h IM	2
	then 500 mg q 12 h IM	2–4
	or gentamicin 1 mg/kg q 8 h IV	4–6
	2. Vancomycin 500 mg q 6 h IV plus either	4–6
	streptomycin 500 mg q 12 h IM	4–6
	or gentamicin 1 mg/kg q 8 h IV or IM	4–6
Staphylococcus aureus‡	1. Nafcillin 1.5 gm q 4 h IV	4
	2. Vancomycin 500 mg q 6 h IV	4
	3. Cephalothin 2 gm q 4 h IV	4
	4. Nafcillin 1.5 gm q 4 h IV plus	4
	gentamicin 1 mg/kg IV or IM	1
Staphylococcus epidermidis	1. Vancomycin 500 mg q 6 h IV plus	6
	gentamicin 1 mg/kg q 8 h IV or IM plus	2
	rifampin 300 mg q 12 h PO	6
	2. Penicillin 2.5 mU q 4 h IV	6
	or nafcillin 1.5 gm q 4 h IV	6
	or cephalothin 2 gm q 4 h IV plus	6
	gentamicin 1 mg/kg q 8 h IM or IV plus	2
	rifampin 300 mg q 12 h PO	6
Streptococcus pneumoniae	1. Penicillin 2.5 mU q 4 h IV	4
	2. Cephalothin 2 gm q 4 h IV	4
	3. Vancomycin 500 mg q 6 h IV	4
GRAM-NEGATIVE ORGANISMS		
Pseudomonas	1. Ticarcillin 3 gm q 4 h IV	4–6
	or piperacillin 3 gm q 4 h IV	4–6
	or ceftazidime 2 gm q 8 h IV plus	4–6
	tobramycin 2.5–3.0 mg/kg q 8 h IV	
Escherichia coli§	1. Ampicillin 2 gm q 4 h IV	4–6
	2. Cephalothin 2 gm q 4 h IV	4–6
	3. Cefotaxime 2 gm q 4 h IV	4–6
Serratia marcescens§	1. Cefotaxime 2 gm q 4 h IV	6
	2 Ticarcillin 3 gm q 6 h IV plus	6
	amikacin 3–5 mg/kg q 8 h IV or IM	
Haemophilus spp.§	1. Ampicillin 2 gm q 4 h IV	4
	2. Ampicillin 2 gm q 4 h IV plus	4
	gentamicin 1 mg/kg q 8 h IM or IV	2
	3. Cefotaxime 2 gm q 4 h IV	4

*Antibiotic doses for 70-kg adult with normal renal function. Choices 1 to 4 throughout are in descending order of preference.

†For enterococci highly resistant to streptomycin, use gentamicin.

‡If organism is sensitive to penicillin G, substitute penicillin G 2 mU q 4 h IV for nafcillin.

§The recommendation for cefotaxime is based only on *in vitro* sensitivity data.

Adapted, with permission, from Chambers HF, Mills J: Management of infective endocarditis and its complications. In Scheinman MM (ed): Cardiac Emergencies. Philadelphia, W. B. Saunders Co., 1984, p. 236.

not be ignored; focal abscesses (including cerebral) should be surgically drained if they cannot be sterilized. In patients with IE who have arteriovenous shunts for purposes of hemodialysis, the source of infection is almost always the shunt; surgical excision is required for cure. Surgical drainage is carried out in patients with pericardial effusion; needle pericardiocentesis is contraindicated (unless cardiac tamponade is present), owing to the possibility of mediastinitis.

Early surgery to excise an infected valve and surrounding tissue is recommended in patients with acute valvular disruption (see Chapter 6) with or without refractory congestive heart failure, recurrent systemic or pulmonary septic emboli (anticoagulation is not indicated), prosthetic valve endocarditis with or without dehiscence, development of AV block, and occurrence of cardiac rupture (e.g., sinus of Valsalva aneurysm rupture, ventricular septal defect formation). Occasionally, recurrent bacteremia in the absence of a source of infection constitutes an indication for valve exploration and possible replacement.

Outcome

Prognosis will depend on the complications that occur during the infection. The valvular disorders that remain after treatment predispose the patient to recurrent endocarditis, and antibiotic prophylaxis should be used prior to any procedure in which entry into the blood stream is anticipated. If surgery has not been performed for valvular insufficiency, the course of the patient with this lesion resembles that of patients with chronic valve insufficiency of any etiology. Patients who have had valve replacement follow a course similar to that in patients with valve replacement for any reason.

"Early onset" prosthetic valve endocarditis (within 60 days of surgery) is usually due to *Staphylococcus aureus* or gram-negative rods and is associated with a mortality of 60–90 percent; early reoperation is usually advised. "Late onset" prosthetic valve endocarditis is often due to *Streptococcus viridans*; it has a better prognosis (mortality 25–40 percent) and can be managed medically in many patients. If the late-onset prosthetic valve endocarditis is caused by nonstreptococcal organisms, however, the mortality is 90 percent without reoperation. Dehiscence is higher with aortic valve prostheses as compared with mitral valve prostheses.

Patients who have had tricuspid valvectomy develop right ventricular failure with high central venous pressures and progressive hepatic damage; tricuspid valvuloplasty or valve replacement is thus usually undertaken.

Patients who have had recurrent septic pulmonary emboli may

develop pulmonary hypertension, which can cause disabling pulmonary symptoms as well as aggravate right ventricular failure.

RECOMMENDED READING

Angrist AA, Oka M: Pathogenesis of bacterial endocarditis. JAMA 183:249, 1963.

Applefeld MM, Woodward TE: Infective endocarditis: a clinical overview. Curr Probl Cardiol 2:1, 1977.

Arnett EN, Roberts WC: Valve ring abscess in active infective endocarditis: frequency, location, and clues to clinical diagnosis from the study of 95 necropsy patients. Circulation 54:140, 1976.

Boyd AD, Spencer FC, Isom OW, et al: Infective endocarditis: an analysis of 54 surgically treated patients. J Thorac Cardiovasc Surg 73:23, 1977.

Chambers HF, Mills J: Management of infective endocarditis and its complications. In Scheinman MM (ed.): Cardiac Emergencies. Philadelphia, W. B. Saunders Co., 1984, p. 232.

Cohen PS, Maguire JH, Weinstein L: Infective endocarditis caused by gram-negative bacteria: A review of the literature, 1945–1977. Prog Cardiovasc Dis 22:205, 1980.

Coleman DL, Horwitz RI, Andriole VT: Association between serum inhibitory and bactericidal concentration and therapeutic outcome in bacterial endocarditis. Am J Med 73:260, 1982.

Davis RS, Strom JA, Frishman W, et al: The demonstration of vegetations by echocardiography in bacterial endocarditis: an indication for early surgery. Am J Med 69:57, 1980.

Dinuble MJ: Surgery in active endocarditis. Ann Intern Med 96:650, 1982.

Dismukes WE, Karchmer AW, Buckley MJ, et al: Prosthetic valve endocarditis. Circulation 48:365, 1973.

Gregoratos G, Karliner JS: Infective endocarditis: diagnosis and management. Med Clin North Am 63:173, 1979.

Kloster FE: Infective prosthetic valve endocarditis. In Rahimtoola SH (ed.): Infective Endocarditis. San Francisco, Grune & Stratton Inc., 1978, p. 291.

Perry EL, Fleming RG, Edwards JE: Myocardial lesions in subacute bacterial endocarditis. Ann Intern Med 36:126, 1952.

Pesanti EL, Smith IM: Infective endocarditis with negative blood cultures: an analysis of 52 cases. Am J Med 66:43, 1979.

Pruitt AA, Rubin RH, Karchmer AW, et al: Neurologic complications of bacterial endocarditis. Medicine 57:329, 1978.

Reid CL, Rahimtoola SH: Infective endocarditis: role of echocardiography, cardiac catheterization, and surgical intervention. Mod Concepts Cardiovasc Dis 55:16, 1986.

15. Hemodynamic Monitoring

Nora F. Goldschlager

INTRODUCTION

Hemodynamic monitoring by means of intravascular catheters is extremely useful in the diagnosis and management of many cardiovascular and pulmonary disorders. The data derived from pulmonary artery catheterization (Tables 15–1 and 15–2) cannot be predicted from the physical examination, electrocardiogram (ECG), or chest roentgenogram. The pressure and flow information obtained from invasive monitoring is complemented by knowledge of intracardiac volumes, which can be measured by isotropic angiography or two-dimensional echocardiography or both. Intraarterial pressure is more accurate than noninvasive sphygmomanometry in patients who are obese, hypotensive (in which the disparity in measured blood pressure can be as high as 50 mm Hg), peripherally vasoconstricted, or severely hypertensive.

INDICATIONS

Invasive monitoring is indicated in patients with (1) shock of any etiology (see Chapter 8); (2) acute myocardial infarction (MI) with ischemic pain and/or congestive heart failure (CHF) unresponsive to therapy; (3) unstable angina refractory to medical management; (4) suspected right ventricular MI; (5) suspected mechanical complication of MI such as interventricular septal or papillary muscle tip rupture; (6) pulmonary edema of unclear etiology (cardiogenic vs. noncardiogenic); (7) pulmonary hypertension, to document its active or passive nature; (8) pericardial effusion with signs of tamponade; (9) acute or chronic valvular disease causing hemodynamic embarrassment; (10) requirement for intraaortic balloon counterpulsation. Hemodynamic monitoring is also indicated in many patients with cardiac disease who are scheduled for major noncardiac surgery and in those who require specific therapeutic interventions such as volume loading (in which the central venous pressure is an unreliable indicator of left ventricular filling pressure), afterload reducing

104

TABLE 15–1. NORMAL RIGHT HEART PRESSURES (mm Hg)

Right atrium	0–8
Right ventricle	25/0–8
Pulmonary artery	25/8–12
Pulmonary artery wedge	8–12

and/or inotropic agents, intravenous (IV) nitroglycerin, and IV antihypertensive agents. An indwelling arterial catheter also allows frequent arterial blood samples to be expeditiously obtained.

CONTRAINDICATIONS

Relative contraindications to arterial cannulation are poor collateral circulation, severe atherosclerotic disease, which can predispose to misleading pressure tracings and values as well as to arterial dissection, and inadequate monitoring facilities and nursing support.

General contraindications to percutaneous venous cannulation are anticoagulant therapy or bleeding diathesis (venous cutdown under direct vision is preferred) and the presence of thrombophlebitis. Subclavian vein cannulation should be avoided in patients with chronic obstructive or bullous lung disease, owing to the possibility of pneumothorax. Internal

TABLE 15–2. HEMODYNAMIC PARAMETERS DERIVED FROM INVASIVE MONITORING

$$LVSWI = SI\ (MAP - PAWP) \times 0.0136$$

$$RVSWI = SI\ (\overline{PA} - RAP) \times 0.0136$$

$$SVR = \frac{MAP - RAP}{\dot{Q}_T}$$

$$TPR = \frac{\overline{PA}}{\dot{Q}_T}$$

$$PVR = \frac{\overline{PA} - PAWP}{\dot{Q}_T}$$

$$Shunt\ Quantitation = \dot{Q}_P/\dot{Q}_S$$

$$\dot{Q}_P = \frac{\dot{V}O_2}{Ao_{O_2} - PA_{O_2}}$$

$$\dot{Q}_S = \frac{\dot{V}O_2}{Ao_{O_2} - (SVC + IVC)\ o_2}$$

LVSWI = left ventricular stroke work index; SI = stroke index; MAP = mean arterial pressure; PAWP = pulmonary artery wedge pressure; RVSWI = right ventricular stroke work index; PA = pulmonary artery; RAP = right atrial pressure; $\dot{Q}_T$ = cardiac output; SVR = systemic vascular resistance; TPR = total pulmonary resistance; PVR = pulmonary vascular resistance; $\dot{Q}_P$ = pulmonary flow; $\dot{Q}_S$ = systemic flow; $\dot{V}O_2$ = oxygen consumption; Ao = aorta; SVC = superior vena cava; IVC = inferior vena cava.

jugular venous cannulation is relatively contraindicated if there is known or suspected high-grade atherosclerotic carotid arterial obstruction because of the risk of embolization, should the artery be inadvertently punctured, or cerebrovascular symptoms if arterial compression is required. In patients with disrupted skin integrity (burns, Stevens-Johnson syndrome), a vein sufficiently remote from the lesions should be selected.

TECHNIQUE

Seldinger Technique of Vessel Cannulation

A Seldinger needle with an obturator (which is removed when the vessel is entered) or a thin-walled needle is inserted into the vessel after the appropriate landmarks are identified. A guide wire (straight or J-shaped) is threaded through the needle, well into the vessel, after which the needle is withdrawn. Using a number 11 scalpel blade tip, a puncture is made through the dermis to allow passage of the larger catheters. A vessel dilator and sheath are then passed over the guide wire into the vessel, and the guide wire and dilator are removed, leaving the sheath, through which is passed the monitoring catheter.

Arterial Cannulation

The radial artery is most commonly utilized, owing to its accessibility, low associated infection and thrombosis rates, and stability without impeding patient movement. The nondominant hand should be used whenever possible, and aseptic precautions taken. Adequacy of collateral flow must first be ascertained by the modified Allen test, in which, with the patient's hand and forearm elevated, both radial and ulnar arteries are compressed while the patient clenches and unclenches his or her fist several times until the hand blanches. The hand is lowered, opened, and relaxed. Release of the ulnar artery should be followed within six seconds by palmar erythema. If color returns to the hand after more than six seconds, inadequate collateral flow from the ulnar artery exists, and the contralateral artery should be evaluated.

To cannulate the vessel, the wrist is hyperextended over a rolled towel and the radial artery palpated along its course throughout the procedure. The hand is immobilized with tape. The skin is anesthetized with 1 percent xylocaine, after which an 18- or 20-gauge needle with overlying catheter is introduced into the artery and the catheter threaded into the artery while the needle is kept immobile. Alternatively, a guidewire can be advanced through the needle well into the artery and the catheter then passed over the wire into the vessel. Occasionally, transient arterial spasm (5–10 percent incidence) occurs; this is much less commonly observed with radial (or dorsalis pedis) than with brachial artery cannulation. Should cannulation not be accomplished, the artery should be compressed for 5–10 minutes to avoid hematoma formation before another attempt is made. After the catheter is secured to the skin, the system is connected via extension tubing to a three-way stopcock and thence to a pressure transducer; patency is assured by a continuous or pulsed infusion of small amounts of heparin and saline.

If the femoral artery is used, percutaneous cannulation is accomplished using the techniques described above. Because of a high incidence of thrombosis and infection, strict aseptic technique should be employed. If the femoral artery is not successfully cannulated, firm pressure must be applied for 15 minutes to avoid hematoma formation. Distal pulses as well as color and temperature of the foot and leg must be checked daily.

Pulmonary Artery Catheterization

The balloon-tipped flow-directed pulmonary artery catheter is used almost exclusively for percutaneous pulmonary artery (PA) catheterization. Triple-lumen catheters that have proximal and distal ports as well as thermistors for cardiac output determinations should be used routinely. Some catheters have electrodes placed at specific distances from the catheter tip and from each other so that atrial, ventricular, and atrioventricular (AV) sequential cardiac pacing can be performed; stability of the electrodes to insure an adequate electrode-myocardium interface is often problematic in critically ill patients, and separate pacing catheters are usually required in pacemaker-dependent patients.

The pulmonary artery catheter is inserted using sterile precautions. Integrity of the balloon tip should always be tested prior to insertion by injection of 2 cc of air through it while it is submersed in water; a heparin-saline solution should be used to flush the system. The pressure transducer should also be tested for expected function.

The preferred insertion route is the right internal jugular vein because of both easy accessibility and stability without impeding of patient movement. The subclavian vein is also readily accessed, and these routes have essentially replaced the femoral vein approach (which usually requires fluoroscopy for catheter placement) and cutdown procedures on the antecubital vein. For internal jugular vein cannulation using the anterior approach (Fig. 15–1), the patient is placed in the Trendelenburg position to avoid air embolism, unless central venous pressure is clearly elevated or clinical symptoms preclude it. After local anesthesia and with the

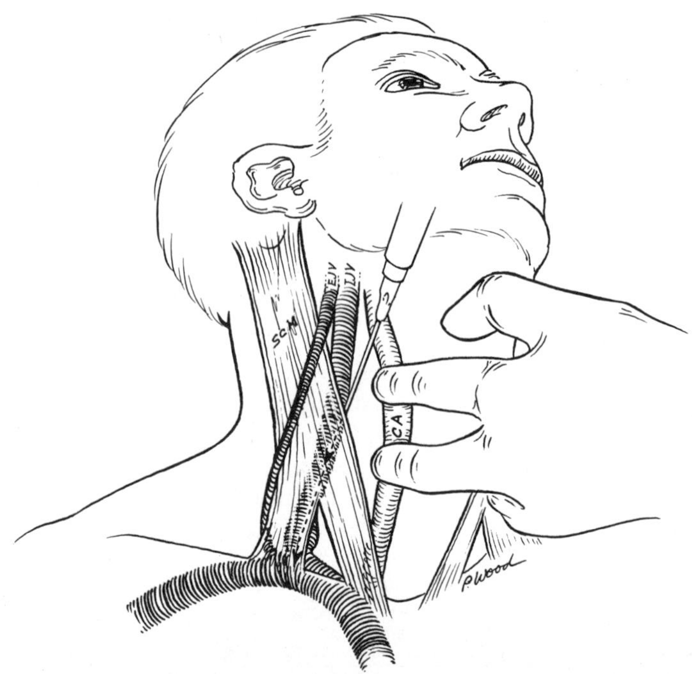

FIGURE 15–1. Anterior approach to internal jugular vein cannulation. See text for further explanation. SCM = sternocleidomastoid muscle; EJV = external jugular vein; IJV = internal jugular vein; CA = carotid artery.

carotid artery being palpated along its course, an 18-gauge thin-walled needle attached to a small syringe is inserted under the medial border of the sternocleidomastoid muscle at a 30-degree angle to the skin and aimed at the ipsilateral nipple. With the medial approach (Fig. 15–2), the needle is inserted near the apex of a triangle formed by the two heads of the sternocleidomastoid muscle and is aimed at the ipsilateral nipple (or slightly medially if access is not achieved). The skin puncture site should be about 3 fingersbreadth above the clavicle if the medial approach is used. With the posterior approach (Fig. 15–3), the needle is inserted underneath the lateral border of the sternocleidomastoid muscle about 5 cm above the clavicle and directed anteriorly toward the suprasternal notch at a 30–45-degree angle to the horizontal planes. Suction is applied to the syringe to allow blood to come into it once the vein is entered. The modified Seldinger technique is then used to cannulate the vessel, the pulmonary artery catheter being advanced through the vascular sheath.

For subclavian vein cannulation, the patient is placed in the Trendelenburg position to avoid air embolism. A rolled sheet or towel is placed underneath the shoulders. Vessel access is achieved by inserting the

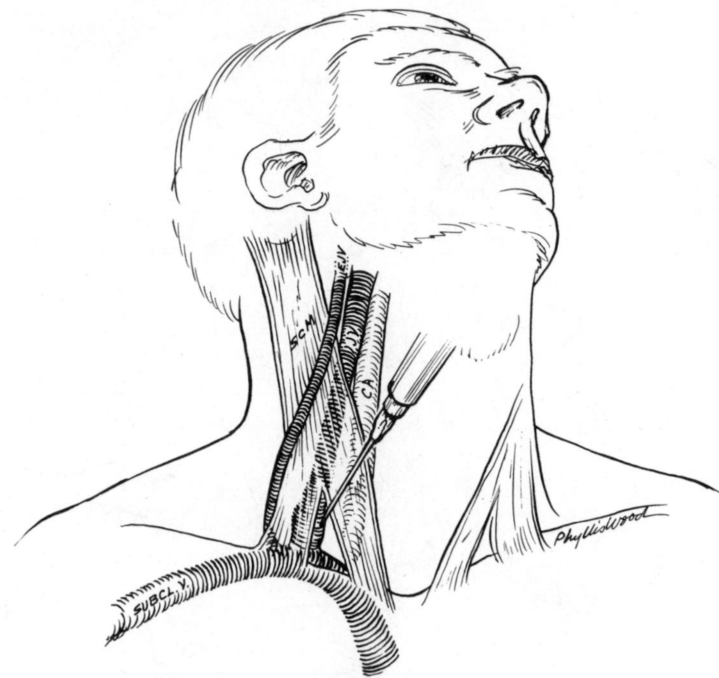

FIGURE 15–2. Medial approach to internal jugular vein cannulation. See text for further explanation. SCM = sternocleidomastoid muscle; EJV = external jugular vein; IJV = internal jugular vein; CA = carotid artery; SUBCL. V. = subclavian vein.

cannulation needle and catheter through the skin slightly medial to the midclavicular line, 1–2 cm caudal to the clavicle. The needle is advanced parallel to the anterior chest wall just under the clavicle, aiming for the suprasternal notch. When blood is obtained, the Seldinger technique is used to cannulate the vessel.

Advancement of the pulmonary artery catheter should always be accompanied by continuous ECG monitoring and by pressure monitoring from the distal port. To guide placement, markers are present every 10 cm from the catheter tip. The right atrium is usually reached by 10 cm and the pulmonary artery by 40–50 cm. Premature ventricular beats and nonsustained ventricular tachycardia are not infrequently encountered as the catheter traverses the inflow and outflow tracts of the right ventricle; rapid placement eliminates the dysrhythmia, hend antidysrhythmic agents are not indicated. Pressure monitoring through the distal port is required for verification of catheter location (Fig. 15–4); the pressure tracings should be undamped and the contours and values reasonable (Table 15–1). When the catheter is in the right atrium, the balloon is inflated and the catheter passed into the right ventricle and the pulmonary artery. Once the tip

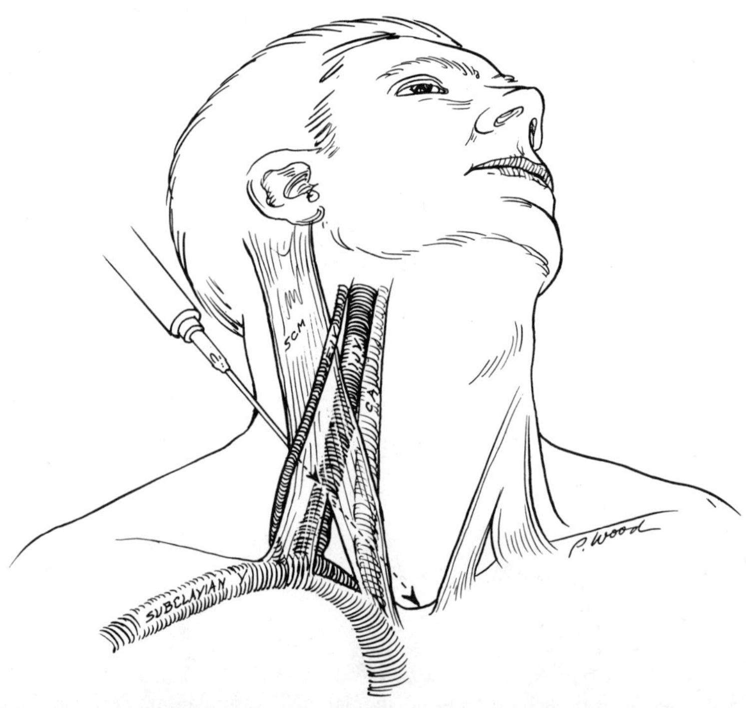

FIGURE 15–3. Posterior approach to internal jugular vein cannulation. See text for further explanation. SCM = sternocleidomastoid muscle; EJV = external jugular vein; IJV = internal jugular vein; CA = carotid artery; SUBCLAVIAN V. = subclavian vein.

has entered the right ventricle, if more than 15 cm of catheter is advanced and the pulmonary artery has still not been reached, the catheter is probably coiled in the right atrium (or ventricle), and withdrawal and repositioning should be undertaken. Ventricularized pulmonary artery pressure tracings indicate a right ventricular outflow tract position and further catheter advancement is required. When a pulmonary artery "wedge" (more properly called "occlusion") pressure tracing is obtained, the balloon is deflated and the catheter secured to the skin. Fluoroscopic guidance is indicated if proper positioning is not achieved within a reasonable period of time or if persistent ventricular dysrhythmias are present. Baseline blood samples for oxygen content may be obtained from the vena cava, right atrium, and pulmonary artery; a chest roentgenogram should be obtained after catheter placement and daily thereafter. The sterile dressing should be changed daily.

COMPLICATIONS

Arterial Cannulation

Major complications include thrombosis (up to 40 percent incidence suggested by Doppler techniques), embolism, hematoma, and infection

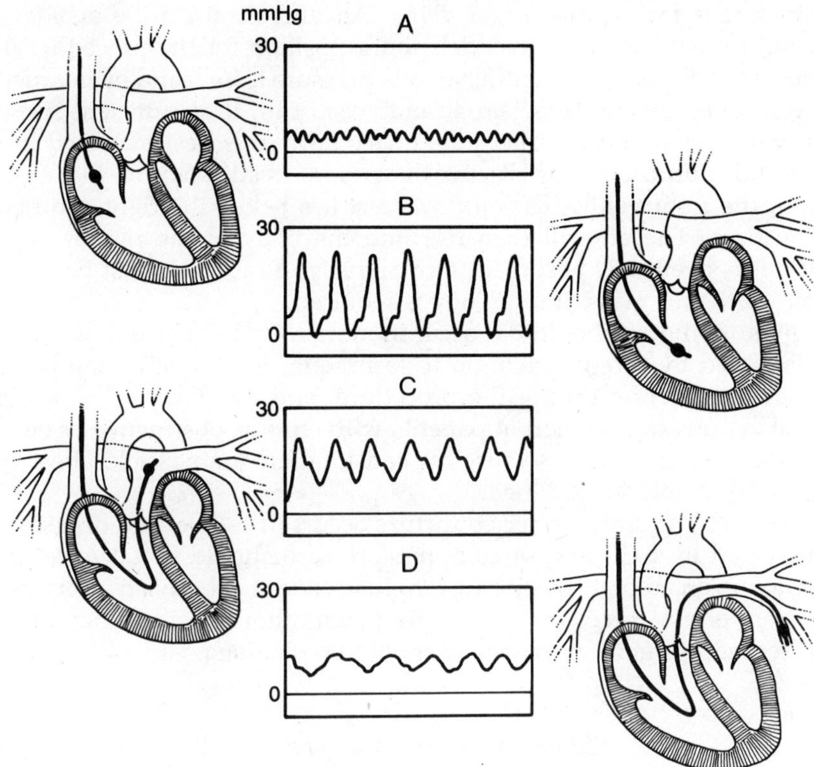

FIGURE 15–4. Pressure tracings obtained from pulmonary artery catheter in the right atrium (A), right ventricle (B), pulmonary artery (C), and "wedge" position (D). (Reproduced, with permission, from Luce JM, Tyler ML, Pierson DJ: Intensive Respiratory Care. Philadelphia, W. B. Saunders Co., 1984, p. 252.)

(4 percent incidence). The incidence of infection rises if the catheter is left in place for four days or longer. Thrombosis is related to large cannula size, prolonged duration of use (beyond 48 hours), low cardiac output, and use of pressor agents. Whereas thrombosis is not usually associated with disabling sequelae, infection can result in bacteremia or endovascular infection, with serious consequences. Arterial dissection and arteriovenous fistula formation have been reported but are rare.

Internal Jugular and Subclavian Venous Cannulation

Thrombosis, embolism, and infection also complicate venous cannulation. Infection may be prevented by strict aseptic technique and short duration of use; catheters should be changed every 3–5 days. Thrombosis occurs but is rare in the larger veins. Air embolism can be avoided by placing the patient in the Trendelenburg position for the procedure (this is especially important if central venous pressure is low) and by instruction to avoid deep inspirations. An air embolism can, if of sufficient size, act as a mass lesion and obstruct pulmonary flow. It is best managed in the absence of fluoroscopy by placing the patient head down on his left side so that the right ventricular outflow tract lies below the right ventricular inflow tract. The air will then rise into the body of the right ventricle, where it is eventualy absorbed. Occasionally, a catheter must be used to break up the air mass; fluoroscopy is required.

Pneumothorax should not occur in more than 1–2 percent of patients. It is avoided by careful attention to technique, by discontinuing positive pressure ventilation during the procedure, and by avoiding, if possible, central venous cannulation in patients with chronic obstructive or bullous lung disease. If it occurs, surgical consultation for possible chest tube placement should be obtained.

Inadvertent carotid artery puncture occurs in 1–5 percent of cases and is managed by 5–10 min of compression; care should be taken to avoid symptoms of cerebral hypoperfusion. Inadvertent subclavian artery puncture can occur rarely, with resulting hemothorax which can be life-threatening. Surgical consultation should be obtained.

Pulmonary Artery Catheterization

Pulmonary infarction (incidence, 5–7 percent) can occur as a result of the catheter being positioned too far distally in the left or right pulmonary arteries and by leaving the balloon inflated for periods exceeding 60 seconds. If the monitored pressure tracings suggest a wedged position, the catheter has probably migrated, and pullback is required.

Significant dysrhythmias are rarely life-threatening, tend to occur in patients predisposed to develop them (such as those with acute myocardial infarction or congestive heart failure), and usually resolve when stable catheter position is achieved. Ventricular salvoes (3–5 consecutive premature ventricular contractions [PVCs]) occur in 30 percent, nonsustained ventricular tachycardia in 20 percent, and sustained ventricular tachycardia in 3 percent. Ventricular fibrillation has been reported but is decidedly rare.

Rarer complications include aseptic valvular vegetations, pulmonary artery rupture due to balloon overinflation or advancement with the balloon deflated, cardiac tamponade due to catheter passage with the balloon deflated, pulmonary artery thrombosis, and avulsion of portions of the tricuspid valve. Shearing off of the electrodes during withdrawal of a multipurpose catheter through the sheath has been reported; prevention is achieved by use of an 8.5F sheath and by withdrawal of the sheath prior to withdrawal of the catheter. The balloon should always be inflated during passage of the catheter and always deflated during withdrawal. Transient right bundle branch block and complete AV block in patients with preexisting left bundle branch block occur with an overall incidence of about 5 percent; in patients with left bundle branch block in whom semielective pulmonary artery catheter placement can be performed, consideration should be given to prior insertion of a temporary ventricular pacing catheter.

RECOMMENDED READING

Armstrong PA, Baigrie RS: Hemodynamic Monitoring in the Critically Ill. Philadelphia, Harper & Row Publishers, Inc., 1979, p. 39.

Buchbinder N, Ganz W: Hemodynamic monitoring—invasive techniques. Anesthesiology 45:146, 1976.

Criley JM, Ross RS: Cardiovascular Physiology. Oldsmar, Tampa Tracings, 1971.

Gillies IDS, Morgan M, Sykes MK: The nature and incidence of complications of peripheral artery puncture. Anesthesia 34:506, 1979.

Kelly TF Jr, Morris GC Jr, Crawford ES, et al: Perforation of the pulmonary artery with Swan-Ganz catheters. Ann Surg 191:686, 1981.

Pace NL: A critique of flow-directed pulmonary arterial catheterization. Anesthesiology 47:455, 1977.

Puri VK, Carlson RW, Bander JJ, et al: Prospective study of 116 critically ill patients, comparing percutaneous vs. cut-down approaches for arterial, central venous and pulmonary artery catheters. Crit Care Med 8:495, 1980.

Sprung CL, Pozen RG, Rozanski JJ, et al: Advanced ventricular arrhythmias during pulmonary artery catheterization. Am J Med 72:203, 1982.

Swan HJC, Ganz W: Use of balloon flotation catheters in critically ill patients. Surg Clin North Am 55:501, 1975.

Swan HJC, Ganz W: Complications of flow-directed balloon-tipped catheters. Ann Intern Med 91:494, 1979.

16. Temporary Transvenous Cardiac Pacing

Nora F. Goldschlager

INTRODUCTION

Temporary cardiac pacing may be used therapeutically or prophylactically. It may be a life-saving procedure in many critically ill patients. The pacing system consists of a pacing lead(s) and a single or dual chamber (atrioventricular [AV] sequential) pulse generator.

INDICATIONS

Temporary pacing is indicated in all patients with symptomatic or hemodynamically compromising bradycardias of any etiology; in patients with acute anterior wall myocardial infarction (MI) who develop Type II AV block, new onset bifascicular block with or without PR interval prolongation, or alternating bundle branch block, who are at high risk (38–50 percent) for development of paroxysmal complete AV block during the infarction; in patients with polymorphic ventricular tachycardia (see Chapter 3) due to congenital long QT interval, hypokalemia, hypomagnesemia, and Type I antidysrhythmic agent (quinidine, procainamide, disopyramide) toxicity; and in symptomatic patients with permanent pacemakers who are awaiting pulse generator replacement. Rapid atrial pacing should be considered in some patients with paroxysmal reentrant supraventricular tachycardia and atrial flutter in order to terminate the rhythm; burst ventricular pacing has been used in selected patients with recurrent, refractory ventricular tachycardia.

Ventricular pacing is used in most clinical circumstances, owing to the ease of placement; however, atrial or AV sequential pacing is recommended in patients with right ventricular MI for optimum hemodynamic function, and atrial pacing is recommended in patients with polymorphic ventricular tachycardia for rhythm control.

CONTRAINDICATIONS

Temporary pacing is not indicated in patients with asymptomatic bradycardia (unless acute inferior wall MI is present and the patient is at

114

risk for AV block), in patients with anterior wall MI and unifascicular block, or in moribund patients with electromechanical dissociation. Transthoracic pacing is now obsolete, having been replaced by transchest devices.

Technique

Sterile technique is mandatory. The percutaneous transvenous routes for electrode catheter insertion are the antecubital, internal jugular, subclavian, and femoral veins. Stability of the pacing catheter is optimal with use of the internal jugular or subclavian veins; in addition, patient movement is less impeded and the incidence of phlebitis is lower using these approaches. Fluoroscopic guidance should be used with antecubital and femoral vein approaches in order to facilitate lead placement, and whenever stiff catheters are used; it is recommended in all cases in which an atrial lead is employed. Care should be taken to avoid inadvertent arterial cannulation. Pneumothorax, not uncommon when the subclavian vein approach is used, can be avoided by placing the patient in the Trendelenburg position during the procedure. Temporary balloon-tipped flow-directed pacing catheters are prepackaged as a complete set, including scout needle and cannula; flotation catheters facilitate rapid placement at the bedside. Larger, stiffer catheters require introduction through an appropriate-sized sheath, with fluoroscopic guidance. If passage of the catheter is difficult, a guide wire may be introduced through the cannula, the cannula removed, the sheath placed over the guide wire, which is then removed, and the catheter advanced through the sheath. Pacing catheters have markers at 10-cm intervals; if the jugular or subclavian veins are used, the approximate distance from the insertion site to the right ventricular apex is 35–45 cm. If satisfactory position is not obtained at this distance, the catheter should be pulled back to the level of the right atrium or superior vena cava (about 20 cm from the insertion site) and advanced again, since coiling in the right atrium is probably present.

To verify the position of the tip of the electrode catheter during its insertion, the intracardiac electrogram from the distal (tip) electrode is continuously recorded by connecting this electrode wire to the V_1 lead of an electrocardiogram (ECG) machine by means of an alligator clamp and recording from the "V" position of the ECG; a surface ECG lead should be simultaneously recorded in order to verify whether a given intracardiac signal represents a P wave (or other atrial wave) or a QRS complex. When a ventricular signal with a current of injury appears, position is probably satisfactory and myocardial stimulation threshold may be measured. The location of the catheter is then evaluated by anteroposterior and trans-bed lateral chest roentgenogram obtained immediately after placement and daily thereafter. Since significant migration of the catheter tip may occur without appreciable change in the roentgenogram, it is not an entirely reliable guide. Right ventricular apical position of the pacing lead is suggested radiographically by an anteriorly and inferiorly directed lead tip, which lies to the left of the spine near the left cardiac border. Right ventricular outflow tract position is suggested by an anteriorly and superiorly directed lead tip, which overlies the spine; leads in this position are unstable and require repositioning. A 12-lead ECG should always be recorded while the patient is paced, immediately after placement, and daily thereafter for comparison purposes. The paced QRS complexes should have a superiorly directed frontal plane axis and a left bundle branch block pattern.

COMPLICATIONS

Important complications of temporary cardiac pacing include sensing problems (undersensing or oversensing), failure to capture, myocardial penetration, and cardiac tamponade. Sensing problems resulting in "failure" to sense (undersensing) may be due to malposition of the temporary catheter(s), to poor intracardiac signal quality, or to generator malfunction. Generator malfunction is only rarely the cause of pacemaker-related problems in the critical care setting. Pacing catheter position is evaluated as described above (see *Technique*). The most common cause of sensing problems in critically ill patients is the suboptimal nature of the intracardiac signal. Borderline signals are recorded in patients with acute MI, myocardial ischemia, acidosis, alkalosis, ventricular dilatation, myocardial cellular edema, and drug and/or electrolyte abnormalities. Ectopic impulses arising in ventricular tissue are often not sensed because of their poor quality, a situation that can lead to repetitive ventricular beating. Unless life-threatening pacemaker-related dysrhythmias occur as a result of unsensed spontaneous complexes, sensing problems can be managed by careful observation alone. It must be emphasized that intracardiac signals "seen" by the catheter electrodes have no relationship to surface ECG complexes; thus, complexes that are either not sensed or signals that are sensed inappropriately (oversensed), cannot be predicted from the surface ECG. Undersensing is managed by turning the sensitivity setting of the pulse generator to full demand (clockwise) position. Unipolarization of the bipolar temporary generator to augment the intracardiac signal can also be tried: The negative terminal of the pulse generator is connected to one of the intracardiac lead electrodes and the positive terminal to a surface (skin) electrode; the free end of the unused lead electrode is encased in rubber to prevent accidental conduction of current directly into the heart.

It is advisable to record both the bipolar and unipolar (from each electrode) signals daily in order to assess changes in signal magnitude so that optimal sensitivity settings may be selected on the pulse generator. The bipolar signal is recorded by connecting the intracardiac leads to the right and left arm electrodes of the ECG machine and recording Lead I. Since most temporary pulse generators are bipolar, the bipolar signal is the sensed signal and should be measured daily. Oversensing (sensing of unwanted signals), with resulting pauses in paced rhythm, can result from sensing of atrial electrical activity if the pacing lead is positioned near the tricuspid valve, from sensing of T waves, and from sensing of voltage transients caused by lead wire fracture, environmental interference, or signals originating in the generator itself. Not uncommonly, movement of the extension cables that are sometimes used to connect the generator to the electrode catheter produces electrical signals that can be sensed by and inhibit the generator. Oversensing is managed by turning the sensitivity setting towards the asynchronous position (counterclockwise) until the unwanted signals are no longer sensed.

Failure to capture may be due to lead malposition or to an increase in myocardial stimulation threshold. Common causes of increased stimulation threshold are hyperkalemia, myocardial necrosis, acidosis, shock, and high concentrations of Type I antidysrhythmic agents (quinidine, procainamide, disopyramide). (Flecainide, a newer antidysrhythmic agent, is associated with high pacing thresholds in recommended doses.) Failure to capture may be intermittent or complete and may take the form of Type I (Wenckebach) or Type II exit block; it is frequently a harbinger of electromechanical dissociation. The current output should be increased until consistent capture occurs. Correction of hemodynamic and drug and electrolyte abnormalities should be undertaken. Lead position should be checked and the catheter repositioned if necessary. In urgent situations, intravenous steroids (e.g., 40 mg methylprednisolone) or low-dose isoproterenol may temporarily restore pacing function.

Myocardial penetration or frank perforation into the pericardial space may not *per se* be dangerous to the patient, although it is considered a complication of temporary pacing. Penetration is usually accompanied by a pericardial friction rub (which may be present even though actual perforation has not occurred) and often by a squeaking systolic sound or murmur. A change in configuration of paced QRS complexes is often, but not always, seen. No treatment is required. However, if chest pain and/ or failure to sense or to pace or both are present, the diagnosis should be established by recording unipolar electrograms from both distal and proximal intracardiac electrodes (which will show an epicardial complex [resembling V4–5] rather than an endocardial complex) and, if doubt still remains, by two-dimensional echocardiography, which can more precisely localize the position of the catheter tip. The pacing lead must then be repositioned: Merely pulling it back to the ventricular endocardium does not suffice, as it tends to migrate out the same tract; the lead should be pulled back to the right atrium and then repositioned. Fluoroscopic guidance may be required. If cardiac tamponade has occurred in association with myocardial perforation, urgent pericardiocentesis should be performed (see Chapter 13).

During passage of the pacing catheter, ventricular extrasystoles or rapid ventricular tachycardia may occur. This is usually due to catheter abutment at the right ventricular inflow or outflow tracts. Rapid manipulation of the pacing lead into proper position will eliminate the ectopy; use of lidocaine should be avoided. Since significant ventricular ectopy may indicate lead malplacement, its position should be verified by chest roentgenogram and a paced 12-lead ECG. Repositioning with fluoroscopic guidance may be necessary to achieve a stable position at which ventricular ectopy is not problematic.

Other complications are the same as those for any intravascular catheter and include venous thrombosis, pulmonary embolism (usually clinically silent), and infection.

DISCONTINUATION OF TEMPORARY PACING

When pacing is no longer required, the catheter can be removed without fluoroscopy. Rapid removal is recommended in order to avoid ventricular extrasystoles, which are often encountered around the area of the right ventricular inflow tract.

RECOMMENDED READING

Barold SS, Gaidula JJ: Failure of demand pacemaker from low-voltage bipolar ventricular electrograms. JAMA 215:923, 1971.

Chamorro H, Rao G, Wholey MH: Superior vena cava obstruction syndrome. A complication of transvenous pacemaker implantation. Radiology 126:377, 1978.

Chatterjee K, Davies G, Harris A: Fall of endocardial potentials after acute myocardial infarction. Lancet 1:1308, 1970.

Furman S: Pacemaker emergencies. Med Clin North Am 63:113, 1979.

Furman S, Hurzeler P, DeCaprio V: Cardiac pacing and pacemakers. III. Sensing the cardiac electrogram. Am Heart J 93:794, 1977.

Furman S, Hurzeler P, Mehra R: Cardiac pacing and pacemakers. IV. Threshold of cardiac stimulation. Am Heart J 94:115, 1977.

Gay RJ, Brown DF: Pacemaker failure due to procainamide toxicity. Am J Cardiol 34:728, 1974.

Goldschlager N, Sudduth B: Pacemaker emergencies. In Scheinman MM (ed): Cardiac Emergencies. Philadelphia, W. B. Saunders Co., 1984, p. 152.

Hughes HC, Tyers FO, Torman HA: Effects of acid-base imbalance on myocardial pacing thresholds. J Thorac Cardiovasc Surg 69:743, 1975.

Misra KP, Korn M, Ghahramani AR, et al: Auscultatory findings in patients with cardiac pacemakers. Ann Int Med 74:245, 1971.

Mond HG, Stuckey JG, Sloman G: The diagnosis of right ventricular perforation by an endocardial pacemaker electrode. PACE 1:62, 1978.

Morgan G, Ginks W, Siddons H, et al: Septicemia in patients with an endocardial pacemaker. Am J Cardiol 44:221, 1979.

Preston TA: Electrocardiographic diagnosis of pacemaker catheter displacement. Am Heart J 85:445, 1973.

Van Durme JP, Heyndrickx G, Snoeck J, et al: Diagnosis of myocardial perforation by intracardiac electrograms recorded from the indwelling catheter. J Electrocardiol 6:97, 1973.

17. Intraaortic Balloon Counterpulsation

Nora F. Goldschlager

INTRODUCTION

Intraaortic balloon counterpulsation (IABC) is a form of mechanical circulatory assist; it is palliative only, and thus it is best used as a temporizing measure until more definitive therapy can be provided.

IABC is synchronized with the cardiac cycle to reduce blood pressure in the ascending aorta during ventricular systole (thus reducing resistance to ejection) and to augment it during ventricular diastole. Diastolic augmentation of coronary arterial flow as well as reduction in left ventricular afterload and preload (of which ventricular diastolic pressure is an index) are thereby accomplished. The reduction in afterload during systole, and in preload, serve to reduce myocardial oxygen (O_2) consumption relative to available O_2 supply; the augmentation in coronary perfusion pressure may serve to increase O_2 supply directly (although the point is disputed in studies of regional myocardial blood flow). The measured blood pressure will be determined by the volume of blood moved and by the stiffness of the peripheral vasculature as well as by the counterpulsation itself.

Hemodynamic improvement with IABC is determined by the favorable alterations in loading conditions of the left ventricle: As afterload is reduced, stroke volume increases; preload is reduced *pari passu* with the increase in stroke volume as well as by the IABC itself. The enhanced stroke volume results in amelioration of tachycardia, improved cardiac output (by as much as 20 percent) and urine output, and alleviation or actual abolishment of ischemic cardiac pain.

INDICATIONS

IABC may be indicated in patients with severe but potentially reversible cardiac dysfunction such as intractable unstable angina and myocardial infarction complicated by postinfarction angina, congestive failure, hypotension, and mechanical problems such as ruptured interventricular sep-

120

tum and mitral papillary muscle tip. IABC has also been used in the management of patients with lethal intractable ventricular dysrhythmias unresponsive to pharmacologic therapy. IABC is often employed in patients after cardiac surgery when weaning from cardiopulmonary bypass has been difficult and low cardiac output persists.

Contraindications

Since IABC provides diastolic augmentation of aortic flow to the level of the aortic root, it is contraindicated in patients with aortic regurgitation. Cardiogenic shock that is not improved within 12–24 hours of initiation of IABC is generally a contraindication to its continued use. Patients with aortofemoral bypass grafts cannot undergo arterial cannulation, and thus IABC cannot be used (unless it is performed surgically); severe peripheral vascular disease is not an absolute contraindication, however. Since anticoagulation is required during IABC, patients in whom this is contraindicated cannot undergo it.

Technique

The balloon catheter is inserted percutaneously through an intraarterial sheath into the femoral artery and advanced retrograde to the level of the subclavian artery. Fluoroscopic guidance should be used whenever feasible to facilitate optimum catheter positioning. Single- and double-lumened catheters are available, the latter being preferred for its central lumen through which a guide wire can be inserted and pressure monitored once the system is in place. Helium is generally used to inflate the balloon during ventricular diastole. Ventricular diastole is synchronized to the end of the T wave of the electrocardiogram (ECG). The balloon is deflated during ventricular systole, which is synchronized to the beginning of the QRS complex (or to the pacing stimulus in patients with ventricular pacemakers). The volume of the balloon is 30–40 ml. The timing of balloon inflation must be precise so as to provide optimum augmentation in diastole but more importantly so as to avoid the occurrence of ventricular systole against the increased afterload caused by a partially inflated balloon. Figure 17–1 demonstrates timing guidelines.

Anticoagulation with heparin is required, although low-molecular weight dextran has occasionally been used in patients with a contraindication to heparin. The balloon should not be inactive for more than 15-20 minutes in order to avoid thrombosis.

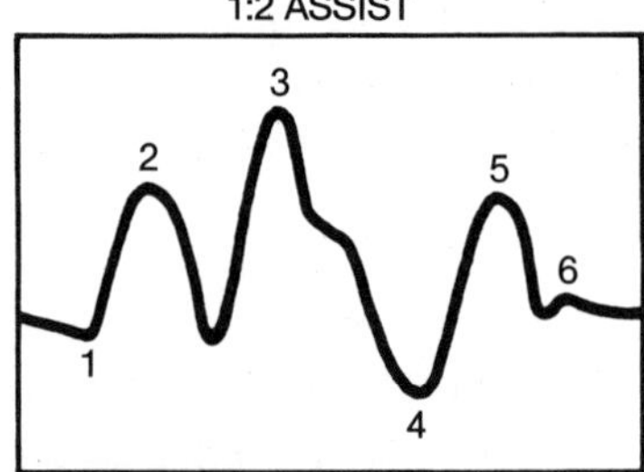

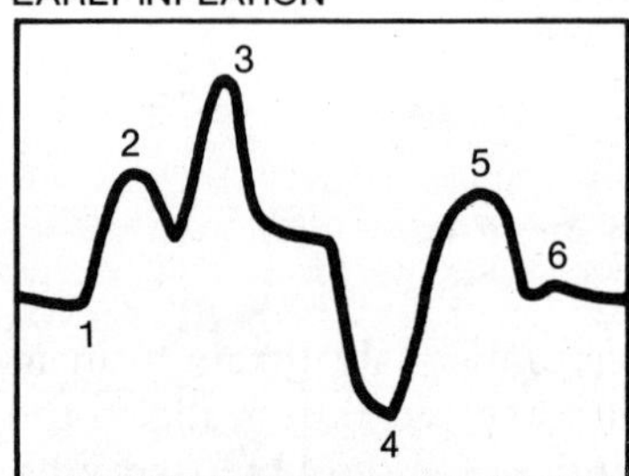

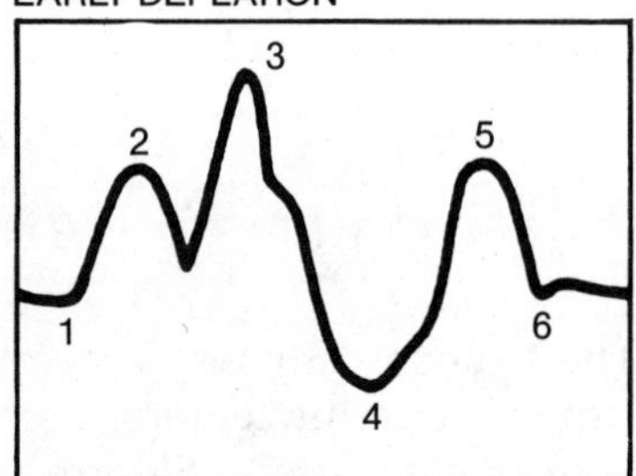

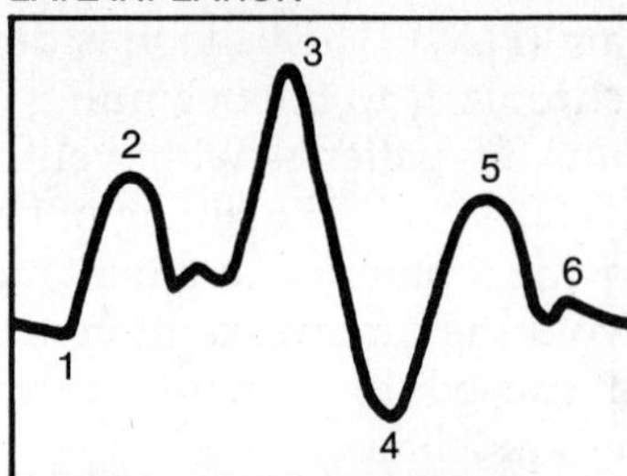

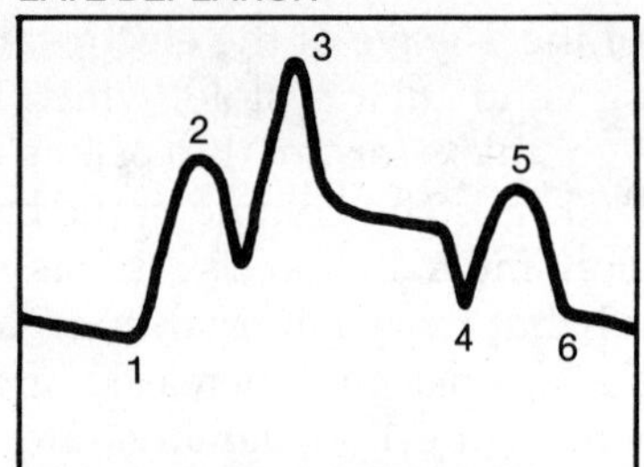

FIGURE 17–1. Timing guidelines for intraaortic balloon counterpulsation (IABC). CO = cardiac output; MVO_2 = myocardial oxygen consumption.

Weaning

Weaning from IABC consists of reducing the percentage of assisted cardiac cycles (e.g., from 1:1 to 1:2, 1:4, and 1:8). Clinical and hemodynamic deterioration will recur minutes to hours later in patients who cannot sustain cardiac function without support. Many patients undergo cardiac catheterization and proceed directly to surgery while on IABC. If definitive therapy such as coronary artery bypass grafting or angioplasty can be offered, there is no reason to wean the patient from IABC. In patients who are not operative candidates but in whom prognosis is not extremely poor (such as those with cardiogenic shock, in which mortality continues to approach 70–80 percent), IABC can be continued for up to four weeks if tolerated and if complications do not ensue. In all patients, once the arterial pressure is supported, inotropic and vasodilator therapy may be given as required.

Complications

Up to 10–15 percent of patients experience complications during IABC, depending in part on patient selection and on operator and nursing skill. Major complications include aortic trauma and dissection, hemorrhage due to the required anticoagulation, ischemia of the leg in which the balloon catheter is placed, infection, and thromboembolism. Aortic dissection may be underestimated clinically; its incidence is reduced by using a double-lumened balloon catheter, which allows a guide wire to be inserted into the aorta to the level of the subclavian artery before the catheter itself is placed.

If ischemia develops in the leg in which the catheter is placed (which occurs in 15–20 percent of patients), removal of the system with insertion in the opposite femoral artery must be accomplished. Occasionally, iliofemoral bypass procedures are required. Patients with low cardiac output and low arterial pressure who also have peripheral vascular disease are particularly prone to ischemic complications. Prophylactic antibiotics are not given.

RECOMMENDED READING

Baron DW, O'Rourke MF: Long-term results of arterial counterpulsation in acute severe cardiac failure complicating myocardial infarction. Br Heart J 38:285, 1976.
Bolooki H: The effects of counterpulsation with an intra-aortic balloon on cardiovascular dynamics and metabolism. In Bolooki H (ed): Clinical Application of Intra-Aortic Balloon Pump. Mount Kisco, Futura Publishing Co., Inc., 1977, p. 15.

DeWood MA, Notshe RN, Hensley GR, et al: Intraaortic balloon counterpulsation with and without reperfusion for myocardial infarction shock. Circulation 61:1105, 1980.

Gold HK, Leinbach RC, Sanders CA, et al: Intra-aortic balloon pumping for ventricular septal defect or mitral regurgitation complication acute myocardial infarction. Circulation 47:1191, 1973.

Hauser AM, Gordon S, Gangadmar V, et al: Percutaneous intraaortic balloon counterpulsation: clinical effectiveness and hazards. Chest 82:422, 1982.

Kantrowitz A, Wasfie T, Freed PS, et al: Intraaortic balloon pumping 1967 through 1982: analysis of complications in 733 patients. Am J Cardiol 57:976, 1986.

McEnany MT, Kay HR, Buckley JM, et al: Clinical experience with intra-aortic balloon pump support in 728 patients. Circulation 58(Suppl. 1):1, 1978.

Scheidt S, Collins M, Goldstein J, et al: Mechanical circulatory assistance with the intraaortic balloon pump and other counterpulsation devices. Prog Cardiovasc Dis 25:55, 1982.

Scheidt S, Wilner G, Rubenfire M, et al: Intraaortic balloon counterpulsation in cardiogenic shock. Report of a cooperative clinical trial. N Engl J Med 288:979, 1973.

Willerson JT, Curry GC, Watson JT, et al: Intraaortic balloon counterpulsation in patients in cardiogenic shock, medically refractory left ventricular and/or recurrent ventricular tachycardia. Am J Med 58:183, 1975.

Williams D, Korr K, Gerwirtz H, et al: The effect of intraaortic balloon counterpulsation on regional blood flow and oxygen consumption in the presence of coronary artery stenosis in patients with unstable angina. Circulation 66:593, 1982.

18. Cardioversion

Nora F. Goldschlager

INTRODUCTION

Synchronized direct current (DC) cardioversion is the application of electrical energy to the myocardium for the purposes of changing an abnormal cardiac rhythm to a normal one. It may be used emergently or electively. By delivering a shock of sufficient strength, a critical mass of myocardial tissue is depolarized simultaneously, allowing emergence of the dominant, normal rhythm to occur.

INDICATIONS

Urgent cardioversion should be performed in any patient with a tachydysrhythmia (other than sinus or digitalis-toxic rhythms) that is sufficiently rapid as to result in hemodynamic embarrassment or that has not responded to antidysrhythmic medication, and results in clinical deterioration. Elective and semielective cardioversion is performed in patients whose tachydysrhythmia is hemodynamically reasonably well tolerated, whatever its mechanism (it is important to note that ventricular tachycardia may cause no symptoms and be unassociated with hypotension). Rapid rate or mechanism of tachycardia alone are thus insufficient indications to cardiovert immediately.

CONTRAINDICATIONS

DC cardioversion is contraindicated in patients with tachydysrhythmias that result from digitalis toxicity, in those in whom the dysrhythmia is unsustained, in patients with long-standing atrial fibrillation, atrial fibrillation with normal or slow ventricular rate in the absence of use of atrioventricular (AV) nodal blocking agents, and in those with multifocal atrial tachycardia (see Chapter 3).

Digitalis toxic tachydysrhythmias include ectopic atrial tachycardia, usually with 2:1 AV block (this rhythm may also be seen in patients with end-stage heart disease in the absence of digitalis toxicity), sustained ventricular tachycardia, and bidirectional tachycardia. A serum level of digoxin that is in the "toxic" range is not *per se* a contraindication to proceeding with cardioversion unless the rhythm is itself the result of digitalis toxicity. Thus, patients with atrial fibrillation whose ventricular rate has been slowed with digoxin often have serum levels of digoxin that are well above the "therapeutic" range; such patients may undergo cardioversion without problems, and discontinuing digoxin therapy prior to the procedure is not warranted.

Patients with multifocal atrial tachycardia should not undergo cardioversion, as this rhythm is usually due to severe chronic obstructive pulmonary disease or endocrine-metabolic disorders, and attempts at cardioversion are almost always unsuccessful. Moreover, multifocal atrial tachycardia is usually a well-tolerated rhythm, whatever its rate. Patients with long-standing atrial fibrillation (duration greater than 1½–2 years) are not candidates for cardioversion, as the success rate is nil.

Patients with known sinus node dysfunction and paroxysmal supraventricular tachycardias should be cardioverted with caution, if at all, since postconversion asystole or marked bradycardia may occur; temporary cardiac pacing can be employed in such patients. Patients with atrial fibrillation whose ventricular rate is controlled or slow and who are not receiving AV nodal blocking agents (verapamil, diltiazem, β-blocking agents, digitalis) should be suspected of having underlying sinus node dysfunction; cardioversion should not be performed in these patients unless a temporary transvenous pacing system is in place.

In general, patients with tachydysrhythmias (usually supraventricular) that are associated with underlying structural or inflammatory heart disease should not undergo cardioversion until these conditions have been effectively treated, in order to both achieve and maintain sinus rhythm. Patients who are scheduled for cardiac catheterization or cardiac surgery should not be cardioverted, as their dysrhythmia is likely to recur during these procedures.

TECHNIQUE

Cardioversion should always be performed with the patient anesthetized, unless there is loss of consciousness associated with the tachydysrhythmia. For elective procedures, the patient should be fasting for at least six hours. An intensive care unit (ICU) in which blood pressure and electrocardiogram (ECG) monitoring can be carried out and cardiopulmonary resuscitation performed if required, is the proper setting for all elective cardioversions. The patients should remain under observation until awake and until the rhythm is stable. A 12-lead ECG should be performed before and after the cardioversion.

The cardioverting paddles are placed at the level of the cardiac apex at the midaxillary line and just below the right clavicle at the second and third right intercostal space or anteroposteriorly at the second and third right intercostal space and at the angle of the left scapula. There is no documented advantage of one configuration over the other, although anecdotal reports suggest that anteroposteriorly placed paddles can be more successful in obese patients and in those with obstructive lung disease.

The cardioverting shock should be precisely synchronized to the R wave of the ECG (the earlier and tallest portion of the QRS complex in patients with bundle branch block) in order to avoid ventricular fibrillation. If fibrillation occurs, immediate defibrillation should be carried out. It should be remembered that the delivered shock is about 80–90 percent of the stored energy.

Low energy levels are chosen to convert atrial flutter (10–50 J to start, with increments of 25–50 J if initially unsuccessful). Low energy levels should also be used in cases of ventricular tachycardia occurring in the setting of acute myocardial infarction (5-25 J to start, with increments of 50 J if initially unsuccessful). Atrial fibrillation and paroxysmal reentrant supraventricular tachycardia almost always require shock strengths of 150–300 J initially. Chronic recurrent ventricular tachycardia unassociated with acute ischemia generally requires 150–200 J. The minimum amount of current should be used to convert the rhythm.

If the patient is not already receiving antidysrhythmic drugs, these should be started prior to cardioversion and continued if sinus rhythm is restored. The choice of drug and duration of therapy will depend upon the rhythm and the specific clinical setting in which it occurs.

In patients with permanent pacemakers, the cardioverting paddles should be placed along an imaginary line perpendicular to the implanted electrodes, if possible, in order to avoid damage to the lead electrode or myocardial burns or both. The paddles should not be placed within 5 to 10 cm of the pacemaker generator. Abnormalities of pulse generator function, including misprogramming and failure to capture, owing to current drain, can occur; generator pacing and sensing functions, including telemetric capability in generators with this feature, should be completely assessed postconversion, as should capability to receive commands from a programmer.

COMPLICATIONS

The major complications of cardioversion are bradycardia, bradycardia-dependent tachycardia, another tachydysrhythmia (which is often short-lived and may not need specific therapy), ventricular fibrillation, systemic embolism, and chest burns. Ventricular fibrillation occurs in up to 5 percent of patients and is almost always due to improper synchronization of the cardioverting shock to the R wave of the ECG. Embolism occurs in 1–2 percent of all patients undergoing cardioversion and is related to the presence of a large left atrium or ventricle or both from any cause. Patients at high risk for embolism (cardiomyopathy, mitral valve disease, thrombus demonstrated by echocardiography) should be anticoagulated before the procedure; routine anticoagulation is not recommended. Myocardial trauma of clinical significance does not occur, although transient ST-segment elevation and small rises in creatine kinase (CK) can rarely be seen; myocardial fraction (MB) is usually normal, however, and should not confound the diagnosis of myocardial infarction, even if multiple shocks have been given.

An occasional patient may develop postconversion hypotension, low cardiac output, and pulmonary edema. The reasons are unclear but may have to do with autonomic discharge; management is supportive.

RECOMMENDED READING

Chun PKC, Davia JE, Donohue DJ: ST-segment elevation with elective DC cardioversion. Circulation 63:220, 1981.

Ditchey RV, Karliner JS: Safety of electrical cardioversion in patients without digitalis toxicity. Ann Int Med 95:676, 1981.

Ewy GA: Influence of paddle-electrode location and size on success of cardioversion (letter). N Engl J Med 306:174, 1982.

Kerber RE, Jensen SR, Grayzel J, et al: Elective cardioversion: influence of paddle-electrode location and size on success rates and energy requirements. N Engl J Med 305:658, 1981.

Lown B: Electrical reversion of cardiac arrhythmias. Br Heart J 29:469, 1967.

Mann DL, Maisel AS, Atwood JE, et al: Absence of cardioversion-induced ventricular arrhythmias in patients with therapeutic digoxin levels. J Am Coll Cardiol 5:881, 1985.

McCarthy P, Varghese PJ, Barritt DW: Prognosis of atrial arrhythmias treated by electrical countershock therapy: a three year follow-up. Br Heart J 31:496, 1969.

Ovsyshcher IA, Ilia R, Wanderman KL: Conduction disturbance and ST elevation following cardioversion. Isr J Med Sci 20:736, 1984.

Selzer A, Kelly JJ, Johnson RB, et al: Immediate and long-term results of electrical conversion of arrhythmias. Prog Cardiovasc Dis 9:90, 1966.

19. Defibrillation

Nora F. Goldschlager

INTRODUCTION

The principle of electrical termination of ventricular fibrillation is to deliver a current of sufficient intensity so as to depolarize and render refractory a critical mass of fibrillating myocardium. Fibrillation is characterized by highly disorganized, random, continuous waves of excitation traveling through a critical mass of excitable myocardial tissue. The refractory period of the excitable muscle cells, the velocity of propagation of the excitation wave fronts, and the mass of myocardial tissue involved determine whether or not the fibrillation will be maintained.

After defibrillation, when the myocardium has recovered excitability, it can accept a normal stimulus to depolarize and contract. The magnitude of the defibrillating current required to terminate the abnormal rhythm will depend upon the resistance of the subject (usually between 25 and 125 ohms) and the mass of involved myocardium. Thus, higher energies may be required for thick-chested, emphysematous, or markedly obese individuals and possibly also for patients with myocardial hypertrophy.

TECHNIQUE

The defibrillating electrodes may both be placed on the precordium (one at the upper right sternal border and the other at the apex of the left ventricle) or anteroposteriorly (one at the upper right sternal border and the other at the angle of the left scapula).

Delivery of defibrillating shocks to the patient may be begun at relatively low levels (100 J) with or without increases in shock strength with successive attempts or may commence at higher energy levels with intent to convert the rhythm with the first shock; although the total energy delivered to the patient by these means may be higher using one method versus the other, measurable detriment to myocardial pump function (elevation in the myocardial fraction of creatine kinase and postdefibrillation dysrhythmias as well as scintigraphic evidence of myocardial necrosis) with either method has not been demonstrated. The actual energy delivered to the patient at a particular energy output setting is in fact a fraction of the selected setting, averaging 80–85 percent.

The chance of successful defibrillation decreases in the presence of cardiovascular collapse due to acidosis, hypoxia, local ionic imbalance, especially involving potassium, and continued ischemia and necrosis. Thus, relatively high defibrillating shocks should be used at the outset (200 J or greater). In 67 percent of patients who have ventricular fibrillation for two minutes or less, ventricular defibrillation is successful; the success rate is 50 percent if the fibrillation is present for more than two minutes. If vigorous resuscitative efforts are carried out continuously prior to defibrillation, late successful defibrillation (after 30 minutes and more) can occur.

POTENTIAL COMPLICATIONS

Digitalis lowers the amount of energy required for defibrillation (as well as the threshold for induction of ventricular fibrillation); thus, in a digitalized patient, lower initial shock strengths (sometimes on the order of 5–10 J) are recommended. Cardioversion of tachydysrhythmias in digitalized patients does not result in postconversion digitalis–toxic dysrhythmias unless the original rhythm is a digitalis-toxic one; in these cases, cardioversion should be avoided if at all possible or performed at the lowest allowable energy setting.

DEFIBRILLATION IN PATIENTS WITH CARDIAC PACEMAKERS

Pacemaker generators are designed so that the sensing and pacing circuitry is protected from excessive electrical energy, but on occasion the protective mechanisms may fail, resulting in pulse generator malfunction.

Guidelines for electroversion in patients with pacemakers include adequate separation between defibrillator paddles, avoidance of paddle placement within 3 to 5 inches of the pulse generator, and insuring that the dipole created by the defibrillatory paddles is perpendicular to an imaginary line between the catheter electrode and the generator in unipolar pacing systems, or between the two catheter electrodes in bipolar pacing systems.

Abnormalities of pulse generator function following defibrillation include failure to capture owing to current drain, myocardial burns due to high current flow along the pacing lead, and unwanted programming of, for example, automatic (standby) rate in some programmable units.

The pacemaker malfunction may be transient, with restoration of normal function within a short period of time, or it may be more permanent, warranting early pulse generator replacement. Sensing problems after defibrillation may be due to pulse generator malfunction but are usually related to the electromechanical effects of the dysrhythmia itself or defibrillation-related myocardial injury or both, resulting in distortion of intracardiac signals, making them suboptimal for sensing.

The integrity of all programmable parameters of the pacing system should be tested as soon as the patient's condition is stabilized. In pulse generators having the capability of transmitting stored information by telemetry, interrogation may reveal a change from previously programmed parameters, signifying misprogramming by the defibrillation procedure; the interrogation command itself may be faulty in defibrillation patients. Failure of pulse generator function to return to normal within a reasonable period of time mandates generator replacement.

RECOMMENDED READING

Adgey AAJ, Campbell NPS, Webb SW, et al: Transthoracic ventricular defibrillation in the adult. Med Instrum 12:17, 1978.

Aylward P, Blood R, Tonkin A: Complications of defibrillation with permanent pacemaker *in situ*. PACE 2:462, 1979.

Barold SS, Ong LS, Scovil J, et al: Reprogramming of implanted pacemaker following external defibrillation. PACE 1:514, 1978.

Chambers W, Miles R, Stratbucker R: Human chest resistance during successive countershocks. Med Instrum 12:53, 1978.

Gascho JA, Crampton RS, Cherwek ML, et al: Determinants of ventricular defibrillation in adults. Circulation 60:231, 1979.

Giedweyn JO: Pacemaker failure following external defibrillation. Circulation 44:293, 1971.

Kerber RE, Sarnat W: Factors influencing the success of ventricular defibrillation in man. Circulation 60:226, 1979.

Koning G, Geuze RH, Meinema AJ: Electrical requirements of defibrillation. Br Heart J 42:493, 1979.

Machin JW: Thoracic impedance of human subjects. Med Biol Eng Comput 16:169, 1978.

Tacker WA, Galioto FM, Giuliani E, et al: Energy dosage for human transchest electrical ventricular defibrillation. N Engl J Med 290:214, 1974.

Pulmonary Disorders

20. Upper Airway Obstruction

David J. Pierson

DEFINITION

Obstruction of the upper airway (which may be considered to extend from the nose and mouth to the tracheal bifurcation) is most likely to be life-threatening when it occurs below the hypopharynx, where the effective cross-sectional diameter of the air passage becomes smaller. The site of obstruction may be either extrathoracic or intrathoracic. Clinically, such obstruction may range from asymptomatic (as in mild postintubation tracheal stenosis detectable only by imaging studies) to rapidly fatal (as in asphyxia from aspiration of a large piece of food—the "café coronary"), as determined by the nature of the obstruction, its severity, the rapidity of its development, and the patient's underlying state of cardiopulmonary health.

Commonly encountered causes of life-threatening upper airway obstruction are listed in Table 20–1. Their relative frequencies vary in different practice settings. Acute epiglottitis is common in children but was previously considered to be a rare, benign disorder in adults; however, recent studies reveal that acute epiglottitis occurs in as many as 10 adults per million in the adult population each year and has a higher mortality rate in adults than in children.

PATHOPHYSIOLOGY

How a lesion obstructing the upper airway affects respiratory function depends upon whether the obstruction is constant or varies throughout the respiratory cycle, and, in the latter instance, whether the obstruction is inside or outside the thorax (Table 20–2). Acute pulmonary edema may develop during acute upper airway obstruction or upon its abrupt relief.

DIAGNOSIS

Sudden total or near-total obstruction of the upper airway produces severe distress, stridor, progressive cyanosis, and rapid loss of conscious-

135

TABLE 20–1. CAUSES OF LIFE-THREATENING UPPER AIRWAY OBSTRUCTION

EXTRATHORACIC OBSTRUCTION
Aspirated foreign body
   Complete or near-complete airway occlusion ("cafe coronary")
   Partial airway obstruction
Submucosal hemorrhage and edema (head/neck trauma)
Spontaneous retropharyngeal hemorrhage (anticoagulant therapy)
Acute epiglottitis
Acute angioedema
   Allergic hypersensitivity
   Hereditary C1 esterase inhibitor deficiency
Neoplasm
Goiter
Adenotonsillar hypertrophy
Bilateral vocal cord paralysis
Cricoarytenoid arthritis

INTRATHORACIC OBSTRUCTION
Tracheal neoplasm
Extrinsic compression (lymph nodes; tumor; abscess)
Submucosal hemorrhage (trauma; biopsy; other instrumentation)
Tracheal stenosis
Tracheomalacia

ness. Its hallmark is the universal sign of choking (Fig. 20–1), accompanied by strenuous respiratory efforts but little or no air movement.

Less severe upper airway obstruction causes highly variable symptoms and signs. Wheezing and dyspnea are common and are accentuated or brought on by exertion. Breathing may be noisy at rest, and this often varies with body position. Inspiratory stridor is characteristic in extrathoracic obstruction and is increased by hyperventilation or forced inspiration. The voice may be hoarse or altered in its character, particularly in epiglottitis or croup. In intrathoracic upper airway obstruction, the physical findings are often nonspecific, and patients are commonly misdiagnosed as having obstructive lung disease (lower airway obstruction).

When symptoms are present, the upper airway obstruction must be considered substantial, since early or mild obstruction is both asymptomatic and difficult to detect physiologically. Manipulation of the airway should be avoided, and the patient should be kept calm. Lateral soft-tissue roentgenograms of the neck have long been the diagnostic procedure of choice for epiglottitis, although recent data suggest that, in adult patients, indirect laryngoscopy is acceptably safe and more sensitive. When the clinical picture of upper airway obstruction is less acute and acute epiglottitis is not suspected, fiberoptic bronchoscopy permits visualization of the hypopharynx, vocal cords, and trachea, although the instrument should not be passed through an area of airway compromise.

Physiologic assessment of upper airway obstruction that is subacute or not immediately life-threatening is best accomplished using readily-available pulmonary function tests (Table 20–2). Expiratory air flow is

TABLE 20–2. PHYSIOLOGIC CHARACTERISTICS OF EXTRATHORACIC
AND INTRATHORACIC UPPER AIRWAY OBSTRUCTION

	VARIABLE EXTRATHORACIC OBSTRUCTION	VARIABLE INTRATHORACIC OBSTRUCTION	FIXED EXTRA- OR INTRATHORACIC OBSTRUCTION
Inspiration	$P_{atm} > P_{aw}$ Airway collapses Obstruction worsens	$P_{aw} > P_{pl}$ Airway expands Obstruction decreases	Airway diameter fixed Obstruction constant
Expiration	$P_{aw} > P_{atm}$ Airway expands Obstruction decreases	$P_{pl} > P_{aw}$ Airway collapses Obstruction worsens	Airway diameter fixed Obstruction constant
FIV_1	Reduced	Normal	Reduced
FEV_1	Normal	Reduced	Reduced
Flow-volume loop	Inspiration flattened Expiration normal	Inspiration normal Expiration flattened	Inspiration flattened Expiration flattened
Clinical examples	Vocal cord paralysis Croup	Tracheal tumor Tracheomalacia	Tracheal stenosis Goiter

FEV_1 = forced expiratory volume in the first second; FIV_1 = forced inspiratory volume in the first second; P_{atm} = atmospheric pressure; P_{aw} = airway pressure; P_{pl} = pleural pressure.

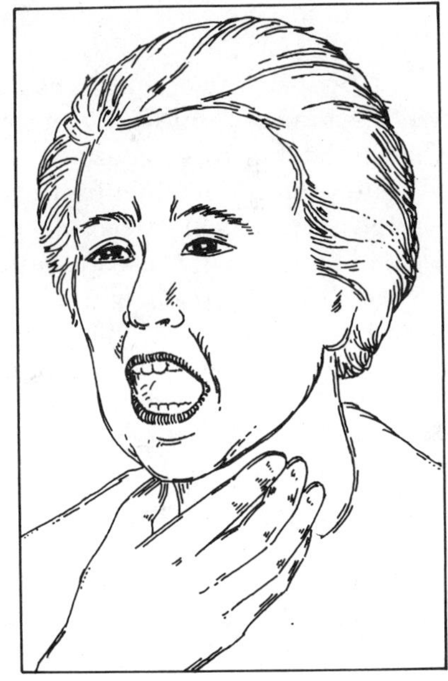

FIGURE 20–1. Universal sign of choking, as seen most commonly in upper airway occlusion by aspirated food ("café coronary"). (Reproduced, with permission, from Luce JM, Tyler ML, Pierson DJ: Intensive Respiratory Care. Philadelphia, W. B. Saunders Co., 1984, p. 273).

traditionally quantitated using the forced expiratory volume in the first second (FEV_1). This will detect clinically significant fixed obstruction, regardless of its location, and variable intrathoracic obstruction but will miss variable extrathoracic obstruction, in which the functional abnormality is present mainly during inspiration. Although not routinely performed, the forced inspiratory volume in the first second (FIV_1) is easy to do and readily detects variable extrathoracic obstruction.

The "gold standard" for evaluating upper airway obstruction is the flow-volume loop, which plots forced expiratory and inspiratory airflow vs. lung volume between total lung capacity and residual volume. Effects of the different forms of upper airway obstruction on the flow-volume loop are summarized in Table 20–2.

Blood cultures should be obtained whenever acute epiglottitis is suspected because, when positive (in 25–50 percent of cases), they identify the causative organism and also signify the presence of a greater risk for development of severe upper airway obstruction.

Arterial blood gas values are insensitive as indicators of the severity or progression of upper airway obstruction. Acute respiratory acidosis is a late sign, portending an immediate threat of cardiorespiratory arrest and should not be used as a threshold criterion for endotracheal intubation.

MANAGEMENT

Upper airway occlusion by aspirated food will cause death by asphyxia within minutes, unless the obstructing foreign body is removed. Manual thrusts to the lower chest or upper abdomen (the Heimlich maneuver) are the primary treatment and can be delivered with the patient in either upright (Fig. 20–2) or supine position. An initial series of four thrusts should be given. If these measures are not successful, the clinician should sweep the oropharynx with the index finger in an attempt to dislodge the object and then repeat the sequence or administer four back blows.

In acute epiglottitis and other settings in which partial upper airway obstruction may progress to asphyxia, assessment and maintenance of airway patency are the first objectives of management. There is no reliable way to predict which patients will do well without intubation. All patients must be observed closely, and the clinician should err on the side of intubating too early rather than the reverse. Life-threatening airway obstruction can develop rapidly; deaths from epiglottitis typically occur in patients who are not admitted to the intensive care unit (ICU) and who are "watched" without airway protection. Fatalities are rare once intubation or tracheostomy has been performed. Whenever possible, intubation should be done semielectively by someone experienced in the procedure,

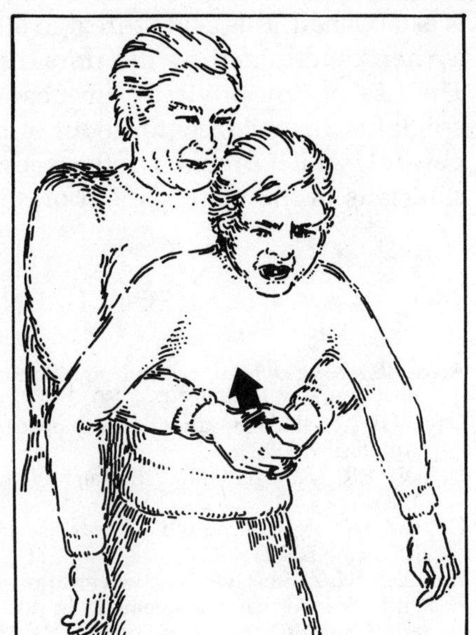

FIGURE 20–2. Administration of manual thrusts (Heimlich maneuver) to clear upper airway. (Reproduced, with permission, from Luce JM, Tyler ML, Pierson DJ: Intensive Respiratory Care. Philadelphia, W. B. Saunders Co., 1984, p. 276.)

and if tracheostomy becomes necessary, this should be carried out in the operating room.

Once intubated, patients generally do not require mechanical ventilation unless the tube is of small diameter in relation to their physical size and activity; otherwise healthy adults usually tolerate a 7.0 mm internal diameter (ID) tube without difficulty. Extubation can usually be accomplished after 3–4 days of appropriate antibiotic therapy; visualization of the epiglottic area and soft-tissue neck films can aid in predicting when it is safe to remove the tube, but personnel and equipment for reintubation should be at hand.

Initial antimicrobial therapy in acute epiglottitis should provide coverage for *Haemophilus influenzae,* pneumococcus, and *Staphylococcus aureus.* Corticosteroids and aerosolized racemic epinephrine are frequently given but are of unproven benefit.

Acute hypersensitivity angioedema responds to nebulized racemic epinephrine or parenteral epinephrine. Hereditary angioedema due to C1 esterase inhibitor deficiency is best managed prophylactically with danazol. Therapy for upper airway obstruction in the other conditions listed in Table 20–1 is determined by the primary process.

OUTCOME

Upper airway obstruction may lead to hypercapnic acidosis, exhaustion, and death if allowed to persist or progress. However, once an airway is established, this acute threat to life is removed, and the overall prognosis is then determined by the primary condition that led to the obstruction. The use of "prophylactic" intubation has reduced the mortality of acute epiglottis in children to about 1 percent; in adults it is currently 5–10 percent, which probably reflects less aggressive use of intubation by many clinicians in the management of this disorder in adults.

RECOMMENDED READING

Acres JC, Kryger MH: Clinical significance of pulmonary function tests: upper airway obstruction. Chest 80:207, 1980.

Davis HW, et al: Acute upper airway obstruction: croup and epiglottitis. Pediatr Clin North Am 28:859, 1981.

Demers RR: Management of the airway in the perioperative period. Respir Care 29:529, 1984.

Gelfand JA, et al: Acquired C1 esterase inhibitor deficiency and angioedema: a review. Medicine 58:321, 1979.

Heimlich JH: A life-saving maneuver to prevent food-choking. JAMA 234:398, 1975.

Kastendieck J: Airway management. In Rosen P, et al (eds): Emergency Medicine: Concepts and Clinical Practice. St. Louis, C. V. Mosby Co., 1983, p. 26.

Levy ML, Ericsson CD, Pickering LK: Infections of the upper respiratory tract. Med Clin North Am 67:153, 1983.

MayoSmith MF, et al: Acute epiglottitis in adults: an eight-year experience in the state of Rhode Island. N Engl J Med 314:1133, 1986.

Miller RD: Obstructing lesions of the larynx and trachea: clinical and pathophysiologic aspects. In Fishman AP (ed): Pulmonary diseases and disorders. New York, McGraw-Hill Inc., 1980, p. 490.

Proctor DF: State of the art: the upper airways. Am Rev Respir Dis 115:97, 315, 1977.

Stauffer JL, Silvestri RC: Complications of endotracheal intubation, tracheostomy, and artificial airways. Respir Care 27:417, 1982.

21. Asthma

David J. Pierson

David J. Pierson

DEFINITION

Asthma is defined as exaggerated responsiveness of the conducting airways to a variety of stimuli, which can trigger widespread airway narrowing and the characteristic symptoms of cough and wheezing. These symptoms, along with accompanying physical signs and diminished airflow on laboratory testing, typically wax and wane over time, either spontaneously or in response to therapy. They may or may not remit completely between attacks.

Asthma occurs either by itself or in combination with emphysema and chronic bronchitis as a component of chronic obstructive pulmonary disease (COPD). "Pure" asthma is most common in children and young adults but occurs in all age groups. Individual cases lie within a broad clinical spectrum from predominantly "extrinsic," with symptoms triggered predictably on exposure to pollens or other allergens, to "intrinsic," without identifiable external precipitating factors. Severe acute asthma, the subject of this chapter, is assessed and managed similarly regardless of underlying clinical type or individual precipitating factors.

Status asthmaticus is an imprecise term used to describe episodes of severe acute asthma that do not respond to initial intensive bronchodilator therapy. The concept of status asthmaticus can now be supplemented and made more objective by direct measurements of severity of airflow obstruction such as one-second forced expiratory flow rate (FEV_1) or peak expiratory flow rate (PEFR).

PATHOPHYSIOLOGY

Asthma is a functional rather than a structural disorder; although the lungs of asthmatic individuals have characteristic pathologic findings that distinguish them from those of normals, these differences are relatively minor. The hallmark of asthma is diffuse airway narrowing due to a combination of three factors: (1) bronchospasm (airway smooth muscle contraction), (2) mucosal edema and other inflammatory changes in the airway walls, and (3) tenacious intraluminal secretions.

Airway narrowing causes airflow obstruction, which leads to air trapping, lung overdistention, increased pulmonary vascular resistance, and right ventricular afterload, as well as large swings in intrathoracic pressure in response to the greatly increased work of breathing. Acute asthma produces hypoxemia through mismatching of ventilation and perfusion. If airway narrowing is not reversed, fatigue and worsening ventilation:perfusion imbalance may lead to acute respiratory acidosis, often accompanied by metabolic acidosis; exhaustion and death from asphyxia or cardiac dysrhythmia may follow.

EVALUATION

Either FEV_1 or PEFR can be used in assessing acute asthma, as studies have shown them to be clinically equivalent for this purpose. These values can be obtained in virtually any conscious patient, and equipment for their measurement should be readily available in every clinical facility that sees patients with acute asthma. Patients seen urgently in clinics or emergency rooms should be evaluated, treated, and either discharged or admitted to the hospital within 1–2 hours, not the 3–6 hours or longer commonly seen in the past.

Table 21–1 classifies acute asthma in three categories of severity according to initial FEV_1 or PEFR measurement. The degree to which the initial value improves over the first 30–60 minutes of therapy predicts the reversibility of the attack; patients with values still in the "severe" category after initial treatment should be admitted to the hospital.

Bedside indicators of the severity of asthma include the following:

• Tachypnea, severe dyspnea, inability to lie recumbent, inability to speak whole phrases or sentences

• Disturbance of mental state (irritability, noncooperation, inappropriate responses to questions, confusion, drowsiness, coma)

• Grossly overexpanded chest, absence of wheezing, use of accessory muscles of respiration

TABLE 21–1. ASSESSMENT OF THE SEVERITY OF ACUTE ASTHMA

FEV_1		PEFR		
Absolute Value (L)	Percent of Predicted Value	Absolute Value (L/min)	Percent of Predicted Value	SEVERITY
>2.0	>60	>200	>60	Mild to moderate
1.0–2.0	30–60	80–200	30–60	Moderately severe
<1.0	<25–30	<80	<25–30	Severe

FEV_1 = one-second forced expiratory volume (measured by portable spirometer); PEFR = peak expiratory flow rate (measured by hand-held portable peak-flow meter).

- *Pulsus paradoxus* (inspiratory disappearance of systolic Korotkoff sound) greater than 10–15 mm Hg
- Sinus tachycardia (usually reflecting the asthma, not the drugs used in treating it); hypo- or hypertension
- Ineffective cough, diaphoresis, exhaustion, dehydration

Arterial blood gases (ABGs) during acute asthma attacks typically show mild-to-moderate hypoxemia and acute respiratory alkalosis; an elevated or rising systemic arterial carbon dioxide tension ($PaCO_2$), accompanied by a fall in arterial pH below normal in the setting of continued respiratory distress, is an ominous sign that indicates the need for mechanical ventilation unless it can be rapidly reversed. ABGs are insensitive measures of the severity of an asthma attack, although patients with hypercapnia virtually always have FEV_1 or PEFR values below 25–30 per cent of the predicted value.

A chest roentgenogram should be obtained in severe acute asthma that does not respond rapidly to therapy, in order to look for pneumonia, atelectasis (from mucous plugging of main airways), or extraalveolar air (pneumomediastinum or pneumothorax).

Electrocardiographic signs seen in severe acute asthma include right axis deviation, clockwise rotation, right bundle-branch block, ST-T wave changes, P-pulmonale, and signs of right ventricular strain such as dominant R in V_1 and dominant S in V_5–V_6. Although characteristic, these changes are highly variable and may be absent.

Clinicians frequently underestimate the severity of acute asthma. Studies of asthma fatalities show that patients who die have typically had asthma for many years, have had previous attacks requiring hospitalization, have had poor symptom control in recent days or weeks, and have not had the severity of their asthma measured objectively using FEV_1 or PEFR.

Management

Patients with severe acute asthma must be assessed and managed individually rather than in "cookbook" fashion; however, certain basic principles of the initial approach can be generalized and are outlined in Table 21–2.

Patients with asthma tend not to be susceptible to suppression of ventilatory drive by supplemental oxygen as is true with some COPD patients. In addition, the hypoxemia of acute asthma may require more supplemental oxygen for reversal than is seen in COPD. Thus, oxygen at 2–4 L/min by nasal prongs (preferred by most patients over masks when acutely dyspneic) may be given initially without ABG measurement.

β-Agonist bronchodilators administered by aerosol are at least as

Table 21–2. Initial Steps in Assessment and Management of Severe Acute Asthma

1. Brief history and physical examination
2. Measurement of FEV_1 or PEFR (see Table 20–1)
3. Arterial blood gas measurement if
   a. FEV_1 or PEFR <25–30 percent of predicted value, or
   b. disturbance of mental state is present, or
   c. patient fails to improve after steps 4–8 below
4. Oxygen (2–4 L/min by nasal prongs, or 28–35 percent by mask)
5. Inhaled β_2–agonist bronchodilator (via MDI or nebulizer)
6. Subcutaneous terbutaline or epinephrine if patient cannot be given inhaled bronchodilator as above; use cautiously if over age 40 or if cardiovascular disease is present
7. Intravenous or oral bolus of corticosteroids
8. Intravenous aminophylline if assessment indicates severe attack, if patient has not improved markedly with steps 4–6, and if no contraindication is present
9. Intravenous fluids, 1 L in initial 2 hr, 2–4 L in 24 hr

FEV_1 = one-second forced expiratory volume; PEFR = peak expiratory flow rate; MDI = metered-dose (canister) inhaler.

effective in acute asthma as epinephrine or terbutaline given subcutaneously, and it is not necessary to use both routes unless the patient has difficulty inhaling the aerosol. The inhaled route produces fewer side effects (see Chapter 39 for dosages and administration of individual β-agonist drugs).

Recent studies contradict the earlier notion that corticosteroids have no clinical effect in the first 4–6 hours after administration, and they support the use of these agents immediately in severe asthma. Other recent work suggests that oral administration is as effective as intravenous unless the patient is unable to swallow or requires gastric suction. Optimum dosage for each available preparation has not been established; many clinicians use 200 mg hydrocortisone or 40 mg methylprednisolone as an initial intravenous bolus and repeat this every 4–6 hr. Some advocate much larger doses (e.g., 250 mg methylprednisolone) in very severe cases or when no improvement is seen after 24 hours at lower doses. As discussed in Chapter 39, the short-term use of corticosteroids, even in high doses, is without significant side effects in the majority of patients.

Intravenous aminophylline, long a mainstay of therapy for acute asthma in the United States, is more toxic and less efficacious than the other agents listed in Table 21–2 and in many geographic areas is reserved for cases that fail to respond to β-agonist bronchodilators and corticosteroids. Guidelines for administration of aminophylline are given in Chapter 39.

Anticholinergics such as ipratropium and atropine are as effective as β-agonists in some asthmatics, especially in those who also have chronic bronchitis, and they may be used concomitantly with these agents. Ether, halothane, and ketamine have been reported anecdotally to be effective

TABLE 21–3. SEVEN PRINCIPLES OF ASTHMA MANAGEMENT

1. Repeated asthma attacks in individual patients tend to be similar and to respond similarly to therapy.
2. The longer an asthma attack lasts, the more severe it becomes; the more severe an attack, the longer it will last.
3. The duration of an asthma attack and its response to therapy are partly determined by the event or factors precipitating the attack (e.g., an attack accompanying a respiratory infection will not resolve until the infection resolves).
4. Regardless of what precipitated the attack, the therapy is essentially the same (e.g., an attack of psychogenic origin requires drug therapy as does any other).
5. Add therapies, don't substitute them (e.g., if additional drugs—corticosteroids, anticholinergics—are indicated by the severity of the attack, continue all previous therapies when starting these drugs).
6. Don't cut back on therapy (unless toxicity is present) until the patient improves (e.g., don't taper the corticosteroid dose until the attack breaks, even if it has been continuing for a week).
7. Monitor airway function objectively (e.g., with FEV_1 or PEFR) as well as by following symptoms and clinical signs.

FEV_1 = one-second forced expiratory volume; PEFR = peak expiratory flow rate.

bronchodilators in severe, life-threatening asthma unresponsive to maximum therapy with other agents, but the use of these agents has not been studied systematically.

Expectorants are generally unnecessary in acute asthma, and mucolytics such as acetylcysteine should be avoided because they may increase airway hyperreactivity. Antimicrobial agents should be reserved for cases of pneumonia and other proven respiratory tract infections and should not be used routinely. Inhaled corticosteroids and cromolyn are ineffective in acute asthma. Sedatives and narcotics should be used with great caution and are best avoided altogether; morphine is said to be capable of worsening asthma by releasing mediators of bronchoconstriction.

Adequate hydration is important, as most patients with attacks of at least several hours' duration are dehydrated. Venous access should be established with a large-bore needle, both for fluid replacement and for administration of medications.

Endotracheal intubation and mechanical ventilation should be used when acute respiratory acidosis (elevated or rising $PaCO_2$ with pH < 7.25–7.30) is unresponsive to intensive bronchodilator and other therapies; when the patient has severe disturbance of mental state (e. g., increasing drowsiness, combativeness, or coma) that interferes with management; or when progressive exhaustion and persistent severe airflow obstruction occur despite several hours of intensive therapy. A high-capability ventilator should be used, and inspiratory flow rate should be adjusted to maximize expiratory time. Tidal volume should be no more than 10–12 ml/kg, and minute ventilation should be adjusted so as to relieve acute respiratory acidosis but to avoid alkalemia. Other aspects of ventilator care are the same as those used with other patients.

Seven general principles applying to the care of any patient with acute asthma are listed in Table 21–3.

OUTCOME

Several thousand children and adults die from asthma in the United States each year. Every episode of asthma is potentially reversible, however, and hence virtually all fatalities from this disorder should be considered preventable.

Asthma deaths are of two types—those that occur suddenly outside the hospital, and those that occur in the hospital in the setting of a prolonged, intractable attack. Common factors in both types are failure of both patient and physician to appreciate the attack's severity and a lack of objective measurements of airway function. Causes of death in asthma include dysrhythmias, pneumothorax, asphyxia due to progressive airflow obstruction and respiratory acidosis, the injudicious use of sedatives and narcotics, adverse reactions to β-blocking drugs, and, rarely, hypersensitivity to hydrocortisone, aspirin and related drugs, and other agents.

RECOMMENDED READING

Acute asthma [editorial]. Lancet 1:131, 1986.

Advances in the diagnosis and treatment of asthma. Chest 87(Suppl. 1), 1985.

Benatar SR: Fatal asthma. N Engl J Med 314:423, 1986.

Edelson JD, Rebuck AS: The clinical assessment of severe asthma. Arch Intern Med 145:321, 1985.

Fanta CH, Rossing TH, McFadden ER, Jr: Treatment of acute asthma: is combination therapy with sympathomimetics and methylxanthines indicated? Am J Med 80:5, 1986.

Harrison BD, et al: Need for intravenous hydrocortisone in addition to oral prednisolone in patients admitted to hospital with severe asthma without ventilatory failure. Lancet 1:181, 1986.

Littenberg B, Gluck EH: A controlled trial of methylprednisolone in the emergency treatment of acute asthma. N Engl J Med 314:150, 1986.

Petty TL: Status asthmaticus. In Petty TL (ed): Intensive and Rehabilitative Respiratory Care. Philadelphia, Lea & Febiger, 3rd edition, 1982, p. 207.

Rebuck AS, Read J: Assessment and management of severe asthma. Am J Med 51:788, 1971.

Scoggin CH, Petty TL: Clinical Strategies in Adult Asthma. Philadelphia, Lea & Febiger, 1982.

Shim CS, Williams MH Jr: Evaluation of the severity of asthma: patients vs physicians. Am J Med 68:11, 1980.

Strunk RC, et al: Physiologic and psychological characteristics associated with deaths due to asthma in childhood. JAMA 254:1193, 1985.

Symposium on asthma. Clin Chest Med 5:555, 1984.

Westerman DE, et al: Identification of the high-risk asthmatic patient: experience with 39 patients undergoing ventilation for status asthmaticus. Am J Med 66:565, 1979.

22. Chronic Obstructive Pulmonary Disease

David J. Pierson

DEFINITION

Chronic obstructive pulmonary disease (COPD) is defined clinically as the coexistence of long-standing respiratory symptoms (dyspnea and/or productive cough) with spirometrically demonstrable airflow obstruction, the latter indicated by a reduced ratio of one-second forced expiratory volume (FEV_1) to forced vital capacity (FVC). Pathophysiologically, COPD may also be thought of as a variable combination of emphysema, chronic bronchitis, and "reversible obstructive airways disease," or asthma.

Emphysema is irreversible by definition, and even partial reversal of chronic bronchitis ultimately requires cessation of exposure to its irritant source—cigarette smoke. The asthmatic component is thus the one most directly amenable to medical therapy in the short run; Chapters 21 and 39 cover this aspect of COPD management. As discussed here, management of the patient with an acute exacerbation of COPD consists primarily of intensifying and optimizing the modalities used in long-term care and of nonspecific supportive measures aimed at buying time while these take effect.

PATHOPHYSIOLOGY

Impairment of expiratory airflow is the physiologic hallmark of COPD. It is the result of a loss of lung elastic recoil and is added to by bronchospasm, mucosal inflammation, and airway secretions. Airflow obstruction increases the work required of the respiratory muscles, and hyperinflation due to air-trapping also places these muscles at a mechanical disadvantage.

Hypoxemia in COPD is mainly due to mismatching of ventilation and perfusion ($\dot{V}_A/\dot{Q}$). Alveolar hypoventilation also plays a part when the arterial carbon dioxide tension ($PaCO_2$) is elevated, but right-to-left shunt is not a prominent mechanism in COPD unless a discrete area of pulmonary consolidation is present. Although diffusion limitation is demonstrable in the laboratory, it is not a cause of clinical hypoxemia, even in severe emphysema. Because hypoxemia due to $\dot{V}_A/\dot{Q}$ mismatching, as occurs in COPD, is readily improved by modest elevations in inspired oxygen fraction (FiO_2), low-flow supplemental oxygen is all that is necessary to correct this problem, even in severe exacerbations.

In addition to alleviating hypoxemia, supplemental oxygen also improves cardiac function in these patients by reducing the reflex pulmonary arterial constriction triggered by alveolar hypoxia. Because pulmonary vasoconstriction raises pulmonary vascular resistance, pulmonary arterial pressure, and hence right ventricular afterload, oxygen reduces the work required of the right heart, both in stable cor pulmonale and in an acute exacerbation.

DIAGNOSIS

The term "COPD" is often misapplied to the condition of individuals with restrictive pulmonary disorders or even to cardiac disease causing chronic respiratory symptoms. Some aspects of COPD management would be inappropriate for other conditions; therefore, it is crucial to document the presence of expiratory airflow obstruction, if this has not been done, by measuring FEV_1 or peak expiratory flow rate (PEFR), something that can be accomplished quickly at the bedside in virtually any conscious patient.

Acute respiratory failure exists whenever there is impairment in tissue oxygen delivery or in CO_2 elimination or both that is severe enough and has developed suddenly enough to threaten the life of the individual. In COPD, as in other clinical states, there are certain characteristic signs and symptoms (e.g., dyspnea, tachycardia, confusion, tremor), but none can determine the diagnosis by itself, since arterial blood gas analysis and sometimes hemodynamic assessment are required as well.

As discussed in Chapter 1, hypoxemic acute respiratory failure is present when the systemic arterial oxygen tension (PaO_2) falls acutely to less than 50 mm Hg, assuming normal hemoglobin, cardiac function, and peripheral needs. Ventilatory failure exists when the $PaCO_2$ rises above 50 mm Hg; in acute ventilatory failure, this rise is sufficient to drop arterial pH below about 7.25–7.30. In the patient with COPD and preestablished ("compensated") respiratory acidosis, $PaCO_2$ values of 50, 60, or even 80 mm Hg may be present without acute ventilatory failure so long as coexistent metabolic alkalosis (raised serum bicarbonate) prevents pH from falling below 7.25–7.30. It is crucial that pH, not absolute $PaCO_2$ value, be used to guide therapy.

An acute exacerbation of COPD typically consists of worsening of the patient's usual symptoms (dyspnea, cough, and sputum) in the setting of an apparent upper respiratory infection, an episode of environmental pollution or weather change, or interruption in prescribed medication. The patient feels ill, fever may be present, and the sputum typically becomes yellow or green. All of this suggests a bacterial chest infection, although careful studies have been unable to show convincingly that such is the case in most exacerbations.

In patients ill enough to be admitted to the hospital, assessment should be directed toward detection of causes of acute worsening that require specific therapy, such as pneumothorax, pneumonia, and congestive heart failure. Arterial blood gas analysis is mandatory for both diagnosis and monitoring. Serum electrolyte abnormalities (particularly hypokalemia) are common and should be sought. Sputum Gram stain and bacterial cultures tend not to be helpful unless radiographic evidence of pneumonia is present, the patient has recently been hospitalized, or there has been recent treatment with multiple antibiotics.

MANAGEMENT

Fatalities in acute exacerbations of COPD commonly involve failure to appreciate the severity of the illness and occur characteristically when such patients are admitted to the ward instead of to the intensive care unit (ICU) or are transferred out of the ICU prematurely. It is a mistake to assume that if the patient does not require intubation and mechanical ventilation, ICU care is unnecessary; error should be on the side of caution, particularly during the first 24 hours.

Because most acute exacerbations have no readily identifiable specific etiology and, thus, nothing to monitor in this respect, management is basically empirical, with supportive therapy guided by objective monitoring of cardiorespiratory function.

Controlled Oxygen Therapy. Life-threatening hypoxemia must be treated with supplemental oxygen, even in the presence of respiratory acidosis. Patients' PaO_2 values must never be allowed to remain in the 40s because of fear of worsening CO_2 retention. Because some patients with long-standing hypoxemia may be susceptible to depression of hypoxic ventilatory drive if PaO_2 is raised above about 65 mm Hg, the initial "target" PaO_2 should be 55–60 mm Hg, which is sufficient to raise blood oxygenation out of the dangerous range without causing respiratory depression in most patients.

Nasal prongs are preferable to masks for this purpose because they are more comfortable for most patients, and they tend to stay on, making administration continuous. Therapy should begin with 1–2 L/min rather than a higher flow in order to avoid inadvertent hyperoxia. A pediatric flowmeter is helpful in adjusting oxygen flows below 2 L/min (see Chapter 34).

Drug Therapy. Because the asthma component of COPD is the one most amenable to acute intervention, all patients should be assumed to have a reversible component and be treated with bronchodilators and corticosteroids. The former should start with inhaled β_2–agonists such as albuterol or metaproterenol (see Chapter 39) and should include theophylline if toxicity is not already present and no contraindications exist. Theophylline therapy must be monitored with serum levels in this setting.

Short-term (3 days) administration of corticosteroids such as methylprednisolone (2 mg/kg/24 hr in 4–6 doses/24 hr), followed by tapering after several days, hastens physiologic improvement and is without adverse effects in the great majority of patients. Antibiotics may be helpful, even in the absence of pulmonary infiltrates, although this is controversial.

Respiratory stimulant drugs such as doxapram and progesterone increase the patient's desire to breathe without augmenting the capacity and should not be used. Sedatives and hypnotics must be given with extreme caution and under very close observation; they are best avoided unless the patient is receiving mechanical ventilation.

Management of Secretions. This consists of four modalities: liquification, which can best be accomplished by hydrating the patient systemically rather than by giving "bland" aerosols; therapeutic cough, aided by appropriate positioning of the patient and repeated encouragement; chest physiotherapy, consisting of postural drainage and chest percussion; and airway suctioning, using the nasotracheal route or, in rare cases, via an endotracheal tube inserted for this purpose. Secretion management is empirical and should be tailored to individual circumstances; few patients need all of these measures. In addition, acutely dyspneic patients tolerate postural drainage poorly.

Endotracheal Intubation. Because intubation interferes with mucociliary clearance, abolishes effective cough, provides an avenue for nosocomial infection, and eliminates speech, it is especially onerous for the patient with COPD and should be avoided if this is possible. In fact, of patients with exacerbations causing acute respiratory failure, 10 percent or fewer will actually require intubation and mechanical ventilation if avoidance of their use is made a conscious goal. As discussed in Chapter 33, intubation should only be required to relieve upper airway obstruction, to facilitate secretion removal (very rare), or to permit mechanical ventilation.

Mechanical Ventilation. The indications for mechanical ventilation as listed in Chapter 35 apply to patients with severe COPD as well as to other individuals. It should be stressed that in acute ventilatory failure (severe acute respiratory acidosis), it is the pH, not the $PaCO_2$ value, that determines whether ventilatory support is needed. Initiating mechanical ventilation in a patient whose hypercapnia is "compensated" by a high serum bicarbonate with pH above 7.25–7.30 increases the risk of complications and invites difficulty in weaning.

If the COPD patient requires mechanical ventilation following surgery or for other reasons, adjustments in the usual settings are necessary in order to avoid air trapping, cardiovascular compromise, and barotrauma. These adjustments include using a lower tidal volume (10 ml/kg or less) and rapid peak inspiratory flow rates (80–100 L/min) to allow as much time as possible for exhalation.

Whether intermittent mandatory ventilation (IMV) or assist-control mode (AMV) should be used is partly a matter of personal preference. However, IMV requires the patient's respiratory muscles to continue working, something that may be at cross-purposes with the goals for mechanical ventilation in this setting, and many clinicians prefer to use AMV, employing sedation if necessary to control hyperventilation.

"Auto-PEEP" (described in Chapter 35) is a common occurrence when patients with COPD are ventilated, and steps should be take to avoid or minimize it. These include using high-peak inspiratory flow rates and low-compressible-volume circuit tubing, in order to minimize inspiratory cycle duration and to allow more time for exhalation.

Weaning from Mechanical Ventilation. A primary goal should be to make the period of ventilatory assistance as short as possible. One reason for this is that weaning, as described in Chapter 35, becomes more troublesome the longer the patient is ventilated. The principles outlined in Chapter 35 become less and less applicable with prolonged ventilation, and such factors as severity of underlying illness, number of organ systems impaired, nutrition, and mental status become primary determinants of whether weaning can be accomplished. In such cases, the clinician's focus must switch from daily attempts to discontinue ventilatory support to a several-week, global attempt to improve the patient's overall condition. Psychological support, nutritional guidance, and exercise, including ambulation with assistance several times daily if this is achievable, can be key aspects of a successful regimen.

OUTCOME

With current management techniques, most patients (70–80 percent) will survive an exacerbation of COPD resulting in acute respiratory failure. Studies have demonstrated that this survival rate is largely independent of whether intubation and mechanical ventilation are employed, underscoring the importance of avoiding these measures and their complications, if possible.

Although the short-term outlook is favorable, it is less encouraging thereafter, with about half the patients succumbing to complications of

COPD within about 2 years. Acute mortality increases with each succeeding episode, and the intervals between them tend to shorten. This information may be helpful in counseling patients while they are clinically stable, so that the appropriateness of intubation, mechanical ventilation, and other vigorous measures in subsequent exacerbations can be decided in advance.

RECOMMENDED READING

Albert RK, et al: Controlled clinical trial of methylprednisolone in patients with chronic bronchitis and acute respiratory insufficiency. Ann Intern Med 92:753, 1980.

Hudson LD: Evaluation of the patient with acute respiratory failure. Respir Care 28:542, 1983.

Hudson LD: Management of chronic obstructive pulmonary disease: state of the art. Chest 85(Suppl.):76S, 1984.

Hudson LD: Prognosis: immediate and long-term sequelae of acute respiratory failure. Respir Care 28:663, 1983.

Light RW: Conservative treatment of hypercapnic acute respiratory failure. Respir Care 28:561, 1983.

Morganroth ML, et al: Criteria for weaning from prolonged mechanical ventilation. Arch Intern Med 144:1012, 1984.

Petty TL: Critical care for chronic airflow limitation: emphysema, chronic bronchitis, and cystic fibrosis. Semin Respir Med 3:263, 1982.

Pierson DJ: Chronic obstructive pulmonary disease and bronchiectasis. In Rakel RE (ed): Conn's Current Therapy 1985. Philadelphia, W. B. Saunders Co., 1985, p. 96.

Pierson DJ: Exacerbation of chronic bronchitis and emphysema: ventilatory management. In Kacmarek RM, Stoller JK (eds): Current Respiratory Care Techniques and Therapy. Burlington, Ontario, B.C. Decker, Inc., 1987 (in press).

Pierson DJ (ed): Respiratory Intensive Care. Dallas, Daedalus Press (American Association for Respiratory Care), 1986.

Recent advances in the management of obstructive airways disease. Chest 88(2)(Suppl.):75S, 1985.

Rosen RL: Acute respiratory failure and chronic obstructive lung disease. Med Clin North Am 70:895, 1986.

Scott LR, Benson MS, Pierson DJ: Effect of inspiratory flowrate and circuit compressible volume on auto-PEEP during mechanical ventilation. Respir Care 31:1075, 1986.

Shibel EM: Acute respiratory failure with hypercapnia. In Shibel EM, Moser KM (eds): Respiratory Emergencies. St. Louis, C.V. Mosby Co., 1977, p. 85.

Special issue: Continuing care of the ventilator-dependent patient. Respir Care 31:266, 1986.

23. Pulmonary Embolism

David J. Pierson

DEFINITION

Pulmonary embolism (PE) occurs when clots from peripheral veins dislodge, travel through the right side of the heart and are impacted in the pulmonary arterial tree. This common entity (at least a half-million instances occur in the United States each year) is also one of clinical medicine's most unsettled and frustrating disorders, with most aspects of its diagnosis and therapy embroiled in controversy.

PATHOPHYSIOLOGY

Although thromboemboli can originate in the veins of the arms, in the heart, or elsewhere, in 95 percent of instances they are formed in the deep veins of the lower extremities. Thrombus formation classically requires stasis, vascular wall injury, and hypercoagulability. The clinical conditions that favor these factors, and hence predispose to both deep venous thrombosis (DVT) and PE, are listed in Table 23–1.

Occlusion of a portion of the pulmonary arterial bed increases pulmonary arterial pressure and dead space ventilation, and these effects are believed responsible for most of the clinical picture of PE. Vasoactive substances released from the thrombus and other factors may also be involved. In normal individuals, occlusion of at least 50 percent of the arterial bed is necessary to raise pulmonary arterial pressure and cause systemic hypotension; however, correspondingly less is required to cause physiologic impairment when there is preexisting cardiac or pulmonary disease.

Because oxygen can reach the pulmonary parenchyma via the bronchial circulation and alveolar air in addition to via the pulmonary arterial system, infarction of lung tissue is relatively infrequent. About 10 percent of episodes of PE involve infarction, but this incidence is increased three-fold when the patient has underlying cardiopulmonary disease.

DIAGNOSIS

Because the clinical manifestations of PE are nonspecific and highly variable, and the laboratory tests for establishing its presence are either nonspecific or invasive, the nature and thoroughness of evaluation will be dictated mainly by the strength of clinical suspicion in a given case. Short of pulmonary angiography, which is the "gold standard" but unnecessary in many patients, the clinician must rely on a series of relative probabilities rather than on any truly quantitative measure.

The history is the main determinant of clinical probability. PE is unlikely in the absence of dyspnea, tachycardia, and one or more of the predisposing factors listed in Table 23–1. Although the symptoms are variable, the most common is sudden, unexplained dyspnea. Apprehension and cough are present in about half of all patients. Chest pain is less common; massive PE can produce severe, oppressive substernal discomfort, and pulmonary infarction is commonly associated with pleuritic pain. Hemoptysis is typical of infarction but can also occur in its absence in patients with underlying heart disease. Massive or submassive PE can also present with syncope.

On physical examination, tachycardia is the most common finding. The chest may be clear or show scattered crackles; wheezing is uncommon. Fever (usually 38–39°C) may be present without other evidence of infection. Classic cardiac findings such as prominent jugular venous a waves, right ventricular lift and gallop, and loud pulmonic closure sound, are infrequent and suggest a massive embolus.

Chest roentgenograms are abnormal in most cases, but all findings are nonspecific. Atelectasis, a raised hemidiaphragm, localized infiltrates, pleural effusion, and areas of relatively hypovascular parenchyma may all be seen. Nonspecific changes are also the most common electrocardiographic findings; typically, the classic signs—right axis deviation, P-pulmonale, right bundle-branch block, and the $S_1Q_3T_3$ triad—are present only in massive PE, and they may be transient.

TABLE 23–1. CLINICAL RISK FACTORS FOR PULMONARY EMBOLISM

1. Previous documented pulmonary embolism
2. Conditions associated with venous stasis
    a. Congestive heart failure; atrial dysrhythmias; mural thrombus; acute myocardial infarction
    b. Chronic lower extremity deep venous insufficiency
    c. Immobilization or paralysis, especially recent
    d. Pregnancy and the postpartum period
    e. Chronic obstructive pulmonary disease
    f. Obesity
3. Conditions associated with venous injury
    a. Major surgery, especially orthopedic procedures on the hip or knee, open prostatectomy, or major intraabdominal procedures
    b. Trauma, especially involving the pelvis, hips, or lower extremities
    c. Burns
4. Conditions associated with hypercoagulability
    a. Carcinoma
    b. Polycythemia rubra vera; hemolytic anemia
    c. Exogenous estrogens

Arterial blood gases show hypoxemia (or at least an increased alveolar-to-arterial oxygen gradient [P(A − a)O$_2$] in most instances, commonly with mild hypocapnia, but they may also be normal in proven PE. Routine blood studies and enzymes are of little help, although the absence of either fibrin degradation products or soluble fibrin complexes is said to make the diagnosis unlikely. Pleural fluid, when present, is often grossly bloody, and may be either exudative or transudative.

A properly performed, multiple-view perfusion lung scan that is normal essentially rules out acute PE; similarly, a high-probability scan in a patient with a normal chest roentgenogram and a highly suggestive history establishes the diagnosis. Many patients, however, have findings between these extremes. Ventilation lung scanning increases the diagnostic yield, but in most instances, radionuclide studies can only be interpreted as low-, intermediate-, or high-probability, and the clinician must decide on the likelihood of PE by using this information in combination with the relative clinical probability of its occurrence in this patient.

Pulmonary angiography is the definitive diagnostic study in PE. It is invasive, has definite hazards for the patient, must be performed correctly, and may not be readily available in all centers. However, the greater the importance to the patient that the diagnosis be made accurately, the more important it is to perform the procedure. It should always be done when thrombolytic therapy or vena caval interruption is planned. Digital subtraction angiography, although promising, must be more extensively validated in clinical practice before it can be recommended routinely.

Establishing the diagnosis of DVT can be extremely valuable, in that its presence in a patient with suggestive history and laboratory findings makes the diagnosis of PE very likely. Clinical examination is of little value in detecting DVT, as are Doppler studies, because of marked operator variability. Impedance plethysmography is noninvasive, safe, and readily available, and establishes the diagnosis if the abnormality is unilateral; a normal study effectively excludes proximal DVT. Radiofibrinogen studies take 24 hours to perform and are less accurate in detecting proximal thrombi but serve to complement impedance plethysmography. Together, they may be as accurate as ascending contrast venography, which, although the "gold standard," is invasive and may itself cause DVT.

MANAGEMENT

Intravenous heparin is the mainstay of therapy, and should be begun immediately (provided there are no major contraindications) as soon as the diagnosis of DVT or PE is strongly considered; it can be stopped if evaluation fails to establish the diagnosis. Heparin is administered in full

TABLE 23–2. INDICATIONS FOR VENA CAVAL INTERRUPTION

1. Recurrent physiologically significant embolization despite adequate anticoagulation
2. Documented pulmonary embolus in a patient in whom anticoagulation is contraindicated
   a. Current or very recent major bleeding
   b. Recent cerebrovascular accident, neurosurgical procedure, or spinal injury
   c. Recent major surgical procedure or trauma
   d. Intracranial neoplasm
   e. Severe systemic hypertension (diastolic >110 mm Hg)
3. Complication of anticoagulation requiring its discontinuation in a patient with documented pulmonary embolism
4. Septic pulmonary embolism (after institution of appropriate antibiotic therapy and control of septic focus)
5. Documented chronic recurrent embolization with cor pulmonale

anticoagulating doses for 7–10 days, with once-daily monitoring as soon as the appropriate dose is established, and is discontinued after tapering over 1–2 days (see Chapter 83). Thereafter, whether anticoagulation (with low-dose subcutaneous heparin or oral warfarin) is used, and for how long, depend upon the nature of the predisposing conditions that led to acute pulmonary embolism and whether they have resolved.

Heparin prevents further thrombus formation but does not dissolve clots that are already present. Its use in acute DVT or PE is thus predicated upon the assumption that the patient will survive the present episode if additional embolization can be prevented. If the physiologic impact of the current embolic event is such that the patient's survival is immediately threatened, the therapeutic options include thrombolytic therapy, vena caval interruption, and pulmonary embolectomy. It has not been established conclusively that any of these actually improve survival or reduce morbidity among those who do survive, but most clinicians opt for some therapy in addition to heparin when it appears that the patient with documented PE is likely to die otherwise. Thrombolytic therapy, which is increasingly used in patients with PE, is discussed in Chapter 83.

Indications for vena caval interruption are listed in Table 23–2. Several techniques and devices are available for this procedure; the Kim-Ray Greenfield and Mobin-Uddin filters are most widely used. Pulmonary embolectomy is the most controversial of the aggressive treatments: It has been argued that patients who are so ill as to justify embolectomy cannot be saved by the procedure, and that those who survive probably did not need it. However, surgery is probably justified as a heroic measure in patients with refractory hypotension, in whom other measures have failed or cannot be used.

PREVENTION

DVT and PE can be prevented in several high-risk groups. Patients scheduled for elective major abdominal, thoracic, or gynecologic procedures should receive subcutaneous heparin (5000 units every 8–12 hr), beginning shortly before the operation and contining until they are fully ambulatory. This therapy should also be given to patients with acute myocardial infarction complicated by congestive heart failure, chronic venous insufficiency, and previous episodes of DVT or PE. The elderly and the obese should also receive prophylactic heparin during periods of immobilization in the hospital.

· OUTCOME

In the United States, some 50,000 persons die suddenly each year from PE, and perhaps another 100,000 succumb to this disorder in other circumstances. Mortality may exceed 30 percent in undiagnosed cases, but it is about 10 percent when treatment is undertaken. Massive PE with hypotension is fatal in approximately 25 percent of cases. Most emboli resolve clinically in individuals who survive, and long-term morbidity is uncommon.

RECOMMENDED READING

Bell WR, Bartholomew JR: Pulmonary thromboembolic disease. Curr Probl Cardiol 10:1, 1985.

Benotti JR, Dalen JE: The natural history of pulmonary embolism. Clin Chest Med 5:403, 1984.

Coon WW: Venous thromboembolism: prevalence, risk factors, and prevention. Clin Chest Med 5:391, 1984.

Del Campo C: Pulmonary embolectomy: a review. Can J Surg 28:111, 1985.

Fulkerson WJ, et al: Diagnosis of pulmonary embolism. Arch Intern Med 146:961, 1986.

Goodman PC: Pulmonary angiography. Clin Chest Med 5:465, 1984.

Greenfield LJ: Vena caval interruption and pulmonary embolectomy. Clin Chest Med 5:495, 1984.

Hull RD, et al: Pulmonary angiography, ventilation lung scanning, and venography for clinically suspected pulmonary embolism with abnormal perfusion lung scan. Ann Intern Med 98:891, 1983.

Hyers TM: Antithrombotic therapy for venous thromboembolism. Clin Chest Med 5:479, 1984.

Kinasewitz GT, George RB: Management of thromboembolism: anticoagulants, thrombolytics, or surgical intervention? Chest 86:106, 1984.

Mansour M, Chang AE, Sindelar WF: Interruption of the inferior vena cava for the prevention of recurrent pulmonary embolism. Am Surg 51:375, 1985.

Moser KM: Pulmonary thromboembolism. In Braunwald E, et al (eds): Harrison's Textbook of Internal Medicine. New York, McGraw-Hill, Inc., 11th edition, 1987, p. 1105.

Rosenow EC III, Osmundson PJ, Brown ML: Pulmonary embolism. Mayo Clin Proc 56:161, 1981.

Vogelsang GB, Bell WR: Treatment of pulmonary embolism and deep vein thrombosis with thrombolytic therapy. Clin Chest Med 5:487, 1984.

Wilson JE III: Pulmonary embolism. In Wyngaarden JB, Smith LH Jr (eds): Cecil Textbook of Medicine. Philadelphia, W. B. Saunders Co., 17th edition, 1985, p. 426.

24. Pneumonia

David J. Pierson

DEFINITION

Pneumonia is an infection of the lung parenchyma; in this chapter, it is discussed in three general categories: (1) community-acquired infection, (2) hospital-acquired (nosocomial) pneumonia, and (3) acute or subacute pulmonary infiltrates in the immunocompromised host. Successful management of this condition, particularly in the last two categories, requires close cooperation among primary physician, infectious diseases consultant, microbiologist, and skilled nursing and respiratory care staffs.

Aspiration pneumonia and other pulmonary conditions related to aspiration of gastric and mouth contents are discussed in Chapter 26.

PATHOPHYSIOLOGY

Table 24–1 lists the most common infecting agents in community-acquired pneumonia as determined by the underlying health status of the host. Most cases affecting otherwise healthy individuals are viruslike illnesses (prodromal symptoms, dry cough, little systemic toxicity) and are caused by viruses and *Mycoplasma*; in contrast, pneumococcal pneumonia in healthy hosts, as well as all the types listed for other hosts in the table, tend to produce a more severe bacterialike illness (sudden onset, productive cough, chest pain, leukocytosis). Legionellosis can display either of these clinical pictures. It is unusual for the gram-negative rods listed in Table 24–1 to be drug-resistant in community-acquired pneumonia.

Hospital-acquired pneumonia is a more serious illness in that it develops in patients who are by definition already ill; its causative organisms are often more virulent and tend to be more difficult to treat, and it is usually slower to resolve and associated with more complications than is community-acquired pneumonia. Risk factors for development of this condition are listed in Table 24–2; in general, the more seriously ill the patient and the more invaded by procedures and support systems, the more likely is life-threatening nosocomial infection to occur.

Organisms most likely to cause hospital-acquired pneumonia include

TABLE 24–1. MOST LIKELY ETIOLOGIES OF COMMUNITY-ACQUIRED PNEUMONIA*

CLINICAL SETTING	INFECTIOUS AGENT
Normal, healthy host	Viruses *Mycoplasma pneumoniae* *Streptococcus pneumoniae* *Legionella pneumophila*
Recent influenza	*Streptococcus pneumoniae* *Staphylococcus aureus* *Haemophilus influenzae*
Old age; residence in nursing home or other institution	*Streptococcus pneumoniae* *Klebsiella* spp. *Staphylococcus aureus* *Haemophilus influenzae*
Chronic obstructive pulmonary disease; chronic bronchitis	*Streptococcus pneumoniae* *Haemophilus influenzae*
Chronic alcoholism	*Streptococcus pneumoniae* *Klebsiella* spp. *Staphylococcus aureus* *Haemophilus influenzae*

*Except for pneumonia in the normal host, the causative agents shown apply to patients with a clinical "bacterial syndrome" (see text). Drug-resistant gram-negative bacilli are unusual in the setting of community-acquired pneumonia. Aspiration pneumonia is discussed in Chapter 26.

Klebsiella species, *Escherichia coli*, *Staphylococcus aureus*, and *Pseudomonas aeruginosa*. Less common are other enteric gram-negative bacteria, *Haemophilus influenzae*, *Streptococcus pneumoniae*, mouth anaerobes, *Legionella pneumophila*, and *Aspergillus* species.

Causes of pulmonary infiltrates and respiratory symptoms in the immunocompromised host are partly determined by the nature of the immune defect. Patients with impaired cell-mediated immunity, as in the acquired immunodeficiency syndrome (AIDS), the lymphomas, organ transplantation, and high-dose corticosteroid therapy, are particularly prone to infection with viruses of the herpes group (especially cytomegalovirus), *Pneumocystis carinii*, *Cryptococcus neoformans*, *Nocardia*, and *Legionella*. In contrast, usual organisms causing pneumonia in patients with granulocytopenia include gram-negative bacilli, staphylococci, and fungi such as *Aspergillus*, *Mucor*, and *Candida*.

TABLE 24–2. RISK FACTORS FOR HOSPITAL-ACQUIRED PNEUMONIA*

Endotracheal intubation/tracheostomy
Admission to intensive care unit
Current/recent antibiotic therapy
Surgery/trauma
Chronic obstructive pulmonary disease, heart failure,
  or other underlying cardiopulmonary disease
Immunosuppression
Advanced age

*Listed in approximate order of importance

TABLE 24–3. MOST COMMON ETIOLOGIES FOR PULMONARY INFILTRATES
IN PATIENTS WITH ACQUIRED IMMUNODEFICIENCY SYNDROME*

Pneumocystis carinii
Cytomegalovirus
Mycobacterium avium-intracellulare
Bacteria
    Haemophilus influenzae
    Group B *Streptococcus* sp.
    Streptococcus pneumoniae
    Staphylococcus aureus
    Legionella pneumophila
Fungi
    Candida spp.
    Cryptococcus neoformans
    Others
        Histoplasma capsulatum
        Coccidioides immitis
Mycobacterium tuberculosis
Epstein-Barr virus
Toxoplasma gondii

*Most common infecting/infesting agents are shown in boldface; relative frequencies of all the agents listed vary in different geographic locations.

Pneumocystis and bacteria (gram-negative rods, staphylococci, *Legionella*) typically produce rapidly progressing pulmonary infiltrates in immunocompromised patients, whereas *Aspergillus* species and *Mucor* cause a less aggressive, more subacute clinical picture. Cytomegalovirus infections can produce either of these patterns. Pneumonias due to *Nocardia*, *Cryptococcus*, and mycobacteria tend to be more insidious in onset and progression.

The infective agents most commonly responsible for pulmonary infiltrates in patients with AIDS are listed in Table 24–3.

DIAGNOSIS

Patient assessment should address several questions: (1) Does the patient have pneumonia, or another condition (pulmonary thromboembolism, pulmonary edema, atelectasis, carcinoma) that can produce fever, sputum, leukocytosis, and pulmonary infiltrates? (2) What is the most likely etiologic agent? (3) Are there complications such as bronchial obstruction, atelectasis, parapneumonic effusion or empyema, or lung abscess? Attention should be focused on assessing the patient's overall condition, a major determinant of prognosis, and on the adequacy of cough and the clearance of respiratory tract secretions.

Diagnostic options for determining the etiology of pneumonia are listed in Table 24–4. History, physical examination, and routine blood studies are valuable in indicating how ill the patient is but cannot provide

TABLE 24–4. DIAGNOSTIC METHODS AND PROCEDURES IN PNEUMONIA

Clinical diagnosis
   History and physical examination
   Chest roentgenogram
   Blood leukocyte count and differential
Sputum evaluation
   Smears/stains
   Cultures
Blood culture
Immunodiagnostic studies
Transtracheal aspiration
Transthoracic needle aspiration
Fiberoptic bronchoscopy
   Aspiration
   Protected-brush catheter
   Bronchoalveolar lavage
   Transbronchial biopsy
Open lung biopsy

a specific diagnosis. Along with the sputum Gram stain, they can suggest likely candidates, but this is, typically, only as firmly as the etiologic agent can be identified before therapy is initiated. Serologic studies are of little help to the clinician making initial management decisions, although they can provide later confirmation of an assumed diagnosis; faster immuno-diagnostic techniques for sputum and other specimens are becoming available. Positive blood cultures confirm the identity of an infecting agent but occur in a minority of patients, and these findings are not immediately at hand.

In every case of pneumonia, a primary objective is to obtain lower respiratory secretions for culture and microscopic examination. In uncomplicated cases in which the patient can expectorate an adequate sputum specimen that can be processed immediately, this may be sufficient. However, in seriously ill patients and those with other risk factors, more invasive studies are usually required.

Transtracheal aspirates have high sensitivity, but specificity is low in patients who have been intubated, who have previously undergone nasotracheal suctioning, or who have chronic bronchitis; obtaining them is associated with significant morbidity, particularly when that duty is in inexperienced hands. Transthoracic needle aspiration has similar yields but also carries a substantial complication rate and cannot be done in patients with bleeding diathesis or in those who are uncooperative, very tachypneic, or mechanically ventilated.

Fiberoptic bronchoscopy can provide respiratory tract specimens less traumatically in many patients (see Chapter 37). Suctioned specimens are of limited value because of contamination, but protected-catheter specimens (in bacterial pneumonia) and broncho-alveolar lavage (especially in *Pneumocystis* but also in viral and fungal pneumonia) have high accuracy

TABLE 24–5. INITIAL EMPIRIC ANTIBIOTIC THERAPY FOR PNEUMONIA*

CLINICAL SETTING	INITIAL THERAPY
Community-acquired pneumonia	
Normal healthy host	
"Viral syndrome"	Erythromycin 1 g IV (or 500 mg PO) q 6 h (Tetracycline)
"Bacterial syndrome"	Penicillin G 1.2–2.4 million units IV (or equivalent IM or PO) per day (Erythromycin) (Tetracycline)
Recent influenza	Cefamandole 2 g IV q 6 h
Old age; residence in nursing home or other institution	Cefamandole 2 g IV q 6 h
Chronic obstructive pulmonary disease; chronic bronchitis	Ampicillin or amoxicillin 2 g IV q 6 h (Cefamandole)
Chronic alcoholism	Cefamandole 2 g IV q 6 h
Hospital-acquired pneumonia†	
Gram-positive bacteria	A semisynthetic penicillin or a cephalosporin
Gram-negative bacteria other than *Pseudomonas*	An aminoglycoside *plus* a cephalosporin or a broad-spectrum penicillin
Gram-negative bacilli, *Pseudomonas* suspected	An aminoglycoside *plus* carbenicillin or ticarcillin
Immunocompromised Host (Non-AIDS)	
Diffuse bilateral infiltrates‡	An aminoglycoside *plus* a cephalosporin *plus* trimethoprim-sulfamethoxazole
Focal infiltrate§	An aminoglycoside *plus* a cephalosporin, +/− erythromycin, +/− amphotericin B
Acquired Immunodeficiency Syndrome (AIDS)	
Diffuse bilateral infiltrates‖	Either trimethoprim-sulfamethoxazole or pentamidine for presumed *Pneumocystis carinii*

*Alternative drugs are shown in parentheses.

†Recent sensitivity patterns of a hospital should be taken into account when selecting the initial antibiotic coverage.

‡All patients who can tolerate the procedure should have a tissue diagnosis established within 48 hours.

§All patients who do not improve clinically within 48–72 hours and who can tolerate the procedure should have a tissue diagnosis established.

‖A specific diagnosis should be sought in most instances.

if obtained correctly. In the experience of most centers, transbronchial biopsy improves the yield in immunocompromised patients but also increases morbidity.

Because of the large numbers of organisms present in patients with AIDS and pneumonia due to *Pneumocystis carinii*, many centers routinely begin treatment and collect two or three induced sputum specimens to search for the organisms before proceeding to bronchoscopy. Blind transnasal catheter lavage has also been reported to be efficacious in *Pneumocystis* pneumonia in AIDS.

In non-AIDS patients with severe immunosuppression, such as after bone marrow transplantation, open lung biopsy is the surest method for establishing the etiology of pneumonia and is therefore preferred in many centers over transbronchial biopsy. Although more invasive, open biopsy offers better hemostasis than closed procedures in patients with thrombocytopenia.

MANAGEMENT

Because firm identification of the etiologic agent is seldom available in the initial 24–48 hours, the clinician must have a management strategy based on the clinical presentation of the patient. Particularly in the area of hospital-acquired pneumonia, considerable variation may be encountered among consultants as to the best initial therapy, and it is useful to be familiar with local experience. Suggested initial antibiotic regimens are shown in Table 24–5. The empiric therapy in the table is intended only as initial treatment, pending results of microbiologic and other studies.

Adjunctive therapy for pneumonia includes supplemental oxygen to raise the systemic arterial oxygen tension (PaO_2) to 60 mm Hg or higher and chest physiotherapy (chest percussion and postural drainage), which will facilitate secretion clearance in patients who have difficulty clearing their airways. The latter include those with severe chronic respiratory disease and copious secretions, those with neuromuscular disorders that interfere with cough, and those who are immobilized. There is no evidence that intermittent positive-pressure breathing (IPPB), other aids to intermittent lung inflation, mucolytic agents, or bland aerosols are beneficial in the therapy of pneumonia.

OUTCOME

The mortality of community-acquired pneumonia requiring hospitalization is between 10 and 20 percent and is highest in individuals with severe underlying disease. Nosocomial pneumonia is a frequent cause of death among terminally ill patients and is fatal in as many as half of all cases, reflecting the gravity of the underlying illness. In immunocompromised patients, any pneumonia is typically more virulent and harder to treat than in other settings, and the acute mortality rate is correspondingly higher.

RECOMMENDED READING

Bradsher RW Jr: Overwhelming pneumonia. Med Clin North Am 67:1233, 1983.

Donowitz GR, Mandell GL: Empiric therapy for pneumonia. Rev Infect Dis 5(Suppl. 1):S40, 1983.

Fanta CH, Pennington JE: Fever and new infiltrates in the immunocompromised host. Clin Chest Med 2:19, 1981.

Grant IH, Armstrong D: Management of infectious complications of acquired immunodeficiency syndrome. Am J Med 81(1A)59, 1986.

Long SS: Treatment of acute pneumonia in infants and children. Pediatr Clin North Am 30:297, 1983.

Matthay RA, Moritz ED: Invasive procedures for diagnosing pulmonary infection. Clin Chest Med 2:3, 1981.

Parrino TA, et al: The management of pneumonia. Adv Intern Med 30:113, 1984.

Pennington JE (ed): Respiratory Infections: Diagnosis and Management. New York, Raven Press, 1983.

Podnos SD, Toews GB, Pierce AK: Nosocomial pneumonia in patients in intensive care units. West J Med 143:622, 1985.

Sande MA, Hudson LD, Root RK (eds): Respiratory Infections. New York, Churchill Livingstone, Inc., 1986.

Stulbarg MS: Problems in diagnosing pneumonia. West J Med 140:594, 1984.

Tobin MJ, Grenvik A: Nosocomial lung infection and its diagnosis. Crit Care Med 12:191, 1984.

Toews GB: Nosocomial pneumonia. Am J Med Sci 291:355, 1986.

Verghese A, Berk SL: Bacterial pneumonia in the elderly. Medicine 62:271, 1983.

25. Hemoptysis

David J. Pierson

DEFINITION

Hemoptysis means coughing up blood and implies that this blood has arisen in the lower respiratory tract. The expectorated material may be frank blood or sputum with visible blood in it. However, the rusty sputum of pneumococcal pneumonia and the pink froth of acute pulmonary edema are not usually thought of as hemoptysis. Hemoptysis that is of sufficient volume to cause death from asphyxiation (more than 600 ml/24 hr) has a mortality rate of at least 25 percent and has different diagnostic and therapeutic implications from those of lesser degrees of bleeding.

PATHOPHYSIOLOGY

Bleeding may occur anywhere in the lower respiratory tract, and its anatomic source may be a pulmonary artery, a pulmonary vein, a bronchial artery, or an extrapulmonary systemic artery. Hemorrhage in the last two of these may be rapidly fatal, owing to the high perfusion pressure in the systemic circulation; but massive hemoptysis also occurs in bleeding from the pulmonary circuit.

There are significantly more than 100 reported causes of hemoptysis, and virtually any disorder of the cardiorespiratory system or of blood coagulation can cause this symptom. However, the list of usual etiologies is much shorter. In developed countries, more cases are due to bronchitis than to any other single mechanism. Bronchiectasis, lung cancer, and pneumonia (particularly when due to *Klebsiella*, *Staphylococcus*, or influenza virus) are other common etiologies. Tuberculosis is another frequent cause, and in North America, cases are equally divided between active infection and old, inactive disease; saprophytic infection with fungi (i.e., fungus ball due to *Aspergillus*) increases the likelihood of hemoptysis in the latter. Hemoptysis occurs in about 20 percent of diagnosed cases of pulmonary embolism and is more common in presumed infarction and in the presence of concomitant cardiac disease.

DIAGNOSIS

Hematemesis can sometimes be confused with hemoptysis if an accurate history cannot be obtained. Useful aids for distinguishing the two include the sequence of events (hemoptysis is preceded by coughing, hematemesis by vomiting), the character of the expectorated material (blood from the lungs is frothy, often bright red, and neutral or alkaline on pH testing; blood from the stomach is not frothy, is usually dark red or brown, and is often acid), and the rate of clearing (hemoptysis is usually followed by hours or days of red-streaked sputum). Blood from the lungs contains leukocytes and macrophages, whereas that from the stomach usually contains food particles.

Although the list of possible causes is extensive, in any individual patient, two or three most likely etiologies are usually suggested by the history and clinical circumstances. The most likely causes in five commonly encountered patient groups are listed in Table 25–1. Other considerations that influence the probability of different diagnoses include geographic factors (tuberculosis in developing countries; paragonimiasis in Southeast Asia; coccidioidomycosis in the U.S. Southwest), population base, coexistent disease (pulmonary infarct in chronic heart failure; coagulopathy and opportunistic infection in immunosuppression), and associated symptoms (cancer and tuberculosis with anorexia and weight loss; pneumonia and bronchiectasis with fever and purulent sputum; pulmonary infarction with phlebitis and pleuritic pain).

The results of initial diagnostic studies constitute another variable. If the chest roentgenogram reveals a mass or evidence of atelectasis, neoplasm is the most likely diagnosis. Fibrotic changes, especially with cavity formation, suggest tuberculosis. Fluid-filled cystic spaces, thickened bronchial walls, and "dirty" lung markings in the lower lobes are common findings in bronchiectasis, and similar signs may be present in cystic fibrosis.

Massive hemoptysis has different usual causes from hemoptysis of lesser magnitude (Table 25–2). In this condition, identification of the

TABLE 25–1. MOST FREQUENT CAUSES OF HEMOPTYSIS IN DIFFERENT PATIENT GROUPS

HEALTHY NONSMOKER UNDER AGE 40	"HEALTHY" CIGARETTE SMOKER	CHRONIC OBSTRUCTIVE PULMONARY DISEASE	OLD TUBERCULOSIS (or other granulomatous lung disease)	CHRONIC ALCOHOLISM
Bronchitis	Bronchitis	Lung cancer	Bronchiectasis	Tuberculosis
Pneumonia	Lung cancer	Bronchitis	Tuberculosis	Consequences
Pulmonary	Pneumonia	Bronchiectasis	Lung cancer	of aspiration:
infarct			Aspergillosis	Lung abscess
Benign			Bronchitis	Necrotizing
neoplasm				pneumonia
Vascular				Empyema
disorder				Foreign body
				Lung cancer
				Bronchiectasis
				Trauma

TABLE 25–2. DIFFERENTIAL DIAGNOSIS OF LIFE-THREATENING HEMOPTYSIS*
(>600 ml/24 hr)

INFLAMMATORY AND SUPPURATIVE PROCESSES
Tuberculosis
Bronchiectasis
Necrotizing pneumonia
Lung abscess
Fungus ball; other fungal infections
Cystic fibrosis
NEOPLASMS
Lung cancer
Bronchial adenoma
TRAUMA
Blunt
Penetrating
Iatrogenic
VASCULAR DISORDERS
Bronchovascular/arteriovenous fistula
Congenital/traumatic/neoplastic
Mitral stenosis
Aortic arch aneurysm
Vascular prostheses

*Entities in boldface account for >90 percent of cases.

etiology must take a secondary role so that efforts can be focused on preventing asphyxiation and stopping the bleeding.

While the chest roentgenogram is useful in suggesting likely diagnoses, more definitive identification of the cause is usually necessary, and bronchoscopy is the procedure of choice if sputum examination and other clinical findings do not confirm this. Patients with hemoptysis should undergo bronchoscopy if they are over 40 years of age, if they have a significant cigarette-smoking history, if there is an abnormality on chest roentgenogram that suggests a neoplasm, if a specific diagnosis other than carcinoma is suggested clinically (e.g., aspirated foreign body), or if the hemoptysis persists for more than 1 week.

Other diagnostic procedures include bronchography, which is used less often now than in past decades but is valuable in assessing patients with bronchiectasis prior to elective surgery. Computerized tomography and magnetic resonance imaging do not often contribute new information to the work-up.

In as many as half of all instances of hemoptysis, depending on the practice environment and patient population, no cause is found despite evaluation as described above. Numerous studies have demonstrated that such "idiopathic" or "cryptogenic" hemoptysis is benign and that patients can safely be followed without further diagnostic procedures; less than one percent are subsequently found to have carcinoma or some other potentially fatal condition.

In massive hemoptysis, rigid bronchoscopy is preferable to the use of the fiberoptic instrument because of the greater ability of the former to remove clots and large volumes of blood.The two most useful diagnostic procedures in life-threatening hemoptysis are bronchial angiography and radionuclide scans. Bronchial angiography is usually used in conjunction with attempts to embolize the bleeding vessel; it requires considerable technical expertise but can provide anatomic information about the bleeding site. Radionuclide scans have had less widespread use and give only a general localization of the bleeding source. Both procedures can identify a bleeding site only in the presence of ongoing hemorrhage.

MANAGEMENT

Table 25–3 outlines an overall management approach to massive hemoptysis and lists the various specific maneuvers that have been used in attempts to stop the bleeding. Selective bronchial intubation, endobronchial balloon tamponade, and other techniques for isolating the bleeding lobe or lung are only temporary measures, but the bleeding often stops once initial control has been achieved. Although it requires technical expertise and carries the risk of paraplegia and other complications, bronchial artery embolization has been highly successful in several series.

Iced-saline lavage has been used successfully by one group to stop massive pulmonary hemorrhage. Favorable results have been reported

TABLE 25–3. MANAGEMENT OF LIFE-THREATENING HEMOPTYSIS

1. Assessment and monitoring of the patient
    a. Intensive care unit
    b. Blood loss (quantitate expectorated blood)
    c. Blood volume/fluid status (central line)
    d. Blood pressure/arterial blood gases (arterial line)
2. Early consultation with thoracic surgeon
3. General supportive measures
    a. Strict bed rest with bleeding side down
    b. Mild sedation (without abolishing cough reflex): Morphine 2 mg or diazepam 5 mg IV
        q 4–6 h
    c. Endotracheal tube and suction apparatus at bedside
    d. Blood (4–6 units) typed/crossmatched for transfusion
4. Localization of bleeding site
    a. Chest roentgenograph
    b. Bronchoscopy (rigid preferred if actively bleeding)
    c. Radionuclide scan
    d. Bronchial arteriography
5. Available options for control of bleeding
    a. Selective bronchial intubation
    b. Intubation with double-lumen endotracheal tube
    c. Endobronchial balloon tamponade
    d. Iced saline lavage via rigid bronchoscope
    e. Bronchial arterial embolization
    f. Surgical resection of bleeding lung tissue

using intravenous vasopressin, conjugated estrogens, and coagulants, but experience is limited and anecdotal.

Surgical resection of the bleeding lung tissue is definitive but technically impossible in many patients such as those with severe chronic obstructive pulmonary disease or diffuse disease such as necrotizing pneumonia. Operative mortality correlates with continued bleeding at the time of the procedure, and if surgery is to be done, the hemorrhage should first be stopped using selective bronchial intubation or some other maneuver. Even in patients who have had bleeding sites identified during previous episodes, it is important to localize the involved area prior to lung resection.

OUTCOME

Acute mortality exeeds 75 percent when hemorrhage continues at more than 600 ml/16 hr during medical management. With current management techniques, the originally reported mortality of 50 percent with bleeding of 600 ml/24 hr can probably be reduced by half, but massive hemoptysis is still a severe threat to life. In other settings, the underlying cause, rather than the hemoptysis itself, determines both management and long-term outlook.

RECOMMENDED READING

Adelman M, et al: Cryptogenic hemoptysis. Clinical features, bronchoscopic findings, and natural history in 67 patients. Ann Intern Med 102:829, 1985.

Bobrowitz ID, Ramakrishna S, Shim Y-S: Comparison of medical vs surgical treatment of major hemoptysis. Arch Intern Med 143:1343, 1983.

Conlan AA: Massive hemoptysis—diagnostic and therapeutic implications. Surg Annu 17:337, 1985.

Conlan AA, et al: Massive hemoptysis. J Thorac Cardiovasc Surg 85:120, 1983.

Crocco JA: Massive hemoptysis. NY State J Med 85:573, 1985.

Gong H Jr, Salvatierra C: Clinical efficacy of early and delayed bronchoscopy in patients with hemoptysis. Am Rev Respir Dis 124:221, 1981.

Haponik EF, et al: Radionuclide localization of massive pulmonary hemorrhage. Chest 86:208, 1984.

Jackson GV, Savage PJ, Quinn DL: Role of fiberoptic bronchoscopy in patients with hemoptysis and a normal chest roentgenogram. Chest 87:142, 1985.

Lyons HA: Differential diagnosis of hemoptysis and its treatment. Basics RD 5(2):1, 1976.

Remy J, et al: Treatment of hemoptysis by embolization of bronchial arteries. Radiology 122:33, 1977.

Saw EC, et al: Flexible fiberoptic bronchoscopy and endobronchial tamponade in the management of massive hemoptysis. Chest 70:589, 1976.

Strickland B: Investigating hemoptysis. Br J Hosp Med 35:246, 1986.

Trento A, et al: Massive hemoptysis in patients with cystic fibrosis: three case reports and a protocol for clinical management. Ann Thorac Surg 39:254, 1985.

Uflacker R, et al: Bronchial artery embolization in the management of hemoptysis: technical aspects and long-term results. Radiology 157:637, 1985.

Wedel M: Massive hemoptysis. In Moser KM, Spragg R (eds): Respiratory Emergencies. 2nd edition. St. Louis, C.V. Mosby Co., 1982.

26. Aspiration

David J. Pierson

Definition

Aspiration of solid or liquid material produces several clinical syndromes, the presentation of which depends upon what is aspirated, its quantity, and the patient's underlying cardiorespiratory status. These syndromes include foreign body aspiration, aspiration pneumonitis, aspiration-related bacterial pneumonia, lung abscess and empyema, lipoid pneumonia, and drowning. The first four are among the most common disorders encountered in respiratory medicine. The several forms of lipoid pneumonia are subacute or chronic conditions and are not considered here; drowning is discussed in Chapter 93.

Pathophysiology

Foreign body aspiration produces asphyxia if the airway is occluded, regardless of the nature of the aspirated material. This happens most often with eating ("café coronary"), especially in the presence of acute alcohol intoxication or sedation (see Chapter 20). Inhalation of smaller objects is common in children but is also seen in adults; the clinical picture depends on the nature of the object (vegetable matter may produce intense inflammation), where it lodges (lower lobes are most common), the degree to which it compromises respiratory function, and how long after the event the patient is seen.

Aspiration pneumonitis, originally described during parturition under general anesthesia (Mendelson's syndrome), is an acute inflammatory response to the inhalation of gastric contents. Depending upon the quantity of material aspirated, it often produces noncardiac pulmonary edema clinically indistinguishable from other forms of adult respiratory distress syndrome (ARDS, Chapter 27). Although it is commonly held that aspiration of stomach acid at pH <2.5 is necessary for this syndrome, studies have shown this not to be the case; aspiration of gastric contents at pH 5.9 can produce diffuse lung injury if the inhaled material contains food particles.

Conditions predisposing to aspiration and thus to aspiration pneumonitis and the conditions described below include depressed consciousness of any etiology, anesthesia and surgery, neuromuscular disease, gastric outlet obstruction, esophageal reflux, repeated vomiting, and the presence of medical devices such as nasogastric and uncuffed tracheostomy tubes.

Most bacterial pneumonias are technically aspiration-induced, in that the infecting organisms gain access to the lower respiratory tract through inhalation of material from the upper airway. However, by convention, aspiration-related bacterial pneumonia means a lower respiratory infection following contamination with a substantial quantity of mouth contents. This syndrome clinically resembles bacterial pneumonia in other settings (see Chapter 25) and typically occurs one to several days after the aspiration episode. Pneumococci and mixed aerobic/anaerobic organisms are most commonly found when the aspiration has occurred outside the hospital, whereas in-hospital or institutional aspiration more often involves bacteria typical of nosocomial infections.

Lung abscess and empyema also follow inhalation of mouth organisms, although the episode of aspiration is frequently not recalled. These conditions are seen most often in chronic alcoholics, in individuals with epilepsy or a history of loss of consciousness for other reasons, or in bronchial obstruction by tumor or foreign body. Causative organisms are typically those capable of necrosing lung parenchyma: *Klebsiella pneumoniae*, other enteric gram-negative rods, *Staphylococcus aureus*, and anaerobes. The frequency with which mouth anaerobes are recovered on culture is a function of the collecting and processing techniques.

DIAGNOSIS

The clinical picture of foreign body aspiration is variable. Patients are often either aware of having inhaled something or have experienced an episode of sudden coughing and choking. In some, however, symptoms of cough and dyspnea are present without a definite moment of onset. Occasionally there are no new symptoms. Physical examination may reveal signs of consolidation or, less commonly, a localized wheeze. Most foreign bodies are radiolucent; the chest radiograph may show infiltrates, atelectasis, or postobstructive hyperlucence but is often normal. Accurate diagnosis requires bronchoscopy in an appropriate clinical setting.

The sequence of vomiting, choking and coughing, and progressive respiratory dysfunction makes the diagnosis of aspiration pneumonitis obvious; in instances without such an obvious sequence or in which the aspiration has been less massive, the clinician is left with excluding other causes of ARDS and such disorders as pulmonary embolism, pneumothorax, and bacterial pneumonia. Physiologic assessment, particularly of oxygenation, is the key to successful management. The results of routine laboratory studies are usually not helpful, and the chest roentgenogram is highly variable and poorly correlated with the clinical course. Most commonly the latter shows perihilar or basilar infiltrates, which may progress bilaterally to produce the typical pattern of noncardiac pulmonary edema.

Diagnosis in bacterial pneumonia following aspiration is no different from evaluation of this disorder in other settings (see Chapter 25); nosocomial and resistant pathogens are more likely if the patient has been treated "prophylactically" with antibiotics or corticosteroids.

The presence of a lung abscess is usually obvious from the chest roentgenogram and the clinical setting; evaluation focuses on ruling out an obstructing carcinoma or foreign body if these are clinically suggested and on assuring that adequate endobronchial drainage is present (indicated by sputum expectoration and presence of an air-fluid level in the abscess). Identification of the specific organisms involved is usually less important in lung abscess than in pneumonia and empyema, as this information seldom alters the choice of antibiotic used.

Most important in evaluation of a pleural empyema is to establish its presence as quickly as possible, so that physical drainage can be established. Initial antibiotic selection will also depend on the results of a Gram's stain of the fluid in conjunction with evaluation of sputum cultures and of the clinical setting.

Management

When aspiration is witnessed, initial therapy centers on establishing and clearing the patient's airway. Nasotracheal or orotracheal suctioning may help to remove some of the aspirated material, but lavage with more than a few milliliters of fluid may make the injury worse rather than better. Instilling or aerosolizing bicarbonate solution is of no value, as the injury is immediate and gastric acid is rapidly neutralized by airway secretions. Bronchoscopy is often performed to look for and remove large particles of food after massive aspiration of gastric contents but is usually unhelpful in this setting.

Management must center on support of oxygenation and appropriate fluid replacement. Despite decades of empiric therapy, no well-designed study has demonstrated clinical benefit from corticosteroids following aspiration, and routine use in this setting increases the likelihood of antibiotic-resistant superinfection. Similarly, antibiotics should not be administered routinely, but should be selected, as in other instances of pneumonia, when fever, purulent sputum, and leukocytosis develop 1 or more days after aspiration.

Assuming that adequate communication with the airways exists, lung abscess should be treated with either penicillin G (initially 1 million units IV q 4 h) or clindamycin (initially 600 mg IV q 8 h). Although it may take several days, a positive clinical response is usual, even in the presence of bacteria that appear resistant on laboratory sensitivity testing. After initial therapy, the same drug should be continued orally; resolution often takes many weeks.

Empyema is treated with prompt drainage and with antimicrobials selected according to sensitivity testing. Repeated needle aspiration may be sufficient when the fluid is thin with no loculations, but tube thoracostomy is necessary in most cases; when the inflammatory response is exuberant and thick pus or multiple loculations are present, additional chest tubes or an open drainage procedure will be required.

OUTCOME

Mortality is high following aspiration because it tends to occur in individuals with serious underlying health impairment. Although reported mortality rates vary, about one fourth to one half of all cases end fatally. Death rates from aspiration pneumonitis are highest in the elderly, when shock or profound hypoxemia are present, and when secondary bacterial pneumonia develops. Prognosis in survivors is determined mainly by the underlying condition that predisposed to aspiration.

RECOMMENDED READING

Bartlett JG, Finegold SM: Anaerobic infections of the lung and pleural space. Am Rev Respir Dis 110:56, 1974.

Bartlett JG, Gorbach SL: The triple threat of aspiration pneumonia. Chest 68:560, 1975.

Bynum LJ, Pierce AK: Pulmonary aspiration of gastric contents. Am Rev Respir Dis 114:1129, 1976.

Crapo JD: Physical, chemical, and aspiration injuries of the lung. In Wyngaarden JB, Smith LH Jr (eds): Cecil Textbook of Medicine. 17th edition. Philadelphia, W.B. Saunders Co., 1985, 2287.

Johanson WG Jr, Harris GD: Aspiration pneumonia, anaerobic infections, and lung abscess. Med Clin North Am 64:385, 1980.

Levison ME, et al: Clindamycin compared with penicillin for the treatment of anaerobic lung abscess. Ann Intern Med 98:466, 1983.

Luce JM, Pierson DJ: Corticosteroids and antibiotics in the adult respiratory distress syndrome: a review. Semin Respir Med 2:151, 1981.

McCammon RL: Prophylaxis for aspiration pneumonitis. Can Anaesth Soc J 33(3 part 2):S47, 1986.

Newman GE, Effman EL, Putman CE: Pulmonary aspiration complexes in adults. Curr Probl Diagn Radiol 11:1, 1982.

Schwartz DJ, et al: The pulmonary consequences of aspiration of gastric contents at pH values greater than 2.5. Am Rev Respir Dis 121:119, 1980.

Wynne JH, Modell JH: Respiratory aspiration of stomach contents. Ann Intern Med 87:466, 1977.

27. Adult Respiratory Distress Syndrome

David J. Pierson

DEFINITION

The adult respiratory distress syndrome (ARDS) was first defined as the combination of acute dyspnea, severe hypoxemia, diffuse pulmonary infiltrates, and decreased lung compliance, occurring in a clinical setting that did not otherwise explain these findings. A more precise definition, developed to facilitate research on ARDS but also useful clinically, is the following: (1) The ratio of arterial oxygen tension to inspired oxygen function (PaO_2/FIO_2) < 150 mm Hg (e.g., PaO_2 less than 90 mm Hg on FIO_2 = 0.60), (2) infiltrates in all lung fields on chest roentgenogram, (3) pulmonary artery wedge pressure (PAWP) < 18 mm Hg (if available), and (4) no other clinical explanation for these findings.

PATHOPHYSIOLOGY

ARDS is not so much a specific disease as a characteristic clinical state, and it has been associated with more than 100 separate disease entities. Each of these disorders can be categorized as producing generalized lung injury by one of three mechanisms: inhalation- or airway-borne injury (as in aspiration of gastric contents, near-drowning, and smoke inhalation), blood-borne injury (as in sepsis syndrome and multiple long-bone fractures), or mechanical injury to the lung (as in pulmonary contusion).

Whatever the initiating clinical event or process, it leads to a diffuse inflammatory response in the lung, in which complement activation, alveolar macrophages, and polymorphonuclear leukocytes play important roles. High-permeability (noncardiogenic) pulmonary edema and refractory hypoxemia typical of right-to-left intrapulmonary shunt are prominent features. However, although pulmonary dysfunction is its initial hallmark, ARDS is a multisystem disorder in which the ultimate outcome is related more to sepsis and dysfunction in other organs than it is to respiratory failure.

Table 27–1 lists the most important clinical risk factors for the development of ARDS. Sepsis syndrome (defined by the clinical features shown in the table, not simply as a positive blood culture) is the most prominent of these not only in the incidence but also in the mortality of ARDS. In general terms, the likelihood of developing ARDS, given one of the risk factors other than sepsis syndrome in Table 27–1, is about 20 percent; with two of them it is 40 percent, and with three risk factors present simultaneously, it is as high as 60 percent. Sepsis syndrome itself is associated with development of ARDS in about 40 percent of patients.

DIAGNOSIS

In general, the more critically ill or injured a patient, the more likely is the development of ARDS. However, despite numerous studies aimed at identifying blood elements or other markers to predict development of the disorder in an individual patient, there is at present no reliable means of specifying risk beyond the clinical settings listed in Table 27–1.

ARDS is diagnosed as defined above, and physiologic assessment focuses on oxygenation. Although arterial blood gas values are used in the definition, it is important to remember that oxygen transport ($\dot{D}O_2$) is more important than PaO_2 in the assessment. As noted in Chapter 1, $\dot{D}O_2$ is the product of arterial oxygen content (which considers both PaO_2 and the quantity and function of available hemoglobin) and cardiac output. It is not necessary to measure or calculate these factors directly in all cases of ARDS, but they must always be kept in mind.

TABLE 27–1. MAJOR CLINICAL RISK FACTORS FOR ARDS

1. Sepsis syndrome, defined as follows:
   A. Two or more of the following:
      1. Temperature >39°C or <36°C
      2. Leukocyte count <3000 or >12,000 cells/mm³
      3. Leukocyte differential with >10 percent immature granulocytes
      4. Blood culture positive for commonly accepted pathogen
      5. Known or strongly suspected source for systemic infection from which a known pathogen has been cultured
   B. *And* one or more of the following:
      1. Continuing, otherwise unexplained metabolic acidosis, with base deficit >5 mEq/L
      2. Systemic vascular resistance <800 dynes/s/cm⁻⁵
      3. Unexplained hypotension, with systolic blood pressure <90 mm Hg for >2 hr
2. Documented aspiration of gastric contents
3. Near-drowning
4. Pulmonary contusion
5. Multiple long-bone (femur; tibia; humerus) or unstable pelvic fractures
6. Multiple emergency transfusions (>10 units in 6 hr)
7. Hypotension, with systolic blood pressure <90 mm Hg for >2 hr

How invasively to assess and monitor patients with ARDS will vary according to the patient's underlying state of health, the severity of cardiorespiratory dysfunction, and the clinician's basic management approach. Indications for insertion of a pulmonary artery (Swan-Ganz) catheter are discussed in Chapters 15 and 36.

MANAGEMENT

At present, management in ARDS remains supportive. Once the patient has been placed at increased risk by the factors in Table 27–1, there is no convincing evidence that development of the full-blown syndrome can be prevented or modified. Similarly, despite hundreds of investigations during two decades, there is no convincing evidence that the natural history of the disorder can be interrupted or its course ameliorated by positive end-expiratory pressure (PEEP), drugs, or any other therapy. Management must therefore concentrate on the support of tissue oxygenation and the prevention of complications.

PEEP is the mainstay of therapy to improve oxygenation in ARDS; its use in this condition is described in Chapter 36. Using the clinical approach taken in this book, the goals of PEEP therapy in ARDS are to attain clinically acceptable oxygen transport at an FIO_2 of 0.60 or less, at least in the initial 2–4 days of management, and to avoid pulmonary barotrauma. With this approach, PEEP levels of 10–20 cm H_2O are commonly employed, and Swan-Ganz catheters are often used in monitoring.

With the possible exception of the fat embolism syndrome, corticosteroids are not helpful in any setting of ARDS. Antimicrobial agents are also not indicated as primary treatment and should be used only for documented or strongly suspected specific infections. The pulmonary parenchyma is not homogeneously involved in ARDS; moving the patient into the prone position may improve oxygenation, although this response is usually only temporary. Extracorporeal membrane oxygenation (ECMO) has been proven ineffective in decreasing the mortality of severe ARDS.

OUTCOME

Despite technologic advances, the widespread use of PEEP, invasive hemodynamic monitoring, and other measures, the mortality of ARDS (60 percent) has not changed since the syndrome was first described 20 years ago. Most deaths within the first 3 days of illness are related to the precipitating event or underlying disease process. Beyond 3 days, fatalities in ARDS are mainly due to sepsis syndrome and multiple organ failure, with only 15–20 percent due to intractable respiratory failure. Persistent sepsis syndrome without an identified primary source has a particularly poor prognosis in this condition.

Although lung biopsy in patients with severe ARDS commonly shows varying degrees of fibrosis, most individuals who survive return to clinically normal cardiorespiratory function. However, perhaps one third have some exercise limitation or demonstrate an increased alveolar to arterial oxygen difference ($P[A-a]O_2$) on exercise testing, and both restrictive and obstructive ventilatory defects may be found. Up to 2 years may be required for full recovery of pulmonary function.

RECOMMENDED READING

Andreadis N, Petty TL: Adult respiratory distress syndrome: problems and progress. Am Rev Respir Dis 132:1344, 1985.

ARDS: a clinical view. Editorial. Lancet 2:439, 1986.

Ashbaugh DG, et al: Acute respiratory distress in adults. Lancet 2:319, 1967.

Baumann WR, et al: Incidence and mortality of adult respiratory distress syndrome: a prospective analysis from a large metropolitan hospital. Crit Care Med 14:1, 1986.

Bell RC, et al: Multiple organ system failure and infection in adult respiratory distress syndrome. Ann Intern Med 99:293, 1983.

Fowler AA, et al: Adult respiratory distress syndrome: risk with common predispositions. Ann Intern Med 98:593, 1983.

Fowler AA, et al: Adult respiratory distress syndrome: prognosis after onset. Am Rev Respir Dis 132:472, 1985.

Hudson LD: Prognosis: Immediate and long-term sequelae of acute respiratory failure. In Pierson DJ (ed): Respiratory Intensive Care. Dallas, Daedalus Press (American Association for Respiratory Care), 1986, p. 25.

Hyers TM, Fowler AA: Adult respiratory distress syndrome: causes, morbidity, and mortality. Fed Proc 45:25, 1986.

Maunder RJ: Clinical prediction of the adult respiratory distress syndrome. Clin Chest Med 6:413, 1985.

Maunder RJ, Hudson LD: The adult respiratory distress syndrome. In Current Pulmonology 1986. Chicago, Year Book Medical Publishers, Inc., 1986, p. 97.

Montgomery AB, et al: Causes of mortality in patients with the adult respiratory distress syndrome. Am Rev Respir Dis 132:485, 1985.

Pepe PE, et al: Clinical predictors of the adult respiratory distress syndrome. Am J Surg 144:124, 1982.

Rinaldo JE, Rogers RM: Adult respiratory distress syndrome: changing concepts of lung injury and repair. N Engl J Med 306:900, 1982.

Truog WE: ARDS in children: a critical care challenge. J Respir Dis 7:104,1986.

28. Nonpenetrating Chest Trauma

David J. Pierson

DEFINITION

Patients may sustain blunt trauma to the chest in motor vehicle accidents; by being kicked or struck in the chest; in falls against objects or the ground, or into water from a height; in explosions; and in numerous other ways. The injuries involved are often more serious than they appear on initial assessment, and they are likely to be encountered by any clinician who sees patients in the intensive care unit (ICU). Preexisting cardiopulmonary disease renders thoracic trauma of any kind more serious.

PATHOPHYSIOLOGY

Nonpenetrating chest injuries are usually the result of sudden deceleration and may affect any organ or tissue in the thorax. Rib fractures are the most common injury, usually occurring in the middle of the chest, frequently in the posterior axillary line. They are often multiple but may not be apparent on the chest roentgenogram unless posterior or lateral. Lower rib fractures are associated with injuries to the kidneys, spleen, or liver, whereas involvement of the first three ribs or scapula is a frequent marker for injury to the aorta or major airways. Because they cause pain and splinting, rib fractures impair lung inflation and secretion clearance and thus predispose to atelectasis and pneumonia.

Fracture of two or more adjacent ribs in two places each may produce a flail chest—a segment of chest wall that moves paradoxically with spontaneous respiration. This is most likely to happen with anterior and lateral fractures and often involves sternocostal fractures or separations that are not visible on the chest roentgenogram. Rarely, there may be so many fractures as to completely disrupt the integrity of the thorax; in such cases ("stove-in-chest"), ventilation may be so impaired as to require mechanical support. In most cases, however, flail *per se* is not an indication

178

for mechanical ventilation; it is the underlying pulmonary dysfunction that determines whether this will be necessary.

Injuries involving the pleural space include pneumothorax and hemothorax. The latter is usually caused by laceration or avulsion of intercostal vessels by the sharp edges of fractured ribs, but the bleeding source may be any structure in the chest, including the heart or great vessels. Chapter 29 discusses the pathophysiology and management of traumatic pneumothorax.

A pulmonary contusion is an area of bleeding into the lung parenchyma caused by disruption of small blood vessels that produces a zone of diffuse infiltrate on the chest roentgenogram. It causes hypoxemia due to ventilation-perfusion mismatching and right-to-left shunt. For unknown reasons, pulmonary contusion is also a major predisposing factor for development of the adult respiratory distress syndrome (ARDS). Contusion occurs more readily in young individuals, whose chest walls are more compliant than those of older people and tend to transmit the force of a blow rather than to absorb it; thus, lung contusion often occurs without rib fracture in younger patients.

A localized tear or laceration in the lung may produce a pulmonary hematoma, characterized roentgenographically by a sharply demarcated mass-like density. Unlike a contusion, this lesion usually does not become visible on the chest roentgenogram for 1–3 days after the accident and causes little, if any, physiologic effect. It may take weeks or months to resolve and may leave a permanent scar.

Tracheobronchial injuries are uncommon but serious. They usually occur within a few centimeters of the carina, where the airway is less firmly tethered and thus more susceptible to shear forces during deceleration; these injuries range from a barely visible submucosal tear to through-and-through transection of trachea or main bronchus. Tracheobronchial injuries usually produce large air leaks, often with failure of collapsed lung tissue to reexpand under chest tube suction, and there may be bleeding into the airway. Early diagnosis and repair are essential, even in smaller tears, as these can lead to stricture formation, chronic atelectasis, and bronchiectasis.

Injury to the thoracic aorta, a common cause of death at the accident scene, may be missed in patients who survive and are evaluated in the hospital. The heart and pericardium may be injured in several ways, the most common of which is myocardial contusion. This may produce infarction, cardiac rupture, conduction abnormalities, and various dysrhythmias, as discussed in Chapter 7. Pericardial tamponade is infrequent after blunt chest trauma but must be recognized promptly for successful decompression to be accomplished.

Diaphragmatic injury, including rupture of one hemidiaphragm with eventration of abdominal contents into the chest, is more often seen with penetrating than with blunt trauma, usually in patients with multiple, serious injuries. It is commonly discovered at exploratory laparotomy.

The fat embolism syndrome consists of hypoxemia, dyspnea, restlessness, confusion, petechiae (on conjunctivae, axillae, and upper torso), and bilateral, diffuse infiltrates on chest roentgenogram in patients who have sustained long-bone fractures or, rarely, other trauma. The syndrome results from liberation of fat into the circulation; its deposition diffusely in the lungs, brain, and elsewhere; and its subsequent enzymatic breakdown into more toxic form. The syndrome may range from mild hypoxemia and transient confusion to full-blown ARDS. Most patients with long-bone fractures have abnormal arterial oxygenation on admission, but the syndrome itself characteristically does not develop until 1–3 days after the injury.

DIAGNOSIS

Table 28–1 sumarizes the relative frequency, timing of presentation, and means of diagnosis of the different forms of blunt chest trauma. Pneumothorax, rib fractures, air leak resulting from tracheobronchial disruption, and upper mediastinal widening from aortic rupture are generally evident on admission. Flail chest is diagnosed by bedside observation, rather than by chest roentgenogram; it may not appear for hours or days, until paradoxical chest wall motion is accentuated by decreased pulmonary compliance accompanying contusion or pneumonia. Hemothorax of 1000 ml or more may not be evident on initial films, especially if the patient cannot be placed upright; its presence should be suspected if one lung field is less lucent than the other or if there are multiple rib fractures.

A pulmonary contusion should be present roentgenographically within a few hours after the injury and should be located beneath an area of chest wall that was involved in the trauma. Pulmonary hematomas are more sharply circumscribed and do not appear for one or more days.

The diagnosis of fat embolism syndrome is straightforward when long-bone fracture is the only injury and the clinical manifestations are typical, but it may be only a diagnosis of exclusion in the presence of multiple trauma and other potential causes for ARDS. Petechiae are often absent or obscured by dressings, and fat droplets may be detected in body fluids with any long-bone fracture.

MANAGEMENT

Rib fractures should not be bandaged tightly or splinted with "rib belts," especially in the elderly, as this predisposes to atelectasis and

TABLE 28–1. CLINICAL PRESENTATION AND DIAGNOSIS OF NONPENETRATING CHEST INJURIES

INJURY	RELATIVE FREQUENCY AS SEEN IN ICU	USUAL TIME OF CLINICAL PRESENTATION	METHOD OF DIAGNOSIS
Rib fracture	+ + + +	Immediate to several days	CXR (may not show anterior fractures); physical exam
Flail chest	+ +	Immediate to several days	Physical exam; (CXR)
Pneumothorax	+ + +	Immediate	CXR; physical exam if tension
Hemothorax	+ + +	Immediate	CXR; thoracentesis
Pulmonary contusion	+ +	Within first 6–24 hours	CXR (diffuse infiltrate under area of trauma); clinical setting; ABG
Pulmonary hematoma	+	1–3 days after injury	CXR (localized mass lesion); clinical setting
Tracheobronchial injury	+	Immediate	Clinical setting (air leak; lung collapse; bleeding); bronchoscopy
Aortic injury	+	Immediate (recognition may be delayed)	CXR (mediastinal widening; indistinct aortic knob; pleural fluid); angiography
Cardiac contusion	+ +	First 24 hours	ECG; two-dimensional echocardiography; clinical setting
Diaphragm injury	+	Immediate (recognition may be delayed)	CXR; clinical setting; laparotomy
Fat embolism syndrome	+ +	1–3 days after trauma	Clinical setting; physical exam; ABG

ICU = intensive care unit; CXR = chest roentgenogram; ABG = arterial blood gases; ECG = electrocardiogram.

pneumonia; instead, the patient should be given small doses of narcotics and, if necessary, intercostal nerve blocks for the first few days. Patients with flail chest require ventilatory support (with continuous, not intermittent, mechanical ventilation) if they meet the criteria described in Chapter 35 but not otherwise; the older regimen of volume-cycled ventilation until all paradoxical chest wall motion ceases causes unnecessary complications and prolongs hospitalization. Intercostal blocks can also be highly efficacious in flail chest.

Traumatic hemothorax of sufficient size to be evident on chest roentgenogram should always be drained with a large-bore chest tube. Indications for thoracotomy include a very large initial accumulation of blood (> 2000 ml) or continued bleeding at 200 ml/hr or more. However, most patients do not need chest exploration, and, in contrast with the situation in penetrating chest trauma, a repairable lesion is less often found in blunt trauma.

Pulmonary contusion requires supplemental oxygen and careful monitoring for development of ARDS but has no specific treatment. No therapy is required for pulmonary hematoma. Tracheobronchial injuries require immediate surgical repair as do aortic disruption and rupture of the diaphragm. The management of myocardial contusion is discussed in Chapter 7.

The management of fat embolism syndrome is essentially that of ARDS in any setting, although the use of pharmacologic doses of corticosteroids is better supported in this condition than in others associated with ARDS. Early corticosteroid therapy in high-risk patients may prevent the syndrome or decrease its severity.

OUTCOME

Outcome in nonpenetrating chest trauma is primarily determined by the nature and severity of the individual injuries sustained and by the complications occurring during management. Patients with severe underlying cardiopulmonary disease have a poorer prognosis than those who are otherwise healthy, and the elderly survive serious injury less well than the young.

RECOMMENDED READING

Blunt trauma to the heart. Editorial. Lancet 2:724, 1986.

Carrico CJ: Pulmonary response to injury. Bull NY Acad Med 55:174, 1979.

Eichelberger AAR, Randolph JG: Thoracic trauma in children. Surg Clin North Am 61:1181, 1981.

Estrera AS, Platt MR, Mills LJ: Traumatic diseases of the pleura. In Chrétien J, Hirsch A (eds): Diseases of the Pleura. New York, Masson Publishers, 1983, p. 301.

Estrera AS, Platt MR, Mills LJ: Traumatic injuries of the diaphragm. Chest 75:306, 1979.

Goodman LR, Putman CE: The SICU chest radiograph after massive blunt trauma. Radiol Clin North Am 19:111, 1981.

Gossling HR, Donohue TA: The fat embolism syndrome. JAMA 241:2740, 1979.

Guenter CA: Chest trauma. In Guenter CA, Welch MH (eds): Pulmonary Medicine. 2nd edition. Philadelphia, J. B. Lippincott Co., 1982, p. 511.

Kirsch MM, Sloan H: Blunt Chest Trauma: General Principles and Management. Boston, Little, Brown & Co., Inc., 1977.

Oreskovich MR, Carrico CJ: Trauma: management of the acutely injured patient. In Sabiston DC Jr (ed): Textbook of Surgery. 13th edition. Philadelphia, W. B. Saunders Co., 1986, p. 294.

Schonfeld SA, et al: Fat embolism prophylaxis with corticosteroids: a prospective study in high-risk patients. Ann Intern Med 99:438, 1983.

Shackford SR, Virgilio RW, Peters RM: Selective use of ventilator therapy in flail chest injury. J Thorac Cardiovasc Surg 81:194, 1981.

Shires GT (ed): Principles of Trauma Care. 3rd edition. New York, McGraw-Hill, Inc., 1985.

Wilson RF, Murray C, Antonenko DR: Nonpenetrating thoracic injuries. Surg Clin North Am 57:17, 1977.

Wiot JF: Tracheobronchial trauma. Semin Roentgenol 18:15, 1983.

29. Pneumothorax

David J. Pierson

Definition

Pneumothorax is defined as air in the pleural space. Simple, or primary, spontaneous pneumothorax occurs typically in slender young males and usually does not produce serious physiologic impairment; it is seldom seen in the intensive care unit (ICU). When spontaneous pneumothorax occurs in a patient with underlying pulmonary disease, it is known as secondary, or complicated pneumothorax, which may cause acute clinical deterioration and death. This condition responds less well to therapy than simple pneumothorax and is associated with more frequent complications.

Iatrogenic pneumothorax occurs when the lung is punctured during attempted subclavian vein catheterization or percutaneous lung aspiration, when a bronchus is perforated during transbronchial biopsy, other bronchoscopic procedures, or errant nasogastric tube insertion, or if the lung is overdistended during anesthesia, cardiopulmonary resuscitation, or mechanical ventilation. In chest injuries, traumatic pneumothorax may result from direct laceration or from alveolar rupture due to high momentary pressure gradients.

When pleural air accumulates under pressure—as when a flap of tissue permits air to enter the pleural space during deep breathing, coughing, or positive-pressure breaths but prevents it from leaving—a tension pneumothorax is created. Intrapleural pressures greater than 15–20 cm H_2O displace the mediastinum and compromise venous return to the heart, creating a true medical emergency that is rapidly fatal if not relieved. Tension pneumothorax can develop in each of the above settings but is rare in primary pneumothorax.

Pathophysiology

Several mechanisms can introduce air into the pleural space. Most common is the rupture of one or more alveoli, which allows air to enter the peribronchial interstitium and to dissect either distally to the visceral pleura or proximally to the hilum and then via the mediastinum into the pleural cavity. The second of these mechanisms is felt to be the usual one. Air may also enter from outside the body as a result of penetrating chest trauma or through a thoracentesis or pleural biopsy needle.

Perforation of the esophagus commonly leads to hydropneumothorax. Gas-forming bacteria in a pleural empyema may also produce enough air to create an air-fluid level on chest radiograph. In addition, free peritoneal or retroperitoneal air may occasionally dissect into the chest and produce a pneumothorax.

Pneumothorax during mechanical ventilation may be a manifestation of disease or it may be of iatrogenic origin. It is especially likely to occur in the adult respiratory distress syndrome (ARDS), in aspiration or necrotizing pneumonia, or in obstructive lung disease and is made more likely by right mainstem bronchial intubation and by the use of high tidal volumes. Alveolar rupture (barotrauma) is common in ARDS, in which positive end-expiratory pressure (PEEP) is used; whether this is due to the PEEP or to the underlying disease is unclear, but barotrauma may be more frequent when high peak lung inflation volumes are reached.

DIAGNOSIS

Pneumothorax typically produces sudden, sharp, pleuritic chest pain, which becomes a dull, continuous ache after several hours. This picture is most common in primary pneumothorax, and the diagnosis should also be considered when these symptoms appear following thoracentesis, central venous catheter insertion, or other procedure. Dyspnea occurs in primary or iatrogenic pneumothorax when it is large and in secondary pneumothorax of any size. Pneumothorax is one cause for acute respiratory distress in a patient receiving mechanical ventilation ("fighting the ventilator"), and clinicians must be attuned to this possibility.

The physical findings of pneumothorax are characteristic—diminished chest movement, tactile fremitus, and breath sounds, and increased percussion resonance on the side of the abnormality—but are often unimpressive, especially in acutely ill patients with injuries or other findings. Tension pneumothorax, on the other hand, typically presents dramatically, with severe dyspnea, tachypnea, tachycardia, hypotension, cyanosis, neck vein distention, and tracheal deviation away from the affected side, in addition to the findings previously mentioned.

On chest roentgenogram, the most definitive sign of pneumothorax is identification of the visceral pleural surface bordered by a hyperlucent area without lung markings. The diagnosis can be difficult in the presence of bullae or generalized emphysema, when there are skin folds, bedding, or other external material on the film, and when optimal technique cannot be used, as frequently occurs in the ICU.

Quantitation of a pneumothorax (e.g., "30 percent") is difficult and arbitrary, depending on the patient's position, on the point at which the film was taken between total lung capacity and residual volume, and on the subjective impression of the viewer.

Tension pneumothorax is diagnosed clinically rather than by roentgenogram; roentgenographic evidence of mediastinal deviation, reversal of the diaphragmatic curve, and enlargement of one hemithorax are characteristic but can occur without physiologically significant tension. In patients on mechanical ventilators, the sudden onset of respiratory distress, along with findings of subcutaneous emphysema, absent breath sounds on one side, and signs of mediastinal shift, should prompt immediate therapy without waiting for roentgenographic confirmation of the diagnosis.

MANAGEMENT

The goals of treatment for pneumothorax in any clinical setting are to relieve tension if present, to fully reexpand the lung, to stop any residual air leak, and to prevent recurrence. Tension pneumothorax is a true emergency, and if a thoracostomy tube is not immediately at hand, a large-bore needle should be inserted in an upper anterior or anterolateral intercostal space; this should always be followed by tube thoracostomy as soon as this can be accomplished.

Reexpansion of the affected lung will occur spontaneously, so long as no further air leakage occurs, but reabsorption can take many weeks, depending on how much air is in the pleural space. In the ICU, the only pneumothoraces that can safely be observed without treatment are small iatrogenic ones that cause no symptoms or physiologic compromise in patients not receiving mechanical ventilation.

Needle aspiration may be sufficient in many cases of primary and iatrogenic pneumothorax, and an intracath connected to a Heimlich (flutter) valve is also used by many clinicians in patients with these conditions in order to avoid the morbidity of tube thoracostomy. However, most pneumothoraces encountered in the ICU should be drained with a chest tube: This is mandatory in traumatic and secondary pneumothoraces, no matter how small. Management of chest tubes and their drainage systems is discussed in Chapter 38.

Venting the chest to water seal may be sufficient; the question of whether additional chest tube suction is beneficial is unsettled: its use is routine in most American hospitals but rare in Britain. Suction (10–20 cm H_2O) should be applied if the lung fails to expand fully with water seal.

The initial bronchopleural air leak following spontaneous, iatrogenic, or traumatic pneumothorax usually seals spontaneously in 1 to several days after the lung has been fully reexpanded. Measures to diminish the leak and to facilitate its closure when this does not occur are discussed in Chapter 30.

Primary spontaneous pneumothorax recurs in 40–50 percent of individuals. Once there has been a second episode, more than 60 percent of patients have a third, and without specific therapy, 80 percent will suffer a fourth. Although experienced clinicians disagree about the timing of specific therapy to prevent recurrence, this is most comonly undertaken after the second episode.

Therapeutic measures to close the pleural space and prevent recurrence include chemical pleurodesis (injection of a drug or other foreign substance into the pleural cavity to produce inflammation and subsequent adhesions), and surgical abrasion or ablation of the pleural tissues. Tetracycline (20 mg/kg) is the drug of choice for pleurodesis. Although it may be innocuous in malignant pleural effusion, tetracycline causes severe pain when administered for recurrent pneumothorax and must be given with either local (150 mg lidocaine in 50 ml volume 10 min before the tetracycline) or systemic (ketamine 0.2–0.75 mg/kg IV) analgesia.

The tetracycline is suspended in 50 ml fluid and injected through the chest tube into the pleural cavity; some clinicians follow this with an additional 50 ml to rinse in any drug adhering to the tube. The chest tube is then clamped for 2 hours. Turning the patient to various positions during this period may facilitate intrapleural distribution of the drug, after which the chest tube is unclamped and connected to 20 cm H_2O suction.

Current surgical therapy to prevent recurrent pneumothorax consists of thoracotomy with abrasion of the visceral pleura using a gauze sponge; this produces inflammation and adhesions, which render the two pleural surfaces inseparable. Parietal pleurectomy, a more extensive procedure, is now used less often than previously. Operative treatment is necessary if chemical pleurodesis fails, if the lung cannot be reexpanded, or if leakage of air persists for more than 7–10 days after spontaneous pneumothorax. Surgery may be necessary earlier in airline pilots, professional divers, and those who live in remote areas than in other patients.

OUTCOME

Conservative measures suffice in the great majority of cases of simple and spontaneous pneumothorax and in iatrogenic pneumothorax when mechanical ventilation is not required. Secondary spontaneous pneumothorax responds less well to treatment and is more often associated with recurrence, persistent air leak, failure of the lung to reexpand, and empyema. In trauma and ARDS, the mortality and morbidity are mainly those of the primary disorder; in ARDS, persistent bronchopleural air leak is a marker for high mortality.

RECOMMENDED READING

Black LF: The pleural space and pleural fluid. Mayo Clin Proc 47:493, 1972.

Chiles C, Ravin CE: Radiographic recognition of pneumothorax in the intensive care unit. Crit Care Med 14:677, 1986.

DeMeester TR, Lafontaine E: The pleura. In Sabiston DC Jr, Spencer FC (eds): Gibbon's Surgery of the Chest. 4th edition. Philadelphia, W.B. Saunders Co., 1983, p. 361.

DeVries WC, Wolfe WG: The management of spontaneous pneumothorax and bullous emphysema. Surg Clin North Am 60:851, 1980.

Dines DE, Payne WS, Bernatz PE: Pneumothorax. In Chrétien J, Hirsch A (eds): Diseases of the Pleura. New York, Masson Publishers, 1983, p. 342.

Jenkinson SG: Pneumothorax. Clin Chest Med 6:153, 1985.

Kernodle DS, DiRaimondo CR, Fulkerson WJ: Re-expansion pulmonary edema after pneumothorax. South Med J 77:318, 1984.

Pavlin DJ, et al: Re-expansion hypotension: a complication of rapid evacuation of prolonged pneumothorax. Chest 89:70, 1986.

Pierson DJ: Pneumomediastinum. In Murray JF, Nadel JA (eds): Textbook of Respiratory Medicine. Philadelphia, W. B. Saunders Co., 1988.

Riordan JF: Management of spontaneous pneumothorax. Br Med J (Clin Res) 289:71, 1984.

Rohlfing BM, Webb WR, Schlobohm RM: Ventilator-related extraalveolar air in adults. Radiology 121:25, 1976.

Simple aspiration of pneumothorax. Editorial. Lancet 1:434, 1984.

So S, Yu D: Catheter drainage of spontaneous pneumothorax: suction or no suction; early or late removal? Thorax 37:46, 1982.

Stephenson LW: Treatment of pneumothorax with intrapleural tetracycline. Chest 88:803, 1985.

Weeden D, Smith GH: Surgical experience in the management of spontaneous pneumothorax. Thorax 38:737, 1983.

30. Bronchopleural Fistula

David J. Pierson

DEFINITION

Air commonly continues to leak into the pleural space after placement of a chest tube in treatment of pneumothorax, although these leaks usually stop spontaneously in hours to a few days as the injury heals. When they do not, the condition is known as persistent bronchopleural air leak, or bronchopleural fistula (BPF). The latter term also applies to spontaneously developing communications between the airways and the pleural space, as seen in malignancy, tuberculosis, and suppurative lung infections, or when a bronchial stump breaks down following pulmonary resection.

BPF is a particularly troublesome problem when it occurs during mechanical ventilation. In this setting, BPF can result in incomplete lung expansion, the loss of part of each delivered tidal volume, inability to maintain positive end-expiratory pressure (PEEP), factitious ventilator cycling, and acute respiratory acidosis. Continued leakage of air may also spread bacteria from the upper airways, with resultant pleural infection.

PATHOPHYSIOLOGY

During positive-pressure ventilation, high airway pressures and suction through the chest tube conspire to perpetuate the air leak by maintaining a high pressure gradient between bronchus and pleural cavity. Anything that tends to augment this gradient will thus increase the leak and, presumably, delay closure of the fistula; such factors include a prolonged inspiratory phase, end-inspiratory pause, large tidal volumes, high levels of PEEP, expiratory retard, and excessive suction pressures.

Gas that passes through the airways and out through a BPF during mechanical ventilation is not simply wasted, as might be supposed. Studies have shown that, at least in the adult respiratory distress syndrome (ARDS), the leaked gas does participate in gas exchange. When carbon dioxide (CO_2) production is measured in this setting for metabolic assessment or to determine the cause of a high minute ventilation, it is important to collect gas from the chest tube as well as from the endotracheal tube. Unlike in the case of CO_2 production, however, dead-space ventilation (VD/VT) may be determined accurately in ARDS using expired gas collection and arterial PCO_2 measurement and does not require collecting leaked gas.

DIAGNOSIS

By definition, BPF during mechanical ventilation is present whenever gas continues to bubble from the chest tube 24 hours or more after its insertion. The diagnosis is also readily apparent in most other settings, such as suppurative pneumonia with pyopneumothorax and postpneumonectomy break-down of the bronchial stump.

A characteristic physical finding in BPF is the "leak squeak," a unique sound heard when auscultating over the site of the leak while the patient performs a Valsalva maneuver. Large leaks produce a low-pitched squeak, smaller leaks a higher-pitched sound. The "leak squeak" has been used to localize a BPF during sequential occlusion of individual bronchi with the bronchoscope; when the involved bronchus is plugged, the squeaking noise diminishes sharply or ceases. Radionuclides have also been used successfully to localize air leaks.

How much gas is lost through a BPF during mechanical ventilation may be estimated in several ways, the simplest but the least accurate of which is to observe each inspiratory burst of bubbles through the water seal of the collection system. For leaks in excess of 100–200 ml/breath, the difference between inspired and exhaled tidal volume, measured at the endotracheal tube with a hand-held spirometer, gives clinically acceptable quantitation.

More precise, direct measurement can be achieved by collecting the leaked gas in a large spirometer under the same suction pressure as that used in the collection system or by placing a pneumotachograph in-line in the pleural collection system. This is the only accurate means of quantitating leaks of less than about 2 L/min, although portable hand-held spirometers such as the Wright Respirometer and the Bourns LS–75 are acceptably accurate for larger leaks.

One commercial pleural drainage unit incorporates a compound bubble chamber that is calibrated to indicate leak volume. This is of little clinical help, however, because it registers only instantaneous leak flow at a given moment, while virtually all leaks are pulsatile with the respiratory cycle.

Some quantitation of the air leak can be helpful in adjusting ventilator settings and performing other maneuvers in an attempt to minimize the leak, as discussed below. It can also help to track the progression and healing of the lesion, although such measurements need not be of laboratory precision.

Regardless of the quantity of gas leaked from a BPF, whether it constitutes a threat to the patient in the short run is assessed physiologically, using arterial blood gases and other measures of the adequacy of tissue oxygenation and alveolar ventilation. Even a leak of several hundred ml/breath poses no acute threat to the patient so long as oxygenation and CO_2 removal are adequate, the latter indicated not so much by the arterial PCO_2 value but by an arterial pH greater than about 7.30.

MANAGEMENT

The basic goals of management for BPF during mechanical ventilation are to maintain adequate gas exchange, to keep the lungs fully expanded, and to minimize the pressure gradient between the airways and the chest tube. These are primarily supportive measures undertaken while the underlying pulmonary process improves.

A number of exotic and sometimes hazardous measures have been used in attempts to decrease leak size, and the literature contains many anecdotal (and typically very short-term) accounts of success. The most widely used of these measures has been high-frequency jet ventilation, but they also include applying PEEP to the chest tube, occluding the chest tube during the ventilator's inspiratory cycle, synchronized or asynchronous independent lung ventilation using a double-lumen endotracheal tube, and various attempts to plug the leak directly.

However, in the largest reported series to date, only 2 of 39 patients seen during a 4-year period developed respiratory acidosis (pH <7.30) that could not be controlled with manipulations of conventional ventilator

TABLE 30–1. MANAGEMENT OF PERSISTENT BRONCHOPLEURAL AIR LEAK DURING MECHANICAL VENTILATION

1. Use the lowest number of mechanical breaths compatible with adequate ventilation (spontaneous ventilation if possible; IMV at a low rate is preferable to continuous ventilation).
2. Reduce effective (returned) tidal volume to 10 ml/kg or less.
3. Minimize inspiratory time (keep I:E low; high inspiratory flow rate; no inflation hold).
4. Avoid expiratory retard.
5. Avoid or minimize PEEP.
6. Use the lowest effective chest tube suction.
7. Explore positional differences.
8. Sedate patient, with or without paralysis, if spontaneous movements accentuate the leak.
9. Treat the underlying cause of respiratory failure, while maintaining nutritional and respiratory care support.

IMV = intermittent mandatory ventilation; I:E = ratio of inspiration to expiration; PEEP = positive end-expiratory pressure.

Reproduced, with permission, from Luce JM, Tyler ML, Pierson DJ: Intensive Respiratory Care. Philadelphia, W.B. Saunders Co., 1984, p. 170.

settings. Situations demanding experimental or other unconventional measures for controlling BPF are thus rare, and management should therefore focus on adjustments in customary ventilator care, as summarized in Table 30–1. Only when these measures fail to maintain physiologically acceptable oxygenation and alveolar ventilation should other techniques such as high-frequency jet ventilation be tried.

Persistent BPF following spontaneous pneumothorax in patients who do not require ventilatory assistance may respond favorably to chemical pleurodesis with tetracycline, as discussed in Chapter 29, providing the lung is fully reexpanded. BPF in tuberculosis usually occurs in patients with other debilitating conditions requiring prolonged chest tube drainage in addition to multiple-drug chemotherapy. Operative procedures may be necessary to establish complete drainage.

Postpneumonectomy BPF has a substantial mortality, and its surgical management is difficult. If stump breakdown occurs very early in the postoperative period, reexploration and direct repair may be successful. Later in the course, however, more extensive procedures such as the interposition of pedicle flaps of omentum or muscle may be necessary, and prolonged pleural drainage is often required.

OUTCOME

It is not known whether development of a BPF in and of itself worsens the prognosis of acute respiratory failure, but this complication identifies a group of patients whose in-hospital mortality is very high—on the order of 67 per cent. When the leak complicates trauma, the outlook is more favorable than in other conditions, especially ARDS. Development of an air leak late in the course of respiratory failure indicates a particularly bad prognosis, as do very large leaks (>500 ml/breath).

In general, resolution of BPF parallels the course of the underlying acute respiratory failure. In ARDS particularly, healing of the leak is unlikely to occur until the general condition of the patient improves.

RECOMMENDED READING

Baldwin JC, Mark JBD: Treatment of bronchopleural fistula after pneumonectomy. J Thorac Cardiovasc Surg 90:813, 1985.

Benson MS, Bishop MJ, Pierson DJ: Determination of dead-space ventilation and CO_2 production in the presence of gas leak from bronchopleural fistula complicating ARDS. Respir Care 31:398, 1986.

Bishop MJ, Benson MS, Pierson DJ: Carbon dioxide excretion via bronchopleural fistulas in patients with adult respiratory distress syndrome. Chest 91:400, 1987.

Donath J, Khan FA: Tuberculous and post-tuberculous bronchopleural fistula: ten-year clinical experience. Chest 86:697, 1984.

Krumpe PE, Hadley J, Marcum RA: Evaluation of bronchial air leaks by auscultation and phonopneumography. Chest 85:777, 1984.

Larson RP, Capps JS, Pierson DJ: A comparison of three devices used for quantitating bronchopleural air leak. Respir Care 31:1065, 1986.

Lillington, T, Stevens R, DeNardo G: Bronchoscopic location of broncho-pleural fistula with xenon-133. J Nucl Med 23:322, 1982.

Lowe RE, et al: Scintimaging of bronchopleural fistula: a simple method of diagnosis. Clin Nucl Med 9:10, 1984.

Pierson DJ: Persistent bronchopleural air leak during mechanical ventilation. In Pierson DJ (ed): Respiratory Intensive Care. Dallas, Daedalus Press, 1986, p. 175.

Pierson DJ, Horton CA, Bates PW: Persistent bronchopleural air leak during mechanical ventilation: a review of 39 cases. Chest 90:321, 1986.

Powner DJ, Grenvik A: Ventilatory management of life-threatening bronchopleural fistulae: a summary. Crit Care Med 9:54, 1981.

Ritz R, Benson M, Bishop MJ: Measuring gas leakage from bronchopleural fistulas during high-frequency jet ventilation. Crit Care Med 12:836, 1984.

Stephenson LW: Treatment of pneumothorax with intrapleural tetracycline. Chest 88:803, 1985.

Steiger Z, Wilson RF: Management of bronchopleural fistulas. Surg Gynecol Obstet 158:267, 1984.

31. Tuberculosis

David J. Pierson

Definition

Tuberculosis is a chronic bacterial infection caused by *Mycobacterium tuberculosis* and spread by the respiratory route. Clinical disease usually involves the lung, but the pleura, lymph nodes, central nervous system, and a variety of other tissues may be affected. Although commonly fatal if left untreated, tuberculosis can be clinically cured in the great majority of cases if appropriate antituberculous drugs are used and if they are taken correctly by the patient.

Other species of mycobacteria are common in the environment, and although they do not spread person-to-person, some can cause clinical disease. Among these, the one most important in critical care is *Mycobacterium avium-intracellulare*, which causes progressive pulmonary disease and frequently disseminates via the bloodstream in patients with suppressed cell-mediated immunity, particularly those with the acquired immunodeficiency syndrome (AIDS).

Pathophysiology

A person becomes infected with *M. tuberculosis* by inhaling the organism in the form of "droplet nuclei," particles consisting of tubercle bacilli exhaled in droplets by someone with active disease, the moisture in the droplets having evaporated. Deposited in the alveoli, the organisms proliferate, spread to the regional lymph nodes, and within several weeks disseminate hematogenously. In most instances, cell-mediated immunity to the organism develops at about this time. This makes the person tuberculin skin test reactive (PPD-positive), halts further bacterial replication, and prevents development of clinical disease, although living tubercle bacilli remain in many areas of the body.

Subsequently, often many years after the initial infection, cell-mediated immunity to tuberculosis may weaken, allowing the organisms to proliferate and clinical illness to develop. This sequence produces insidiously progressive, chronic disease, usually affecting the upper zones of the lungs. However, especially in immunocompromised patients, dissem-

193

inated, more clinically acute disease may develop, and deviation from the classic picture of pulmonary tuberculosis is common.

DIAGNOSIS

Tuberculosis produces highly variable symptoms, signs, and laboratory manifestations. The classic presentation of pulmonary tuberculosis consists of weeks or months of cough, hemoptysis, night sweats, and weight loss, along with cavitary upper-lobe infiltrates on chest roentgenogram. However, patients may present with many combinations of symptoms or with no symptoms at all, and the roentgenographic pattern may vary from subtle, streaky opacities in the lung apices to diffuse infiltrates or a generalized miliary pattern.

The diagnosis of tuberculosis requires demonstration of the organism on culture from sputum, other body fluids, or tissue. Because of the slow growth of *M. tuberculosis*, several weeks are required for confirmation of the diagnosis by conventional methods, and additional weeks are often necessary to establish sensitivities to antituberculous agents. However, the Bactec radiometric culture system, which permits detection of mycobacterial growth within 2–4 days in many cases, and by 5–6 days even when few organisms are present, is becoming more widely available. *M. tuberculosis* can be distinguished from other mycobacteria in another 3–5 days. This technique enables the suspected diagnosis of tuberculosis to be confirmed much earlier than in the past and greatly reduces the number of cases in which bronchoscopy or biopsy will be required.

Although not established with certainty, a strong presumptive diagnosis of active tuberculosis can be made if "acid-fast bacilli" can be demonstrated on special stains of sputum or other specimens. Techniques commonly used include the Ziehl-Neelsen stain or methods using fluorochrome dyes, auramine, or rhodamine.

MANAGEMENT

Isolation. Intensive care unit (ICU) patients with suspected active pulmonary or laryngeal tuberculosis should be placed in tuberculosis isolation: private room with special ventilation, if available, and mask if the patient is coughing without covering the mouth. Health care personnel should wear masks when entering the room if the patient cannot or will not cover the mouth when coughing or sneezing. Masks should be worn during collection of sputum and other specimens. Gowns and gloves are unnecessary.

Tuberculosis is not spread by ingesting the organism or by contact

TABLE 31–1. ANTITUBERCULOUS DRUGS

DRUG	BRAND NAME	USUAL DAILY DOSE	METHOD OF DELIVERY	TOXICITY
Isoniazid	INH, Nydrazid, others	300 mg (5 mg/kg)	Oral Intra-muscular	Hepatitis (0.5–2.0 percent); elevated transaminase (10 percent); peripheral neuropathy; rash; fever
Rifampin	Rifadin, Rimactane	600 mg	Oral	Hepatitis; influenzalike syndrome; thrombocytopenia
Streptomycin	—	0.75–1.0 g	Intra-muscular	Auditory nerve damage; vestibular nerve damage; nephrotoxicity
Ethambutol	Myambutol	15 mg/kg	Oral	Optic neuritis
Pyrazinamide	—	1.5–2.0 g (20–35 mg/kg)	Oral	Hepatitis; hyperuricemia
Ethionamide	Trecator-SC	1.0 g	Oral	Hepatitis
Cycloserine	Seromycin	1.0 g	Oral	Depression; psychosis; personality changes; convulsions
p-Aminosalicylic acid	Teebacin	12 g	Oral	Diarrhea; hepatitis; hypersensitivity reactions
Kanamycin	Kantrex	1.0 g	Intra-muscular	Auditory nerve damage; nephrotoxicity; vestibular nerve damage
Capreomycin	Capastat	1.0 g	Intra-muscular	Auditory nerve damage; vestibular nerve damage; nephrotoxicity

with clothing, dishes, or other objects. One cannot catch tuberculosis from ventilators, tubing, pulmonary function apparatus, or other respiratory care equipment.

Extrapulmonary nonlaryngeal tuberculosis poses little if any threat of person-to-person transmission. Patients with suspected pulmonary tuberculosis whose sputum is smear-negative on two or three examinations of good-quality specimens do not pose a significant infection threat to others, even if their cultures subsequently prove to be positive.

Chemotherapy. Because of the presence of small numbers of organisms that are naturally resistant to any individual drug, active tuberculosis must always be treated with at least two antituberculous drugs. Treatment must be continued for at least several months because of the organism's slow growth and long periods of inactivity. It was formerly taught that some forms of tuberculosis required treatment with three or more drugs, but today recommended treatment regimens for extrapulmonary tuberculosis no longer differ from those for pulmonary disease.

Table 31–1 lists the main antituberculous drugs currently in use, along with their daily dosages and main side effects. Isoniazid and rifampin, both of which are bactericidal, are the most potent agents available.

Streptomycin and the other "injectables" can only be given parenterally; isoniazid is available in intramuscular as well as oral form, but the other agents in Table 31–1 are available only as oral preparations.

The currently recommended drug regimen for initial treatment of tuberculosis consists of isoniazid (300 mg daily) and rifampin (600 mg daily) for 9–12 months. Several others are available, including short-course regimens, which are effective only under close patient supervision. At present, the recommended short-course schedule is to give four drugs (isoniazid [300 mg], rifampin [600 mg], pyrazinamide [2 g], and either streptomycin [1 g] or ethambutol [15 mg/kg]) daily for 2 months, followed by either isoniazid and rifampin daily for four months, or isoniazid, rifampin, and streptomycin twice weekly for 6 months, at the same doses as above. The last of these regimens is suited to closely supervised therapy for patients whose full compliance cannot be assured.

Patients with tuberculosis may require ICU admission because of miliary or meningeal disease, intravascular coagulation, hemoptysis, or severe reactions to drugs. More commonly, individuals with known or undiagnosed tuberculosis are admitted to the ICU because of other illness. Unless required for these or other reasons, hospitalization is unnecessary for management of tuberculosis in the presence of adequate chemotherapy. Once begun on appropriate drugs, inpatients with pulmonary tuberculosis become noninfectious to others after 7–10 days and can be taken out of isolation.

OUTCOME

With the drug regimens described above, cure can be achieved in at least 95 percent of otherwise healthy individuals with active tuberculosis. The most common reason for therapeutic failure is noncompliance with the drug regimen. Tuberculous meningitis has a worse prognosis than pulmonary and most other forms: Even with appropriate therapy, 10–20 percent of cases are fatal, and this increases to more than 50 percent if the patient is comatose at the onset of treatment.

RECOMMENDED READING

Addington WW, et al: Non-drug issues related to the treatment of tuberculosis. Chest 87(Suppl. 2):125S, 1985.

Bass JB, et al: American Thoracic Society, medical section of the American Lung Association: Treatment of tuberculosis and tuberculosis infection in adults and children. Am Rev Respir Dis 134:355, 1986.

Daniel TM: Tuberculosis. In Braunwald E, et al (Eds): Harrison's Principles of Internal Medicine. 11th edition. New York, McGraw-Hill, Inc., 1987, p. 625.

Dutt AK, Moers D, Stead WW: Short-course chemotherapy for extrapulmonary tuberculosis. Nine years' experience. Ann Intern Med 104:7, 1986.

Gangadharam PR: Isoniazid, rifampin, and hepatotoxicity. Am Rev Respir Dis 133:963, 1986.

Garner JS, Simmons BP: CDC guidelines for isolation precautions in hospitals. Infection Control 4(Suppl. 4):245, 1983.

Hawkins CC, et al: *Mycobacterium avium* complex infections in patients with the acquired immunodeficiency syndrome. Ann Intern Med 105:184, 1986.

Horsburgh CR Jr, et al: Disseminated infection with *Mycobacterium avium-intracellulare*: A report of 13 cases and a review of the literature. Medicine 64:36, 1985.

Katz I, Rosenthal T, Michaeli D: Undiagnosed tuberculosis in hospitalized patients. Chest 87:770, 1985.

Mandell GL, Sande MA: Drugs used in the chemotherapy of tuberculosis and leprosy. In Gilman AG, et al (Eds): Goodman and Gilman's The Pharmacological Basis of Therapeutics. 7th edition. New York, Macmillan Publishing Company, 1985, p. 1199.

Molavi A, LeFrock JL: Tuberculous meningitis. Med Clin North Am 69:315, 1985.

Neff TA: Bronchoscopy and Bactec for the diagnosis of tuberculosis. Am Rev Respir Dis 133:962, 1986.

Russell MD, Torrington KD, Tenholder MF: A ten-year experience with fiberoptic bronchoscopy for mycobacterial isolation. Impact of the Bactec system. Am Rev Respir Dis 133:1069, 1986.

Snider DE Jr, et al: Standard therapy for tuberculosis 1985. Chest 87(Suppl. 2):117S, 1985.

32. Respiratory Monitoring

David J. Pierson

INTRODUCTION

Respiratory monitoring is the continuous or repetitive performance of clinical observations or measurements pertaining to respiratory function during evaluation and management of critically ill patients. In this context, monitoring extends to the function of ventilators and other apparatus supporting respiration in addition to measurements made on patients. The general purposes of respiratory monitoring are listed in Table 32–1. Respiratory variables that can presently be monitored, directly and with reasonable accuracy and convenience, are shown in Table 32–2.

Although the recent explosion in monitoring technology has expanded the clinician's capabilities, it has also brought unnecessary cost, overuse, and the introduction of new "parameters" based not on physiologic need but on what can readily be measured electronically. The first principle of monitoring should be not to collect data or make measurements unless they are clinically needed. Except for vital signs, intake and output, and weight, monitoring of intensive care unit (ICU) patients should not be "routine." Instead, what is measured should be tailored to each patient's individual situation, with the type and frequency of assessments adjusted according to the clinical course.

The measurements listed in Table 32–2 are mainly noninvasive. They complement the more invasive monitoring techniques discussed in Chapter 15, which are also important in respiratory monitoring.

INDICATIONS AND CONTRAINDICATIONS

Any patient with a cardiorespiratory disorder who is sufficiently ill to require admission to the ICU needs close observation for the purposes listed in Table 32–1. However, which measurements to make and how frequently to make them should be determined by each patient's clinical condition rather than by technical capability. Collection of unnecessary data is not only wasteful of resources but also leads to further unnecessary measurements and unwise changes in management. Before looking at the

198

TABLE 32–1. PURPOSES OF RESPIRATORY MONITORING

1. To assess the adequacy of oxygenation and alveolar ventilation
2. To follow the course of acute respiratory illness
3. To assess the need for intubation and mechanical ventilation
4. To assess the performance of a mechanical ventilator or other support device and its effects on the patient
5. To detect readiness for, to predict success in, and to evaluate the outcome of ventilator weaning and extubation
6. To evaluate a patient's metabolic or nutritional state

results of monitoring measurements, the clinician should have in mind the reason for making them and how they will affect management.

TECHNIQUES

Oxygenation. The systemic arterial oxygen tension (PaO_2) is the "gold standard" for assessing arterial oxygenation. However, because for monitoring it requires either repeated arterial punctures or an indwelling arterial catheter, several techniques have been introduced as substitutes. Transcutaneous PO_2 is used for monitoring in neonates and may reflect arterial values in older patients who are hemodynamically stable, but it has not proved sufficiently reliable in critically ill adults to be used instead of repeated PaO_2 measurements. End-tidal expired oxygen monitoring, although easy to perform, does not reliably track arterial oxygenation,

TABLE 32–2. RESPIRATORY VARIABLES THAT CAN BE DIRECTLY AND CONVENIENTLY MONITORED IN PATIENTS IN THE INTENSIVE CARE UNIT

	CONTINUOUS	INTERMITTENT
Nonintubated Patient	Respiratory rate Tidal volume* SaO_2	Vital capacity and FEV_1 Maximum inspiratory force Minute ventilation Arterial blood gases Expired gases
Intubated, Spontaneously Breathing Patient	Respiratory rate Tidal volume SaO_2	Vital capacity Maximum inspiratory force Minute ventilation Arterial blood gases Inspired and expired gases
Intubated, Mechanically Ventilated Patient	Respiratory rate Tidal volume SaO_2 Peak and mean airway pressures Inspired and expired gases	Vital capacity Maximum inspiratory force Spontaneous and delivered minute ventilation Static airway pressures Arterial blood gases Inspired and expired gases

*Semiquantitative
SaO_2 = systemic arterial hemoglobin oxygen saturation

and direct tissue PO_2 measurements, although theoretically attractive, have not proved feasible for clinical monitoring.

Ear and finger oximetry are now widely available and can provide continuous measurements of systemic arterial oxygen saturation (SaO_2). Oximetry is most useful for detecting desaturation, as occurs during sleep, suctioning, activity, position changes, or transport, or for monitoring oxygenation in patients with PaO_2 values consistently below 60–65 mm Hg; because PaO_2 values higher than this fall on the flat portion of the hemoglobin saturation curve (see Fig. 1–1) and changes in them will not be reflected in changes in SaO_2, oximetry is less helpful for monitoring well-oxygenated patients.

How best to assess arterial oxygenation when the inspired oxygen fraction (FiO_2) varies is controversial. Calculation of right-to-left shunt (on $FiO_2 = 1.0$) or venous admixture (on $FiO_2 < 1.0$) is used routinely by some clinicians but can be cumbersome at the bedside and requires mixed venous blood and hence an indwelling pulmonary artery (Swan-Ganz) catheter. The alveolar-to-arterial PO_2 difference ($P[A-a]O_2$), calculated using the alveolar gas equation, usually requires an assumed rather than measured value for the respiratory quotient (R) but can also be used for this purpose. See Chapter 1 for further details.

More simple, and acceptably accurate for bedside use when FiO_2 is between 0.30 and 0.70, is the ratio PaO_2/FiO_2. For example, a PaO_2 of 80 mm Hg on an FiO_2 of 0.40 gives a PaO_2/FiO_2 ratio of 200 mm Hg, which suggests the same state of oxygenation as a PaO_2 of 120 mm Hg on an FiO_2 of 0.60. Some clinicians use the ratio PaO_2/PAO_2 for quick bedside assessment of impairment in arterial oxygenation, although estimating PAO_2 requires use of the alveolar gas equation and making an assumption about R.

Ventilation. Expired minute ventilation ($\dot{V}E$) can be measured directly using a bedside or hand-held spirometer via a mouthpiece or a connector to an endotracheal tube. Alveolar ventilation ($\dot{V}A$) cannot be measured directly but is reflected by the $PaCO_2$. When $\dot{V}E$ is elevated, the physiologic cause must be either alveolar hyperventilation, increased dead space ventilation (VD/VT), and/or increased CO_2 production ($\dot{V}CO_2$), and distinguishing among these is easily accomplished at the bedside. Expired gas is collected for 3 minutes in a large bag, simultaneous to the drawing of an arterial blood gas specimen. Alveolar hyperventilation is gauged by the severity of hypocapnia, and $\dot{V}CO_2$ is determined by the product of expired volume and mixed fraction of expired CO_2 ($F\bar{E}CO_2$). Dead space ventilation is calculated by the formula: $VD/VT = (PaCO_2 - P\bar{E}CO_2)/PaCO_2$, where $P\bar{E}CO_2$ is the PCO_2 in the mixed expired gas.

Transcutaneous PCO_2 measurements are subject to the same limitations as those of transcutaneous PO_2. They may be useful in some instances for following trends or in detecting acute changes, but they cannot be used in adult patients as the sole assessment of $\dot{V}A$. Expired CO_2 monitoring (capnography) is useful in the operating room and in certain other short-term settings. However, although end-tidal PCO_2 approximates $PaCO_2$ in normal individuals, this is not the case in the presence of high VD/VT, severe ventilation:perfusion ($\dot{V}A/\dot{Q}$) mismatching, or expiratory airflow limitation. Changes in these factors, as well as in $\dot{V}A$, can alter end-tidal PCO_2. Thus, patients with severe respiratory insufficiency of any etiology, and patients who are acutely unstable from either a cardiovascular or a respiratory standpoint, are not candidates for continuous end-tidal CO_2 monitoring as a primary surveillance technique.

Pulmonary–Chest Wall Mechanics. Tidal volume (VT) is difficult to measure meaningfully in nonintubated patients but can be monitored readily when an endotracheal tube is in place using a hand-held spirometer. Some ventilators and ventilation monitors calculate average VT by dividing $\dot{V}E$ by respiratory rate. Vital capacity (VC) can be determined in cooperative patients by use of either a mouthpiece or an endotracheal tube and a hand-held spirometer; an inspiratory capacity giving some indication of VC can be obtained in comatose or uncooperative patients who are intubated.

Maximum inspiratory force (MIF), an indicator of inspiratory muscle strength (though not necessarily of endurance), is measured by occluding the airway at end-expiration and using a pressure manometer to quantitate the patient's efforts to breathe in during a preset time period, usually 15 seconds or longer.

Compliance measures the change in pressure required to produce a given volume change: $C = \Delta V/\Delta P$. In the ICU, separation of lung from chest wall compliance is difficult, and the compliance of the total respiratory system is used. Dynamic respiratory system compliance (CDYN) is a measure of the maximum airway pressure (PMAX) required to deliver a given VT to a ventilated patient minus the amount of PEEP also used to expand the lungs: $CDYN = VT/(PMAX - PEEP)$. PMAX and CDYN reflect the resistance in airways and ventilator tubing as well as the compliance characteristics of the patient's lungs and chest wall.

Static respiratory system compliance (CSTAT) is a measure of the airway pressure (PSTAT) required to hold the lungs and chest wall at end-inspiration. PSTAT is determined by momentarily preventing exhalation after delivery of a ventilator breath. The amount of PEEP being used should again be subtracted: $CSTAT = VT/(PSTAT - PEEP)$. A normal value is 60–90 ml/cm H_2O. Because they are made in the absence of gas flow, measurements of PSTAT and CSTAT reflect only the compliance of the lungs and chest wall and are not affected by airway resistance.

Although single measurements of compliance provide some information, serial determinations are more clinically helpful. Plotting PDYN or PSTAT against different VTs can help to detect changes in airway resistance, pneumothorax, and other clinical events and can also assist in selecting the best V_T to use in a given patient. Serial determination of C_{STAT} during a PEEP trial (see Chapter 35) can help to avoid alveolar rupture.

Ventilators of recent manufacture can provide numerous other "indices" and "parameters" of ventilatory mechanics, although these sometimes reflect what can be measured rather than what is physiologically needed; which of these devices will prove to be of real help in patient management remains to be established.

Respiratory Muscle Function. Although the function of the diaphragm and other respiratory muscles is now known to be crucially important in ventilatory management and acute respiratory failure, reliable, convenient monitoring by techniques that are applicable clinically in the ICU has been slow to come. Maximum inspiratory force, VC, and maximum voluntary ventilation are rough assessments that can be made intermittently. Asynchronous movement of the thorax and abdomen during spontaneous breathing is a sign of inspiratory muscle fatigue, and can be observed at the bedside. Respiratory inductive plethysmography using the Respitrace has been done in some centers for noninvasive, semiquantitative monitoring of V_T and breathing pattern.

COMPLICATIONS

Respiratory monitoring is mainly noninvasive and so carries less risk of complications than does hemodynamic monitoring (see Chapter 15).

RECOMMENDED READING

Bone RC: Monitoring respiratory function in patients with the adult respiratory distress syndrome. Semin Respir Med 2:140, 1981.

Bone RC: Monitoring ventilatory mechanics in acute respiratory failure. Respir Care 28:597, 1983.

Clemmer TP, Gardner RM: Data gathering, analysis, and display in critical care medicine. Respir Care 30:586, 1985.

Dantzker DR, Gutierrez G: Assessment of tissue oxygenation. Respir Care 30:456, 1985.

Dantzker DR, Tobin MJ: Monitoring respiratory muscle function. Respir Care 30:422, 1985.

Fallat RJ: Respiratory monitoring. Clin Chest Med 3:181, 1982.

Gonzalez H, et al: Accuracy of respiratory inductive plethysmograph over wide range of rib cage and abdominal compartmental contributions to tidal volume in normal subjects and in patients with chronic obstructive pulmonary disease. Am Rev Respir Dis 130:171, 1984.

Gottfried SB, et al: Noninvasive monitoring during mechanical ventilation. Am Rev Respir Dis 131:414, 1985.

Hudson LD: Diagnosis and management of acute respiratory distress in patients on mechanical ventilators. In Moser KM, Spragg RG (eds): Respiratory Emergencies. 2nd edition. St. Louis, C.V. Mosby Co., 1982 p. 201.

Hudson LD: Monitoring critically ill patients: Conference summary. Respir Care 30:628, 1985.

Luce JM, Tyler ML, Pierson DJ: Intensive respiratory care. Philadelphia, W.B. Saunders Co., 1984, p. 240.

Marini JJ, Rodriguez RM, Lamb V: Bedside estimation of the inspiratory work of breathing during mechanical ventilation. Chest 89:56, 1986.

Neff TA: Monitoring alveolar ventilation and respiratory gas exchange. Respir Care 30:413, 1985.

Thorson SH, et al: Variability of arterial blood gas values in stable patients in the ICU. Chest 84:14, 1983.

33. Endotracheal Intubation

David J. Pierson

INTRODUCTION

Airway management is one of the basic clinical components of critical care medicine. It requires not only good manual skills but also a clear understanding of the physiology, indications, and hazards of endotracheal intubation.

INDICATIONS

The five indications for intubation are (1) to provide a closed system for mechanical ventilation and/or therapy with positive end-expiratory pressure; (2) to deliver a higher inspired oxygen fraction (FIO_2), with greather reliability during transport or patient agitation, than can be achieved with nasal cannulae or masks; (3) to relieve or bypass upper airway obstruction; (4) to safeguard the airway against aspiration of gastric contents; and (5) to facilitate tracheobronchial toilet when secretions are excessive or unusually thick or in patients whose cough mechanism is impaired. Of these, the last two are often difficult to translate into clinical practice, as there are no objective guidelines for either assessment of risk or effectiveness of therapy.

Intubation is an integral part of cardiopulmonary resuscitation and is obviously indicated for patients who are not spontaneously breathing. However, adequate airway protection, alveolar ventilation, and arterial oxygenation can nearly always be maintained using correct positioning, an oral airway, and bag-and-mask ventilation in such situations, at least for the few minutes required to summon an anesthetist or other person experienced in intubation. Hurried attempts to establish an airway by those unskilled in the procedure often result in more harm than good to the patient.

CONTRAINDICATIONS

Relative contraindications to endotracheal intubation include cervical spine injury (proven or potential), immobilization of the cervical spine

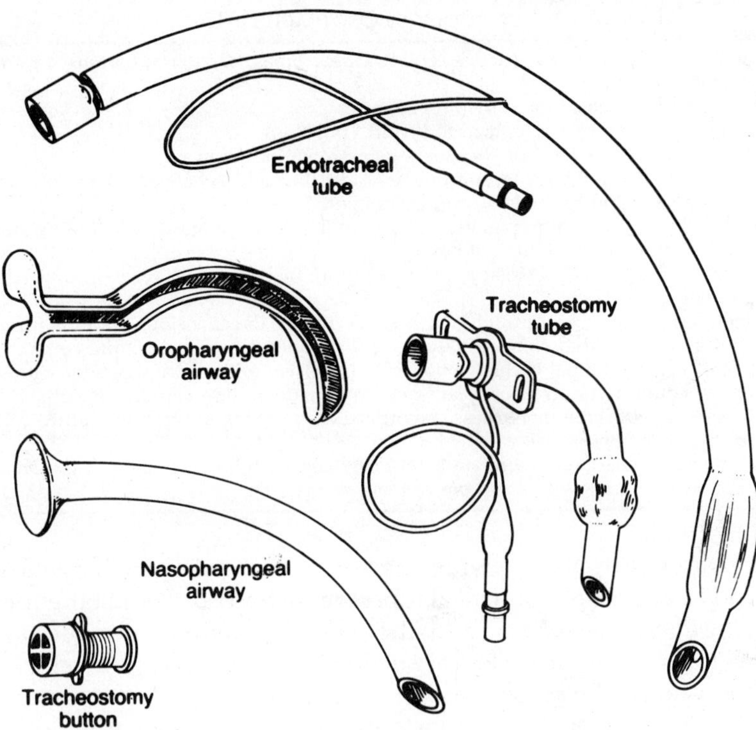

FIGURE 33–1. Five frequently used artificial airways. For further explanation, see text. (Reproduced, with permission, from Luce JM, Tyler ML, Pierson DJ: Intensive Respiratory Care. Philadelphia, W. B. Saunders Co., 1984, p. 112.)

(halo, cast, tongs, or other appliances; arthritis or ankylosis), and inability to open the mouth (mandibular fracture or wiring; muscle spasm as in convulsion, trismus, or tetanus; temporomandibular joint abnormalities). It may be technically impossible to intubate the upper airway in the presence of mechanical obstruction (foreign body, tumor, edema), severe maxillofacial trauma, bilateral vocal cord paralysis or laryngospasm, or laryngeal or subglottic stenosis from previous intubation, in which cases tracheostomy may be required. Similarly, loose or excessively carious teeth, dental prostheses that are difficult to remove, anatomic abnormalities such as micrognathia or macroglossia, and a history of difficulty on previous intubation make the procedure relatively contraindicated.

TECHNIQUES

Several types of airway devices are commonly used (Fig. 33–1). Those that occupy the nose and mouth without passing the vocal cords include

TABLE 33–1. TECHNIQUE OF OROTRACHEAL INTUBATION

1. Assemble equipment: laryngoscope, endotracheal tubes, suction apparatus, oral airway or bite block, and tape.
2. Position the patient appropriately (Fig. 33–2*A*):
   a) Lift angles of jaw and extend neck ("sniff" position);
   b) Elevate head above level of shoulders using towel or pillow.
3. Using the left hand, insert laryngoscope blade through right side of mouth, moving tongue anteriorly and to the left; identify epiglottis.
4. Lift mandible, tongue, and epiglottis anteriorly (curved laryngoscope blade tip proximal to epiglottis, straight blade tip just beyond epiglottis), to expose epiglottis and arytenoids (as shown in Fig. 33–2*B*). Pressure on cricothyroid helps to bring cords into view and to seal esophagus.
5. Insert endotracheal tube through vocal cords under direct vision, starting from right corner of mouth to avoid obscuring view, and advance tube 5 cm beyond cords.
6. Inflate cuff using minimal occlusive volume, and listen with stethoscope over lungs and stomach to confirm endotracheal placement and bilateral lung ventilation.
7. Secure airway with tape or harness, recording cm marking at teeth for future reference and adjustment if necessary.
8. Obtain portable chest roentgenogram to verify correct tube placement. Tube should be pulled back if its tip is within 3–4 cm of main carina.

the oropharyngeal airway, which serves to maintain oropharyngeal patency and to protect endotracheal tubes, bronchoscopes, and other devices passed through the mouth; and the nasopharyngeal "trumpet," which can greatly facilitate nasotracheal suctioning. Endotracheal tubes traverse the larynx and can be passed through either mouth or nose or occasionally through a tracheostomy. Tracheostomy tubes come in a variety of styles; Figure 33–1 shows a polyvinyl chloride tube with low-pressure, high-volume cuff, which is generally used in the intensive care unit.

A tracheostomy button is a short, straight cannula that extends from the skin to the anterior surface of the trachea, used to maintain stomal patency as an intermediate step during decannulation, or for patients requiring only intermittent (e.g., nocturnal) ventilatory support. It cannot be used for mechanical ventilation and is less than optimal as a route for suctioning.

Orotracheal intubation is preferable to the nasotracheal route for emergent intubation. Larger tubes can be passed through the mouth than through the nose, thus permitting better suctioning and also fiberoptic bronchoscopy if needed (which requires a tube of 8.0 mm ID or greater) as well as decreasing the patient's work of breathing. However, oral tubes are more uncomfortable, more difficult to stabilize, and interfere more with oral hygiene than do nasotracheal tubes.

Table 33–1 outlines the procedure for orotracheal intubation, and Figure 33–2 illustrates the proper position and glottic landmarks for its correct performance. It is crucial that the operator remain calm during the procedure. If the patient is awake and time permits, atropine (0.6 mg IM) and topical anesthesia with nebulized lidocaine should be given; sedation and paralysis may be necessary if the patient is agitated.

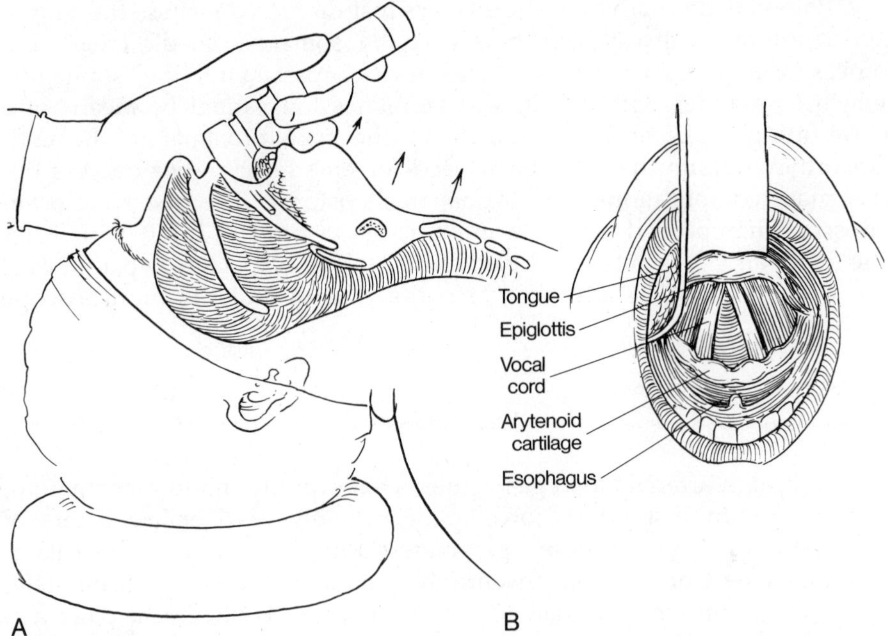

FIGURE 33–2. *A*, Orotracheal intubation, using a curved laryngoscope blade. The blade's tip is placed between the base of the tongue and the epiglottis. (When a straight blade is used, its tip is advanced beyond the base of the tongue, over the epiglottis, so that both are lifted in the direction of the arrows.) *B*, Operator's view of patient's airway, showing the primary landmarks, prior to insertion of the endotracheal tube.

For the initial attempt, a tube of 8.5 or 9.0 mm ID for average-sized men and 8.0 mm for women should be used. If a stylette is employed, it must not be allowed to extend beyond the distal end of the tube. The initial intubation attempt should not be prolonged beyond about 1 minute; if it is unsuccessful, the tube should be withdrawn and adequate ventilation and oxygenation reestablished using bag and mask before another attempt is made.

Nasotracheal tubes are less uncomfortable for the patient but are harder to insert than orotracheal tubes. Smaller in diameter and longer, nasal tubes create more airway resistance, and make suctioning more difficult and less effective than oral tubes. Tracheostomy permits normal oral hygiene, and enables patients to eat and, in some instances, to speak. It eliminates the risk of laryngeal injury (unless the patient has already had a long endotracheal intubation) but is also a surgical procedure, and carries a higher overall complication rate than the other forms of intubation. Whenever possible, tracheostomy should be performed in the operating room, over an endotracheal tube.

Potential alternatives to the airways just discussed include the esophageal obturator airway, which is used by some paramedic crews and others for temporary intubation. This device is passed into the esophagus, which it occludes with a cuff, and ventilates the patient by means of a close-fitting mask and perforations in the tube proximal to the cuff. Cricothyroidotomy has also been used for emergency airway access but has more complications than formal tracheostomy. The fiberoptic bronchoscope has proved useful in many cases of difficult intubation: After the lower airway is entered, the endotracheal tube, previously placed over the bronchoscope, is advanced into the trachea and the bronchoscope withdrawn.

EXTUBATION

Although arterial blood gas values, vital capacity, minute ventilation, and maximum inspiratory force are commonly used as predictors of successful extubation, these "parameters" in fact pertain to ventilator weaning (see Chapter 35), an entirely separate process. Unfortunately, there are at present no analogous tests to predict whether a patient is ready for extubation. In general, extubation (or decannulation, in the case of tracheostomy) is appropriate when the original indication for intubation has resolved and the patient is otherwise stable.

Extubation should be an elective procedure, performed when adequate personnel and equipment are available in case reintubation becomes necessary. The longer the patient has been intubated, the more carefully the appropriate time must be selected; such extubation attempts should not be undertaken in the middle of the night.

Supplemental oxygen is administered by nasal cannulae, and the trachea and oropharynx are cleared of secretions, using suction. The extubation sequence is explained to the patient. After the patient takes or is given a deep breath, the tube cuff is rapidly deflated and the tube quickly withdrawn while the patient coughs or exhales forcefully. Adequacy of ventilation is assessed by physical examination, and oxygenation is checked using oximetry or an arterial blood gas measurement within 15–30 minutes. The patient should not be left unattended until it is clinically evident that reintubation will not be required.

COMPLICATIONS

Both endotracheal intubation and tracheostomy bypass the mechanical defenses of the upper airway, grossly contaminate it, and remove its natural humidification system. Intubated patients are thus vulnerable to

TABLE 33–2. COMPLICATIONS OF ENDOTRACHEAL INTUBATION, TRACHEOSTOMY, AND ARTIFICIAL AIRWAYS

ENDOTRACHEAL TUBE	TRACHEOSTOMY
During Intubation Patient discomfort Trauma (dental; facial; naso- or oropharynx) Esophageal intubation Laryngeal trauma; laryngospasm Intubation of right main stem bronchus (atelectasis; barotrauma) Hypoxemia Dysrhythmias; cardiac arrest Cervical spine/cord injury	*During Tracheostomy* Hemorrhage Injury to thyroid or recurrent laryngeal nerve Pneumothorax; subcutaneous and mediastinal emphysema Tracheoesophageal fistula Dysrhythmias; cardiac arrest
While Tube is in Place Patient discomfort Mechanical problems (tube; cuff) Laryngeal injury Hemorrhage Tracheal injury (cuff; tube tip) Necrosis of nose, lip, or gum Sinusitis; otitis media Pneumonia; sepsis Self-extubation	*While Tracheostomy is in Place* Patient discomfort Mechanical problems (tube; cuff) Hemorrhage Tracheal injury (cuff; tube tip) Pneumothorax; subcutaneous and mediastinal emphysema Pneumonia; sepsis Self-decannulation
During Extubation Patient discomfort Laryngospasm; laryngeal edema Glottic injury Aspiration Dysrhythmias; cardiac arrest	*During Decannulation* Patient discomfort Difficult removal Dysrhythmias; cardiac arrest
After Extubation Hoarseness; vocal cord paralysis Dysphagia; aspiration Laryngeal stenosis; granuloma Tracheal stenosis (site of cuff or tube tip) Tracheomalacia	*After Decannulation* Cutaneous scar; keloid Persistent stoma tract Dysphagia; aspiration Tracheal stenosis (site of cuff, tube tip, or stoma) Tracheomalacia

Adapted, with permission, from Stauffer JL, Silvestri RC: Respir Care 27:417, 1982.

aspiration of mouth and gastric contents, nosocomial pneumonia and sepsis, and inspissation of respiratory tract secretions. In addition, a large number of other complications, many of them potentially fatal, are associated with intubation, tracheostomy, and the use of artificial airways (Table 33–2).

RECOMMENDED READING

Applebaum EL, Bruce DL: Tracheal intubation. Philadelphia, WB Saunders Co., 1976.

Demers RR: Management of the airway in the perioperative period. Respir Care 29:529, 1984.

Dunkin LJ: How to intubate. Br J Hosp Med 23:77, 1980.

Fluck RR Jr, et al: The esophageal obturator airway—a review. Respir Care 27:1373, 1982.

Kastendieck J: Airway management. In Rosen P, et al (eds): Emergency Medicine: Concepts and Clinical Practice. St. Louis, CV Mosby Co., 1983, p. 26.

Luce JM, Tyler ML, Pierson DJ: Intensive Respiratory Care. Philadelphia, WB Saunders Co., 1984, p. 111.

Pierson DJ (ed): Respiratory Intensive Care. Dallas, Daedalus Press (Am Assoc Respir Care), 1986.

Rosenbaum SH, et al: Use of the fiber-optic bronchoscope to change endotracheal tubes in critically ill patients. Anesthesiology 54:169, 1981.

Shapiro BA, et al: Clinical Application of Respiratory Care. 3rd edition. Chicago, Year Book Medical Publishers, Inc., 1985, p. 213.

Stauffer JL, Silvestri RC: Complications of endotracheal intubation, tracheostomy, and artificial airways. Respir Care 27:417, 1982.

Taryle DA, et al: Emergency room intubations—complications. Chest 75:541, 1979.

34. Supplemental Oxygen Therapy

David J. Pierson

Introduction

As described in Chapter 1, tissue oxygenation may be inadequate because of failure of ventilation, arterial oxygenation, oxygen transport, or tissue oxygen uptake. Impairment in oxygenation of arterial blood is the most frequently encountered of these disorders and may itself result either from low systemic arterial oxygen tension (PaO_2) (due either to low fractional inspired oxygen [FIO_2] or to inadequate oxygen uptake by the lungs) or from other causes of low arterial oxygen content (CaO_2). Although commonly due to hypoxemia (low PaO_2), inadequate CaO_2 can also exist despite normal PaO_2 if there is insufficient available hemoglobin for carrying of oxygen in the blood (Fig. 34–1). Failure of oxygen transport may be due to low CaO_2 or to low cardiac output ($\dot{Q}T$). It should be apparent that supplemental oxygen therapy can correct only some instances of inadequate oxygenation, specifically those characterized by a low PaO_2.

This chapter covers oxygen administration by nasal prongs, masks, and endotracheal tubes during spontaneous ventilation. Positive end-expiratory pressure (PEEP) therapy, with or without mechanical ventilation, another key modality in the treatment of inadequate oxygenation, is discussed in Chapter 36.

Indications

Oxygen is a potent, potentially hazardous, expensive drug. It should be administered only when clearly indicated, and its effects must be monitored appropriately. The chief indication for supplemental oxygen is hypoxemia. Figure 34–1 shows how rapidly arterial oxygen saturation (SaO_2), and hence CaO_2, drops off as PaO_2 falls progressively below 50–55 mm Hg and also illustrates why a PaO_2 value of less than 50 mm Hg is commonly used to define acute failure of oxygenation. From the same curve, it is evident that hypoxemia can largely be corrected if PaO_2 can be

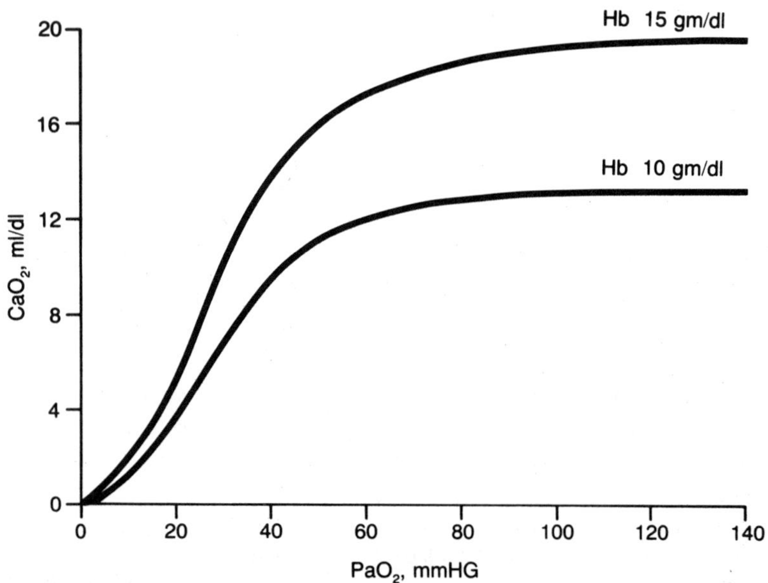

FIGURE 34–1. Differences in arterial oxygen content (CaO$_2$), attainable at PaO$_2$ values up to 140 mm Hg, with blood hemoglobin values of 15 vs 10 gm/dl. (Reproduced, with permission, from Luce JM, Tyler ML, Pierson DJ: Intensive Respiratory Care. Philadelphia, W. B. Saunders Co., 1984, p. 225.)

raised above about 60 mm Hg and that increases in PaO$_2$ above about 80 mm Hg cause little further improvement in SaO$_2$ or CaO$_2$.

Generally speaking, supplemental oxygen should be given whenever PaO$_2$ is consistently below 50–55 mm Hg. As mentioned below, some patients with chronic obstructive pulmonary disease (COPD) and other conditions characterized by chronic hypoxemia may suffer adverse consequences if PaO$_2$ is raised acutely above 50–55 mm Hg. For all other hypoxemic patients, the goal is to raise PaO$_2$ above 60 mm Hg, usually into the range of 60–90 mm Hg. From the clinical standpoint, values higher than 90 mm Hg do not imply further improvement in CaO$_2$, and to achieve them may require administration of high FiO$_2$ or other maneuvers that are unnecessarily hazardous.

Supplemental oxygen is also used to prevent hypoxemia in specific circumstances in which its occurrence is likely. These include endotracheal intubation, bronchoscopy, and endotracheal suctioning (particularly in patients with marginal initial oxygenation). Some patients who are not hypoxemic while awake or at rest may be given supplemental oxygen during sleep or exercise if they are shown to develop significant hypoxemia at these times.

Supplemental oxygen at high FiO$_2$ (as close to 100 percent as possible) is used in carbon monoxide poisoning, in which it displaces the carbon monoxide from hemoglobin in direct proportion to PaO_2. It is also used in dysbarism (see Chapter 96) to facilitate gas absorption from body cavities and tissues and to hasten elimination of certain anesthetic gases following surgery. These are the only situations in which raising PaO_2 above about 90 mm Hg is unequivocally beneficial from the clinical standpoint. Supplemental oxygen is also commonly given, in the absence of hypoxemia, to patients with acute myocardial infarction, sickle-cell crisis, and moderate attacks of bronchial asthma; although the mechanisms for claimed benefit are uncertain, use of the drug appears safe in these situations.

CONTRAINDICATIONS

Because of its cost and potential hazards, supplemental oxygen should only be used when clear indications are present. However, it should not be withheld because of the fear of adverse effects (see subsequent section). Acute hypoxemia (PaO_2 <50 mm Hg) is a threat to life and must not be allowed to continue for fear of CO_2 retention or other complication. Oxygen should not be administered intermittently to acutely hypoxemic patients, as this can produce a cycle of progressive hypoventilation and hypoxemia.

TECHNIQUES

Supplemental oxygen can be given by three basic techniques: low-flow, controlled administration; high-FiO_2 oxygen by mask; and via endotracheal intubation. Of these techniques, the first is used in conditions in which hypoxemia is due to mismatching of ventilation and perfusion ($\dot{V}A/\dot{Q}$) and/or alveolar hypoventilation as seen, for example, in COPD and asthma. Hypoxemia is relatively easy to correct in these conditions and requires only a modest increase in FiO_2. In addition, especially in patients with severe COPD in acute exacerbation, a major goal is to avoid raising PaO_2 beyond approximately 55–65 mm Hg. Thus, low-FiO_2 supplemental oxygen needs to be delivered continuously and at a constant rate.

Nasal Prongs (Cannulae). This is the preferred technique because of better patient acceptance and because oxygen delivery can continue during eating, expectoration, etc. Flow can be varied between 0.5 and 5 or 6 L/min, depending upon the flowmeter used, which represents a range of FiO_2 roughly between 0.24 and 0.40 in most patients. The fact that the exact FiO_2 is unknown is clinically irrelevant so long as flow remains constant and the resultant PaO_2 is measured. Humidification is of little value at flows below 4 L/min but can decrease nasal drying and discomfort above this level.

Venturi Masks. These utilize Bernouilli's principle to dilute supplemental oxygen with room air and to emit a constant FiO_2 that can range between 0.24 and 0.50. Because of variable additional air entrainment and, more important, because they are difficult to wear properly over a period of hours, the actual FiO_2 in the patient's trachea is no more certain with Venturi masks than with nasal prongs. Most patients prefer nasal prongs for comfort, and masks must be removed intermittently, interrupting oxygen delivery.

High-FiO$_2$ Oxygen by Mask. Severe hypoxemia due to right-to-left shunt and very low $\dot{V}A/\dot{Q}$ areas, as is seen in pneumonia and both cardiogenic and noncardiogenic pulmonary edema, generally requires a higher FiO_2 than can be attained using nasal prongs or Venturi-type masks. Short of endotracheal intubation, the options available to the clinician are simple masks, partial-rebreathing (reservoir) masks, and nonrebreathing masks.

At the highest oxygen flow available from a single outlet in most hospitals, simple and partial-rebreathing masks can produce effective FiO_2 values up to perhaps 0.60, depending upon the patient's minute ventilation and breathing pattern. With a tight-fitting nonrebreathing mask and a relatively low minute ventilation, effective FiO_2 values up to 0.90–0.95 can be achieved; these decline progressively as the patient's inspiratory minute volume increases above about 15 L and as the mask ceases to fit tightly. Patients given oxygen via nonrebreathing mask need to be watched closely in case it becomes disconnected from the oxygen source, because the one-way inlet valves of these masks create the potential for suffocation, particularly if the mask is strapped tightly in place and the patient is too weak to remove it.

Supplemental Oxygen via Endotracheal Tube. Unless the condition requiring high FiO_2 can be reversed or substantially improved within a few hours, oxygen delivery by mask will likely prove inadequate, and endotracheal intubation will be necessary. A cuffed endotracheal tube and a postendotracheal tube expiratory extension that prevents room air entrainment effectively create a closed inspiratory circuit through which any FiO_2 from 0.21 (room air) to 1.0 can be delivered to the patient. Because the protective apparatus of the upper airway is bypassed, gases administered through an endotracheal tube must be filtered and completely humidified. When endotracheal intubation is done for oxygenation rather than mechanical ventilation, the patient should breathe through a T-piece or "blow-by" circuit rather than through a ventilator because the latter can substantially increase the work of breathing.

Monitoring

The adequacy of arterial oxygenation cannot reliably be assessed by physical examination. Arterial blood gases should be measured whenever supplemental oxygen therapy is initiated, modified, or discontinued, and whenever there is a significant change in the patient's clinical condition. Measurements of SaO_2 by ear or pulse oximetry can sometimes substitute for PaO_2 values when the latter are below 60–65 mm Hg but are less helpful for quantitating changes when the hemoglobin is more completely saturated, and they cannot be used to detect concomitant changes in $PaCO_2$.

Complications and Hazards

Suppression of Hypoxic Ventilatory Drive. Chronically hypoxemic patients whose ventilation is driven primarily by hypoxia may develop dangerous acute respiratory acidosis if this stimulus is abruptly relieved, particularly during acute exacerbations. Practically speaking, this is most likely to occur in patients with severe COPD and established CO_2 retention whose initial PaO_2 of 40–50 mm Hg is raised acutely to 60–90 mm Hg. This complication is rare in clinically stable patients.

Supplemental oxygen should never be withheld from a hypoxemic patient for fear of acute CO_2 retention; instead, it is wisest to start with a low flow of nasal oxygen (e.g., 0.5 L/min) and to sequentially increase this at 20–30 minute intervals until the PaO_2 is above 50 mm Hg. The $PaCO_2$ may rise by 4–8 mm Hg, but this generally does not produce life-threatening acidemia and is preferable to continued severe hypoxemia.

Absorption Atelectasis. Pulmonary ventilation is not completely uniform, and the washout of nitrogen from poorly ventilated alveoli during 100 percent oxygen breathing may lead to their collapse as oxygen is taken up by the blood faster than it can be replaced. This process increases the alveolar-to-arterial oxygen difference ($P[A - a]O_2$) in normal individuals and may worsen hypoxemia in those with lung disease; it is increased by areas of focal airway obstruction. The clinical importance of absorption atelectasis in patients who require FIO_2 values of 0.9–1.0 because of profound hypoxemia is unclear.

Pulmonary Oxygen Toxicity. Exposure of normal animals or humans to high FIO_2 produces a syndrome that resembles the adult respiratory distress syndrome (ARDS) both clinically and pathologically. Patients who require high FIO_2 because of severe hypoxemia appear to be less susceptible than normal individuals, although this theory is controversial, and the clinical applicability of available data, much of it from experiments on animals, is uncertain.

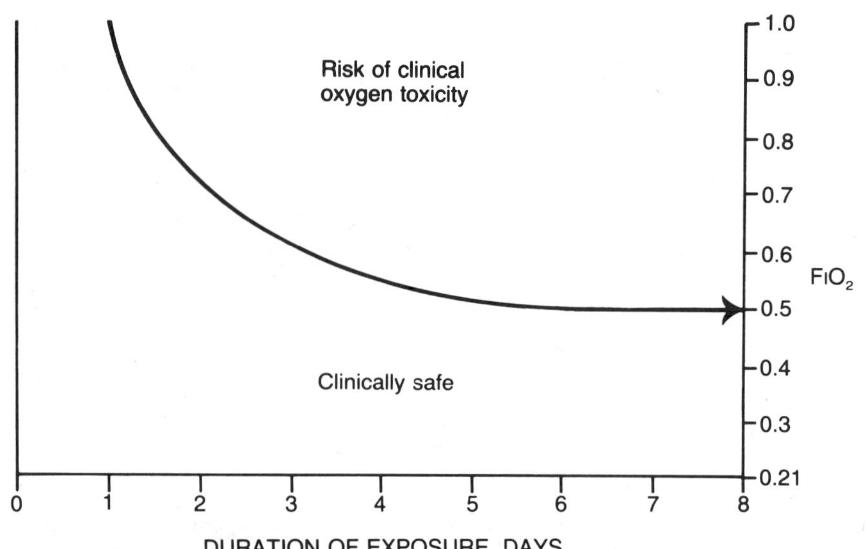

FIGURE 34–2. Pulmonary oxygen toxicity: general relationship between the fraction of inspired oxygen (FIO_2), duration of exposure, and risk of clinically significant oxygen toxicity. (Reproduced, with permission, from Luce JM, Tyler ML, Pierson DJ: Intensive Respiratory Care. Philadelphia, W. B. Saunders Co., 1984, p. 213.)

Figure 34–2 shows a curve relating FIO_2 and the duration of exposure to the clinical risk of parenchymal pulmonary oxygen toxicity during treatment for acute respiratory failure. In the area beneath the curve, the risk of oxygen toxicity is considered clinically acceptable. If possible, patients should not be exposed to 100 percent oxygen for more than 24 hours; if the FIO_2 can be reduced below 0.7 within 2–3 days, the risk of oxygen toxicity is low, and 0.5 appears to be clinically safe for many weeks. Sufficient oxygen should be administered to keep PaO_2 between 60–90 mm Hg, utilizing PEEP (see Chapter 36) and other measures as required, and doing everything possible to reverse the primary process creating the need for supplemental oxygen therapy.

Fire and Explosion. Oxygen supports combustion but is not inherently explosive. Facial burns among patients who smoke while receiving nasal oxygen are not uncommon, but more serious injuries are rare. Major accidents involving hospital oxygen systems are exceedingly uncommon.

RECOMMENDED READING

Anthonisen NR: Home oxygen therapy in chronic obstructive pulmonary disease. Clin Chest Med 7:673, 1986.
Jenkinson SG: Oxygen toxicity in acute respiratory failure. Respir Care 28:614, 1983.

Luce JM, Tyler ML, Pierson DJ: Intensive Respiratory Care. Philadelphia, W.B. Saunders Co., 1984, p. 207.
McPherson SP: Respiratory Therapy Equipment. 2nd edition. St. Louis, C.V. Mosby Co., 1984.
Pierson DJ: The toxicity of low-flow oxygen therapy. Respir Care 28:889, 1983.
Ryerson GG, Block AJ: Oxygen as a drug: Chemical properties, benefits and hazards of administration. In Burton GG, Hodgkin JE (eds): Respiratory Care. A Guide to Clinical Practice. 2nd edition. Philadelphia, J.B. Lippincott Co., 1984, p. 395.
Shapiro BA, et al: Clinical Application of Respiratory Care. 3rd edition. Chicago, Year Book Medical Publishers, Inc., 1985, p. 176.
Timms RM, et al: Selection of patients with chronic obstructive pulmonary disease for long-term oxygen therapy. JAMA 245:2514, 1981.
West GA, Primeau P: Nonmedical hazards of long-term oxygen therapy. Respir Care 28:906, 1983.
Winter PM, Miller JN: Carbon monoxide poisoning. J Am Med Assoc 236:1502, 1976.

35. Mechanical Ventilation

David J. Pierson

INTRODUCTION

Despite an ever-expanding variety of new techniques and devices, the basic needs of patients with acute respiratory failure and, with few exceptions, the principles of mechanical ventilation, have not changed during the last 20 years. Whichever brand of ventilator or operating mode is selected, patients can be managed effectively and safely if the clinician keeps these basic needs and principles in mind.

Although different basic types of ventilators are available, management of acute respiratory failure is best done with a positive- rather than a negative-pressure machine and volume- (or time-) rather than pressure-cycling. The patient must be endotracheally intubated (see Chapter 33) and may require therapy with positive end-expiratory pressure (see Chapter 36). The management outlined in this chapter pertains to patients with acute respiratory failure rather than to individuals receiving temporary postoperative ventilation.

INDICATIONS AND CONTRAINDICATIONS

In keeping with this book's emphasis on the physiologic basis for management, Table 35–1 summarizes the indications for mechanical ventilation according to six basic mechanisms. A seventh indication commonly used is "prophylactic" mechanical ventilation, the initiation of ventilatory support when a patient does not meet any criterion in the table but is considered to be at high risk for developing one or more. This indication is difficult to state objectively and results in much unnecessary therapy; instead of "prophylactic" mechanical ventilation, most clinicians recommend close observation of the patient and deferral of ventilatory support until it is more clearly justified.

Three special clinical settings deserve mention. Deliberate hyperventilation to lower intracranial pressure in patients with closed head injury is discussed in Chapter 73; if such patients are not already hyperventilating, keeping the systemic arterial carbon dioxide tension ($PaCO_2$) between 25 and 30 mm Hg during the first 12–24 hours after injury, followed by

218

TABLE 35–1. INDICATIONS FOR MECHANICAL VENTILATION

Basic Physiologic Impairment	Best Available Indicators	Approximate Normal Range	Values Indicating Need for Ventilatory Support
Inadequate alveolar ventilation (acute ventilatory failure)	$PaCO_2$, mm Hg	36–44	(Acute increase from normal or patient's baseline)
	Arterial pH	7.36–7.44	<7.25–7.30
Inadequate lung expansion	Tidal volume, ml/kg	5–8	<4–5
	Vital capacity	60–75	<10
	Respiratory rate, breaths/min (adults)	12–20	>35
Inadequate respiratory muscle strength	Maximum inspiratory force, cm H_2O	80–100	<25
	Maximum voluntary ventilation, L/min	120–180	<2 × resting ventilatory requirement
	Vital capacity, ml/kg	60–75	<10–15
Excessive work of breathing	Minute ventilation necessary to maintain normal $PaCO_2$, L/min	5–10	>15–20*
	Dead space ratio, percent	0.25–0.40	>0.60
	Respiratory rate, breaths/min (adults)	12–20	>35
Unstable ventilatory drive	Breathing pattern; clinical setting	—	—
Hypoxemia (acute oxygenation failure)†	Alveolar-to-arterial PO_2 gradient breathing 100 percent O_2, mm Hg	25–65	>350
	Intrapulmonary right-to-left shunt fraction, percent	<5	>20–25
	PaO_2/FIO_2, mm Hg	350–400	<200

*May be less in the presence of severe airflow obstruction.

†Usually accompanied by one or more of the above. When present as an isolated abnormality, acute oxygenation failure may not require mechanical ventilation (see Chapters 34 and 36).

gradual resumption of normocapnia over another 24 hours, may improve prognosis and hasten neurologic recovery. Hyperventilation has not been proven helpful in stroke or localized intracranial processes. Traumatic flail chest was formerly a separate indication for mechanical ventilation; however, this has been disproven; the same criteria should be used in patients with flail chest as for others with acute respiratory failure (see Chapter 28). Finally, patients with status asthmaticus or acute exacerbations of chronic obstructive pulmonary disease (COPD) seldom require mechanical ventilation if they are managed appropriately; however, the indications for initiating mechanical ventilation shown in Table 35–1 apply in these as in other conditions.

Because of its hazards and expense, mechanical ventilation is contraindicated whenever the conditions discussed above and listed in Table 35–1 are not met.

TECHNIQUES

Mode. Figure 35–1 shows diagrammatically the features of the three most commonly used ventilatory modes in comparison with spontaneous breathing (SV). With intermittent mandatory ventilation (IMV), the ventilatory burden is meant to be shared by patient and machine: The clinician

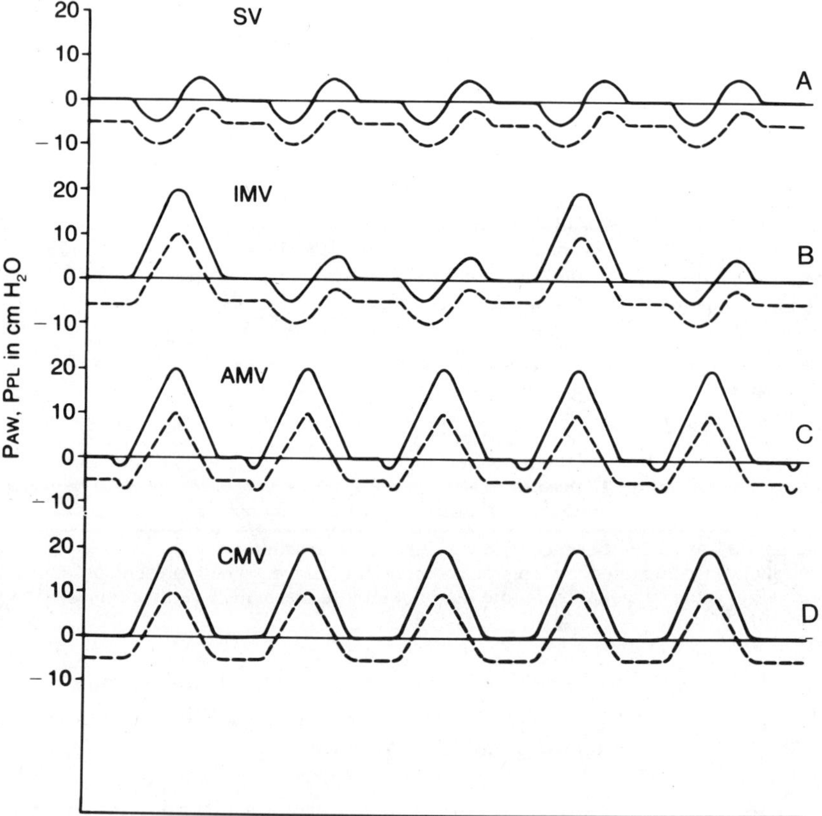

FIGURE 35–1. Conceptual illustration of the three main modes of mechanical ventilation, compared with spontaneous ventilation. Solid lines indicate airway pressure (PAW) and dashed lines, pleural pressure (PPL). SV = spontaneous ventilation; IMV = intermittent mandatory ventilation; AMV = assisted mechanical ventilation, or assist-control mode; CMV = controlled mechanical ventilation (or IMV with rate sufficiently fast that patient takes no intervening spontaneous breaths). (Reproduced, with permission, from Luce JM, Tyler ML, Pierson DJ: Intensive Respiratory Care. Philadelphia, W. B. Saunders Co., 1984, p. 199.)

provides part of it by setting a fixed ventilator frequency and tidal volume, but the patient is expected to take spontaneous breaths between the machine-delivered breaths. Advocates of IMV believe that these spontaneous breaths (which are usually small and rapid) maintain respiratory muscle tone, prevent respiratory alkalosis, and facilitate weaning, although objective attempts to prove these assertions scientifically in patients with acute respiratory failure have been unsuccessful.

With controlled mechanical ventilation (CMV) and assisted mechanical ventilation (AMV), or assist-control mode, all breaths are provided by the ventilator, using a fixed tidal volume. With AMV, the patient can increase the cycling frequency by generating negative proximal airway pressure. AMV and IMV are appropriate for patients who are awake and capable of initiating some breaths on their own; CMV is appropriate only for comatose patients or others who cannot attempt to breathe spontaneously.

High-frequency ventilation is an experimental mode that provides 60–2400+ breaths/min, using small tidal volumes and several techniques. High-frequency ventilation should not be used routinely in the management of acute respiratory failure; despite several theoretical advantages it has not yet proven to be either more effective or more safe than conventional mechanical ventilation in this setting.

Inspired Oxygen Fraction (FIO_2). It is best to err on the side of giving too much rather than too little oxygen in initial ventilator setup. An FIO_2 setting should be chosen arbitrarily if previous systemic arterial blood gas (ABG) values are unavailable, and this should be adjusted according to ABG results obtained 15–20 minutes later. The FIO_2 should be kept sufficient to maintain satisfactory arterial blood oxygen content; if this FIO_2 is considered potentially toxic, therapy with positive end-expiratory pressure (PEEP) may be necessary (see Chapter 36).

Tidal Volume. Ventilator breaths of 12 ml/kg ideal body weight (range 10 to 15) will provide adequate lung inflation to prevent absorption atelectasis without overdistending most patients' lungs. However, smaller tidal volumes are advisable in patients with severe hyperinflation (COPD; status asthmaticus) and when high levels of PEEP are used. The old-fashioned technique of using "physiologic" tidal volumes (5–8 ml/kg) with intermittent sighs of 1.5–3.0 times tidal volume is still used in some centers, but sighs should probably be avoided in the two situations just mentioned, because of the risk of barotrauma.

Inspiratory Flow Rate and Pattern. Modern ventilators offer several inspiratory pressure-flow patterns, but clinically important differences among them are generally not apparent. Whichever pattern is used, sufficient expiratory time must be provided to permit complete exhalation prior to the next breath. This is especially important in patients with airflow obstruction or when minute volumes greater than 15–20 L/min are required. In such settings, "auto-PEEP" (raised alveolar pressure, with the same adverse effects as deliberately applied PEEP, owing to air-trapping on successive breaths) is common and should be checked for routinely by momentarily occluding the expiratory arm of the ventilator circuit when the next delivered breath is due. Dyspneic patients tend to prefer rapid peak inspiratory flow rates, and we routinely use 70 L/min or higher when initiating mechanical ventilation; using rapid inspiratory flows will permit inspiratory duration to be kept well below that of expiration.

Alarms and Safety Settings. Inspiratory flow interruption or "pop-off" pressure should be set about 10 cm H_2O higher than the current peak inspiratory pressure, so that a sudden decrease in compliance (as with pneumothorax or plugged airway) can be detected early. When AMV is used, the ventilator's back-up cycling rate should be set only 2–4 breaths/min below the patient's current triggered rate, so that cessation of triggering (as with oversedation or change in neurologic function) will not produce acute respiratory acidosis.

WEANING

In respiratory care, "weaning" means the process of switching a patient from mechanically supported to spontaneous ventilation. For most postoperative patients and for many recovering from an episode of acute respiratory failure, this simply means substituting a blow-by or "T-piece" circuit for the ventilator, rather than a stepwise or gradual process. However, weaning should always be done with appropriate monitoring and according to an established protocol (Table 35–2).

There has been much controversy over whether patients should be weaned by the traditional T-piece technique or by IMV. In the latter, the number of ventilator breaths is sequentially reduced, so long as the patient does not become acidemic, until all breaths are spontaneous. While either method is probably fine for most patients, IMV weaning requires more blood gas measurements and tends to take longer. The T-piece method described in Table 35–2 is especially helpful when patients have marginal ventilatory reserve or have required mechanical ventilation for a week or more. In such instances, a series of short training periods on the T-piece, interspersed by periods of adequate rest on the ventilator, is usually successful over one to several days. The training periods are progressively increased in length as the patient tolerates more and more time off the ventilator; it is sometimes advantageous to return the patient to the ventilator at night for a few days once he or she is able to be on the T-piece throughout the day. Intensive nutritional and other general support

TABLE 35–2. WEANING FROM MECHANICAL VENTILATION

---

1. Satisfy some preset criteria (these or others) before starting weaning
   a. Disorder that precipitated need for mechanical ventilation has improved
   b. FIO_2 requirement for acceptable PaO_2 is 0.5 or less
   c. Ventilatory demand is manageable: minute ventilation no more than 10–12 L/min for normal $PaCO_2$
   d. Patient's own ventilatory mechanics are adequate for this need
       i. Spontaneous vital capacity at least 10 ml/kg
       ii. Maximum inspiratory force at least 20–25 cm H_2O
       iii. Patient can double resting minute ventilation during brief voluntary hyperventilation
2. Choose an appropriate time for the attempt at weaning
   a. Adequate support personnel available
   b. No other procedures or manipulations of the patient scheduled during the period of the weaning attempt
3. Eliminate or minimize respiratory depressants
   a. Narcotics and other systemic analgesics
   b. Sedatives
4. Suction airway as needed
5. Place patient in semiupright position if possible
6. Switch patient from mechanical to spontaneous ventilation at the same or 0.1 higher FIO_2 via one of the following:
   a. Separate blow-by (T-piece) circuit
   b. Ventilator*
7. Monitor patient
   a. Bedside observation and reassurance
   b. Arterial blood gas measurement after 20–30 minutes
   c. Continue spontaneous ventilation if both of the following:
       i. PaO_2 acceptable (>80 percent of preweaning value with acceptable SaO_2)
       ii. Arterial pH at least 7.30 and stable
   d. Assess patient for extubation (see Chapter 33)

---

*Breathing through the ventilator circuit with rate = zero may markedly increase the work of breathing, depending on the ventilator and the other apparatus used. A T-piece is preferable for patients with marginal ventilatory reserve.

are crucial in such cases, as is increased physical activity, including ambulation if this is feasible.

Failure to Wean. Inability of a patient to meet the criteria set forth in Table 35–2 or to tolerate a trial of spontaneous ventilation is a clinical problem that should be approached physiologically in a fashion similar to that used in assessing the need for mechanical ventilation (see Table 35–1). Acute respiratory acidosis (increase in $PaCO_2$ such that arterial pH falls abruptly to less than 7.30 units) means that the patient cannot match CO_2 production ($\dot{V}CO_2$) with alveolar ventilation. This may be because of inadequate respiratory muscle strength (manifested by low spontaneous vital capacity and maximum inspiratory force), in which case drugs (neuromuscular blocking agents; aminoglycosides), electrolyte disorders (hypophosphatemia; hypomagnesemia; hypokalemia), a primary neuromuscular disorder, or malnutrition may be responsible. It may be because ventilatory demand is excessive for the patient's present capabilities, as suggested by rapid, shallow respirations and subjective respiratory distress. Possible causes of excessive minute ventilation requirement include elevated $\dot{V}CO_2$ (sepsis; fever; agitation; shivering; excessive carbohydrate intake), a high dead space fraction (VD/VT) (due to ARDS; COPD; pulmonary embolism), or both; these may be distinguished by collecting a 3-minute expired-gas sample and an ABG specimen while the patient is on the ventilator and calculating $\dot{V}CO_2$ and VD/VT. Insufficient ventilatory drive is manifested by poor ventilatory effort (rather than by respiratory distress) and rapidly rising $PaCO_2$ when the patient is off the ventilator. Its most frequent causes are respiratory alkalosis (either absolute or relative to the patient's baseline elevated value) and metabolic alkalosis (from overzealous gastric suction, diuretics, or bicarbonate administration); both of these may be present. Other possible causes for inadequate respiratory drive are the administration of sedatives, narcotics and other depressant drugs, malnutrition, and, rarely, a primary disorder of ventilatory control.

Failure to wean because of hypoxemia is typically due to inadequate lung expansion, with worsening of ventilation:perfusion ($\dot{V}A/\dot{Q}$) mismatching and right-to-left shunt, accompanied by increased oxygen consumption during the trial. Continuous positive airway pressure (CPAP) (see Chapter 36) may be indicated in some instances. Severe hypoxemia as a reason for failure to meet the criteria for initiating weaning generally implies that the patient's respiratory failure has not yet improved enough for weaning to be attempted.

COMPLICATIONS

Fighting the Ventilator. Patient agitation and distress during mechanical ventilation develop because of incorrect setup of the machinery for the patient's metabolic or psychologic needs, because of an acute change in the patient's medical condition, because the airway has become obstructed by secretions or by something else, or because the ventilator is malfunctioning. Sudden distress in a patient who previously tolerated mechanical ventilation should be approached as an emergency. The patient should be taken off the ventilator and hand-ventilated; if this does not solve the problem, a rapid bedside examination of the patient should be undertaken. Only after such an evaluation and confirmation that no sudden change in ABG values has occurred should sedatives be administered. Reassurance and calmness on the part of the clinician are also of considerable help in this situation.

Respiratory Alkalosis. The tendency of some patients to hyperventilate and to become alkalemic is a major problem for the clinician managing mechanical ventilation. It was hoped that IMV would prevent or correct this problem, but studies have shown this not to be the case. IMV increases work of breathing and may thus cause a "compensating" element of acute respiratory acidosis in patients who cannot keep up with their ventilatory needs; however, this is hardly physiologic management. Patients usually hyperventilate because of dyspnea, so that the best approach is to search for the cause of the dyspnea, which may be hypoxemia, bronchospasm, pain, or anxiety.

Patients with underlying chronic respiratory acidosis, as in severe COPD, must not be allowed to become alkalemic during mechanical ventilation. If this happens they will lose their compensating metabolic alkalosis over 2 or 3 days and then be unable to be weaned. This complication can be avoided if arterial pH, not some preconceived "normal" $PaCO_2$, is used to guide mechanical ventilation.

Barotrauma. Alveolar disruption during mechanical ventilation (barotrauma) can result in pneumomediastinum, subcutaneous emphysema, and pneumothorax, the last of which can be an immediate threat to life. Patients especially prone to these complications are those with severe underlying hyperinflation (COPD; asthma; cystic fibrosis), severe diffuse lung injury (ARDS, especially late in the clinical course), or localized airway obstruction (right mainstem bronchial intubation; "ball-valve" tumor; foreign body), and the risk is increased when tidal volumes exceed 12–15 ml/kg or when PEEP levels are more than 15–20 cm H_2O. In such circumstances, equipment for performing emergency tube thoracostomy should be kept at the bedside.

RECOMMENDED READING

Brown DG, Pierson DJ: Auto-PEEP is common in mechanically ventilated patients: a study of incidence, severity, and detection. Respir Care 31:1069, 1986.

High-frequency ventilation. Editorial. Lancet 1(8479):477, 1986.

Hudson LD: Diagnosis and management of acute respiratory distress in patients on mechanical ventilators. In Moser KM, Spragg RG: Respiratory Emergencies. 2nd edition. St. Louis, C.V. Mosby Co., 1982, p. 201.

Hudson LD, Carrico CJ: Ventilatory management. In Shires GT (ed): Principles of Trauma Care. 3rd editon. New York, McGraw-Hill, 1985, p. 488.

Hudson LD, Hurlow RS, Craig KC, et al: Does IMV correct respiratory alkalosis in patients receiving assisted mechanical ventilation? Am Rev Respir Dis 132:1071, 1985.

Kirby RR, Smith RA, Desautels DA (eds): Mechanical Ventilation. New York, Churchill Livingstone, Inc., 1985.

Luce JM: The cardiovascular effects of mechanical ventilation and positive end-expiratory pressure. JAMA 252:807, 1984.

Luce JM, Tyler ML, Pierson DJ: Intensive Respiratory Care. Philadelphia, W.B. Saunders Co., 1984, p. 190.

Pierson DJ (ed): Respiratory Intensive Care. Dallas, American Association for Respiratory Care (Daedalus Press), 1986.

Pierson DJ: Indications for mechanical ventilation in acute respiratory failure. Respir Care 28:570, 1983.

Pierson DJ: Weaning from mechanical ventilation in acute respiratory failure: concepts, indications, and techniques. Respir Care 28:646, 1983.

Pierson DJ, Lakshminarayan S: Postoperative ventilatory management. Respir Care 29:603, 1984.
Sherman CB, Dacey RG, Pierson DJ, et al: The use of hyperventilation in head injury. Respir Care 31:1121, 1986.
Shibel EM: Acute respiratory failure with hypercapnia. In Shibel EM, Moser KM (eds): Respiratory Emergencies. St. Louis, C.V. Mosby Co., 1977, p. 85.
Zwillich CW, et al: Complications of assisted ventilation. Am J Med 57:161, 1974.

36. Positive End-Expiratory Pressure

David J. Pierson

INTRODUCTION

The term positive end-expiratory pressure (PEEP) means airway pressures greater than ambient at end-expiration and is used here in a conceptual rather than in a technical way to refer to any situation in which pressure above atmospheric is present in the patient's airway at end-expiration, whether deliberately applied or occurring endogenously.

Continuous positive-pressure ventilation (CPPV) is PEEP applied during ventilator-delivered breaths. Continuous positive airway pressure (CPAP) is PEEP during spontaneous breaths, with both inspiration and expiration remaining above ambient. Expiratory positive airway pressure (EPAP) is PEEP delivered either by a ventilator or via spontaneous ventilation in which only the expiratory side is above ambient and the patient must generate a subambient pressure to initiate each breath. With EPAP, work of breathing is increased but mean intrathoracic (pleural) pressure is lower than with CPPV or CPAP. These different forms of PEEP are depicted graphically in Figure 36–1. PEEP therapy during intermittent mandatory ventilation (IMV) comprises both CPPV (during the ventilator-delivered breaths) and CPAP (during any spontaneous breaths).

By establishing a higher pressure in the chest at end-expiration, PEEP raises functional residual capacity (FRC) and the amount of air in the lungs throughout the breathing cycle. It may thus open atelectatic alveoli and enlarge toward normal others that have impaired ventilation, resulting in decreased right-to-left shunt and improving the matching of ventilation and perfusion ($\dot{V}_A/\dot{Q}$) throughout the lung. It will also increase the size of already normal or enlarged alveoli, as in COPD or acute lung injury that is localized rather than homogeneous and may rupture these alveoli, producing pneumothorax and other manifestations of barotrauma. By increasing intrathoracic pressure, PEEP may clinically impair venous return to the right side of the heart, especially if the patient is hypovolemic or if PEEP levels greater than 10 cm H_2O are employed.

PEEP's effects are palliative, not therapeutic, in and of themselves.

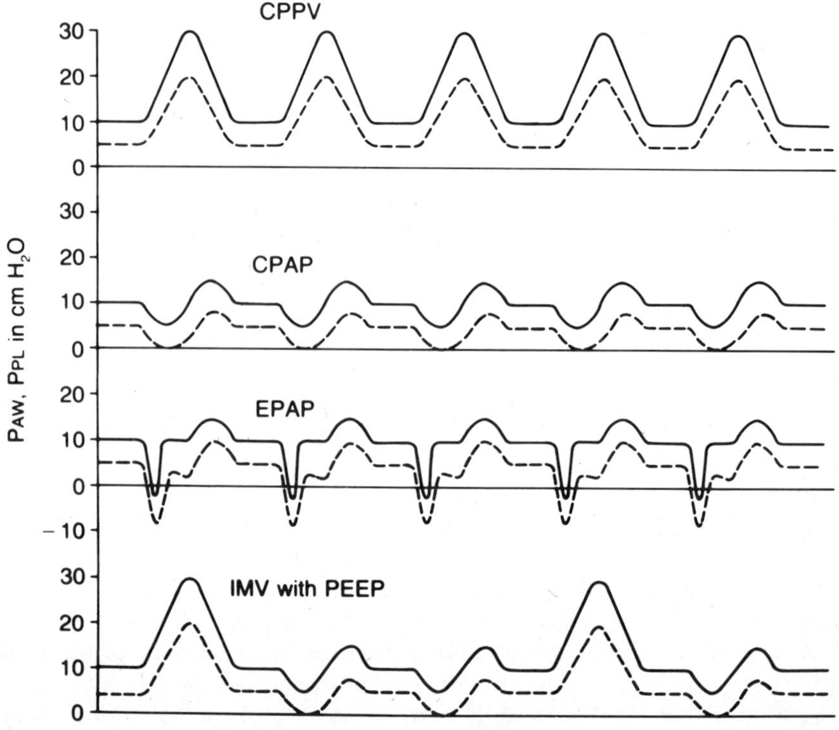

FIGURE 36–1. Conceptual illustration of the four main forms of PEEP therapy. Solid lines indicate airway pressure (PAW), and dashed lines indicate pleural pressure (PPL). CPPV = continuous positive pressure ventilation; CPAP = continuous positive airway pressure; EPAP = expiratory positive airway pressure; IMV = intermittent mandatory (mechanical) ventilation. (Reproduced, with permission, from Luce JM, Tyler ML, Pierson DJ: Intensive Respiratory Care. Philadelphia, W. B. Saunders Co., 1984, p. 217.)

The use of PEEP has not improved survival in ARDS, and currently available evidence does not support any role for high levels of PEEP other than to augment oxygenation while the lung repairs itself. Because of its often life-threatening adverse effects, it thus seems prudent to use PEEP cautiously, with well thought out goals and careful monitoring for both positive and negative effects, and to avoid levels above those necessary to achieve acceptable oxygen delivery.

INDICATIONS AND CONTRAINDICATIONS

A clinical trial of therapy with PEEP is indicated when acute diffuse lung disease is accompanied by severe hypoxemia that is refractory to administration of supplemental oxygen alone. PEEP should be tried in this setting when the systemic arterial oxygen tension (PaO_2) is 60 mm

Hg or less on an inspired oxygen fraction (FiO_2) of 0.6 or more or when the PaO_2/FiO_2 ratio is less than 150 mm Hg in a patient whose condition is deteriorating despite other therapy. The patient should have diffuse infiltrates involving all lung zones on the chest roentgenogram; PEEP must be used with great caution in the presence of a clear chest roentgenogram or if the infiltrates are localized or focal rather than homogeneous throughout the lungs. Hypovolemia is a relative contraindication, and patients who are clinically volume depleted should be monitored very closely if PEEP is used.

PEEP is ineffective in preventing ARDS, even in patients identified as being at increased risk for its development, and it is contraindicated in any patient with normal oxygenation. It has been shown to be ineffective in reducing mediastinal bleeding following cardiac surgery. Because of the dangers of barotrauma and cardiovascular compromise as well as the effectiveness of appropriately applied chest physiotherapy, PEEP is not the treatment of choice for acute lobar atelectasis.

CPAP delivered by mask to a nonintubated patient may be appropriate if the patient is alert and cooperative, if the need for PEEP is expected to be short-lived, if no more than 10 or 15 cm H_2O is to be used, and if there are no other indications for endotracheal intubation. The physiologic effects and complications of CPAP by mask are the same as for PEEP in other settings, and the patient should receive intensive nursing care and monitoring.

CLINICAL APPLICATION

There are several clinical approaches to the use of PEEP in ARDS, and although none is necessarily right or wrong, it is crucial that the clinician have clear-cut goals in mind and employ a level of monitoring and support consistent with the aggressiveness of his approach. The approach given in this book utilizes a "PEEP trial" in every patient and seeks to improve oxygen delivery while avoiding adverse effects of PEEP. Table 36–1 outlines this clinical approach in the management of ARDS. Using this approach, PEEP levels of 10–20 cm H_2O may be necessary, and appropriate hemodynamic monitoring is essential. A flow-directed pulmonary artery (Swan-Ganz) catheter should be used during PEEP therapy if (1) the patient's central volume status is uncertain (hypotension; unexplained tachycardia), (2) there is known severe left-ventricular dysfunction, or (3) a PEEP level exceeding 10 cm H_2O is employed (thus increasing the likelihood that cardiac output will be compromised).

WITHDRAWING PEEP

PEEP should be decreased cautiously once the patient has improved during its use. Premature PEEP reduction often results in clinical deteri-

TABLE 36–1. PROTOCOL FOR THE THERAPEUTIC APPLICATION OF POSITIVE
END-EXPIRATORY PRESSURE (THE "PEEP" TRIAL")

1. Obtain baseline respiratory and hemodynamic data* before initiating PEEP and at each level employed
2. Change only one variable at a time—keep tidal volume, inspired oxygen fraction, ventilator mode, and other settings the same at each level
3. Keep time intervals between PEEP levels short, e.g., 15–30 minutes
4. Apply PEEP in sequential increments, e.g., 5 cm H_2O (smaller increments are acceptable but trial takes longer; larger increments increase likelihood of adverse effects)
5. Monitor for immediate adverse effects at each PEEP level
   a. Hypotension or >20 percent fall in cardiac output
   b. Ectopy or raised intracranial pressure
   c. Fall in respiratory system compliance
6. Once patient has stabilized at new PEEP level (e.g., 15 minutes), repeat baseline respiratory and hemodynamic data as in 1
7. Evaluate overall cardiorespiratory response at each PEEP level used
   a. Favorable: Improved oxygenation, compliance
   b. Unfavorable: Decreased cardiac output, oxygenation, compliance
8. Assess results in light of overall goals for PEEP therapy
   a. If oxygen delivery has improved without adverse effects, leave patient on current PEEP level and reevaluate frequently as needed
   b. If oxygenation is still inadequate, inspired oxygen fraction is unacceptably high, and no adverse effects have occurred, increase PEEP sequentially, applying steps 4–7 above
   c. If oxygen delivery has dropped or compliance has fallen significantly at new PEEP level, return patient to previous level and reevaluate
      i. If deterioration is due to decreased PaO_2, reevaluate indications for PEEP
      ii. If deterioration is due to decreased cardiac output, consider volume loading or administration of pressor drugs
      iii. If compliance has fallen, consider decreasing tidal volume (danger of barotrauma has increased)

---

*Appropriate measures depend on severity of illness and intended aggressiveness of therapy. Respiratory data should include FiO_2, PEEP level, corrected tidal volume, respiratory rate, peak inflation and hold pressures, and arterial blood gas results. Mixed venous oxygen tension and saturation may also be helpful (see Chapter 1). Hemodynamic data may include heart rate, mean arterial pressure, pulmonary artery wedge pressure, and cardiac output.

oration and delayed recovery, and applying specific criteria such as used in the protocol in Table 36–2 can minimize the likelihood of this complication. Further, a 3-minute lowering of the PEEP level by 5 cm H_2O can safely predict whether the patient is ready for this maneuver. Patients whose conditions would allow a more rapid reduction in PEEP than that recommended in the table include those who do not meet the guidelines for a trial of PEEP in the first place, those who have not responded favorably during a PEEP trial, and those with barotrauma or low cardiac output unresponsive to other therapy.

Whether PEEP should be reduced to zero prior to extubation is controversial, and some clinicians prefer to maintain 5 cm H_2O of PEEP as long as the patient is intubated. Although this is probably unnecessary in many patients, it is reasonably safe in the absence of hypovolemia.

TABLE 36–2. PROTOCOL FOR REDUCTION OF POSITIVE END-EXPIRATORY PRESSURE

1. Patient should meet criteria for reducing PEEP
   a. Disease process requiring PEEP has substantially improved
   b. Patient is stable and not clinically septic*
   c. Arterial oxygen tension is 80–100 mm Hg or more on inspired oxygen fraction of 0.5 or less
   d. Above conditions have been met for at least 6–12 hours
2. Obtain baseline respiratory and hemodynamic data, including arterial blood gases,† as per Table 36–1, as clinically indicated
3. Reduce PEEP level by 5 cm H_2O
4. After 3 minutes, obtain a second specimen for arterial blood gas analysis,† and return PEEP to previous level while awaiting results
5. Compare pre-lowering and 3-minute arterial oxygen tension values (assuming $PaCO_2$ is unchanged)
   a. A dramatic fall in oxygen tension (e.g., more than 20 percent) indicates that the patient is not ready for PEEP reduction and should be maintained at the higher PEEP level for at least another 12 hours
   b. Satisfactory oxygenation (e.g., less than 20 percent drop in arterial oxygen tension) on 3-minute specimen indicates that the PEEP may be lowered by 5 cm H_2O, with repeat assessment, as in 2 above, after 1 hour and subsequently as appropriate

*Features suggesting sepsis include tachycardia, fever or hypothermia, leukocytosis, high cardiac output, and low systemic vascular resistance, with or without positive blood cultures.

†Arterial saturation, as monitored by finger or ear oximeter, is a poor estimate of the magnitude of the arterial oxygen tension change unless values drop below about 70 mm Hg. However, oximetry may afford an additional element of safety during PEEP reduction if the initial arterial oxygen tension is in the range of 80 mm Hg.

COMPLICATIONS

PEEP increases intrathoracic pressure and lung volume, and its most immediately life-threatening complications (depression of cardiac output and alveolar disruption) are the direct consequences of these physiologic effects. These complications are sufficiently common that they must be actively sought every time PEEP is used. As mentioned earlier, the degree of invasiveness with which cardiac function is assessed should be dictated by the patient's underlying condition and the aggressiveness of the therapy. Static respiratory system compliance is not an ideal predictor of barotrauma, but it is all we have other than to keep tidal volume below 12–15 ml/kg and to be alert for "auto-PEEP" (see Chapter 35). Other complications of PEEP therapy include possible increased intracranial pressure due to its effects on intrathoracic pressure, impairment of renal function (particularly when this is already compromised), owing to increased renal vein back-pressure, and passive hepatic congestion.

RECOMMENDED READING

Banasik JL, Tyler ML: The effect of prophylactic positive end-expiratory pressure on mediastinal bleeding after coronary revascularization surgery. Heart Lung 15:43, 1986.

Banner MJ, et al: Flow resistance of expiratory positive-pressure valve systems. Chest 90:212, 1986.

Branson RD, Hurst JM, DeHaven CB Jr: Continuous positive airway pressure applied by face mask. Respir Care 30:846, 1985.

Craig KC, Pierson DJ, Carrico CJ: The clinical application of positive end-expiratory pressure (PEEP) in the adult respiratory distress syndrome (ARDS). Respir Care 30:184, 1985.

Gibney RTN, Wilson RS, Pontoppidan H: Comparison of work of breathing on high gas flow and demand valve continuous positive airway pressure systems. Chest 82:692, 1982.

Hudson LD: Ventilatory management of patients with adult respiratory distress syndrome. Semin Respir Med 2:128, 1981.

Kacmarek RM, Dimas S, Reynolds J, et al: Technical aspects of positive end-expiratory pressure. Respir Care 27:1478, 1982.

Luce JM: The cardiovascular effects of mechanical ventilation and positive end-expiratory pressure. JAMA 252:807, 1984.

Luce JM, Tyler ML, Pierson DJ: Intensive Respiratory Care. Philadelphia, W. B. Saunders Co., 1984, p. 216.

Luterman A, et al: Withdrawal from positive end-expiratory pressure. Surgery 83:328, 1978.

Maunder RJ, Rice CL, Benson MS, et al: Managing positive end-expiratory pressure (PEEP): the Harborview approach. Respir Care 31:1059, 1986.

Pepe PE, Hudson LD, Carrico CJ: Early application of positive end-expiratory pressure in patients at risk for the adult respiratory distress syndrome. N Engl J Med 311:281, 1984.

Pierson DJ (ed): Respiratory intensive care. Dallas, Daedalus Press (Am Assoc Respir Care), 1986.

Springer RR, Stevens PM: The influence of PEEP on survival of patients in respiratory failure. Am J Med 66:196, 1979.

Weisman IM, Rinaldo JE, Rogers RM: Positive end-expiratory pressure in adult respiratory failure. N Engl J Med 307:1381, 1982.

37. Bronchoscopy

David J. Pierson

INTRODUCTION

Introduction of the fiberoptic bronchoscope to clinical practice in the early 1970s made direct examination of the airways readily available in a variety of settings, and today this instrument is commonly used in evaluating critically ill patients. Although less often needed today, the rigid bronchoscope has not been replaced by the fiberoptic instrument and finds application in several important critical care settings. Appreciation of the advantages and limitations of each is important in optimal diagnosis and management.

Some of the last decade's enthusiasm for fiberoptic bronchoscopy has been tempered by experimental data showing its limitations in situations in which it has been widely used. Along with this has come an appreciation of its potential hazards: Knowing when *not* to perform bronchoscopy is thus as important to the clinician as a firm understanding of its indications.

INDICATIONS

Table 37–1 lists the main indications for the use of bronchoscopy, including those commonly encountered in critical care. Suspected bronchogenic carcinoma is perhaps the most common indication: A tissue diagnosis can be made in approximately 90 percent of endobronchially visible masses, although the yield in peripheral lesions (40–70 percent, depending on facilities, experience of the operator, and number of biopsies taken) is less.

Many surgeons routinely perform bronchoscopy to visualize the bronchial stump following lobectomy or pneumonectomy. It is also done frequently following burns, smoke inhalation, or other acute inhalation injury, and in patients who have been intubated for prolonged periods. However, how well the findings of such examinations predict the severity of clinical airway injury or otherwise influence therapy remains to be established.

In diffuse lung disease, bronchoscopy can establish a diagnosis of

TABLE 37–1. INDICATIONS FOR BRONCHOSCOPY

Suspected carcinoma or other endobronchial lesion
  Mass or other suggestion of neoplasm on chest roentgenogram
  Localized wheeze; atelectasis; unresolving pneumonia
  Recurrent laryngeal or phrenic nerve paralysis; abnormal cytology
Hemoptysis
  Life-threatening (>600 ml/24 hr) bleeding (rigid scope preferred)
  Age >40 years; cigarette smoking; persistence for >1 week
  Abnormal chest roentgenogram suggestive of neoplasm
  Bleeding from endotracheal or tracheostomy tube
Evaluation for suspected tracheobronchial injury
  Persistent or massive bronchopleural air leak following trauma
  Failure of collapsed lung to reexpand with suction
Foreign body aspiration (rigid scope for large objects or age <12 years)
Airway inspection following lung resection, burns, inhalation injury, or prolonged
  intubation
Difficult intubation
Diffuse lung disease (of limited value—see text)
To diagnose pulmonary infections (see limitations in text)
  Sputum-negative suspected tuberculosis
  Suspected bacterial infection (protected-brush catheter)
  Infiltrates in the immunocompromised host (lavage; biopsy)
Tracheobronchial toilet (overused for this indication—see text)
  Acute lobar atelectasis (when vigorous chest physiotherapy is unsuccessful or cannot be
    used)
  Secretion removal in other settings
Bronchography

tuberculosis, fungal disease, *Pneumocystis carinii* pneumonia, malignancy, and sarcoidosis, but it is inadequate for this purpose in interstitial pneumonitis, occupational disease, and other conditions. Protected-brush catheter specimens are easily obtained, both in spontaneously breathing and in mechanically ventilated patients with suspected bacterial lung infection, but clinical accuracy is still controversial. These specimens are highly sensitive; their specificity varies but may be improved if they are scrupulously obtained and handled and if semiquantitative culture techniques are used. Protected-brush catheter specimens may be most useful in seriously ill patients who are at risk for unusual pathogens, in whom adequate sputum is unobtainable, who do not respond to therapy, or in whom superinfection is suspected.

Fiberoptic bronchoscopy for tracheobronchial toilet is often overused in the intensive care unit (ICU). It is unnecessary in most cases of acute lobar atelectasis if vigorous chest physiotherapy can be performed; it has not been shown to be helpful as a routine measure following surgery or intubation; and it is not needed in pneumonia, bronchiectasis, or lung abscess if the patient can produce sputum spontaneously.

Other recently introduced procedures involving the bronchoscope include transbronchial or transtracheal needle aspiration, which is proving valuable in staging bronchogenic carcinoma and in avoiding unnecessary thoracotomy; neodymium-YAG laser photocoagulation for palliative relief of major airway obstruction in carcinoma; and hematoporphyrin-guided bronchoscopic identification of dysplasia and carcinoma in situ. Bronchoalveolar lavage is being used increasingly in the assessment and monitoring of diffuse lung disease, although its practical value has yet to be proven in most clinical settings.

The rigid rather than the fiberoptic bronchoscope should be used in massive hemoptysis, in which it allows better removal of blood and clots; in aspiration of large (and, some clinicians feel, all major-airway) foreign bodies; and in patients under about age 12. Many also prefer the rigid instrument for biopsy of necrotic tumor masses or suspected bronchial adenomas, both of which may bleed massively.

CONTRAINDICATIONS

Several situations greatly increase the likelihood of serious complications and are thus contraindications to bronchoscopy: This procedure could become necessary in such situations, but the indications would have to be compelling, alternative procedures unavailable, and every precaution taken. These conditions include asthma, severe hypoxemia, unstable arrhythmias, and recent myocardial infarction. Additional contraindications to transbronchial biopsy (and probably to bronchial brushing as well) include uncorrected bleeding diathesis, uremia, pulmonary hypertension, and mechanical ventilation and/or the use of positive end-expiratory pressure (PEEP) therapy. When a tissue diagnosis is imperative in such situations, open lung biopsy is safer and provides greater likelihood of an adequate specimen.

TECHNIQUE

Prior to bronchoscopy the patient should have a chest radiograph, arterial blood gas measurement, electrocardiogram, complete blood count, and coagulation studies. The patient should not eat or drink for 6–8 hours and in most cases should receive 0.4–0.8 mg atropine intramuscularly 30–45 minutes prior to the procedure. Many patients do not need sedation, but a modest dose of meperidine (Demerol) or diazepam is often given as a premedication. The logistics of the procedure, its risks, and potential complications should be explained. All patients should be electrocardiographically monitored and receive supplemental oxygen during the procedure.

Methods for anesthetizing the upper airways vary. The agent of choice is lidocaine, which can be delivered by hand-bulb nebulizer, compressor-driven nebulizer, or intermittent positive-pressure breathing (IPPB) device for 10–15 minutes prior to the procedure. Additional amounts of 1 percent lidocaine, applied directly to the airways through the bronchoscope, will be necessary after passing the vocal cords, particularly when examining the upper lobe bronchi. Adverse effects are uncommon with total delivered doses of 300 mg or less, although larger amounts are sometimes necessary.

Most routine fiberoptic bronchoscopies are performed via the nasal route, although some clinicians prefer to orally intubate the patient with a large-bore endotracheal tube and to pass the scope through this. Examinations during mechanical ventilation and/or PEEP therapy are performed through specially made swivel adapters that prevent loss of airway positive pressure. The ventilator should be adjusted during the procedure to prevent air trapping, pressure limitation, and hypoxemia: Tidal volume and peak inspiratory flow rate may have to be decreased; the inspired oxygen fraction should be increased by at least 0.2 during and for 10–20 minutes following bronchoscopy.

COMPLICATIONS

Although fiberoptic bronchoscopy is generally benign, it has numerous complications; incidence and severity increase the more seriously ill the patient and the more inexperienced the operator. Complications (respiratory depression, uncontrollable agitation, syncope, hypotension, seizures, cardiorespiratory arrest) may occur from premedication and topical anesthesia, from the bronchoscopy itself (bronchospasm, laryngospasm, hypoxemia, dysrhythmias, fever, pneumonia), or from transbronchial biopsy or brushing (pneumothorax, hemorrhage). Pneumothorax occurs after 5 percent of biopsy or brushing procedures and requires a chest tube in about half of these. Bleeding (>50 ml) occurs in 3–5 per cent overall but much more frequently in immunocompromised patients and in those with renal insufficiency.

For rigid bronchoscopy, the complications of the fiberoptic procedure can be added to those related to general anesthesia. Injury to the neck, upper airway, and cervical spine can also occur, although these and other complications are much less likely when the procedure is performed by experienced operators under controlled conditions in the operating room.

RECOMMENDED READING

Chastre J, et al: Prospective evaluation of the protected specimen brush for the diagnosis of pulmonary infections in ventilated patients. Am Rev Respir Dis 130:924, 1984.

Cortese DA: Endobronchial management of lung cancer. Chest 89 (Suppl. 4):234S, 1986.

Dhillon DP, Collins JV: Current status of fiberoptic bronchoscopy. Postgrad Med J 60:213, 1984.

Fulkerson WJ: Current concepts: fiberoptic bronchoscopy. N Engl J Med 311:511, 1984.

Marini JJ, Pierson DJ, Hudson LD: Acute lobar atelectasis: a prospective comparison of fiberoptic bronchoscopy and respiratory therapy. Am Rev Respir Dis 119:971, 1979.

Sackner MA: Bronchofiberscopy (state of the art). Am Rev Respir Dis 111:62, 1975.

Sheldon RL. Flexible fiberoptic bronchoscopy. Primary Care 12:299, 1985.

Snow N, Lucas AE: Bronchoscopy in the critically ill surgical patient. Am Surg 50:441, 1984.

Stover DE, et al: Bronchoalveolar lavage in the diagnosis of diffuse pulmonary infiltrates in the immunosuppressed host. Ann Intern Med 101:1, 1984.

Stover DE, et al: Diagnosis of pulmonary disease in acquired immune deficiency syndrome (AIDS). Role of bronchoscopy and bronchoalveolar lavage. Am Rev Respir Dis 130:659, 1984.

Stradling P: Diagnostic bronchoscopy: a teaching manual. 5th edition. New York, Churchill Livingstone Inc., 1986.

Villers D, et al: Reliability of the bronchoscopic protected-catheter brush in intubated and ventilated patients. Chest 88:527, 1985.

Winterbauer RH, et al: The use of quantitative cultures and antibody coating of bacteria to diagnose bacterial pneumonia. Am Rev Respir Dis 128:98, 1983.

38. Chest Tubes

David J. Pierson

David J. Pierson

INTRODUCTION

Despite the frequency of their use, chest (thoracostomy) tubes and their drainage systems are often confusing and intimidating to clinicians. However, because chest tubes can be life-saving and because their complications are not infrequently serious or fatal, it is crucial that their functions, indications, monitoring, and possible adverse effects be familiar to all who come in contact with them.

INDICATIONS

These vary with local practice as well as with diagnosis. Such variation is greatest in primary spontaneous pneumothorax, in which some clinicians use a chest tube for all but the smallest rim of intrapleural air, while others employ needle aspiration or an intravenous catheter connected to a flutter (Heimlich) valve, unless the pneumothorax cannot be controlled by these measures. Primary spontaneous pneumothorax seldom requires admission to the intensive care unit (ICU), a setting in which most pneumothoraces *do* require chest tube placement.

Spontaneous pneumothorax occurring in the presence of underlying lung disease is more likely to cause symptoms and physiologic impairment and usually requires a chest tube, even when the pneumothorax is small. In iatrogenic pneumothorax, as seen after percutaneous lung aspiration, transbronchial biopsy, or subclavian vein catheterization, chest tube drainage is advisable if the pneumothorax is large (>40 percent) or enlarging on serial films, if symptoms are severe, or if there is impairment of oxygenation or hemodynamics.

Patients with a pneumothorax that develops during mechanical ventilation are at great risk for sudden tension pneumothorax, which can be rapidly fatal; unless weaning can be accomplished immediately, a chest tube should be inserted or kept at the bedside with someone constantly available to insert it. Even a small or loculated pneumothorax may produce physiologic impairment in a critically ill patient, especially in those with adult respiratory distress syndrome (ARDS).

Traumatic pneumothorax should always be drained with a chest tube, as should hemothorax, in order to monitor blood loss and completely remove the blood and clots, reducing the likelihood of empyema and late fibrothorax. For parapneumonic pleural effusions, a chest tube should be placed if empyema is present (frank pus, positive gram stain, or positive bacterial culture in pleural fluid) and should also be considered if the pleural fluid leukocyte count exceeds 15,000–20,000 cells/mm^3, especially in a rapidly expanding effusion. Chest tubes may also be indicated in some malignant pleural effusions, particularly if chemical pleurodesis is planned.

CONTRAINDICATIONS

Many clinicians consider chest tubes to be contraindicated in the presence of an obstructed bronchus: the lung is unlikely to reexpand, and the risk of empyema is increased. Chest tubes are unnecessary in transudative pleural effusions unless these cause physiologic impairment and accumulate rapidly following thoracentesis.

INSERTION

To drain air, the tip of the tube should be seated high in the pleural cavity. Some clinicians use the second intercostal space in the midclavicular line in male patients, and the fourth space, just behind the anterior axillary fold, in females; others use the latter site in either sex for cosmetic reasons. To drain fluid, the tube should be placed posteriorly and directed downward into the pleural gutter. Although some clinicians prefer to use a small-caliber tube for evacuating air, others believe that a larger tube (e.g., size 24–28 F) is associated with fewer complications and prevents having to insert one or more additional tubes because of poor drainage. Fluid, especially blood and empyema fluid, always requires a large-bore tube.

Two basic approaches to chest tube insertion involve operative placement and the use of a trocar. For fluid drainage, the patient should be seated, if possible; for pneumothorax, the supine position is used for an anterior insertion and the lateral decubitus position for an axillary insertion.

Operative Tube Thoracostomy. After cleansing and draping the skin and injecting local anesthetic, the operator makes a 3–4 cm skin incision parallel to the intercostal space, down to and including the fascia overlying the intercostal muscles. The muscle fibers are separated using a blunt-tipped hemostat, the intercostal fascia is incised just superior to the rib, and the parietal pleura is punctured with the hemostat. After enlarging this puncture hole with the index finger, the operator sweeps the finger over the visceral lung surface to lyse any adhesions and then inserts the chest tube (whose distal end has been clamped to prevent air entry into the pleural space), using the hemostat to guide it.

The tube's most proximal drainage hole should be at least 2 cm inside the pleural cavity. A long suture through the skin and around the tube secures the tube to the insertion site, with care taken not to compress the intervening tissues; the site is then covered with a sterile dressing and tape, further securing the tube. This method is more invasive than the trocar technique but is believed by some clinicians to be less likely to injure the lung or to cause serious bleeding.

Trocar Tube Thoracostomy. This method employs a trocar with a sharp stylet, rather than blunt dissection, to traverse the chest wall, once an incision through the skin and subcutaneous tissues has been made. Some chest tubes are prepared and sterilized with the trocar *in situ*, running the length of the tube; with others, the trocar must first be inserted through the chest wall and the chest tube passed through it.

Careful anesthesia can render placement of a chest tube much less painful and distressing for the patient. The selected site is thoroughly infiltrated with 1 percent lidocaine (up to 20 ml may be used), starting with a cutaneous bleb and extending through subcutaneous tissues and intercostal muscle; the parietal pleura must be thoroughly anesthetized, which requires just entering the pleural space with the needle tip and then injecting lidocaine as it is slightly withdrawn.

An incision just large enough for the trocar and chest tube (1–2 cm) is made through the anesthetized skin. This incision should be extended down through the chest wall muscles, nearly to the pleural surface, in order to make passage of trocar and tube easier. Brief, firm pressure with a sterile pad should stop any local bleeding during this procedure. Before the tube is inserted, its connections and the drainage assembly should be checked for completeness and the collection apparatus filled with water if appropriate.

Insertion of the trocar should be done with a rotating movement and should require little force; care must be taken to avoid sudden penetration into the underlying lung. Once the pleural space is entered, the trocar may be used to direct the tube cephalad or caudad within the chest. The trocar is then removed and the chest tube passed through or over it into the chest. The tube should be clamped at the skin, as the distal clamp is released during removal of the trocar. The chest tube should be sutured securely to the skin and a second, purse-string, suture placed and left open for later closure of the skin defect when the tube is removed. A thick bandage helps to seal the insertion site and to anchor the tube to the chest wall.

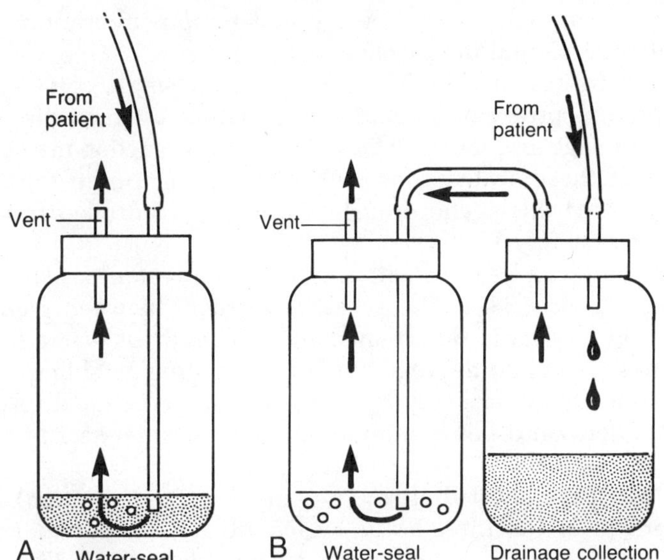

FIGURE 38–1. *A*, One-bottle pleural drainage system. *B*, Two-bottle pleural drainage system. Proximal (right-hand) bottle permits accumulation of pleural drainage fluid without increasing the pressure necessary to vent the pleural space. (Reproduced, with permission, from Luce JM, Tyler ML, Pierson DJ: Intensive Respiratory Care. Philadelphia, W. B. Saunders Co., 1984, p. 164.)

PLEURAL DRAINAGE SYSTEMS

Several of these are available, all having the basic purpose of preventing air from entering the pleural space, while permitting air and fluid to be evacuated. The connecting tubing should be several feet in length in order to allow the patient to move about in bed and to allow the drainage vessel(s) to be situated conveniently; it should be secured to the bottom bed sheet in such a way that it does not form a loop of tubing extending below the mattress.

A Heimlich valve is a short length of collapsible tubing, resembling a Penrose drain, enclosed in a protective sheath, which conducts air from the pleural space to the atmosphere under positive pressure but collapses when there is no air leak. Because it provides no means for collecting fluid drainage, the Heimlich valve is appropriate only for treating pneumothorax.

An "underwater seal" or single-bottle system (Fig. 38–1A) prevents air entry into the pleural space by means of a 2-cm water seal and permits fluid drainage to be collected in the bottle. Its disadvantage is that, as drainage fluid accumulates, the intrapleural pressure required to break the water seal and vent the chest progressively increases. Fluid could also run back into the chest if the bottle were raised—for example, during transport. This system is thus best suited for pneumothorax, or when there is minimal pleural fluid drainage.

A two-bottle system (Fig. 38–1B) works like a single-bottle system but gets around the problem of fluid accumulation by providing separate bottles for drainage and for the water seal. External suction may be applied with either of these systems, as with an Emerson pump (but not with wall suction), but this suction must be precisely controlled from outside the drainage system.

Wall suction can be used with a three-bottle system, as shown in the upper part of Figure 38–2. The pressure gradient between pleural space and collection vessels is determined by the depth of water in the left-hand (farthest distal) bottle; regulated by continuous bubbling of air from the room, the suction applied to the pleural space is equal to the water depth in the left-hand bottle minus the 2 cm of water-seal in the center bottle.

The Pleur-Evac chest drainage system (Fig. 38–2, bottom) is a commercial version of the three-bottle system. If not connected to external suction, it functions as a two-bottle system. Figure 38–3B shows the Argyle Double-seal, another commonly-used commercial system, which is similar to the Pleur-Evac with an additional vented water-seal chamber, equivalent to a fourth bottle. The four-bottle system is diagrammed in Figure 38–3A.

Monitoring and Maintenance

Initial chest tube placement should be checked immediately with a chest roentgenogram, which may require an additional lateral view to assure that it is in the pleural space and not in a fissure. Patency of the system is monitored by observing respiratory fluctuations in the water seal with the suction momentarily turned off; a deep breath or cough by the patient may be required.

Air or liquid should not be introduced into a chest tube. If it becomes occluded, as may happen when there is fresh pleural bleeding or clots, gentle stripping or milking may reestablish patency. Routine stripping of chest tubes has been shown to be unnecessary; because this procedure can generate negative pressures as high as 400 mm Hg within the tube, it should be performed gingerly if used.

Tube Removal

A chest tube should be removed if it is nonfunctional, as it will not vent the chest in case of tension pneumothorax, will permit build-up of

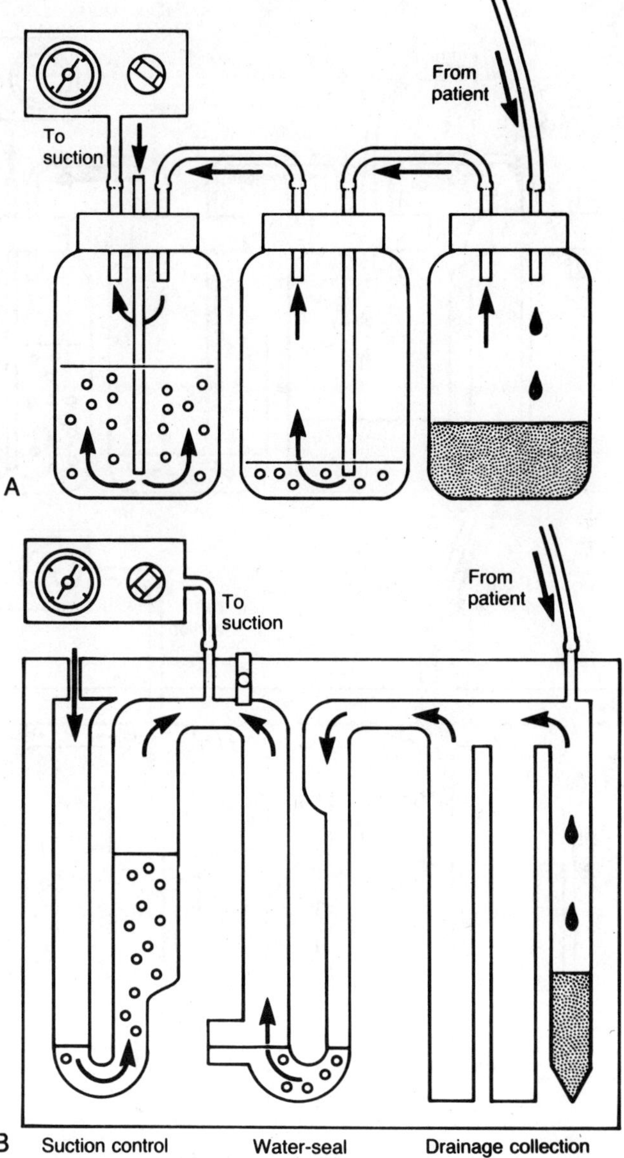

FIGURE 38–2. *A*, Three-bottle pleural drainage system. This permits the use of wall suction to increase the pressure gradient between pleural space and collection bottle. *B*, Pleur-Evac pleural drainage system, a commerical version of the three-bottle system that incorporates a self-contained air vent to prevent pressure build-up within the system. (Reproduced, with permission, from Luce JM, Tyler ML, Pierson DJ: Intensive Respiratory Care. Philadelphia, W. B. Saunders Co., 1984, p. 166.)

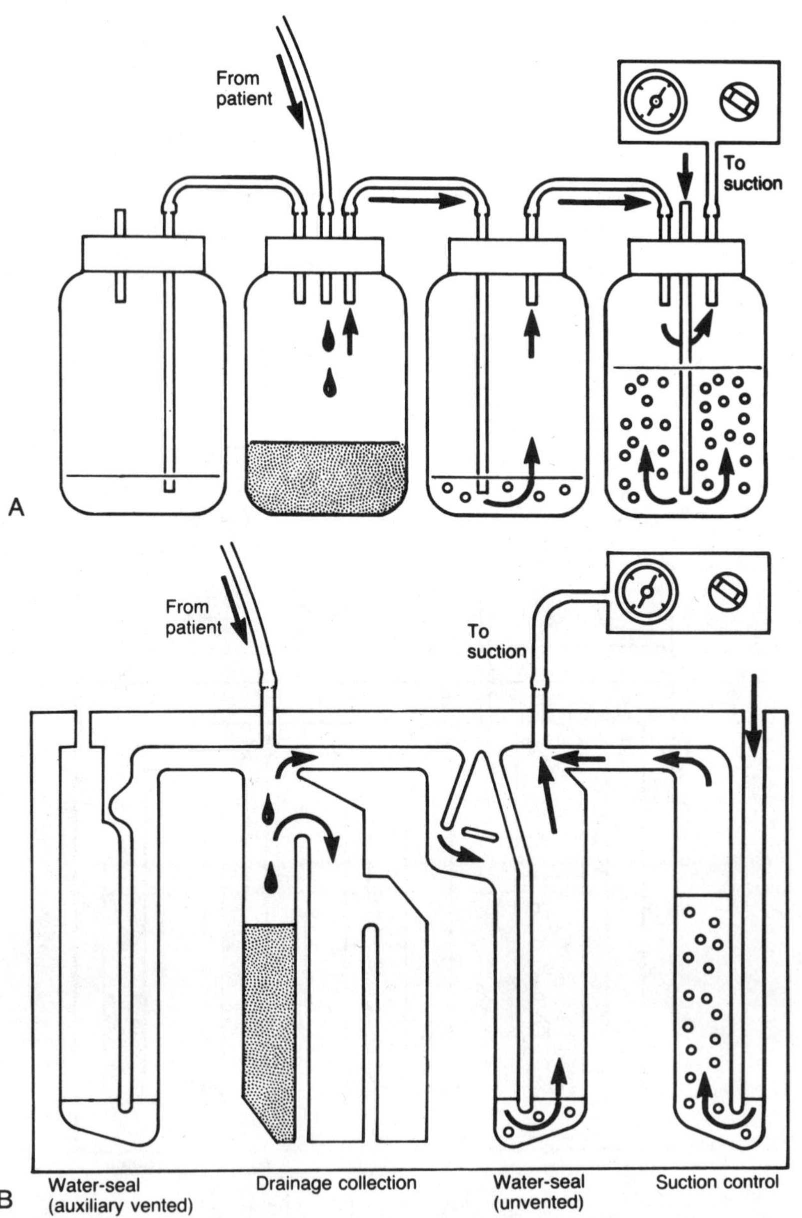

FIGURE 38–3. *A*, Four-bottle pressure drainage system, incorporating a second water seal. *B*, The Argyle double-seal commercial pleural drainage system, which includes a fourth chamber serving as an underwater seal open to air. (Reproduced, with permission, from Luce JM, Tyler ML, Pierson DJ: Intensive Respiratory Care. Philadelphia, W. B. Saunders Co., 1984, p. 167.)

fluid, and may serve as a conduit for the introduction of bacteria. In pneumothorax, whether the patient is breathing spontaneously or is on a ventilator, the tube may be removed when the lung has been fully reexpanded with no air leak for 24–48 hours. Tubes placed in treatment of empyema or hemothorax may be removed when drainage is less than 75–100 ml/day.

The removal procedure should be explained to the patient, whereupon the dressings should be removed, the suture withdrawn, and the tube pulled out quickly while the patient performs a Valsalva maneuver. A sterile dressing serves to occlude the wound and to absorb drainage. As soon as the procedure has been completed, a chest roentgenogram should be obtained to assure that the lung is fully expanded.

COMPLICATIONS

Chest tubes are painful, immobilize the patient, and interfere with nursing care; they should thus be used only when clearly indicated. On initial placement of the tube, the lung may be lacerated or punctured, the tube may come to rest in a fissure (and thus may not function properly), or the most distal drainage hole may remain outside the pleural space (thus causing an apparent air leak or introducing bacteria). Reexpansion pulmonary edema, an incompletely understood phenomenon that may cause severe hypoxemia, is more likely to occur after rapid reexpansion of a lung that has been collapsed for a prolonged period.

The most rapidly fatal complication of a chest tube is tension pneumothorax, which may develop if the tube becomes occluded or kinked in the presence of a persistent bronchopleural air leak. Those caring for a mechanically ventilated patient with an air leak must remain aware of this possibility and must check the tube frequently for patency.

Subcutaneous emphysema is common in patients with chest tubes. Cosmetically unpleasant and often worrisome to those caring for the patient, it is generally harmless and needs no special treatment.

Finally, because a chest tube is a foreign body in direct communication with the skin, pleural space infection is a constant and serious threat, which makes scrupulous wound care and dressing changes of prime importance and emphasizes the importance of removing the tube as soon as it is no longer necessary. Sterility must be preserved in the closed system between pleural space and proximal drainage bottle; if pleural drainage is needed for bacterial culture or other tests, it should be obtained by sterile needle puncture of the tubing rather than by disconnecting it.

RECOMMENDED READING

Duncan C, Erickson R: Pressures associated with chest tube stripping. Heart Lung 11:166, 1982.

Enerson DM, McIntire J: A comparative study of the physiology and physics of pleural drainage systems. J Thorac Cardiovasc Surg 52:40, 1966.
Gilsanz V, Cleveland RH: Pleural reaction to thoracotomy tube. Chest 74:167, 1978.
Griffith GL, et al: Acute traumatic hemothorax. Ann Thorac Surg 26:204, 1978.
Heimlich HJ: Valve drainage of the pleural cavity. Dis Chest 53:282, 1968.
Kersten L: Chest tube drainage system—indications and principles of operation. Heart Lung 3:97, 1974.
Light RW: Pleural diseases. Philadelphia, Lea & Febiger, 1983, p. 243.
Lim-Levy F, et al: Is milking and stripping chest tubes really necessary? Ann Thorac Surg 42:77, 1986.
Luce JM, Tyler ML, Pierson DJ: Intensive Respiratory Care. Philadelphia, W. B. Saunders Co., 1984, p. 156.
Wagaruddin M, Bernstein M: Reexpansion pulmonary edema. Thorax 30:54, 1975.

39. Drugs Used to Improve Pulmonary Function

David J. Pierson

David J. Pierson

INTRODUCTION

This chapter covers drugs used in the intensive care unit (ICU) setting that primarily affect the respiratory system. Before each group of such agents is discussed, some comments applying to all of them are in order.

Drugs such as β-agonist bronchodilators whose desired action is on the airways are safer and more effective if administered directly into those airways by inhalation as opposed to the oral, subcutaneous, or intravenous routes. For equivalent bronchodilatation, only one fifth to one tenth the total dose is necessary by aerosol as compared with oral administration; because most adverse effects of these drugs are related to the total quantity introduced into the body, aerosol administration also minimizes toxicity.

Absorption after subcutaneous or intramuscular injection is unpredictable in critically ill patients, particularly in those with circulatory instability, and intravenous administration is preferable for agents that cannot be given by the inhaled route. Oral administration of drugs such as theophylline and corticosteroids may be appropriate in the ICU, primarily as a step-down maneuver after stabilization or reversal of the acute episode as the patient is being readied for transfer or discharge. However, this does not apply to β-agonists or anticholinergics, for which the inhaled route is always preferable.

Proprietary drug combinations should be avoided for hospitalized patients, and there is also little justification for using more than one drug of a given category simultaneously (for example, both isoetharine and metaproterenol), as this increases the likelihood of adverse effects without evident therapeutic advantage over larger or more frequent doses of either drug by itself.

Drug dosages recommended in this manual are only "best guesses" based on current information about bioavailability, metabolism, and toxicity. They are initial suggestions only, and all drugs given in the ICU should be adjusted individually rather than administered to patients in cookbook fashion. Patients must be monitored for favorable and unfavorable drug effects as long as an agent is being given, especially when a clinical change occurs or other drugs are added or removed.

β-Agonist Sympathomimetic Bronchodilators

Identification and Actions. Sympathomimetics, or adrenergic agonists, include epinephrine and norepinephrine, the natural hormonal transmitters of the sympathetic nervous system, and synthetic drugs of related chemical structure and pharmacologic effects. They differ in the extent to which they stimulate different adrenergic receptors in the lung, heart, and elsewhere. These receptors have been categorized empirically into three types. Stimulation of α receptors produces bronchoconstriction, systemic arterial hypertension, and cardiac ectopy. Tachycardia, ectopy, and some augmentation of blood pressure result from β-1 stimulation. Stimulation of β-2 receptors causes dilatation of bronchial and other smooth muscles and inhibition of the cough reflex and may also lower arterial blood pressure. Thus, the more β-2 stimulation a drug produces in relation to its α- and β-1 effects, the more effective and safe it is as a bronchodilator; currently available agents are more selectively so than those of 20 years ago, but none is completely free from other effects, particularly at high dosage.

Available Preparations (Table 39–1). Epinephrine is the least selectively β-2 of available β-agonist bronchodilators, and is thus the most toxic; paradoxically, it is the only one available without a prescription in the United States. Of the newer, so-called β-2 bronchodilators, which are also longer acting than epinephrine and isoproterenol, isoetharine and metaproterenol are less so than albuterol (salbutamol), terbutaline, and bitolterol. Fenoterol, similar to albuterol, is available in Canada but not in the United States.

Indications and Administration. The drugs of first choice for reversible airflow obstruction (e.g., acute exacerbations of asthma or chronic obstructive pulmonary disease [COPD]) should be β-agonist sympathomimetics because of their high therapeutic index and ease of administration. Table 39–1 summarizes recommended dosages and frequencies of administration of available aerosol agents. Many clinicians routinely exceed these dosages and frequencies when treating severe bronchospasm in patients who can be monitored closely. Note that the quantity of drug recommended for use with a nebulizer is greater than that administered via metered-dose inhaler; this is why patients "refractory" to the latter may respond to the same drug given by powered or hand-bulb nebulizer. There is increasing evidence that, for small children and others who have difficulty using a metered-dose inhaler effectively, the addition of a spacer device between canister and mouth may increase clinical efficacy.

Adverse Effects and Monitoring. Tachycardia, nervousness, palpitation, and generalized central nervous system excitation are the most common adverse effects of sympathomimetic agents and result from their action

TABLE 39–1. β-Agonist Sympathomimetic Bronchodilators for Aerosol Administration

Drug	Brand Names	Relative β-2- Selectivity	Canister: Dose per Activation*	Solution: Recommended Dose†	Duration of Effect‡
Epinephrine	Adrenalin Primatene (Others)	—	0.06–0.20 mg	§	30–90 min
Isoproterenol	Isuprel Medihaler-Iso (Others)	—	0.08–0.13 mg	2.5 mg (0.5 ml of 1:200 solution)	1–2 hr
Isoetharine	Bronkometer Bronkosol	+	0.34 mg	2.5–5.0 mg (0.25–0.50 ml of 1 percent solution)	2–4 hr
Metaproterenol	Alupent Metaprel	+	0.65 mg	10–15 mg (0.2–0.3 ml of 5 percent solution)	2–4 hr
Albuterol	Proventil Ventolin	+ +	0.09 mg	2.5 mg	4–6 hr
Terbutaline	Brethaire Brethine	+ +	0.20 mg	0.25–0.50 mg‖	4–6 hr
Fenoterol¶	Berotec	+ +	0.20 mg	§	4–6 hr
Bitolterol	Tornalate	+ +	0.37 mg	§	4–6+ hr

*Usual dose: two activations.
†Nebulized in 2–3 ml total volume.
‡Varies among individuals.
§Not available.
‖Not approved for this indication in the United States.
¶Available in Canada and Europe but not in the United States.

on α- and β-1 receptors. Tremor, a frequent side effect of the newer agents (especially when given orally), is due to direct stimulation of β-2 receptors in skeletal muscle. Allergy to these agents is exceedingly rare. Other potential adverse effects include tachyphylaxis, which is uncommon and difficult to distinguish from other causes of a poor clinical response, and overuse by patients, which generally reflects deficiencies in overall management rather than in the drug.

Because no quantitative measure of serum levels is available, monitoring for efficacy and toxicity must rely on the patient's clinical responses: symptoms, physical examination, and, where appropriate, serial measurements of peak expiratory flow rate or forced expiratory volume in 1 second (FEV_1). The last two determinations are difficult to obtain in intubated patients but are very helpful in assessing severity, tracking the clinical course, and gauging response to therapy in other patients.

THEOPHYLLINE

Identification and Actions. Methylxanthine compounds, of which theophylline is the chief example used in the ICU, inhibit airway smooth muscle cell cyclic AMP phosphodiesterase and potentiate cellular cyclic AMP levels, although the importance of these actions in the drugs' clinical effects is unclear. Also of uncertain clinical significance are several other effects of theophylline, including alterations in mucociliary clearance and mediator release, increased diaphragmatic contractility and resistance to fatigue, increased respiratory drives, augmentation of right ventricular ejection fraction, and improved cardiac output. In asthma, there is a direct relationship (log-dose, not linear) between serum theophylline level and improvement in FEV_1, although above serum levels of 15–20 µg/mg toxicity increases, and additional improvement is slight in most patients.

Theophylline is metabolized mainly by the liver, and changes in hepatic function affect blood levels dramatically. Many factors alter theophylline metabolism. Drugs such as cimetidine and erythromycin decrease hepatic clearance of theophylline and thus increase blood levels; however, these effects are unpredictable, as they are with acute infectious illness, certain foods, and other drugs; and actual measurement of serum theophylline levels is the only sure monitoring tool, especially in the ICU.

Available Preparations. Aminophylline, oxtriphylline, and other theophylline "salts" are converted in the body to theophylline. Aminophylline is used intravenously (1.2 mg aminophylline = 1.0 mg theophylline) and numerous oral preparations of both aminophylline and theophylline are available.

Indications, Administration, and Monitoring. Theophylline is more toxic and less effective than the β-agonist bronchodilators. However, it is widely used in treating exacerbations of COPD as well as in acute asthma. In acutely ill hospitalized patients, it should be administered intravenously, and this is accomplished in two phases—a loading dose followed by continuous maintenance infusion.

The loading dose is given over 15–30 minutes and is unrelated to hepatic function or other factors that affect clearance rates. Each mg/kg of intravenous aminophylline will increase serum theophylline by approximately 2 µg/ml. Because the desired therapeutic range for initial therapy is 10–15 µg/ml, patients not already receiving theophylline or related compounds should be loaded with 6 mg/kg. For patients previously taking theophylline preparations but with no signs of clinical toxicity, a loading dose of 3 mg/kg may be used. If signs of toxicity are present or if the serum level is already in the upper therapeutic range of 15–20 µg/ml, no loading dose should be given.

Maintenance infusion, which should be begun as soon as the loading dose has been given, should initially be 0.9 mg/kg/hr for children and otherwise healthy young cigarette smokers; 0.6 mg/kg/hr for adult nonsmokers up to age 40; 0.4 mg/kg/hr for older adults with no evidence of liver or cardiac disease (including *cor pulmonale*); 0.1 or 0.2 mg/kg/hr if hepatic or cardiac dysfunction is present. Serum theophylline should be measured 12–18 hours after the loading dose and the maintenance infusion rate adjusted accordingly.

Serum levels must be monitored whenever intravenous aminophylline is used and should also be checked whenever the infusion rate is changed, when the patient is switched to an oral preparation, or when a change in clinical status occurs.

Adverse Effects. Theophylline has a narrow therapeutic range and a low therapeutic index (ratio of therapeutic to toxic blood level), and side effects will occur in as many as half of all patients. These side effects include nervousness, insomnia, anorexia, nausea, vomiting, abdominal discomfort, headache, seizures, and cardiac arrhythmias. The last two seldom occur at serum levels below 30–40 µg/ml unless the patient already has an active seizure focus or preexisting arrhythmias.

When accompanied by signs of toxicity, especially when of rapid onset, serum levels in excess of 30 µg/ml warrant monitoring in the ICU, discontinuation of the drug, and consideration of treatment with activated charcoal. Severe toxicity (seizures or dysrhythmias, with levels over 40 µg/ml) should be treated with agents specific for each manifestation as well as with oral activated charcoal. Hemodialysis may be required less often in such instances with the early administration of activated charcoal.

ANTICHOLINERGICS

Identification, Actions, and Available Preparations. Anticholinergic (antimuscarinic) drugs inhibit the action of acetylcholine on autonomic nerve endings innervated by postganglionic cholinergic nerves. This opposes the actions of the vagus nerve and is thus helpful in preventing or reversing bronchospasm of reflex or irritant origin. Clinically, atropine and related drugs such as ipratropium bromide may be particularly effective as bronchodilators in chronic bronchitis as opposed to allergic asthma. Unlike atropine, ipratropium bromide (Atrovent) can be made available in a metered-dose inhaler as well as in aerosol solution form. Only the metered-dose inhaler form is currently available in the United States.

Indications and Administration. Studies documenting the efficacy of atropine in COPD and asthma have generally been carried out in stable outpatients, and its use in the ICU is currently based largely on inference and analogy. However, in acute exacerbations of COPD requiring hospitalization, an empirical trial of ipratropium may be considered, with efficacy judged either subjectively or through serial measures of FEV_1.

Adverse Effects. Given systemically, atropine causes tachycardia, urinary retention, blurred vision, decreased bowel motility, and drying of respiratory tract secretions. Although topical administration to the respiratory tract by aerosol avoids these side effects in many cases, toxicity is still common, particularly with prolonged administration. Ipratropium has little toxicity.

CORTICOSTEROIDS

Identification and Actions. The corticosteroids are a group of potent natural and synthetic hormones used in conditions characterized by inappropriately severe immune or inflammatory reactions. Their actions are complex and incompletely understood but include decreased exudation and migration of inflammatory cells, protection of cell membranes against damage by a variety of agents, decreased release of vasoactive amines and other mediators, and diminished fluid leakage from blood vessels and edema formation. They also potentiate responsiveness to sympathomimetic agents. Despite these facts, the use of corticosteroid drugs in critical care medicine remains empirical, and the precise indications, mode of action, and ideal dosages for the various available preparations are yet to be established.

Available Preparations. Methylprednisolone (Solu-Medrol), hydrocortisone, and dexamethasone (Decadron) are the most commonly used parenteral preparations. Equivalent dosages of these agents are 4, 20, and 0.75, respectively. Prednisone (Deltasone; others) and prednisolone (Delta-Cortef; others), approximately equal in potency, are the oral preparations generally used. Beclomethasone, flunisolide, and triamcinolone are corticosteroids available in the United States for inhalational use; however, maximum recommended dosages of these agents are only equivalent to about 10 mg prednisone per 24 hours, and for this and other reasons they should not be used in acutely ill patients.

Indications and Administration. In outpatient and long-term therapy, the toxicity of the corticosteroids makes thorough trials of other therapy and documentation of efficacy mandatory. However, the short-term, high-dose administration of these drugs can be thought of differently, with separate indications and less likelihood of adverse effects. Objective documentation of efficacy is difficult to obtain in *status asthmaticus* and severe acute exacerbations of COPD, and empirical treatment is justified. Unless prior episodes have indicated otherwise because of idiosyncratic reactions, acute psychosis, or other unusual toxicity, corticosteroids should be begun as soon as possible in these conditions along with β-agonists, theophylline, and other therapy.

In acute asthma, prednisone or prednisolone, 20–40 mg daily by mouth in one or two doses and tapered after 2 to 4 days once improvement occurs, is often sufficient. Each patient is different, and each tends to respond similarly to therapy in successive episodes; therefore, treatment should be individualized. The more severe an attack, and the longer its duration when treatment is initiated, the larger the doses, and the longer the duration of therapy required to control it.

Status asthmaticus generally requires higher doses and is given intravenously. Hydrocortisone (100 to 1000 mg/24 hr) or methylprednisolone (80 to 1000 mg/24 hr) should be administered every 4 to 6 hours and continued without reduction in dosage until the patient improves. Tapering should follow over several days.

Patients with acute exacerbations of COPD requiring hospitalization should be given methylprednisolone every 6 hours for 3 or 4 days at a dose of 2 mg/kg/24 hr; whether the drug should be tapered over several more days or discontinued abruptly is unknown, although most clinicians prefer the former.

Adverse Effects and Monitoring. Acute effects of corticosteroid use include euphoria and a sense of well-being; restlessness, insomnia, and frank psychosis can occur within a few days of initiating therapy, as can hyperglycemia, peptic ulceration, and upper gastrointestinal bleeding. Long-term toxic effects such as increased susceptibility to bacterial infection, reactivation of previous tuberculosis, myopathy, cataracts, and Cushing's syndrome are very rare with administration for less than two weeks. In the absence of blood level measurements, monitoring must be by clinical response. Serial measurements of peak expiratory flow rate or FEV_1 are helpful but often not feasible in critically ill patients.

CROMOLYN

Disodium cromoglycate is a topical agent administered by inhalation, either in powdered form or in aqueous solution, primarily in the prophylaxis of asthma. Not a bronchodilator, it appears to act by preventing or reducing the release of mediators of bronchoconstriction. It is not generally used in severe exacerbations of asthma or COPD, although it may be useful in the long-term management of these conditions.

MUCOLYTICS AND EXPECTORANTS

Numerous agents [guaifenesin; acetylcysteine (Mucomyst); iodides; others] are available for the purpose of facilitating sputum expectoration. Although they do increase sputum production in many patients, it is unclear whether this is because of facilitated expectoration or increased quantities of sputum, and clinical benefits from the process have been difficult to demonstrate. Although mucolytics and expectorants are widely used in some parts of the world, in North America their use is usually restricted to patients with cystic fibrosis and other conditions producing unusually thick, inspissated secretions. Some clinicians believe that acetylcysteine applied directly onto mucus plugs via the fiberoptic bronchoscope improves the resolution of atelectasis and retained secretions. Hypo- and hypertonic saline can cause bronchospasm, as can acetylcysteine, which is unpleasant for the patient because of its odor and taste. Iodides, acetylcysteine, and other such agents can cause hypersensitivity reactions and tend to become less effective with repeated administration.

Respiratory Stimulants

Respiratory drives and ventilation are depressed by hypothermia, starvation, and anything else that decreases metabolic rate. Similarly, conditions and agents that increase overall metabolic rate stimulate the ventilatory regulation system and increase ventilation. Doxapram (Dopram) and other analeptic agents increase the frequency and depth of respiration through stimulation of respiratory drives; they also increase work of breathing and metabolic demands. Doxapram must be given intravenously, and patients receiving it require careful, continuous monitoring. Used to hasten postanesthetic awakening, it has also been employed by some clinicians to delay or avoid endotracheal intubation in acute respiratory failure. However, controlled studies have not shown doxapram or other respiratory stimulants to affect this or other aspects of acute respiratory failure. Medroxyprogesterone acetate (Provera) stimulates ventilation with long-term administration but has no role in critical care.

Antibiotics

For documented bacterial infections of the respiratory system, appropriate antibiotic therapy is obviously crucial to good patient care. Clinicians wishing to use empirical antibiotic therapy for patients with COPD should use agents with the lowest possible cost and toxicity; amoxicillin, ampicillin, tetracycline, and trimethoprim-sulfa are preferable to erythromycin and more expensive new generation antibiotics.

Whether antibiotics should be given by aerosol for documented respiratory infections in critically ill patients with lung disease is still unproven, although anecdotal experience suggests that this can be effective in some patients. If used, aminoglycosides and other antibiotics given by the airway route should be selected according to sensitivity testing against the patient's infecting organisms; the same drug should be administered systemically, and appropriate blood levels maintained using frequent testing.

RECOMMENDED READING

Albert RK, et al: Controlled clinical trial of methylprednisolone in patients with chronic bronchitis and acute respiratory insufficiency. Ann Intern Med 92:753, 1980.

Cherniack RM (ed): Drugs for the Respiratory System. Orlando, Grune & Stratton, Inc., 1986.

Clarke SW, Newman SP: Therapeutic aerosols 2—Drugs available by the inhaled route. Thorax 39:1, 1984.

Dunlap NE, Fulmer JD: Corticosteroid therapy in asthma. Clin Chest Med 5:669, 1984.

George RB, Payne DK: Anticholinergics, cromolyn, and other occasionally useful drugs. Clin Chest Med 5:685, 1984.

Gilman AG, et al (eds): Goodman & Gilman's The Pharmacological Basis of Therapeutics. Seventh edition. New York, Macmillan Publishing Company, 1985.

I.V. guidelines for theophylline products. FDA Drug Bull 10:2, 1980.

Jenne JW: Theophylline use in asthma: some current issues. Clin Chest Med 5:645, 1984.

Konig P: Spacer devices used with metered-dose inhalers: breakthrough or gimmick? Chest 88:276, 1985.

Paterson JW, Woolcock AJ, Shenfield GM: Bronchodilator drugs: state of the art. Am Rev Respir Dis 120:1149, 1979.

Pierson DJ: Chronic obstructive pulmonary disease and bronchiectasis. In Rakel RE (ed): Conn's Current Therapy 1985. Philadelphia, W.B. Saunders Co., 1985, p. 96.

Pierson DJ: Respiratory stimulants: review of the literature and assessment of current status. Respir Care 18:548, 1973.

Sessler CN, Glauser FL, Cooper KR: Treatment of theophylline toxicity with oral activated charcoal. Chest 87:325, 1985.

Shim C: Adrenergic agonists and bronchodilator therapy in asthma. Clin Chest Med 5:659, 1984.

Ziment I: Respiratory Pharmacology and Therapeutics. Philadelphia, W.B. Saunders Co., 1978.

Renal and Fluid and Electrolyte Disorders

40. Acute Renal Failure

Richard A. Zager

DEFINITION

The term acute renal failure describes a syndrome of sudden reduction in renal function such that daily solute loads are incompletely excreted. This solute retention produces stepwise increments in the blood urea nitrogen (BUN) and creatinine concentrations. Retention of water and non-nitrogenous solutes may produce extracellular fluid volume expansion, hyperkalemia, metabolic acidosis, hyperphosphatemia and hyponatremia. Accumulation of nitrogenous waste products produces uremia, typically manifested by nausea, vomiting, encephalopathy, muscle cramps, a bleeding diathesis and, possibly, pericarditis.

Multiple causes of acute renal failure exist. These are frequently subdivided into three broad categories—prerenal, intrarenal, and postrenal—the common etiologies of which are presented in Table 40–1. Acute renal failure is also subdivided into oliguric (less than 400 ml urine/24 hr) and nonoliguric (more than 400 ml urine/24 hr) forms. However, this distinction has little differential diagnostic utility: Virtually any form of acute renal failure can be either oliguric or nonoliguric in its presentation, and changes in urine flow rates may occur in any given case. The vast majority of cases of acute renal failure have the potential for reversibility, occuring either spontaneously or with appropriate medical interventions. Therapy differs dramatically according to etiology. Therefore, accurate diagnosis is essential.

Diagnostic findings for specific causes of acute renal failure are discussed in the next sections and are presented in Table 40–2. The following represents a diagnostic approach to patients with apparently acute renal disease of uncertain etiology:

Step 1: *Does the patient have acute renal failure or previously undiagnosed chronic renal failure?* The differential diagnostic approach to patients with acute and chronic renal failure differs. Therefore, it is essential to ascertain whether the renal failure is, in fact, acute. This is not a problem if previous assessments of renal function are available. This is usually the case, since a majority of cases of acute renal failure develop in the hospital. Chronic renal disease can be assumed if renal size is reduced, as assessed by abdominal roentgenogram or by renal ultrasound. Since the vast majority

TABLE 40–1. CAUSES OF ACUTE RENAL FAILURE

PRERENAL
  Extracellular fluid volume depletion
  Congestive heart failure
  Hypotension
  Cirrhosis; hepatorenal syndrome
  Drugs: nonsteroidal antiinflammatory agents, angiotensin-covering enzyme inhibitors
INTRARENAL
  Acute glomerulonephritis (AGN)
  Acute vasculopathy (AV)
    Vasculitis
    Obliterative arteriolopathy
      Malignant hypertension
      Hemolytic uremic syndrome
      Thrombotic thrombocytopenic purpura
      Atheroemboli
  Allergic interstitial nephritis (AIN)
  Acute tubular necrosis (ATN)
    Ischemia
    Exogenous nephrotoxins
      Aminoglycosides
      Radiocontrast
      Cisplatin
      Cyclosporin A
      Organic solvents
    Endogenous nephrotoxins
      Rhabdomyolysis (myoglobin)
      Tumor cell lysis (chemotherapy)
      Hemolysis
      Major tissue trauma (tissue "toxins")
POSTRENAL
  Extrarenal obstruction
  Intrarenal obstruction
    Acute urate nephropathy
    Acute myeloma kidney
    Ethylene glycol intoxication

of patients with chronic renal failure are nonoliguric, oliguria suggests an acute etiology. Heavy proteinuria (more than 3 g/24 hr) also suggests chronicity, since this degree of urinary protein excretion is very uncommon in patients with acute renal failure, even when due to acute glomerulonephritis. The sole exception to this is in patients with allergic interstitial nephritis due to nonsteroidal antiinflammatory agents, a condition that may at times manifest the nephrotic syndrome.

Step 2: *Clinical assessment.* The best diagnostic information concerning the etiology of acute renal failure comes from clinical assessment. Modest circulatory insufficiency suggests prerenal azotemia. Conversely, severe hypotension, nephrotoxic drug exposure, sepsis, or trauma suggest acute tubular necrosis. Allergic interstitial nephritis should be suspected when fever, rash, eosinophilia, or eosinophiluria develop at approximately the same time at which the renal dysfunction commenced. Postrenal failure

TABLE 40–2. RENAL FAILURE INDICES

CONDITION	U_{NA}	FE_{NA}	U_{OSM}	$U_{SEDIMENT}$	OTHER
Prerenal failure	<20	<1 percent	>500	Usually normal	Response to treatment
Intrarenal failure					
AGN	V	V	V	RBC casts Proteinuria	
ATN					
Oliguric	>40	>1 percent	<500	"ATN casts"	
Nonoliguric	V	V	<500	± "ATN casts"	
AIN	V	V	V	RBCs Eosinophils	Fever Rash Eosinophilia
Postrenal failure	V	V	V	± RBCs or normal	Ultrasound shows extrarenal obstruction

U = urine; U_{NA} = mEq/L; FE_{NA} = urine/serum Na ÷ urine/serum creatinine × 100 percent; V = variable; ATN = acute tubular necrosis; AIN = acute interstitial nephritis; AGN = acute glomerulonephritis.

is easily excluded by bladder catheterization and/or ultrasonography. For patients who develop acute renal failure in the hospital, two exercises are particularly useful: (1) review all medication exposure to look for nephrotoxins or drugs known to induce allergic interstitial nephritis; (2) identify the day on which the BUN and creatinine first started to rise. A review of the progress notes on this day and the day before frequently reveals the cause of the acute renal failure (e.g., onset of sepsis, surgery, hypotension, radiographic contrast administration).

Step 3: *Confirm diagnostic suspicion by laboratory assessments.* Typical diagnostic findings for the various forms of acute renal failure are presented in Table 40–2. It should be noted that any classic urinary finding may be absent in a particular case of acute renal failure. For example, the urinary sodium (Na^+) concentration may be more than 40 mEq/L, and the urine osmolality may be less than 500 mOsm/L in patients with prerenal azotemia if they have recently received diuretics. Thus, repeated evaluation of these renal diagnostic parameters may need to be made before a definitive diagnosis can be reached.

PRERENAL ACUTE RENAL FAILURE

Definition

The term prerenal azotemia (or prerenal acute renal failure) refers to a decline in renal function that is mediated by an alteration in renal hemodynamics.

Pathophysiology

Most typically, prerenal azotemia is induced by a reduction in renal blood flow due to intravascular volume depletion (e.g., due to blood loss, diuretics, vomiting, diarrhea), congestive heart failure, severe nephrotic syndrome, preferential shunting of blood flow away from the kidney such as occurs with severe cirrhosis or, rarely, bilateral renal artery stenosis. Uncommonly, prerenal azotemia can be induced by drugs that alter intrarenal hemodynamics. These include nonsteroidal antiinflammatory agents and angiotensin-converting enzyme inhibitors. These adverse drug effects typically occur in patients who already have one of the above prerenal factors that is then intensified by adding these agents.

Diagnosis and Management

A preliminary diagnosis of prerenal azotemia is based on clinical assessment. Most often, overt congestive heart failure, liver failure, intravascular volume depletion (weight loss, orthostatic hypotension, bleeding, diuretic usage) are obvious from the history and physical examination. However, in some instances, overt circulatory abnormalities causing prerenal azotemia are not clinically apparent. For example, patients can have classic prerenal azotemia despite the presence of a normal cardiac output as assessed by pulmonary artery catheter. Thus, a diagnosis of prerenal azotemia is most typically confirmed by urine and blood testing. Typically, the urine sodium concentration is less than 20 mEq/L, and the fractional resorption of sodium (FE_{NA}) is less than 1 percent. The urinary sediment is usually normal. The urinary osmolality is typically more than 500 mOsm/L. The BUN/serum creatinine ratio is most often greater than 15/1, reflecting a relative increase in tubular resorption of urea, owing to a decrease in effective renal perfusion. However, it is important to recognize that any of these classic laboratory findings may be absent in a given patient with prerenal azotemia. For example, the urinary sodium may be greater than 20 mEq/L if the patient has recently received diuretics. Similarly, the urinary osmolality may be inappropriately low in patients who have received diuretics or who have an underlying renal concentrating abnormality. Lastly, the BUN/creatinine ratio may be less than 15/1 if the patient has had poor dietary protein intake.

In patients who have a tentative diagnosis of prerenal azotemia but who fail to demonstrate typical laboratory findings, the diagnosis is confirmed by judging their response to appropriate therapeutic interventions. Most typically, a trial of intravenous volume expansion with 1–3 liters of normal saline administered over 3–12 hours is used in patients with presumed volume depletion. It is mandatory that a diagnosis of congestive heart failure be excluded prior to such a volume challenge. In the latter instance, therapy should include measures to alleviate the heart failure, which should result in an improvement in the azotemia. Ultimately, the diagnosis of prerenal azotemia rests upon resolution of the renal insufficiency when appropriate therapeutic interventions are undertaken to improve systemic hemodynamics.

Outcome

As noted earlier, prerenal acute renal failure is most often reversible.

Hepatorenal Syndrome

This term refers to the presence of slowly progressive renal insufficiency in association with severe and usually terminal cirrhosis. It resembles typical prerenal azotemia resulting from renal vasoconstriction but is of uncertain etiology. As with classic prerenal azotemia, it is typically associated with a urinary sodium concentration of less than 20 mEq/L and a urine osmolality in excess of 500 mOsm/L. The urinary sediment is oftentimes normal, or it may show a plethora of muddy brown granular casts, mimicking acute tubular necrosis. These casts presumably result from a detergent action of filtered bile salts on the tubular epithelium. The major distinguishing feature between hepatorenal syndrome and prerenal azotemia is that the former is not responsive to any currently available therapeutic interventions. Diuretics and renal vasodilators (e.g., dopamine, 1–2 μg/kg/min) may induce a transient diuresis, but their use does not result in any sustained improvement in renal function.

The most important intervention to make in patients with hepatorenal syndrome is to exclude reversible factors in the renal failure, such as intravascular volume depletion, nephrotoxin exposure, or urinary tract obstruction. To exclude a reversible prerenal component, a therapeutic trial of intravascular volume expansion with approximately 2–3 liters of normal saline and/or albumin solutions is warranted. However, if no improvement in renal function results, such attempts should be abandoned, since they may exacerbate ascites and portal hypertension. In general, patients with hepatorenal syndrome die of hepatic failure, not of renal failure. Thus, the major therapeutic goal in such patients should be to seek out and correct any reversible components to the underlying hepatic disease.

Intrarenal Acute Renal Failure

Definition

By far the most common cause of acute renal failure due to intrinsic renal disease is acute tubular nerosis (ATN). Unfortunately, this has caused the terms acute renal failure and acute tubular necrosis to be used interchangeably. It is critical to avoid equating these two terms, since this can lead to misdiagnosis and, thus, to inappropriate management. The common causes of acute renal failure due to intrinsic renal disease are considered below.

Pathophysiology and Diagnosis

Acute glomerulonephritis (AGN). AGN can occur either as a *de novo* illness, as a manifestation of a multisystem disease (for example, vasculitis, cancer), or in response to an infectious process (postinfectious GN). The latter is particularly likely to be seen in the intensive care unit (ICU) setting in patients with bacterial endocarditis. A diagnosis of AGN can be made with reasonable certainty by careful urinalysis. Red blood cell casts are observed in the vast majority of cases and usually significant proteinuria (2–4+ by dipstick; 1–3 g/24 hr) will be observed. In patients with postinfectious GN, a depression of the serum C_3 and C_4 complement components is typically observed.

Acute vasculopathy (AV). A variety of disease processes may affect the intrarenal vasculature, resulting in acute renal failure. These diseases can be divided into three broad categories: (1) inflammatory, or vasculitis, most notably, *polyarteritis nodosa;* (2) obliterative arteriolopathies (malignant hypertension, hemolytic-uremic syndrome, thrombotic thrombocytopenic purpura); (3) microscopic atheroembolic renal disease. All of these are notable for their ability to induce multisystem organ involvement, a strong clue to their diagnosis. Inflammatory vasculitis tends to involve glomeruli as well as arteriolar and prearteriolar vessels. Thus, they frequently induce red blood cell cast formation. The obliterative arteriolopathies usually produce a mild-to-severe microangiopathic hemolytic anemia. The diagnosis of atheroembolic renal disease is suggested when renal failure ensues days to weeks after abdominal aortography, the most common cause for showering the renal circulation with microscopic atheromatous plaques.

Acute interstitial nephritis (AIN). This condition is characterized by an acute inflammatory process of the renal interstitium, which leads to an acute reduction of glomerular filtration rate. In the vast majority of instances, it is due to an allergic response to drug administration, especially the beta-lactam antibiotics, nonsteroidal antiinflammatory agents, cimetidine, allopurinol, or selected anticonvulsants. The diagnosis of AIN is suggested by the presence of fever, rash, eosinophilia, eosinophiluria, and hematuria, one of these symptoms being observed in approximately 90 per cent of cases. A definitive diagnosis can be made only by renal biopsy.

Acute tubular necrosis (ATN). ATN accounts for approximately 80 percent of cases of intrinsic acute renal failure. It has traditionally been subdivided into ischemic and nephrotoxic categories, reflecting the presumed etiology. However, in the vast majority of cases, ATN is multifactorial in origin, with many of the factors listed in Table 40–1 being present. The most commonly identified precipitating factors are major tissue trauma (including surgery), nephrotoxic drug exposure (radiographic contrast agents, aminoglycosides), sepsis, and systemic hypotension. Many of these have been shown to exert synergistic toxic effects on the renal tubular epithelium. As in virtually all other causes of acute renal failure, patients with ATN may be either oliguric or nonoliguric, the latter conveying a better prognosis, since the renal injury (and the causes of it) are, in general, less severe. The clinical manifestations of ATN are comparable to those seen in other causes of acute renal failure. However, since these patients are typically critically ill with multisystem organ dysfunction, their course is frequently dominated not by the renal failure but rather by the underlying illnesses that precipitated it.

A diagnosis of ATN is usually based on excluding other causes of acute renal failure and by documenting typical urinary findings (see Table 40–1). In oliguric ATN, the urinary sodium concentration is usually greater than 40 mEq/L, the FE_{NA} is greater than 1 percent, the urinary osmolality is less than 500 mOsm/L, and the urinary sediment reveals "muddy brown" granular casts. Proteinuria is usually trace to 2+, and there is an absence of red blood cell casts. Hematuria is commonly observed, but this reflects the frequent use of Foley catheters in these patients and not the intrinsic renal disorder. The BUN/creatinine ratio is typically less than 15/1, unless the patient is extremely catabolic, bleeding, or receiving large amounts of parenteral amino acid containing hyperalimentation solutions. All of these situations can increase the BUN concentration.

In contrast to oliguric ATN, patients with nonoliguric ATN may have a high or low (less than 20 mEq/L) urinary sodium, and they frequently lack muddy brown granular casts in the urinary sediment. Thus, it is possible for the urinary findings in a patient with nonoliguric ATN to mimic those seen in patients with typical prerenal azotemia. In such cases, a distinction between nonoliguric ATN and prerenal azotemia is based on the clinical setting and on the response of the patient to correction of possible prerenal factors.

Management

Treatment of AGN is directed at its underlying cause and at the general complications of renal insufficiency, which are discussed below. The same is true for AV. No known therapy exists for acute renal failure due to atheroembolic disease other than dialysis. For AIN, treatment with glucocortocoids may hasten the recovery of renal function. However, in most instances, the lesion reverts spontaneously once the offending agent has been withdrawn. The decision to use corticosteroids requires careful evaluation, including a renal biopsy to confirm the diagnosis.

The course of ATN is typically divided into three phases: (1) the induction phase, (2) the maintenance phase, and (3) the diuretic phase. These distinctions are useful since treatment directed at the renal failure differs depending on the stage. The initiation phase denotes the period of evolving tubular injury. In most instances, this is short-lived, and usually occurs within several hours. However, it is during this phase that the best chance of ameliorating the severity of renal injury exists. If there is a clinical suggestion that acute tubular injury may be occurring (e.g., shock, sepsis, recent trauma, radiocontrast exposure), the following are appropriate acute interventions: (1) intravascular fluid volume repletion with saline/blood/colloid solutions to alleviate renal ischemia; (2) treatment of sepsis with appropriate antibiotics; (3) establishment of a diuresis by administering diuretics. The rationale for the latter is that a diuresis may prevent the development of intratubular obstruction due to intraluminal inspissation of necrotic tubular cell debris. In addition, it may facilitate the renal excretion of nephrotoxic compounds. Experimental data suggest that mannitol is the diuretic of choice. Typically, 10–25 grams of 20 percent mannitol are administered intravenously over 15–30 minutes. Prior to its administration, it should be determined that the patient is not in severe heart failure, since hypertonic mannitol will increase extracellular fluid volume. If no diuresis results, intravenous furosemide (in intravenous doses up to 200–400 mg administered over 20–40 minutes) or low-dose dopamine (1–2 μg/kg/min) can be used in an attempt to induce a diuresis. However, there is little data to suggest that the two latter maneuvers exert a protective effect over that which can be achieved with mannitol alone.

The term "maintenance phase" denotes that phase of acute tubular necrosis in which tubular injury has been completed, but a sustained reduction in renal function has resulted. Once this phase has been reached, no known therapeutic intervention has been shown to have any sustained beneficial effect on renal function. Diuretics and renal vasodilators, such as low-dose dopamine, may transiently increase urine flow. However, they rarely make a clinically significant impact on glomerular filtration rate nor do they hasten functional recovery. Thus, treatment of the maintenance phase, which can last from several days to 8 weeks, should be directed at improving the patient's underlying medical/surgical illnesses, avoiding if at all possible further renal injury due to nephrotoxin exposure or additional ischemic events, and treatment with dialysis as necessary. If possible, patients should receive a daily intake of 3000 calories, including 40–50 grams of high biologic value protein because they are hypercatabolic. Fluid and electrolytes are given to replace urinary output, drainage, and insensible losses, the latter approximating 400 ml/day. Hyperkalemia (Chapter 45), metabolic acidosis (Chapter 41), hypocalcemia (Chapter 48), and hyperphosphatemia (Chapter 51) are prevented or treated as they arise. Finally, hemodialysis is employed three to five times per week in order to maintain the BUN concentration below 120 mg/dl.

The recovery phase, also known as the diuretic phase, denotes the period of renal functional recovery. In the oliguric patient, it is heralded by gradual stepwise increments in urine flow followed by a plateauing of the rate of rise of the BUN and creatinine concentrations. This is followed shortly therafter by a slow resolution of the azotemia, which lasts for approximately 5–10 days. In nonoliguric patients, urine flow may or may not increase during this period. The amount of diuresis that occurs is almost always appropriate for the degree of the patient's fluid and solute retention. Therefore, one should not routinely attempt to replace the daily urine output with intravenous fluids. Only if obvious intravascular volume depletion occurs or a failure of continued improvement in renal function develops should saline be administered in an attempt to replace urinary losses. Such a necessity rarely arises. In most instances, the BUN and creatinine concentrations return to normal or near-normal values by the completion of the recovery phase.

Outcome

As discussed earlier, the prognosis of intrarenal failure depends in large part on the underlying disorder. Complete or nearly complete recovery of renal function should be expected in patients with ATN.

Rhabdomyolysis-Induced Acute Renal Failure

Rhabdomyolysis-induced acute renal failure is a form of ATN in which myoglobin release from injured muscles is believed to induce tubular damage. The most common causes for this condition are trauma, excessive exercise, particularly in physically untrained individuals in a hot climate, alcoholism, severe hypophosphatemia, hypokalemia, and, on occasion, excessive muscular work due to convulsions or septic rigors. Frequently, many of these conditions coexist (e.g., alcoholism, phosphate depletion, seizures/sepsis). Myoglobin, which is not nephrotoxic, is believed to be converted to hematin, a nephrotoxic compound, at an acid pH in the tubules, thereby producing tubular necrosis. However, it is more likely that substantial intravascular volume depletion, such as that due to the presence of severe muscle edema, leads to decreased renal perfusion and that this, in concert with hematin and other muscle toxins, produces the acute renal failure.

The diagnosis of rhabdomyolysis-induced acute renal failure is made primarily on the basis of the clinical setting in which the acute failure develops plus the finding of myoglobinuria. The quickest bedside clue to the presence of myoglobinuria is a "4 + blood" reaction by urinary dipstick assessment at a time that microscopic exam reveals no hematuria. This occurs because myoglobin gives a (+) hemoglobin reaction. If massive, myoglobinuria will turn the urine a reddish-brown color. Serum creatine phosphokinase levels are invariably elevated, usually with values in excess of 1000 units.

Treatment during the initiation phase of the disease is intravascular volume expansion to correct the renal hypoperfusion and to induce a diuresis. Sodium bicarbonate is traditionally administered to raise the urine pH to 6.5–7.0, although there are no compelling data to prove that this has any benefit over that achieved by saline alone. Sodium bicarbonate can be administered, but care must be exercised so that intravascular volume overload, metabolic alkalosis, or hyperosmolality do not develop. In other respects, management is the same as that for any other patient with acute tubular necrosis. Dialysis may be needed more often than usual because muscle breakdown exaggerates the degree of azotemia, hyperkalemia, hyperphosphatemia, and metabolic acidosis.

Postrenal Acute Renal Failure

Definition

Postrenal failure is synonymous with acute obstructive nephropathy. As the name implies, it is due to anatomic or functional blockage of the kidneys or urinary tract.

Pathophysiology

Acute urinary tract obstruction most often occurs because of bladder outlet obstruction or functional impairment of bladder emptying. It may also be due to correctable surgical lesions such as involvement of the ureters by tumor. Obstructive nephropathy can also occur at the renal tubular level, caused by the deposition of oxalate crystals (in ethylene glycol poisoning, for example—see Chapter 84), Bence Jones proteins (multiple myeloma), or uric acid crystals (chemotherapy-induced massive tumor cell lysis).

Diagnosis and Management

Initial evaluation of all patients with acute renal failure should include percussion of the suprapubic area to evaluate bladder distention and to determine the postvoid residual urine volume. Because these procedures do not exclude bilateral ureteral obstruction or obstruction of a solitary kidney, renal ultrasound should be performed if obstructive nephropathy is suspected. Urinalysis should be performed for the presence of crystals, and urine protein electrophoresis is used to confirm Bence Jones proteinuria. This is because ultrasound does not reveal obstruction if it is at the tubular level. Other than the general measures cited earlier, the therapy for postrenal failure involves removing the anatomic or functional cause of obstruction.

Outcome

The prognosis is favorable for patients with obstructive nephropathy if the obstruction can be removed within a short period of time.

RECOMMENDED READING

Anderson RJ, Schrier RW: Acute renal failure. In Braunwald E, et al (eds): Harrison's Principles of Internal Medicine. 11th edition. New York, McGraw-Hill, Inc., 1987, p. 1149.

Brenner BM, Lazarus JM (eds): Acute Renal Failure. Philadelphia, W.B. Saunders Co., 1983.

Brezis B, Rosen S, Epstein FH: Acute renal failure. In Brenner BM, Rector FC Jr (eds): The Kidney. 3rd edition. Philadelphia, W.B. Saunders Co., 1986, p. 735.

Dixon BS, Anderson RJ: Nonoliguric acute renal failure. Am J Kidney Dis 6:71, 1985.

Franklin SS, Maxwell MH: Acute renal failure. In Maxwell MH, Kleeman CR (eds): Clinical Disorders of Fluid and Electrolyte Metabolism. New York, McGraw-Hill, Inc., 1980, p. 745.

Goldstein MB: Acute renal failure. Med Clin North Am 67:1325, 1983.

Hou SH, et al: Hospital-acquired renal insufficiency: a prospective study. Am J Med 74:243, 1983.

Kron IL, Joob AW, Van Meter C: Acute renal failure in the cardiovascular surgical patient. Ann Thorac Surg 39:590, 1985.

Myers BD, Moran SM: Hemodynamically mediated acute renal failure. N Engl J Med 314:97, 1986.

Rasmussen HH, Ibels LS: Acute renal failure: multivariate analysis of causes and risk factors. Am J Med 73:211, 1982.

Schrier RW: Acute renal failure: pathogenesis, diagnosis, and management. Hosp Pract 16(3):93, 1981.

41. Acid-Base Disturbances

Susan M. Ott

John M. Luce

INTRODUCTION

When the body is in normal acid-base balance, its intracellular and extracellular fluids are neither excessively acidic nor excessively alkaline. Acid-base status may be quantified in terms of either the serum concentration of hydrogen ions (H^+) or the negative logarithm of that concentration, pH. Normally the H^+ concentration is maintained at around 40 ng/L and the pH at around 7.40 (range 7.38–7.42) by the carbonic acid buffering system, which involves bicarbonate (HCO_3^-) and carbon dioxide (CO_2). Although other buffers, such as hemoglobin and bone, also are important, the carbonic acid buffering system is most useful when diagnosing and treating acid-base disturbances.

Carbonic acid (H_2CO_3) is formed by the hydration of CO_2 in the presence of the enzyme carbonic anhydrase (CA) by the following reaction:

$$CO_2 + H_2O \overset{CA}{\rightleftharpoons} H_2CO_3 \rightleftharpoons H^+ + HCO_3^-$$

The equilibrium equation describing this reaction can be written as follows:

$$H^+ \text{ concentration} = 24 \times \frac{PaCO_2}{HCO_3^- \text{ concentration}}$$

where $PaCO_2$ is the partial pressure of CO_2 in arterial blood.

Normally, the H^+ concentration = 40 ng/L, $PaCO_2$ = 40 mm Hg, and HCO_3^- concentration = 24 mEq/L. When arterial blood gases are sent to the laboratory for analysis, the pH and $PaCO_2$ actually are measured, and the HCO_3^- is calculated using the equilibrium equation. By converting H^+ concentration to pH with Table 41–1 and substituting the numbers recorded by the blood gas laboratory, clinicians can determine whether the blood gas values reported to them are accurate or reflect laboratory error. The calculated HCO_3^- should be within 5 mEq/L of that measured on a chemical electrolyte analysis.

The $PaCO_2$ is regulated primarily by alveolar ventilation, which is

TABLE 41–1. RELATIONSHIP BETWEEN pH AND HYDROGEN ION CONCENTRATION

pH (units)	H^+ CONCENTRATION (ng/L)
7.0	100
7.1	79
7.2	63
7.3	50
7.4	40
7.5	32
7.6	25
7.7	20
8.0	10

H^+ = hydrogen ion concentration.

accomplished by the lungs, whereas the HCO_3^- concentration is regulated primarily by the kidneys. Acid-base balance is maintained by changes in alveolar ventilation and the renal excretion of HCO_3^-. Pulmonary compensation is rapid, whereas alterations in renal excretion take days. There are four primary acid-base disturbances: respiratory acidosis (increased $PaCO_2$), respiratory alkalosis (decreased $PaCO_2$), metabolic acidosis (decreased HCO_3^-), and metabolic alkalosis (increased HCO_3^-). Each primary disturbance normally leads to a secondary compensation, as described in Table 41–2.

Often in intensive care units (ICUs) patients have more than one primary disorder; this situation should be suspected if the body is unable to compensate as expected or if there is an apparent overcompensation due to a second disorder. It must be emphasized that very similar blood gas findings may be seen with different disorders, so the correct diagnosis depends on knowledge of the clinical situation. For example, an HCO_3^- concentration of 18 mEq/L and a $PaCO_2$ of 30 mm Hg could result either from hyperventilation or from renal tubular acidosis. Usually the pH will tend to be acidic in cases of primary acidosis and alkaline in primary alkalosis, but this rule of thumb does not invariably apply.

RESPIRATORY ACIDOSIS

Definition

Respiratory acidosis is an increase in $PaCO_2$ above the normal range of 35–45 mm Hg. This condition also is called hypercapnia.

Pathophysiology

Respiratory acidosis results from and is a reflection of alveolar hypoventilation. Acute respiratory acidosis is a primary disturbance seen in

TABLE 41–2. EXPECTED COMPENSATION FOR PRIMARY ACID-BASE DISTURBANCES

DISTURBANCE	COMPENSATION	
Chronic respiratory acidosis	For each 1 mm Hg rise in $PaCO_2$	$[HCO_3^-]$ rises by 0.35 mEq/L
Chronic respiratory alkalosis	For each 1 mm Hg fall in $PaCO_2$	$[HCO_3^-]$ falls by 0.5 mEq/L
Metabolic acidosis	For each 1 mEq/L fall in $[HCO_3^-]$	$PaCO_2$ falls by 1–1.3 mm Hg
Metabolic alkalosis	For each 1 mEq/L rise in $[HCO_3^-]$	$PaCO_2$ rises 0.6 mm Hg

$[HCO_3^-]$ = bicarbonate concentration; $PaCO_2$ = arterial carbon dioxide tension.

sedative drug overdosage, respiratory arrest, or exacerbation of asthma or chronic obstructive pulmonary disease. Respiratory acidosis may also serve as compensation for metabolic alkalosis, although a $PaCO_2$ over 50 mm Hg for purely compensatory reasons is unusual. Although the acidemia of uncompensated respiratory acidosis generally depresses cardiovascular and cerebral function, hypercapnia may increase cardiac irritability through activation of the sympathetic nervous system; it also increases cerebral blood flow.

Diagnosis

This is made by analysis of $PaCO_2$, which is either above the normal range or, in cases of metabolic acidosis, not as low as expected (see Table 41–2).

Management

The body eventually defends agents respiratory acidosis by renal retention of HCO_3^-. Although acute respiratory acidosis may be treated by the administration of HCO_3^-, increasing alveolar ventilation (by reversing sedative drugs, treatment of pulmonary problems, or initiation of mechanical ventilation) is usually more appropriate.

RESPIRATORY ALKALOSIS

Definition

Respiratory alkalosis is a decrease in $PaCO_2$ below the normal range of 35–45 mm Hg. This condition also is called hypocapnia.

Pathophysiology

Respiratory alkalosis results from and is a reflection of alveolar hyperventilation. It may result from anxiety but also may accompany shock, sepsis, cirrhosis, early pulmonary edema, hypoxia, salicylate intoxication, or overvigorous mechanical ventilation. The alkalemia associated with uncompensated respiratory alkalosis may increase cardiac and cerebral irritability. A low $PaCO_2$ also decreases cerebral blood flow.

Diagnosis

This is made by $PaCO_2$ analysis.

Management

The body's compensation for respiratory alkalosis is metabolic acidosis via renal excretion of HCO_3^-. The treatment of acute respiratory alkalosis is aimed at its underlying cause. This includes reduction of the minute ventilation of alkalemic patients on mechanical ventilators; correction with metabolic acids such as dilute hydrochloric acid or arginine hydrochloride (discussed in the section on metabolic alkalosis) or the administration of acetazolamide (Diamox) to cause metabolic acidosis is rarely required.

Outcome

Acute respiratory alkalosis may evolve into chronic respiratory alkalosis, which is of little consequence if renal compensation occurs.

METABOLIC ACIDOSIS

Definition

Metabolic acidosis is reflected by a fall in the serum HCO_3^- concentration below the normal range of 22–26 mEq/L or by an increased anion gap.

Pathophysiology

Metabolic acidosis results from either the loss of HCO_3^- or the addition of H^+ to the body. It may be separated into two categories, depending on whether or not an anion gap is present. The total number of cations—sodium (Na^+) and potassium (K^+)—and anions—chloride (Cl^-), HCO_3^-, and small amounts of phosphate, sulfate, and other metabolic salts—must be equal for serum to maintain electrical neutrality. A 10 mEq/L difference between Na^+ and ($Cl^- + HCO_3^-$) is usually reported in serum samples sent to the laboratory.

When a new acid enters the body, the H^+ (cation) reacts with HCO_3^- to yield CO_2 and water, and the anion remains behind. As a result, for each mEq of acid added, the HCO_3^- drops by a mEq and the anion gap (the new anions are measured by the laboratory) goes up by approximately one. The causes of metabolic acidosis with an increased anion gap are listed in Table 41–3 and are discussed in the following paragraphs.

Increased lactate production (with or without reduced lactate clearance by the liver and kidney) is the most common cause of increased anion gap metabolic acidosis in the critically ill. Pyruvate is metabolized into lactate during glycolysis, and mild increases in lactate occur in this condition. Severe increases result from tissue hypoxia, which alters the ratio of the enzyme nicotinamide-adenine dinucleotide (NAD) to its reduced form, NADH, and thereby causes increased conversion of pyruvate to lactate. Patients with certain enzyme deficiencies that led to alterations in the ratio of NAD to NADH also may develop lactic acidosis.

Metabolic acidosis with an increased anion gap may also occur in ketoacidosis, a condition seen in diabetics (see Chapter 55) and in alcoholics. Alcoholic ketoacidosis usually occurs when patients have been drinking heavily and not eating. Volume depletion caused by vomiting also occurs in these persons and leads to tissue hypoxia. Ketoacid production depends on the NADH to NAD ratio, as does the production of lactic acid, so often there is a component of lactic acidosis in patients with ketoacidosis. In severe cases, β-hydroxybutyric acid is generated, which is not measured by the laboratory as a ketone. Thus, ketoacidosis may go unnoticed. As patients improve, the β-hydroxybutyric acid is

TABLE 41–3. CAUSES OF METABOLIC ACIDOSIS

INCREASED ANION GAP
Lactic acidosis
Ketoacidosis
Renal failure
Aspirin intoxication
Methanol, ethylene glycol intoxication

NORMAL ANION GAP
Amino acid administration
Diarrhea
Post-treatment diabetic ketoacidosis
Posthyperventilation
Renal tubular acidosis

converted into acetoacetate, which is measured by the laboratory, and can falsely suggest that the ketoacidosis is getting worse. Alcoholic ketoacidosis may be accompanied by metabolic alkalosis because of the vomiting; sometimes the only clue to the acidosis is the high anion gap.

The anion gap increases in renal failure because the kidneys are unable to excrete phosphate, sulfate, and other organic acids.

Salicylic acid itself can contribute to an increased anion gap, but in salicylate intoxication (see Chapter 89), most of the anions come from a combination of lactic acid and organic acids that are released owing to the toxic effects of aspirin on cell metabolism. Salicylate toxicity classically demonstrates a mixed acid-base disturbance; in addition to the metabolic acidosis, there is a respiratory alkalosis. Thus, the patient will hyperventilate more than is necessary to compensate for the acidosis. The actual pH depends on which of the disorders predominates. Methanol and ethylene glycol metabolize into formic and oxalic acid, respectively, which cause the elevated anion gap. Further discussion of these intoxications is found in Chapter 84.

Whereas addition of nonvolatile acids will increase the anion gap, loss of HCO_3^- is accompanied by increases in Cl^-, so the anion gap is not elevated. Thus, a decreased HCO_3^- with a normal anion gap usually represents HCO_3^- loss, as seen in diarrhea, treatment of diabetic ketoacidosis, hyperventilation, and renal tubular acidosis. The exceptions to this occur when hydrochloric acid is added to the body or when the serum albumin concentration is low. If hydrochloric acid is added, there will be added anions, but the addition of Cl^- will not change the anion gap. In some cases, a "normal" anion gap (especially one on the high side of normal) occurs in patients who previously had a low anion gap and then developed a type of acidosis usually associated with a high anion gap. This situation is seen in patients who have low plasma proteins, owing say, to malnutrition, cirrhosis, or the nephrotic syndrome.

Addition of hydrochloric acid does not occur naturally, and it is rarely administered except to treat respiratory alkalosis. However, amino acids such as arginine hydrochloride, which are contained in hyperalimentation solutions, are metabolized to hydrochloric acid by the body; thus, parenteral nutrition fluids can cause metabolic acidosis. If this iatrogenic disease occurs, the composition of the nutrition should be changed or more acetate added to the solution.

Profound diarrhea may also cause metabolic acidosis because the pH of the fluid is alkaline and HCO_3^- is lost. The colon can exchange Cl^- for HCO_3^-. Often the volume loss is then replaced with saline, maintaining the Cl^- but not correcting the acidosis. Treatment should be aimed at stopping the diarrhea or adding HCO_3^- to the replacement solutions.

Metabolic acidosis may persist in patients with ketoacidosis treated with large volumes of saline, although the anion gap becomes normal.

Ketoacids are easily excreted in the urine, especially with an osmotic diuresis. These ketoacids could have been metabolized, regenerating HCO_3^-, but if they are excreted, the potential HCO_3^- is lost. Thus, the acidosis resembles HCO_3^- loss. After several days the kidneys will regenerate HCO_3^- and correct the situation. Some clinicians feel that HCO_3^- is useful as therapy until the acidosis is corrected, although this is debatable.

When patients have sustained respiratory alkalosis for several days, their kidneys compensate by excreting HCO_3^-. The serum HCO_3^- concentration is lower than normal in this situation. If the patients then suddenly stop hyperventilating (or if the mechanical ventilator settings are suddenly changed), they will be left with a low serum HCO_3^-, a normal $PaCO_2$, and metabolic acidosis with a normal anion gap. The urine will initially inappropriately contain HCO_3^-, but the kidneys soon start to conserve it. The problem will correct itself in several days.

The final cause of metabolic acidosis with a normal anion gap is renal tubular acidosis. The kidneys must normally reclaim all HCO_3^- that is filtered and, in addition, must excrete any nonvolatile acids that are consumed or metabolized. Tissue catabolism normally releases about 50–100 mEq of acid each day and more in stressful situations. Whenever renal tubular cells excrete H^+ into the urine, HCO_3^- is generated and secreted back into the blood. Failure of this mechanism leads to renal tubular acidosis (RTA). There are several different forms of RTA, depending on the part of the nephron that is abnormal. Renal tubular acidosis with early renal failure is not strictly considered a RTA, but early in renal failure, the kidneys fail to excrete the necessary acid before the accumulation of anions. Thus, the anion gap is normal. In this situation, the creatinine clearance is not normal. Attempts to classify the patient's condition into one of the usual types of RTA will lead to frustration. As renal failure worsens, the picture will become more typical.

Distal RTA (also called Type I RTA) is characterized by an inability to lower urine pH to less than 5.5 in any circumstance, owing to abnormalities in the distal nephron. This can cause problems in acid excretion because other buffer systems, particularly that of ammonia, depend on a favorable pH in urine. Distal RTA can be caused by inability of cells to secrete H^+, backleak of H^+ into renal cells, or abnormalities in Na^+ transport that secondarily lead to abnormal electrical potential differences not favoring excretion of H^+. However, all these have similar clinical manifestations: a low serum HCO_3^-, acidosis with a normal anion gap, a high urine pH, and hypokalemia. If other types of metabolic acidosis are superimposed on a patient with distal RTA (for example, sepsis with lactic acidosis), then the kidney has no way to compensate, and the acidosis easily becomes severe. Etiologies include medications such as amphotericin and lithium as well as immunologic diseases such as Sjögren's syndrome and primary biliary cirrhosis, myeloma, and nephrocalcinosis. The diagnosis is confirmed if urine pH is above 5.5 when the serum bicarbonate concentration is less than 15 mEq/L, and this form of RTA can be excluded if the urine pH ever drops below 5.5.

Proximal RTA (also known as Type II RTA) is characterized by incomplete reabsorption of HCO_3^- by the proximal tubular cells. Normally the kidneys will resorb all HCO_3^- until a set level is reached, usually 24 mEq/L, beyond which HCO_3^- will be spilled into the urine. In kidneys with proximal RTA, the set point is too low, and HCO_3^- is wasted. The actual point varies with the severity of the disease, but it is uncommon to see a HCO_3^- concentration lower than 15 mEq/L. If the serum HCO_3^- is lower than the set point, owing to superimposed acidosis, the HCO_3^- will all be resorbed, just as in normal kidneys. However, when HCO_3^- is infused to raise the serum HCO_3^- to normal levels, over 15 percent of the filtered HCO_3^- will be excreted. Proximal RTA is usually accompanied by other evidence of proximal tubular damage, such as wasting of phosphate, amino acids, and glucose. Proximal RTA is unusual; etiologies include Fanconi's syndrome, heavy metal intoxication, acetazolamide, outdated tetracycline, multiple myeloma, vitamin D deficiency with secondary hyperparathyroidism, and hereditary fructose intolerance.

Hyperkalemic RTA (also called Type IV RTA) is caused by relatively low renin and aldosterone levels. Aldosterone acts on the distal tubule and normally promotes excretion of K^+ and H^+ with resorption of Na^+. The aldosterone levels may be in the normal range, but they are not sufficient to maintain a normal serum K^+, especially under stress. It is not helpful to measure the levels of these hormones. The diagnosis is usually made when a patient with acidosis and a normal anion gap has hyperkalemia without other causes of acidosis. The urine pH may vary; usually the acidosis is mild. Since the proximal tubules function normally and the distal tubules are able to acidify the urine, its pH may be low; however, it will not be low enough to cure the acidosis. An additional component of the acidosis is the inhibition of ammonia production by hyperkalemia: Since ammonia is an important buffer for removal of acid, the low production contributes to the acidosis. This type of RTA is found most frequently in patients with diseased kidneys, advanced age, and diabetes. It also can be caused by drugs such as spironolactone, amiloride, triamterene, prostaglandin inhibitors, and angiotensin-converting enzyme inhibitors. Urinary obstruction also leads to this type of RTA, which may be reversible after the obstruction is treated.

Diagnosis

Metabolic acidosis is diagnosed by the presence of a low HCO_3^- level. Arterial pH is usually less than 7.40. The identification of specific types depends on the presence or absence of an anion gap, a search for underlying diseases, and the use of toxicologic studies.

Management

Metabolic acidosis will usually resolve when the conditions that underlie it—including hypoxia and ischemia, diabetic or alcoholic ketosis, salicylate or aliphatic alcohol intoxication, injudicious addition of acid to the body, diarrhea, hyperventilation, and RTA—are corrected. When they cannot be corrected, the acidosis should be treated with HCO_3^- if a normal anion gap is present. Treating lactic acidosis with HCO_3^- is difficult, however, and raises the question of whether patients with lactic acidosis should be treated with HCO_3^- at all. Proximal RTA is difficult to treat because the kidneys will dump the additional HCO_3^- and also waste K^+.

The treatment of lactic acidosis depends on its severity and the nature of the underlying disease. If tissue oxygenation is restored, then the lactate is rapidly metabolized by the liver and kidneys, and the problem corrects itself. For example, after a major seizure, the pH may drop as low as 6.9, but within an hour it will be normal. Lactic acidosis may also accompany diabetic ketoacidosis, and it will respond to volume replacement. If shock or circulatory failure led to the lactic acidosis, then rapid recovery can be seen with restoration of the circulation. On the other hand, some patients with sepsis or shock generate large quantities of lactic acid, and if they are not treated their acidosis becomes severe enough to compromise cardiovascular function. Antibiotics or other treatment may not take effect quickly enough to alter the acidosis.

Clinicians should be aware that giving HCO_3^- to treat lactic acidosis may cause rebound alkalosis. Recent studies also suggest that HCO_3^- increases the production of lactic acid. Hypernatremia or volume overload may complicate HCO_3^- therapy. The oxygen dissociation curve shifts to the right in acidosis, facilitating oxygen release to the tissues; if the acidosis is corrected the curve shifts in the opposite direction, so that less oxygen is available to tisues. Finally, the blood-brain barrier is impermeable to HCO_3^- but permeable to the CO_2 generated by HCO_3^-, so acidosis may persist there despite normalization of the systemic pH. All the above reasons should engender reluctance to treat lactic acidosis with HCO_3^-. However, the acidosis itself is also harmful, particularly when the pH is less than 7.20. Hypotension, impaired cardiac contractility, and neurologic impairment may occur. There is currently a debate about when to treat acidosis, but it seems reasonable to suggest that if the pH is below 7.20 in a situation in which the underlying disease is not likely to improve quickly, then HCO_3^- should be given to increase the pH to about 7.20.

The amount of HCO_3^- necessary to increase the serum concentration of HCO_3^- varies widely from patient to patient. As a very rough guide, 44 mEq of HCO_3^- (1 ampule) should raise the serum HCO_3^- of a 70 kg patient by about 1 mEq/L. The pH will depend on both the HCO_3^- concentration and the $PaCO_2$. Thus, after administration of HCO_3^-, arterial blood gases must be measured. If patients are receiving mechanical ventilation, the ventilatory rate should be increased to help normalize the pH. If patients with lactic acidosis show impaired cardiac contractility with hypoperfusion, inotropic agents and afterload-reducing agents should be used. Vasoconstrictors should be avoided because they will increase the lactic acidosis, which will then further impair cardiac contractility and make the heart less sensitive to adrenergic agents. Dichloroacetate has recently been used to treat patients with lactic acidosis; this drug decreases the lactate levels but does not seem to improve overall survival.

Outcome

Disorders such as ischemia and hypoxia that cause metabolic acidosis may be fatal. In fact, an increased lactate level is usually an ominous clinical sign.

METABOLIC ALKALOSIS

Definition

Metabolic alkalosis is manifested by a serum HCO_3^- concentration in excess of the normal range of 22–26 mEq/L.

Pathophysiology

If renal function is normal, the kidneys will excrete all HCO_3^- added to the body, and metabolic alkalosis will not develop. Thus, metabolic alkalosis can only occur when renal failure is present, when HCO_3^- is rapidly administered, or when other factors cause the kidneys to retain HCO_3^-.

Metabolic alkalosis most commonly occurs in patients who have lost H^+ from the stomach either through protracted vomiting or nasogastric suction. The loss of H^+ from the stomach initiates the alkalosis in these persons. Saline depletion occurs concomitantly; this stimulates production of aldosterone, which leads to enhanced resorption of Na^+ and excretion of K^+ and H^+. The urine will thus be acidic, and the serum will remain alkaline. Since relatively more Cl^- than Na^+ is lost, Cl^- deficiency occurs. When the renal tubules try to resorb all the Na^+, they must resorb some anion with it; when Cl^- is unavailable, HCO_3^- accompanies the Na^+ instead, perpetuating the alkalosis. The final urine will have very low Cl^- levels.

Patients may also develop alkalosis from high aldosterone levels. In these persons, the urine Cl^- will not be low, so they are sometimes said to have "Cl^--resistant alkalosis." Cushing's disease, adrenal hyperplasia, adrenal adenoma, or ectopic secretion of adrenocorticotrophic hormone (ACTH) from cancer can lead to high aldosterone levels. Renin-secreting tumors and Bartter's syndrome also cause alkalosis by this mechanism.

Hypokalemia is usually associated with alkalosis that is caused by gastrointestinal loss or hyperaldosteronism. If the serum K^+ concentration is below 2 mEq/L, the hypokalemia itself may contribute to alkalosis. It is thought that the cells may exchange H^+ for K^+. The increased intracellular H^+ concentration is associated with a decreased extracellular H^+ concentration.

Posthypercapnic alkalosis is seen in patients with chronic CO_2 retention. The kidneys compensate by increasing the serum HCO_3^- concentration. If such patients are suddenly placed on mechanical ventilation and their CO_2 is brought to normal, the increased HCO_3^- will be manifested as alkalosis. In several days, the kidneys will readjust and excrete the HCO_3^-. This situation can usually be prevented by appropriate ventilation.

Diagnosis

Metabolic alkalosis is diagnosed by a high HCO_3^- concentration in the appropriate clinical setting.

Management

Metabolic alkalosis can often be prevented or corrected. Alkalosis caused by hypokalemia will respond to supplemental K^+; remember that the serum K^+ concentration does not usually reflect total body K^+, and that considerable amounts of K^+ may be required. When upper gastrointestinal losses are involved, treatment consists of restoring the extracellular volume with normal saline and replenishing whatever K^+ has been lost. Once the volume is normal, the aldosterone levels decline, and the kidneys will excrete the excess HCO_3^-. Histamine II receptor blockers, such as cimetidine and ranitidine, may also be useful in patients with sustained nasogastric losses, since they decrease the acid lost in the gastrointestinal fluid.

TABLE 41–4. SOME MIXED ACID-BASE DISTURBANCES

DISORDER	CLINICAL SETTING	pH	PaCO$_2$	[HCO$_3^-$]	AG
Respiratory acidosis and metabolic alkalosis	COPD and diuretic	Normal to high	High	High	Normal
Respiratory acidosis and metabolic acidosis	Cardiac arrest; sepsis; pneumonia and lactic acidosis; drug overdose with shock and hypoventilation	Very low	High	Low	High
	COPD and any metabolic acidosis	Low	High	Low	Varies
Respiratory alkalosis and metabolic acidosis	Salicylate toxicity Early sepsis: hyperventilation and lactic acidosis	Normal*	Low	Low	High
Metabolic acidosis and metabolic alkalosis	Diarrhea and vomiting	Normal*	Normal	Normal	Normal
	Vomiting or diuretics and any metabolic acidosis	Normal*	Normal	Normal	Varies
Respiratory alkalosis, metabolic acidosis and metabolic alkalosis ("the triple Ripple")	Alcoholism with cirrhosis (hyperventilation) and vomiting and alcoholic ketoacidosis	Normal* to slightly high	Low	Normal to high	High

*If one disorder is more predominant, the ph will more closely resemble that of the predominant disorder.

COPD = chronic obstructive pulmonary disease; GI = gastrointestinal; PaCO$_2$ = arterial carbon dioxide tension; [HCO$_3^-$] = serum bicarbonate concentration; AG = anion gap.

In unusual cases in which the pH is greater than 7.6, complications such as dysrhythmias or seizures may accompany the alkalosis. In these cases, more rapid treatment may be needed. Dilute hydrochloric acid (0.1 N) can be administered cautiously via a central line, or arginine hydrochloride may be given. The number of mEq needed to lower the HCO$_3^-$ concentration by 1 mEq/L will be approximately 50 percent of the body weight (35 mEq in a 70 kg patient). Alternatively, clinicians can administer acetazolamide (250–500 mg BID) to produce a compensatory metabolic acidosis.

Outcome

Metabolic alkalosis is a less compromising problem than metabolic acidosis, in large part because its underlying causes are less severe.

Mixed Acid-Base Disturbances

Critically ill patients often have more than one acid-base disturbance at a time. Often it is difficult to determine which of these are primary and which are secondary complications. Arterial blood gases, anion gap, serum anion and cation concentration, volume status, renal history, medications, and the use of mechanical ventilation must all be taken into account. A sampling of mixed acid-base disturbances is presented in Table 41–4.

RECOMMENDED READING

Gabow PA: Disorders associated with an altered anion gap. Kidney Int 27:472, 1985.
Gennari EJ, Cohen JJ: Renal tubular acidosis. Annu Rev Med 29:521, 1978.
Graf H, Leach W, Arieff AI: Evidence for a detrimental effect of bicarbonate therapy in hypoxic lactate acidosis. Science 227:754, 1985.
Halperin ML, Hammeke M, Josse RG, et al: Metabolic acidosis in the alcoholic: a pathophysiologic approach. Metabolism 32:308, 1983.
Harrington JT: Metabolic alkalosis. Kidney Int. 26:88, 1984.
Kassirer JP: Serious acid-base disorders. N Engl J Med 291:773, 1974.
Madias NE: Lactic acidosis. Kidney Int 29:752, 1986.
Narins RG, Emmett M: Simple and mixed acid-base disorders: a practical approach. Medicine 59:161, 1980.
Orringer CE, Eustace JD, Wunsch CD, et al: Natural history of lactic acidosis after grand mal seizures: a model for the study of an anion-gap acidosis not associated with hyperkalemia. N Engl J Med 297:796, 1977.
Richer LL, Tannen RL: The clinical spectrum of renal tubular acidosis. Ann Rev Med 37:319, 1986.
Stacpoole PW, Harman EM, Curry SH, et al: Treatment of lactic acidosis with dichloroacetate. N Engl J Med 309:390, 1983.

42. Fluid and Electrolyte Therapy

Susan M. Ott

INTRODUCTION

Fluid and electrolyte therapy commonly causes great confusion in the intensive care unit (ICU). This chapter focuses on fluid and electrolyte therapy from the standpoint of volume (saline) and water abnormalities. It covers the basic principles of volume distribution in the body and imbalances of volume and water and presents a general approach to writing fluid orders. Although electrolyte disturbances are discussed, the specific problems of hypernatremia and hyponatremia are covered more fully in Chapter 43 and Chapter 44, respectively.

BASIC PRINCIPLES OF VOLUME DISTRIBUTION

Sixty percent of the weight of an average person is made up of body water. The exact percentage depends on age and amount of fat: infants tend to have a higher percentage of water and fat persons a lower one. For most clinical purposes, however, total body water can be assumed to be 60 percent of the usual weight of the patient. Two thirds of the water is contained within the cells (intracellular) and the other one third is outside of them (extracellular). Of this extracellular fluid, about one fourth is intravascular and the remaining three fourths are interstitial. Therefore, a normal person weighing 70 kilograms will have 42 liters of total body water; 28 liters will be intracellular, about 3.5 liters will be in plasma (normally blood is 60 percent plasma, so blood volume is about 6 liters), and 10.5 liters will be in the interstitial space (Fig. 42–1). The distribution of fluid between the intravascular space and the interstitial space depends on the oncotic pressure of the plasma proteins and the hydrostatic pressure in the blood vessels as well as on the permeability of their vascular walls.

An isotonic fluid is a fluid that will not cause cell volume to change. Therefore, isotonic fluids given intravenously will remain in the extracellular space, and loss of isotonic fluids will come from in the extracellular space. The isotonic fluids used in clinical practice include normal saline,

284

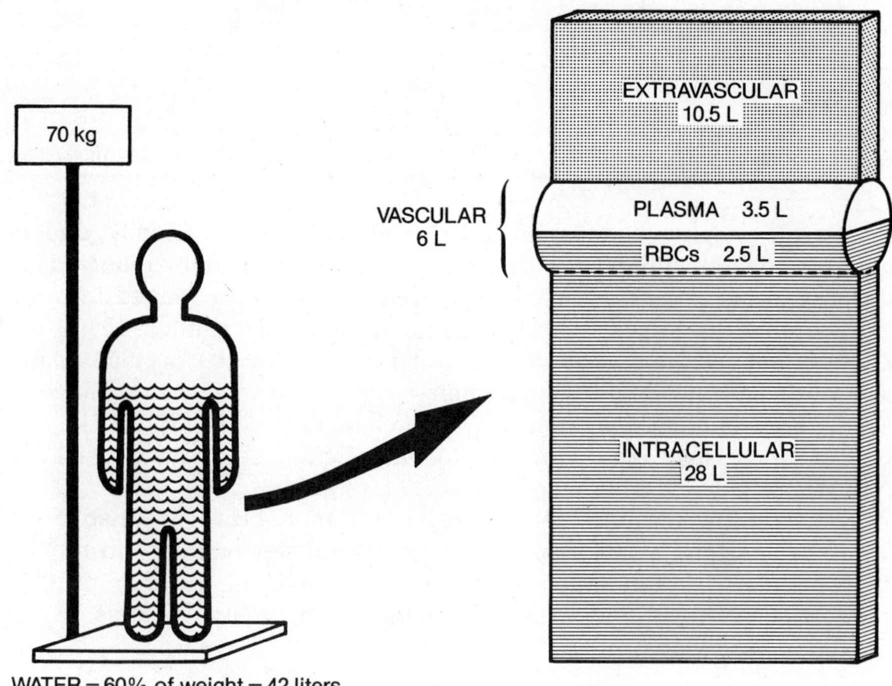

FIGURE 42–1. Normal distribution of body water. See text for explanation.

Ringer's lactate, and plasma (Table 42–1). Dextrose in water may initially behave like an isotonic fluid, but the dextrose is soon metabolized, leaving behind water, which is not isotonic. Note that the gain or loss of normal saline does not change the serum sodium (Na^+) concentration. On the other hand, if water is added to the body, it will evenly distribute throughout the body fluids; two thirds will enter cells and one third will remain extracellular. The cells will swell and the serum Na^+ concentration will decrease when water is added. The reverse happens if water is lost from the body.

The amount of water excess or deficiency can be calculated using the following equation:

Change in water (L) =

$$\frac{\text{Change in serum Na}^+ \text{ concentration}}{\text{Serum Na}^+ \text{ concentration (normally, 140 mEq/L)}} \times 0.6 \times \text{weight (kg)}$$

For example, if the serum Na^+ concentration changes from 140 mEq/L to 130 mEq/L in a patient who weighs 70 kg, then the change in water will be $10/140 \times 0.6 \times 70 = 3.0$ L.

TABLE 42–1. INTRAVENOUS SOLUTIONS

SOLUTION	CONTENTS PER LITER
5 percent dextrose in water	50 g dextrose
Normal saline	9 g NaCl = 3.6 g Na$^+$ = 154 mEq Na$^+$
½ normal saline	4.5 g NaCl = 1.8 g Na$^+$ = 77 mEq Na$^+$
Ringer's lactate	130 mEq Na$^+$, 4 mEq K$^+$, 111 mEq Cl$^-$, 27 mEq lactate

Acute weight changes in critically ill patients are usually due to changes in body fluids; for this reason it is important to follow daily weights in all patients. A change in weight can be partitioned into the sum of changes in water and in isotonic fluid (i.e., saline). Using the above equation, the contribution of water changes can be calculated, and any further unaccounted weight change can be attributed to a change in saline. For example, if a patient's weight changes from 69 kg to 65 kg and his Na$^+$ increases from 140 mEq/L to 145 mEq/L, he will have lost 1.5 L of water (5/140 × 0.6 × 69) and also 2.5 L of saline.

The clinical approach to fluid balance is more clearly defined if the water balance and saline balance are considered separately, even though they often occur simultaneously. In the next section, the four primary fluid problems—volume (i.e., saline) depletion, volume excess, water depletion, and water excess are discussed.

VOLUME (SALINE) DEPLETION

Definition

Volume depletion occurs when extracellular fluid volume is reduced.

Pathophysiology

The most common source of saline loss is the gastrointestinal tract. Many patients are on nasogastric suction and can lose liters of volume daily. Diarrhea may also contribute substantial losses. Urine losses can also lead to volume depletion, especially if a patient is recovering from acute renal failure, has salt-losing nephropathy or diabetes, or is over-treated with diuretics. Excessive sweating, burns, and severe rashes can cause loss of volume. Hemorrhage causes acute volume loss; this will quickly lead to clinical symptoms.

The term third spacing refers to volume that becomes unavailable to the patient but is still inside the body (this is also referred to as transcellular spacing). The third space is inside a layer of epithelial cells separating intravascular fluid from the interstitial spaces; this layer is found inside the gastrointestinal tract or the urinary bladder. Liters of fluid may accumulate in the bowel when there is ileus, and the volume loss will resemble that seen with diarrhea. Ascites or pleural fluid is not the same as third space fluid because it can equilibrate with the rest of the extracellular space. Volume depletion may occur if the ascitic fluid is removed.

Diagnosis

Unless there has been third spacing, volume depletion will result in weight loss. The lost weight will give an estimate of the severity of the problem. Other clinical signs actually reflect decreases in intravascular volume depletion and depend on the rate of loss. Symptoms occur after about 600 ml of volume are lost, but chronic losses may reach several liters before symptoms are noticed. In mild volume depletion, there is tachycardia and vasoconstriction. In more moderate cases, neck veins will be flat, and the central venous pressure and pulmonary artery wedge pressure will be decreased. As volume loss continues, postural blood pressure changes develop, with a drop in the diastolic blood pressure by 10 mm Hg when the patient sits up. Further volume losses lead to further drops in blood pressure and eventually to shock. In severe cases, half of the extracellular volume may be lost (7–8 liters). It should be noted that in some situations (for example, when patients are receiving positive end-expiratory pressure), a normal volume is not sufficient to maintain cardiac output, so the patients may be treated as if they had volume depletion. Laboratory tests are usually not very specific for volume depletion, although a low urine sodium or increasing blood urea nitrogen or hematocrit may be clues.

Management

Since circulating volume is essential for oxygen delivery, it should be restored rapidly. In cases of hemorrhagic shock, blood should be given. Otherwise, isotonic fluids should be administered quickly until the blood pressure or central venous pressure is stabilized. In less severe cases, the losses can be replaced over 6–24 hours. Dextrose in water or ½ normal saline should not be used to treat serious volume depletion because two thirds of the water will enter cells and will not be available to help restore the circulating volume (Table 42–2).

TABLE 42–2. SUMMARY OF INTRAVENOUS FLUID ORDERS

MAINTENANCE	
Use when patient is in good fluid balance	2400 ml water/day + 50–75 mEq Na$^+$/day + 40 mEq K$^+$/day + gastrointestinal losses (same as measured output) + excessive skin and renal losses (same as measured output)
CORRECTIONS	
Volume (saline) depletion only	Normal saline until volume normal, over 2–12 hr, then begin maintenance
Water depletion only	Add 1000–1500 ml 5 percent dextrose in water/day to maintenance
Volume excess only	1000 ml 5 percent dextrose in water/day + diuretics
Water excess only	Subtract 1000–1500 ml 5 per cent dextrose in water/day from maintenance
Volume excess but with intravascular volume depletion	Avoid saline, diuretics Give 1000 dl 5 percent dextrose in water/day Try albumin, red blood cells
Volume excess with water excess	Limit intravenous fluids as much as possible
Volume depletion with water excess	Initially give normal saline, then maintenance, allowing renal water excretion to occur
Volume depletion with water depletion	Restore volume first with normal saline, then maintenance + 1000–1500 ml 5 percent dextrose in water/day

VOLUME (SALINE) EXCESS

Definition

Volume excess occurs when extravascular volume is increased.

Pathophysiology

The most obvious example of volume excess is congestive heart failure. Renal failure also leads to volume excess if salt is not restricted. Many cases of volume excess are iatrogenic and result from the infusion of excess saline. In these forms of volume excess, edema develops owing to increased hydrostatic pressure; in other words, there is excess volume in both the intravascular and the extravascular spaces. In other cases, there is increased total volume in the extravascular space, but the intravascular space is actually depleted. This situation is caused by low oncotic pressure (as in cirrhosis, nephrotic syndrome, or malnutrition) or by increased vascular permeability (as in sepsis or pancreatitis). These cases of abnormal distribution of volume are confusing and are discussed further in the following section.

Diagnosis

Weight gain may be an important sign of volume excess. After patients have accumulated 3–5 liters of extra saline, they will begin to show edema. In the absence of excessive accumulation of volume, even a massive acute shift in distribution of volume from the intravascular to the extravascular space (for example, in an anaphylactic reaction) cannot immediately result in generalized edema since the entire plasma volume is only 3 liters.

When the volume excess occurs in both intra- and extravascular spaces, clinical signs such as elevated neck veins and a high central venous or wedge pressure may develop. The blood pressure may be increased. Patients develop an S3 gallop, and signs of pulmonary edema are present on examination and on the chest roentgenogram.

Management

When both intra- and extravascular volume excesses are present, volume removal is called for (Table 42–2). Diuretics are the mainstay of therapy as long as renal function is adequate. If it is not, fluid removal must be accomplished with dialysis or hemofiltration. It is important to avoid giving saline, which will worsen the situation. Hidden sources of salt, such as in flush solutions or parenteral nutrition, should be sought. The rate of fluid removal depends on the severity of the problem, but usually a loss of 1–2 L/day is optimal. More rapid loss may result in hypotension.

VOLUME EXCESS WITH INTRAVASCULAR VOLUME DEPLETION

Definition

Volume excess and intravascular volume depletion occur when total body Na^+ and water are increased but not in the intravascular compartment.

Pathophysiology

This special case of volume excess deserves further discussion because it is commonly seen in ICU patients and because it is a common source of confusion. The situation arises when there is low oncotic pressure or increased vascular permeability, or both, as occurs with liver failure, sepsis, pancreatitis, or malnutrition. The low serum albumin concentration or high vascular permeability in patients with these disorders causes excess leaking of plasma volume into the extravascular space. This results in signs of volume depletion, and the patients are treated with saline. However, the treatment leads to further accumulation of volume in the extravascular space, and eventually edema is manifest. If more saline is given, more edema develops. But if saline is withheld or diuretics are given, the patients' circulating volume drops and cardiac output declines. Sometimes clinicians get caught in a vicious circle of giving diuretics and saline to no avail.

Diagnosis

Volume excess is diagnosed by an increase in weight, and intravascular volume depletion is diagnosed by hypotension, flat neck veins, and a low central venous or wedge pressure.

Management

Saline should be given only to replace any ongoing saline losses (for example, from the gastrointestinal tract) in patients with volume excess and intravascular volume depletion (Table 42–2). Diuretics should not be administered. If the patient is anemic, transfusions of red blood cells may be helpful in increasing oncotic pressure. Infusions of albumin can be given if the blood pressure or cardiac output falls. All of these are temporizing measures until treatment of the underlying disease corrects the problem of vascular permeability or low oncotic pressure.

WATER DEPLETION

Definition

Water depletion occurs when total body water is reduced. It usually causes hypernatremia (see Chapter 43).

Pathophysiology

The body obligatorily loses 1500 ml of water from the skin, lungs, and kidneys each day, and water depletion will develop if intake is inadequate. This rarely happens in alert patients who have access to water, because their thirst mechanism is active. However, hospitalized patients who are unable to drink or who are not alert may not get enough water. In addition to their usual water losses, there may be excessive losses in the urine or through the skin. Finally, they may lose water as well as saline from the gastrointestinal tract.

Diagnosis

The serum Na^+ concentration can be used to calculate the amount of water depletion. If serum glucose is higher than 200 mg/dl, Na^+ should be corrected by increasing the Na^+ concentration by 1.6 mEq/L for every 100 mg/dl of glucose over the normal level of 100 mg/dl. For example, if the glucose is 300 mg/dl, then 3.2 mEq/L should be added to the Na^+ concentration. Then the degree of water depletion can be calculated using the equation from the beginning of this chapter. This loss of water will also lead to a weight loss. If the weight loss is greater than the calculated water loss, then saline was lost as well.

It is important to remember that saline losses do not change the volume of cells, but water losses cause cell shrinkage. This particularly affects the brain neurons, so that the major symptoms of water depletion are neurologic. Water-depleted patients frequently become agitated, confused, and eventually comatose. If alert, they complain of thirst. Reduced skin turgor and dry mouth are not reliable signs of water depletion in adult patients, although they may be useful in pediatric patients. Water loss does not usually cause symptoms of volume depletion because only a third of the lost water comes from the extracellular space, and the oncotic pressure in the vascular space helps preserve its volume. Only in severe cases of hypernatremia (Na^+ concentration above 160 mEq/L) will circulating volume be compromised (see Chapter 43).

Management

Water depletion should be replaced slowly. Rapid replacement will cause abrupt changes in cell volume that are not well tolerated. This may be particularly true in the brain. When faced with water depletion, the brain neurons may generate so-called idiogenic osmoles to help preserve their volume. If water is given quickly, an excess amount will enter the neurons and cause severe cell swelling that may led to herniation. In treating water depletion, the amount of water lost from the body should be calculated from the equation at the beginning of the chapter and that volume should be given back at an even rate over the next 48 hours. Ongoing losses should be replaced at the rate at which they occur.

Patients with severe water depletion (Na^+ concentration above 160 mEq/L) have a decreased intravascular volume as well. Since it is important to restore their circulating volume, they should first be given normal saline until intravascular volume depletion no longer exists. This can be done over several hours and does not usually require more than 2000 ml of saline. There is no need to give hypertonic saline. Once the vascular volume is restored, the water should be given at a slow rate to correct the loss over 48 hours. Remember to replace ongoing losses as well (Table 42–2).

WATER EXCESS

Definition

Water excess occurs with an increase in total body water. It usually causes hyponatremia (see Chapter 44).

Pathophysiology

The most common reason for water excess in hospitalized patients is the iatrogenic administration of too much water in intravenous solutions. Normal, healthy kidneys are able to excrete excess water loads up to a maximal rate of 20 L/day. However, critically ill patients are often not able to eliminate these excess fluids. Additionally, antidiuretic hormone (ADH) secretion is often stimulated in sick or stressed patients; this will cause the kidneys to retain water. It should be noted that patients would not develop water excess even with very high ADH levels unless water intake exceeded a water loss of about 1500 ml/day.

Diagnosis

As with water depletion, the serum Na^+ concentration is the best indicator of water excess. The equation at the beginning of this chapter should be used after correction for abnormal glucose concentrations, as noted earlier. It must be emphasized that the serum Na^+ concentration reflects water balance, not Na^+ balance. Water excess may easily coexist with Na^+ excess.

The weight will increase in patients with water excess. If the weight is higher than expected from the calculation of water excess, then saline excess is also present. If the weight is lower than expected, there is also a saline deficiency. Water excess does not cause edema; the increased cell water cannot be detected on physical exam. Likewise, signs of volume overload such as elevated neck veins, edema, and high central venous or wedge pressures are not seen unless saline overload is present. The appearance of skin or mucous membranes does not help in the diagnosis of water excess, and most clinical signs are neurologic.

Management

Withholding water is sufficient treatment in most patients with water excess (Table 42–2). Frequently the daily intravenous intake of water is 3–5 liters, and if this can be restricted, no further measures are needed. Clinicians should be aware of the amount of water used to administer medications; often these medicines can be combined or concentrated to avoid giving more water. Sometimes clinicians decide to add Na^+ to the water to avoid water excess. This is not an appropriate treatment; instead of water excess the patient will then develop saline excess. More aggressive treatment of water excess is discussed in Chapter 44.

RECOMMENDED READING

Lindeman RD, Papper S: Therapy of fluid and electrolyte disorders. Ann Intern Med 82:64, 1975.
Narins RG, Jones ER, Stom MC, et al: Diagnostic strategies in disorders of fluids, electrolyte and acid-base homeostasis. Am J Med 72:496, 1982.

43. Hypernatremia

Susan M. Ott

DEFINITION

Hypernatremia is an increase in the serum sodium (Na^+) concentration above the normal range of 135–145 mEq/L. This increase does not necessarily indicate an increase in total body Na^+ or a decrease in total body water, but it does indicate that the serum contains excess Na^+ relative to water.

PATHOPHYSIOLOGY

Hypernatremia results either from an increase in Na^+ or from a decrease in water. An increase in Na^+ may be seen in patients who have ingested excess salt (sodium chloride) or sodium bicarbonate during, say, cardiopulmonary resuscitation. Total body water is usually normal in such patients unless it is increased as the result of water added to dilute the Na^+.

The most common cause of hypernatremia is failure to drink water, seen in patients who cannot obtain water. Usually this is accompanied by thirst, unless there has also been central nervous system damage. Hypernatremia due to water depletion may also result from water loss through the skin, as in excessive sweating, burns, or severe rashes; from the gastrointestinal tract, as with diarrhea or vigorous nasogastric suctioning; and via the urinary tract, as with the administration of osmotic agents such as mannitol, the presence of polyuria due to diabetes mellitus, and the development of diabetes insipidus due to multiple causes.

Diabetes insipidus is a condition of marked polyuria (often up to 10 L/day) in which urine osmolarity is low. Diabetes insipidus is either central, i.e., caused by inadequate levels of antidiuretic hormone (ADH), which normally comes from the pituitary; or nephrogenic, in which case ADH levels are adequate but the renal tubules do not respond. Trauma and surgery, central nervous system tumors, or pituitary sarcoidosis may cause central diabetes insipidus, although half of cases are idiopathic. Nephrogenic diabetes insipidus may result from drugs such as lithium and demeclocycline or from tubular damage due to interstitial nephritis, pyelonephritis, obstructive uropathy, hypercalcemia, multiple myeloma, or sickle cell disease.

Hypernatremia of any cause results in hyperosmolarity because Na^+ is the major extracellular and intravascular ion. Normal serum osmolarity is 285–295 mOsm/L and is calculated by adding 2 times the Na^+ concentration to the glucose concentration divided by 18 and the blood urea nitrogen (BUN) divided by 3. An increase in serum osmolarity will attract water from the intracellular and interstitial spaces to the intravascular extracellular space. This in turn will cause the cells to shrink, producing neurologic sequelae such as stupor and coma. The level of serum osmolarity (and serum Na^+ concentration, if hypernatremia is present) that causes such symptoms varies among patients, but problems should be anticipated if the osmolarity exceeds 310 mOsm/L, which would result from an increase in the serum Na^+ concentration from the normal 135–145 mEq/L to over 150 mEq/L.

DIAGNOSIS

Hypernatremia, by definition, is diagnosed by an increase in the serum Na^+ concentration. It should be suspected in patients who have no access to water. Patients often are confused. Urine output is low with high osmolarity. Diabetes insipidus should be considered in polyuric patients in the appropriate clinical circumstances. As noted earlier, the urine osmolarity is low in diabetes insipidus. Central diabetes insipidus is differentiated from nephrogenic diabetes insipidus by means of the intravenous administration of 0.5 μg of desmopressin: the urine volume should decrease and the urine osmolarity should increase within 1–2 hours of a test dose if central diabetes insipidus is present.

MANAGEMENT

Hypernatremia and hyperosmolarity are treated with water restoration if water loss has occurred. The amount of water needed may be determined by the formula:

$$\text{Water deficit (L)} = \frac{Na^+ \text{ concentration} - 140 \text{ mEq/L}}{140 \text{ mEq/L}} \times 0.6 \times \text{weight (kg)}$$

The replacement should proceed slowly (over 48 hours) to prevent rapid changes in cell volume. Giving water to patients who have received excess Na^+ rather than lost water is potentially hazardous because of the resulting increased intravascular volume, so it should be done carefully. In case of severe water depletion (Na$^+$ concentration greater than 160 mEq/L), there is also decreased intravascular volume. Since it is most important to restore the circulating volume, these patients should first be given normal saline until signs of intravascular volume depletion no longer exist. This can be done over several hours and will usually not require more than 2000 ml. There is no need to give hypertonic saline. Once the vascular volume is restored, the water should be given at a slow rate to correct the loss over 48 hours. Remember to replace ongoing losses as well.

Central diabetes insipidus may be treated with desmopressin. Partial central diabetes insipidus can also be treated with chlorpheniramine, which stimulates the release of ADH. Nephrogenic diabetes insipidus is more difficult to treat, and it may be easier merely to replace urinary water loss if urine volume is less than 4 L/day. Thiazide diuretics such as hydrochlorothiazide may reduce the urine volume by stimulating increased water resorption by the proximal tubules. However, this approach only succeeds if the patient is kept in a state of mild volume depletion, which may be hazardous in the critically ill.

Outcome

Although hyperosmolarity due to hypernatremia may be lethal, modest increases in the serum Na$^+$ concentration usually respond to therapy. The prognosis of diabetes insipidus relates to its underlying cause.

RECOMMENDED READING

Addleman M, Pollard A, Grossman RF: Survival after severe hypernatremia due to salt ingestion by an adult. Am J Med 78:176, 1985.
Feig PU, McCurdy DK: The hypertonic state. N Engl J Med 297:1444, 1977.
Gennari FJ: Serum osmolality: uses and limitations. N Engl J Med 310:102, 1984.
Loeb JN: The hyperosmolar state. N Engl J Med 290:1184, 1974.
Richardson DW, Robinson AG: Diagnosis and treatment: drugs five years later—desmopressin. Ann Intern Med 103:228, 1985.

44. Hyponatremia

Susan M. Ott

DEFINITION

Hyponatremia exists if the serum sodium (Na^+) concentration is less than the normal range of 135–145 mEq/L. A decrease in the serum Na^+ concentration does not necessarily indicate a decrease in total body Na^+ or an increase in total body water, but it does indicate that the serum contains excess water relative to Na^+.

PATHOPHYSIOLOGY (Table 44–1)

The serum Na^+ concentration may be artifactually reduced by the presence of excess lipids or glucose in the serum. Lipids cause artifactual hyponatremia by decreasing the relative proportion of Na^+ in serum. In hyperglycemia, the serum Na^+ concentration will fall, even though there is no change in total body water or saline. The true serum Na^+ concentration in hyperglycemic patients can be determined by adding 1.6 mEq/L of Na^+ for every 100 mg/dl of glucose above the normal level of 100 mg/dl. This represents the Na^+ concentration that would be seen after the glucose level returned to normal.

The causes of true hyponatremia depend on whether patients manifest volume depletion, volume excess, or normal volume status. If volume (saline) is lost from the body and replaced with hypotonic fluid, the serum Na^+ concentration becomes diluted. The saline is actually lost from the extracellular space, but two thirds of the water given as replacement enters cells, so the resultant volume is decreased. Volume depletion, in turn, stimulates the release of antidiuretic hormone (ADH) despite the low serum osmolarity, and the kidneys do not excrete the excess water. The kidneys also resorb all the available Na^+, so the urine Na^+ concentration should be low in the absence of renal disease.

Hyponatremia with volume excess usually occurs in the setting of congestive heart failure, nephrotic syndrome, or cirrhosis, all of which cause edema. With these conditions, total body saline is increased, but total body water is increased even more, producing both saline and water excesses. Faced with an ineffective circulating blood volume, the kidneys

TABLE 44–1. CAUSES OF HYPONATREMIA

	ANTIDIURETIC HORMONE	URINE SODIUM CONCENTRATION
Misleading measurement: hyperglycemia, lipemia	Normal	Variable
With volume depletion		
Nonrenal losses	High	Low
Salt-losing nephropathy	High	High
With volume excess (edema)		
Congestive heart failure, cirrhosis, nephrotic syndrome	Normal to high	Low
With normal volume status		
Massive water drinking	Low	Variable
Water intake in patient with renal failure	Low	No urine
Thiazides	Variable	High
Addison's disease, hypothyroidism	Variable	Variable
Drugs	Normal to high	Variable
Central nervous system disturbances	High	Variable
Surgery	High	Variable
Pulmonary lesions, positive end-expiratory pressure	High	Variable
Malignancies	High	Variable

retain both Na^+ and water. ADH may also be released. The urine Na^+ concentration and volume are low.

The causes of hyponatremia without evident volume disorder may be grouped into those that are not mediated by ADH and those that are. Among the former are massive water drinking (over 20 L/day), usually seen in psychotic patients, which may overwhelm the kidneys' ability to excrete water. Water intake in patients with renal failure may also lead to hyponatremia.

A usually mild form of hyponatremia with normal volume status may also result from thiazide administration. It is thought to be due to an increased proximal resorption of saline that accompanies volume depletion and limits flow to the distal tubule. Thus, a water load cannot be excreted. Occasionally, more severe hyponatremia with resultant seizures develops, owing to an idiosyncratic response to thiazides. Addison's disease may also be associated with hyponatremia because the lack of circulating glucocorticosteroids limits the kidneys' ability to excrete a water load. In addition, hyponatremia may occur with hypothyroidism for unclear reasons.

If a patient has hyponatremia and the serum osmolarity is low but the urine osmolarity is high, evidence for ADH release is present. A normal kidney can dilute the urine to an osmolarity of 50 mOsm/L when there is no ADH. If urine osmolarity is between 50–300 mOsm/L, ADH may be present, or tubular damage may prevent the kidney from making dilute urine. When urine osmolarity is higher than serum osmolarity, ADH is usually present (exceptions occur during glycosuria or after use of roentgenographic dye). Patients with hyponatremia and normal volume status whose urine osmolarity is higher than serum osmolarity are said to manifest the syndrome of inappropriate ADH (SIADH).

Drugs may enhance ADH secretion or may augment its action on the renal cells and thereby produce SIADH. ADH stimulates renal prostaglandin production, which in turn inhibits the action of ADH. Thus, prostaglandin inhibitors such as nonsteroidal antiinflammatory agents will enhance ADH action and contribute to water retention. Other medications that increase ADH or its effect include chlorpropamide, psychotropic agents, angiotensin-converting enzyme inhibitors such as captopril and enalapril, nicotine, oxytocin, narcotics, clofibrate, and vincristine.

Many central nervous system disturbances lead to SIADH. Trauma, tumor, infection, surgery, or psychosis may all cause ADH release. In some cases the hypothalamus resets the body's osmotic regulation, and the serum Na^+ concentration is maintained at a lower level. Hyponatremia due to excess ADH is frequently seen after a wide variety of surgical procedures. Pulmonary disorders such as lung cancer also cause ADH release by unclear mechanisms, as does positive end-expiratory pressure. Finally, tumors, including those of the pancreas, duodenum, ureter, and prostate, may secrete ADH.

DIAGNOSIS

Regardless of its origin, hyponatremia may cause symptoms due to increased swelling of brain cells. The symptoms range from mild confusion or agitation to seizures and coma. Death is seen in a significant number of patients. This is partly due to the fact that the underlying diseases that cause hyponatremia are often serious. The symptoms do not depend on the absolute level of Na^+ as much as on the rate of fall: seizures may be seen when the Na^+ drops quickly from 135 mEq/L to 125 mEq/L, but patients may gradually develop hyponatremia to 100 mEq/L without any symptoms.

The amount of excess water present in hyponatremia patients can be calculated by the following formula:

$$\text{Excess water (L)} = \frac{140 \text{ mEq/L} - Na^+ \text{ concentration}}{140 \text{ mEq/L}} \times 0.6 \times \text{weight (kg)}$$

MANAGEMENT

If the hyponatremia is associated with volume loss, volume replacement, usually with normal saline, is required. In other cases, treatment varies. Although there is general agreement that a serum Na$^+$ concentration below 120 mEq/L should be corrected, debate persists about the rate of therapy. Some evidence suggests that rapid correction can lead to further neurologic difficulties, including central pontine myelinolysis, especially if the hyponatremia is overcorrected. Any drugs that contribute to hyponatremia should be discontinued. Water should be restricted. Medications should be given in as concentrated a form as possible. In patients without symptoms, this is often adequate treatment. Usually about 1000 ml of water is lost daily through the skin and lungs, so water restriction should correct the hyponatremia by about 3 mEq/day. In more severe cases, when the Na$^+$ level has dropped more rapidly or when central nervous system abnormalities exist, more vigorous therapy is probably indicated. This can be done by giving furosemide 1 mg/kg which should cause a diuresis.

The urine Na$^+$ concentration should be measured while furosemide is being given in severely hyponatremic patients. Each hour, the Na$^+$ lost in the urine should be calculated and replaced with hypertonic saline (3 percent saline). Each ml of 3 percent saline contains 0.45 mEq Na$^+$. Thus, for example, if furosemide induces a diuresis of 700 ml of urine with a Na$^+$ concentration of 80 mEq/L, the sodium loss is 56 mEq. The patient should then be given 125 ml of 3 percent saline. The urine flow rate should be approximately 300–600 ml/hr; more furosemide may be given if necessary. At this rate the serum Na$^+$ should correct at about 1–2 mEq/hr. For example, the total amount of water (i.e., urine) that must be removed to increase the Na$^+$ from 115 mEq/L to 125 mEq/L in a patient weighing 75 kg would be $(125 - 115)/115 \times 0.6 \times 75$, or 4 L. A 400 ml/hr correction would take 10 hours (1 mEq/hr). When the serum Na$^+$ concentration reaches 125 mEq/L, this treatment should stop, and the patient should be placed on water restriction until the Na$^+$ is above 130 mEq/L; it is hoped that this conservation effort will reduce neurologic complications. The potassium must also be checked frequently, since it often drops with this therapy.

OUTCOME

Most patients with mild hyponatremia (serum Na$^+$ concentration above 120 mEq/L) respond well to therapy. Severe hyponatremia may be a more hazardous condition for the reasons described.

RECOMMENDED READING

Ashraf N, Locksley R, Arieff AI: Thiazide-induced hyponatremia associated with death or neurologic damage in outpatients. Am J Med 70:1163, 1981.

Ayus JC, Krothapalli RK, Arieff AI: Changing concepts in treatment of severe symptomatic hyponatremia: rapid correction and possible relation to central pontine myelinolysis. Am J Med 78:897, 1985.

Ayus JC, Olivero JJ, Frommer JP: Rapid correction of severe hyponatremia with intravenous hypertonic saline solution. Am J Med 72:43, 1982.

Berl T, Anderson RJ, McDonald KM, et al: Clinical disorders of water metabolism. Kidney Int 10:117, 1976.

Hantman D, Rossier B, Zohlman R, et al: Rapid correction of hyponatremia in the syndrome of inappropriate secretion of antidiuretic hormone: an alternative treatment of hypertonic saline. Ann Intern Med 78:870, 1973.

Narins RG: Therapy of hyponatremia: Does haste make waste? (Editorial.) N Engl J Med 314:1573, 1986.

45. Hyperkalemia

Susan M. Ott

DEFINITION

Hyperkalemia is an increase in the serum potassium (K^+) concentration above the normal range of 3.5–5.0 mEq/L. Severe hyperkalemia is a very urgent problem because the first symptom is often cardiac arrest.

PATHOPHYSIOLOGY

Hyperkalemia can be caused by increased K^+ intake, decreased K^+ excretion, or a shift of K^+ from the cells to extracellular fluid (Table 45–1). In critically ill patients, more than one mechanism is often found.

The first cause of hyperkalemia is increased K^+ load, which is often an iatrogenic problem. For example, too much K^+ may be included in intravenous solution. Unnoticed K^+ may be given in antibiotics or parenteral nutrition solutions. Blood transfusions may also deliver a K^+ load, especially if the blood is old. Excess oral K^+ comes from nutritional supplements, salt substitutes, and excess fruit.

The second cause of hyperkalemia is reduced excretion. Normally, the kidneys carefully regulate the serum K^+ concentration, and excess K^+ is excreted. Renal failure is responsible for most cases of severe hyperkalemia. There are several different forms of decreased K^+ excretion. Renal failure with a decreased glomerular filtration rate is associated with inability to excrete a K^+ load, especially when the urine flow decreases. In acute settings, the rate of rise of the creatinine is more important than the actual value, since filtration may have completely stopped.

Hypoaldosteronism, as seen in Type IV renal tubular acidosis, causes hyperkalemia by several mechanisms: renal excretion of K^+ is diminished, colonic excretion of K^+ is also diminished, and K^+ shifts out of the cells. The colonic excretion of K^+ is not important in most situations, but the colons of patients with chronic renal failure have adapted to excrete a significant part of the usual K^+ intake. This is done without apparent diarrhea, and is probably due to increased aldosterone action on the colon. Thus, aldosterone is important in excretion of K^+ even in a patient without kidneys. Drugs that reduce K^+ excretion include spironolactone,

302

TABLE 45–1. CAUSES OF HYPERKALEMIA

INCREASED POTASSIUM LOAD
  Excess potassium in intravenous fluids or feedings
  Antibiotics such as penicillin
  Blood transfusion
  Salt substitutes and nutritional supplements
DECREASED POTASSIUM SECRETION
  Renal failure
  Hypoaldosteronism
  Drugs: spironolactone, amiloride, triamterene, captopril, enalapril, prostaglandin
    inhibitors, lithium, heparin, cyclosporine
SHIFT OF POTASSIUM FROM CELLS
  Rhabdomyolysis
  Acidosis
  Insulin deficiency
  Hypertonic glucose
  Familial periodic paralysis
  Drugs: propranolol, succinylcholine, digitalis

amiloride, triamterene, angiotensin-converting enzyme inhibitors such as captopril and enalapril, indomethacin, lithium, heparin, cyclosporine, and prostaglandin inhibitors.

The third cause of hyperkalemia is a shift of K^+ out of cells. Since over 90 percent of the body's K^+ is intracellular, the serum K^+ concentration is a poor indicator of total body K^+. Shifts between the cells and the extracellular fluid can cause rapid changes in the serum K^+ concentration. This happens in several situations. Rhabdomyolysis is probably the most extreme case, and patients with extensive muscle injury are at a great risk for hyperkalemia, especially if they also develop acute renal failure. The rhabdomyolysis can be secondary to trauma, to viral syndromes, or to prolonged coma with pressure necrosis of tissue. Acidosis also causes cells to lose K^+, and alkalosis reverses the process.

Several hormones are important in regulation of the serum K^+ concentration. Insulin changes the cellular membrane potential and favors K^+ uptake by cells; this action is independent of glucose transport. Glucose administration without insulin does not shift K^+ into cells; in fact, it does just the opposite. If a bolus of glucose is given to a diabetic, an increase in the serum osmolarity will result. This will lead to a shift in water from the cells and K^+ is carried along, leading to hyperkalemia.

The β-adrenergic sympathetic system is important in protecting the body from a K^+ load. When K^+ is given in the presence of isoproterenol, the serum K^+ does not rise as much as it does without the drug; when K^+ is given in the presence of propranolol, the serum K^+ rises to higher levels than without the drug. A rare cause of hyperkalemia is familial periodic hyperkalemic paralysis, in which K^+ shifts out of the cells for unknown reasons. Drugs that alter the K^+ transport across cells include β-blockers, succinylcholine, and digitalis.

DIAGNOSIS

There are no reliable clinical signs or symptoms of hyperkalemia. In clinical situations in which the K^+ might be high, it must be measured. The major toxicity is cardiac dysrhythmias, and these are usually the first signs that the patient is hyperkalemic. The membrane potential of cells is determined by the ratio of the intracellular to the extracellular K^+ concentration, and any sudden increase in extracellular K^+ will cause depolarization of the membrane. This will eventually result in ventricular fibrillation. Because the ratio of intra- to extracellular K^+ is the important factor, the actual level of serum K^+ that causes toxicity may vary. The rate of rise of K^+ is more important than the absolute level. Patients with chronic renal failure with chronic K^+ elevations have higher intracellular K^+, so that the ratio is near normal.

The best way to recognize if a given level of serum K^+ concentration is dangerous is to examine the electrocardiogram (ECG). The abnormal depolarization of the membrane will be reflected in the tracings, which go through a series of changes: First the T wave becomes symmetrically peaked; when hyperkalemia becomes more severe, the classic peaked T waves become lower and wider; the QRS widens, the P wave gradually disappears, and the tracing looks like a sine wave. It is important for clinicians to remember that severe hyperkalemia can be seen without tall T waves (Fig. 45–1).

MANAGEMENT

If the laboratory report shows hyperkalemia, the ECG should be examined. If there are no changes, measurement of the K^+ level should be repeated because it may be falsely elevated, owing to hemolysis. Mild increases in the K^+ concentration (up to 5 mEq/L or 6 mEq/L, depending on the situation) may not require emergency treatment. Correction of any underlying problem, cessation of offending drugs, and avoidance of K^+ usually solve the problem. Sodium polystyrene sulfonate exchange resins (Kayexalate) may also be used, as discussed later.

If the ECG shows signs of hyperkalemia (usually when the K^+ concentration is above 6 mEq/L) then the patient should be treated urgently and must be followed very closely. Calcium is the most effective fast method of reversing the cardiac toxicity of hyperkalemia. Calcium does nothing to the serum K^+ level, but it acts directly on the cell membrane by increasing the threshold potential. Ten ml of 10 percent calcium gluconate (containing 50 mEq of calcium) given slowly intravenously over about 10 minutes will normalized the ECG within 1–2 minutes.

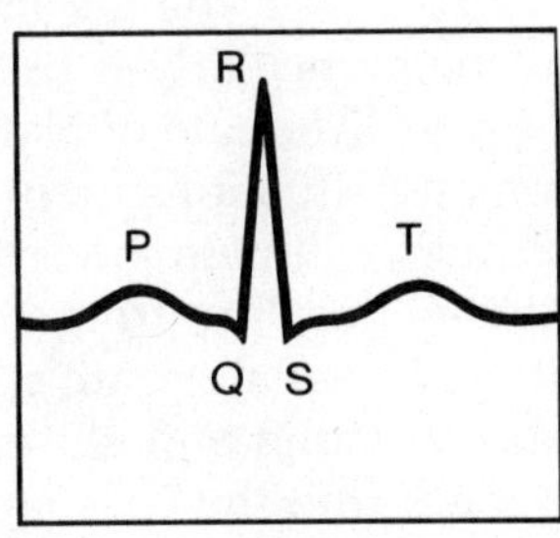

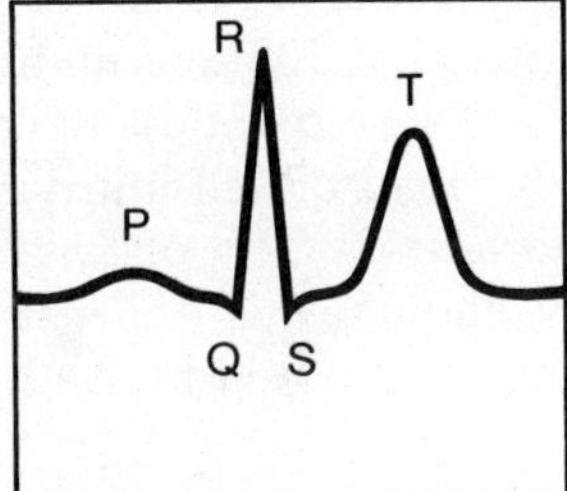

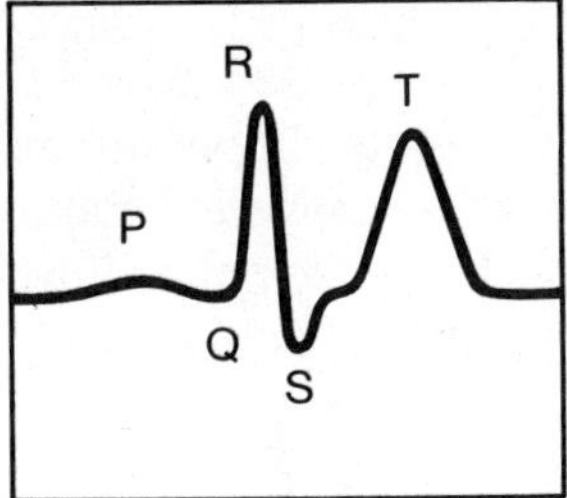

FIGURE 45–1. Progression of electrocardiographic changes in hyperkalemia. The T wave becomes symmetrically peaked, the P wave disappears, and the QRS evolves into a sine wave.

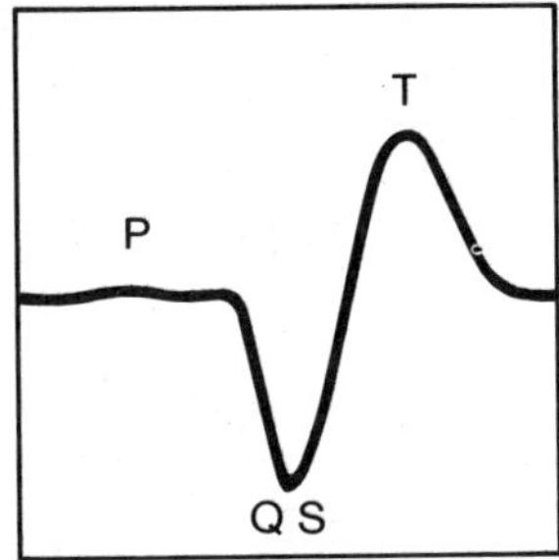

HYPERKALEMIA

However, the effect of calcium is only temporary, and about 15 minutes after the infusion, the ECG will worsen again if nothing is done about the serum K^+ concentration.

To lower the serum K^+, sodium bicarbonate ($NaHCO_3$) should be given, particularly if the patient has acidosis. This will shift the K^+ into the cells. The rate of $NaHCO_3$ infusion will depend on the individual, but in many situations an intravenous infusion of 44 mEq (1 ampule) over 15 minutes will help lower the K^+. The $NaHCO_3$ must be given in a separate intravenous line from that of the calcium to avoid precipitation of the latter. As an alternative to $NaHCO_3$ (or in addition to $NaHCO_3$ in severe cases), insulin and glucose should be administered. The insulin shifts the K^+ back into the cells, and the glucose is given to prevent hypoglycemia. A solution of 500 ml of 10 percent glucose with 15 units of insulin can be infused at 100–200 ml/hr, with adjustments made as necessary.

These maneuvers will shift the K^+ into the cells, but if there has been a K^+ load or cell injury, K^+ must be removed. Exchange resins should be started; 20–30 g of Kayexalate with 25 g of sorbitol can be given orally or by enema; this will usually lower K^+ by about 1 mEq/L. If renal failure has contributed to the hyperkalemia, then dialysis is usually required.

OUTCOME

Acute hyperkalemia should be reversible. However, because this disorder may be a manifestation of severe diseases such as rhabdomyolysis or chronic renal failure, some hyperkalemic patients have a poor overall prognosis.

RECOMMENDED READING

Bia MJ, DeFronzo RA: Extrarenal potassium hemeostasis. Am J Physiol 240:F257, 1981.
Newmark SR, Dluhy RG: Hyperkalemia and hypokalemia. JAMA 231:631, 1975.
Ponce SP, Jennings AE, Madias NE, et al: Drug-induced hyperkalemia. Medicine 64:357, 1985.

46. Hypokalemia

Susan M. Ott

DEFINITION

Hypokalemia is defined as a decrease in the serum potassium (K^+) concentration below the normal range of 3.5–5.0 mEq/L. It may cause weakness, muscle cramping, or cardiac dysrhythmias.

PATHOPHYSIOLOGY

Hypokalemia may be due to inadequate K^+ intake, excess K^+ loss, or shift of K^+ into cells from extracellular fluid (Table 46–1). Obligatory K^+ losses through the skin, gastrointestinal tract, and kidneys normally occur. Although the renal tubules can completely resorb sodium, they cannot do the same for K^+, and 15–40 mEq are lost each day. If patients are given no K^+ supplementation for an extended period, hypokalemia will develop. Occasionally hypokalemia is seen from long-term inadequate oral intake.

Excess K^+ losses can be divided into nonrenal and renal ones. Nonrenal losses may involve either the skin or the gastrointestinal tract. Large amounts of K^+ can be lost in gastrointestinal fluid, especially when there is inflammation, diarrhea, or aggressive nasogastric suctioning. The K^+ concentration in gastrointestinal fluids varies between 10 and 100 mEq/L. K^+ can also be lost in sweat. Occasionally, athletes may ingest salt tablets, which exacerbates the K^+ loss and may produce hypokalemia that is severe enough to cause paralysis or dysrhythmias.

Renal K^+ loss can be secondary to several causes. Whenever there is increased delivery of fluid and sodium to the distal tubule, more K^+ will be excreted in the urine. When the sodium is absorbed from the distal tubule, a negative electric potential is created in the lumen; this attracts K^+ ions. Increased urine flow is seen in diabetes, osmotic diuresis, mannitol administration, postobstructive diuresis, the diuretic phase of acute tubular necrosis, diuresis caused by furosemide and other agents, or overtreatment with saline. Some anions are not easily resorbed, and they will enhance the negative charge in the lumen, which will further increase K^+ transport into the urine. Examples of such nonresorbable anions include sulfate, phosphate, and carbenicillin.

TABLE 46–1. CAUSES OF HYPOKALEMIA

INADEQUATE POTASSIUM INTAKE
EXCESS POTASSIUM LOSSES
    Nonrenal: Burns, gastrointestial losses, sweating
    Renal: States with increased urine flow, diabetes
        Renal tubular acidosis
        Drugs: Sulfate, phosphate, carbenicillin, diuretics,
          amphotericin, heavy metals, cisplatin, licorice
        Hyperaldosteronism
SHIFT OF POTASSIUM INTO CELLS
    Alkalosis
    Refeeding
    Replacement of folate
    Thyrotoxicosis
    Periodic hypokalemic paralysis
    Barium poisoning

Renal tubular acidosis (RTA) is associated with renal K^+ wasting. This is especially true with proximal RTA treated with bicarbonate (HCO_3^-). The HCO_3^- is not resorbed, and the excess amount in the distal nephron acts as a nonresorbable anion. High levels of aldosterone will lead to hypokalemia and alkalosis rather than to acidosis. This occurs secondary to adrenal adenoma, adrenal carcinoma, Cushing's disease, or ectopic adrenocorticotrophic hormone (ACTH) production by tumors. Patients with Bartter's syndrome and renin-secreting tumors also have high levels of aldosterone with hypokalemia. Leukemia may produce a not-yet-identified factor that causes renal K^+ wasting. Hypomagnesemia and hypercalcemia can both be associated with increased K^+ wasting. Drugs that cause renal K^+ wasting include diuretics, antibiotics such as carbenicillin and amphotericin, as well as heavy metals, cisplatin, and licorice.

The last cause of hypokalemia is a shift of K^+ into cells. Alkalosis causes K^+ to shift into cells, which may be responsible for a drop in the serum K^+ concentration. Insulin may also cause such a shift, but it is not usually extensive enough to lead to hypokalemia. In patients who have been starving and are suddenly refed, K^+ enters cells. Also, in patients with a folate deficiency that is replenished, enough K^+ may enter the bone marrow to cause hypokalemia. Thyrotoxicosis may be associated with severe hypokalemia that leads to paralysis; the mechanism for this cellular shift of K^+ is not clear. Patients present with sudden paralysis, often following a carbohydrate meal. A rare entity is periodic hypokalemic paralysis, which is usually familial. Barium poisoning also shifts K^+ into cells.

DIAGNOSIS

Muscle weakness, paralysis, or cramping are the major symptoms seen in hypokalemia. Many cases have no symptoms unless the K^+ drops

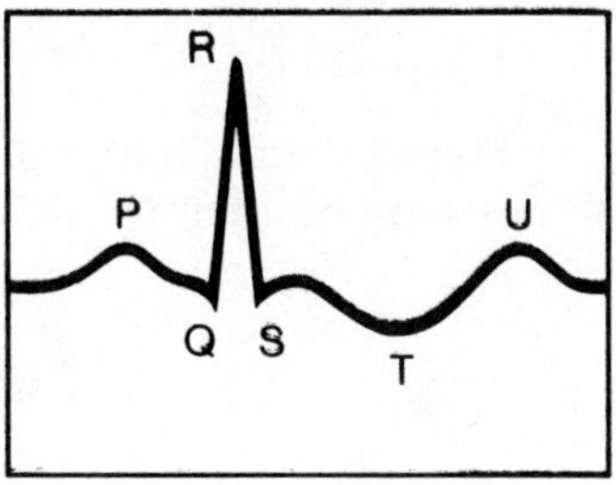

FIGURE 46–1. Electrocardiographic changes in hypokalemia. Note ST depression and prominent U wave.

HYPOKALEMIA

to levels below 3 mEq/L. Cardiac dysrhythmias may then be seen, including ectopic beats, atrioventricular block, ventricular tachycardia, or ventricular fibrillation. The electrocardiogram shows S-T or T-wave depression and U waves (Fig. 46–1).

MANAGEMENT

The underlying cause of hypokalemia should be corrected, and any offending drugs should be discontinued. K^+ should be replaced, but there is no standard rate because the serum K^+ reflects only a small percentage of the total body K^+. Thus, the serum K^+ concentration must be monitored during treatment, and the rate of replacement may need to be adjusted. It is important to realize that a rapid replacement rate can be dangerous and can lead to dysrhythmias. The membrane potential in cardiac cells depends much more on the ratio of intra- to extracellular K^+ than on the absolute serum K^+ concentration. Thus, a rapid rise in extracellular K^+ from low to normal levels may cause ventricular fibrillation.

General guidelines for K^+ replacement follow. First, if the serum K^+ is less than 2 mEq/L, K^+ can be given at a rate of 40 mEq/hr. This amount can be added to a liter of water and infused over 1 hour. If the patient cannot tolerate volume, give 10 mEq potassium chloride in 100 ml water over 15–60 minutes. The serum K^+ concentration should be monitored frequently. K^+ can be replaced at this rate until it is above 2 mEq/L. Only in extraordinary cases should K^+ replacement exceed this rate (for example, when there are huge ongoing gastrointestinal losses) and then only under careful monitoring.

If the K^+ concentration is between 2 and 3 mEq/L, then give approximately 100 mEq/day plus replacement of ongoing losses. If the K^+ concentration is between 3 and 3.5 mEq/L, then give approximately 60 mEq/day plus replacement of ongoing losses. The serum K^+ concentration should be checked every 2–4 hours in severe cases and every 12–24 hours in moderate cases until it becomes normal and stable.

Outcome

Hypokalemia in most cases is a treatable disorder that should respond to appropriate therapy.

RECOMMENDED READING

Bia MJ, DeFronzo RA: Extrarenal potassium homeostasis. Am J Physiol 240 (Renal Fluid Electrolyte Physiol 9):F257, 1981.
Newmark SR, Dluhy RG: Hyperkalemia and hypokalemia. JAMA 231:631, 1975.
Ponce SP, Jennings AE, Madias NE, et al: Drug-induced hyperkalemia. Medicine 64:357, 1985.

47. Hypercalcemia

Susan M. Ott

Susan M. Ott

DEFINITION

Hypercalcemia is defined as an increase in the serum calcium (Ca^{++}) concentration above the normal range of 8.5–10.5 mg/dl.

PATHOPHYSIOLOGY

Extracellular Ca^{++} concentrations are carefully regulated by mechanisms involving Ca^{++} exchange between bone and serum, Ca^{++} absorption by the gut, and renal Ca^{++} handling. Parathyroid hormone, vitamin D sterols, and calcitonin regulate these processes and are usually involved in the hypercalcemic process or its treatment. Hypercalcemia may result from excess Ca^{++} intake, decreased Ca^{++} excretion, increased bone resorption, or decreased bone formation. Often these processes occur concomitantly, and since they are regulated by the same set of hormones, it is sometimes difficult to separate them.

Excess Ca^{++} in total parenteral nutrition solutions or in dietary supplements may occasionally be the cause of hypercalcemia, but usually the excess Ca^{++} is excreted by the kidneys. If renal impairment occurs (which may happen as a result of hypercalciuria), the increased load will contribute to hypercalcemia. Increased Ca^{++} absorption from the intestine occurs with vitamin D toxicity. Patients with this disorder also have marked hypercalciuria; their serum phosphate is normal to high because vitamin D also enhances gastrointestinal phosphate absorption. Vitamin D intoxication may also contribute to increased bone resorption. Sarcoidosis causes hypercalcemia by this mechanism: The granulomatous cells can convert 25-hydroxyvitamin D to the active 1,25-dihydroxyvitamin D form. Other granulomatous disorders and lymphomas may also convert vitamin D, with resulting hypercalcemia.

Increased bone resorption is the most important factor leading to hypercalcemia. Primary hyperparathyroidism associated with increased bone resorption of Ca^{++} is a common cause of hypercalcemia, especially in elderly patients. High levels of parathyroid hormone (PTH) are also seen in syndromes of multiple endocrine adenomas. The serum Ca^{++}

level does not reliably help in the diagnosis of hyperparathyroidism; in early cases, the Ca^{++} is normal, and in severe cases the Ca^{++} may be above 20 mg/dl. Since PTH increases the renal excretion of phosphate, the serum phosphate level is low in primary hyperparathyroidism. This is not a specific finding, however, and patients with critical illnesses often have low phosphate from other causes.

Cancers also commonly cause hypercalcemia, especially squamous cell carcinomas of the head and neck, lung, or breast; cholangiocarcinomas; and hematologic malignancies. The increased bone resorption caused by cancers involves several mechanisms. Direct bony metastases can stimulate local bone resorption. The malignant cells often secrete factors such as prostaglandins as they grow; these lesions can be diagnosed with bone scans. Hematologic malignancies also secrete factors that cause bone resorption; these include osteoclast-activating factor, prostaglandins, and lymphokines. Multiple myeloma should always be suspected in a case of hypercalcemia, especially when there are bone lesions or osteopenia but a negative bone scan. Solid tumors may also cause hypercalcemia by secretion of ectopic hormones. It is very rare to have ectopic PTH secretion, but substances secreted by the malignant cells may activate PTH receptors and simulate PTH action.

Prolonged bed rest, especially in patients with muscle paralysis, causes increased bone resorption and decreased bone formation. These patients have hypercalciuria, and they may develop hypercalcemia. Metabolic acidosis also contributes to bone resorption, but this is not sufficient to cause hypercalcemia; however, it may contribute to the problem. Vitamin A toxicity and thyrotoxicosis are unusual causes of hypercalcemia.

One of the common contributing causes of hypercalcemia is decreased Ca^{++} excretion due to intravascular volume depletion. Under normal conditions, the kidneys can excrete large loads of Ca^{++}, but when there is volume depletion, the calcium is retained. Sodium and Ca^{++} are resorbed in the same manner in the proximal tubule, so when volume depletion enhances sodium resorption, Ca^{++} resorption is also increased. Thus, if there is excess Ca^{++} absorption or bone resorption, hypercalcemia will result. Thiazide diuretics act directly on the distal renal tubule to promote renal resorption of Ca^{++}; thus, the urine Ca^{++} concentration falls; this does not ordinarily lead to hypercalcemia, but it may contribute to it.

Ca^{++} metabolism in patients with renal failure is complex. The most common problem is hypocalcemia due to decreased levels of 1,25-dihydroxyvitamin D. But hypercalcemia may also be seen in patients with renal failure. In acute renal failure caused by rhabdomyolysis, patients are initially hypocalcemic. Often they are treated with Ca^{++}, which precipitates in the muscle. During the recovery phase, this Ca^{++} is released, and hypercalcemia is seen. In some cases, acute renal failure was caused by the hypercalciuria; when the kidneys are no longer able to excrete the excess Ca^{++}, it accumulates in the serum.

Patients with chronic renal failure on dialysis may become hypercalcemic if the Ca^{++} concentration in the dialysate is too high. They may also develop hyperparathyroidism. Vitamin D toxicity may occur, especially when the long-acting preparations of vitamin D are used. Aluminum intoxication also causes hypercalcemia by inhibition of bone formation.

DIAGNOSIS

The symptoms of hypercalcemia vary widely and do not correspond to the serum Ca^{++} level. At levels below 12 mg/dl, there may be no symptoms. Usually, the dignosis is made more accurately by examining the laboratory results rather than the patient. In symptomatic patients, neurologic symptoms vary from confusion to coma, muscles may become weak, and nausea and constipation are frequently seen. The Q-T interval is prolonged on the electrocardiogram, and dysrhythmias may be seen. Renal manifestations include nephrocalcinosis; inability to concentrate urine, leading to polyuria; and potassium wasting, leading to hypokalemia. Hyperparathyroidism is best diagnosed by assaying serum immunoreactive PTH.

MANAGEMENT

The actual level of serum Ca^{++} requiring urgent treatment depends on the clinical situation; in most cases levels above 12 mg/dl require rapid correction. Before starting therapy, make sure that increases in serum proteins due to diseases like multiple myeloma have not spuriously increased serum Ca^{++}, even though ionized Ca^{++} remains normal. Subtract 0.8 mg/dl from serum Ca^{++} to correct for each 1-g/dl increase in serum albumin above 4 g/dl.

If ionized Ca^{++} is truly elevated, normal saline should be given to lower serum Ca^{++}. This will be particularly effective if volume depletion is a factor in the etiology of the hypercalcemia. The proximal renal tubules usually absorb sodium and Ca^{++} in the same manner, so that saline excess, which leads to a saline diuresis, will also lead to a Ca^{++} diuresis. Before concluding that the patient is not responsive to saline, an adequate diuresis must be maintained to the level of 4–6 liters of urine/day.

Often, furosemide is used in order to achieve a large urine volume in hypercalcemic patients. However, clinicians must realize that the diuretics alone do *not* treat the hypercalcemia. Although furosemide may enhance the distal excretion of Ca^{++}, it will not affect the proximal resorption. Thus, a common error is to maintain a patient in a state of mild volume depletion by the use of diuretics, in which case the serum Ca^{++} concentration will remain elevated, even with high urine volumes. To prevent this iatrogenic situation, clinicians must be certain that the patient does not have any volume depletion *before* diuretics are given (a state of mild volume excess is best for eliminating Ca^{++}). Thus, saline should be given first and diuretics used only to help eliminate the extra saline. It also is important to monitor serum sodium and potassium levels during this treatment; potassium may be lost in the diuresis, and the hypercalcemia often causes a form of nephrogenic diabetes insipidus with water loss, leading to hypernatremia. Replacement of potassium or of water is often indicated.

Since vigorous treatment with saline requires such careful attention to fluid balance, it is difficult to maintain for more than a few days, and other treatments aimed at the etiology of the hypercalcemia should also be started. One such therapy is calcitonin, which blocks bone resorption of Ca^{++}. Calcitonin is a safe agent, but its effects last only a few days because there is down-regulation of the calcitonin receptors on bone cells. If corticosteroids are also given, the tachyphylaxis to calcitonin is not seen. 100–400 MRC units/day of calcitonin and 100 mg of hydrocortisone QID should be used. The serum Ca^{++} usually starts to decrease in 4–6 hours.

If the patient has hypophosphatemia, phosphate may be given to decrease the serum Ca^{++}. The Ca^{++}-phosphate product should be kept below 55 mg/dl to prevent metastatic calcifications. In hyperparathyroidism, the serum phosphate is usually low, but in most other forms of hypercalcemia, the phosphate is normal or even elevated, so phosphate therapy is often contraindicated.

Diphosphonates are agents that block bone resorption and are effective in rapidly lowering serum Ca^{++} levels. Several different forms of these medications exist, but unfortunately the most effective ones, clodronate and APD, are not available in the United States. Sodium etidronate (EHDP) is not effective orally, but when given parenterally at 0.5 g/day it lowers serum Ca^{++}. EHDP has more side effects, including osteomalacia, than the other diphosphonates. Initially developed as an antineoplastic drug, WR-2721 has been found to inhibit bone resorption as well as PTH secretion. This double-barrelled agent has been very effective in some preliminary studies.

Once the serum Ca^{++} level has been reduced, the underlying cause of the hypercalcemia should be corrected, if possible. However, unresectable malignancies may not be amenable to therapy, and vitamin D intoxication may take months to resolve. Thus, chronic treatment all too often must be aimed at the hypercalcemia alone rather than at the underlying process. Corticosteroids inhibit the intestinal absorption of Ca^{++} and may suppress some malignancies and granulomatous disease.

Calcitonin and prednisone may be used chronically as well as acutely. Mithramycin blocks bone resorption and may be quite useful. However, its onset of action is delayed by 36–48 hours. This drug may also have side effects, including renal disease, bone marrow suppression, bleeding, and hepatitis. The intravenous dose is 15–25 μg/kg, and the dosing interval varies from several days to 3 weeks, depending on the patient's response. When the drug wears off, serious rebound hypercalcemia may occur.

OUTCOME

The serum Ca^{++} concentration can be lowered somewhat and the symptoms reduced in most hypercalcemic patients. Nevertheless, severe hypercalcemia, especially that caused by cancer, may be very difficult to treat and perhaps should not be treated in certain individuals for whom death due to hypercalcemia may be preferable to other forms of demise. As this example suggests, the overall outcome from hypercalcemia depends largely on its underlying cause.

RECOMMENDED READING

Hirschel-Scholz S, Caverzasio J, Bonjour J-PH: Inhibition of parathyroid hormone secretion and parathyroid hormone-independent diminution of tubular calcium reabsorption by WR-2721, a unique hypocalcemia agent. J Clin Invest 76:1851, 1985.
Jung A: Comparison of two parenteral diphosphonates in hypercalcemia of malignancy. Am J Med 72:221, 1982.
Mundy GR, Martin TJ: The hypercalcemia of malignancy: pathogenesis and management. Metabolism 31:1247, 1982.
Mundy GR, Wilkinson R, Heath DA: Comparative study of available medical therapy for hypercalcemia of malignancy. Am J Med 74:421, 1983.

48. Hypocalcemia

Susan M. Ott

DEFINITION

Hypocalcemia is a decrease in the serum calcium (Ca^{++}) concentration below the normal range of 8.5–10.5 mg/dl. Mild hypocalcemia is a common problem in critically ill patients, and often a specific cause in not identified.

PATHOPHYSIOLOGY

Hypocalcemia may result either from decreased Ca^{++} intake or binding in the body, decreased bone resorption, or increased bone formation. Decreased Ca^{++} intake is seen in poorly nourished patients, including those receiving too little Ca^{++} in parenteral nutrition and in patients with vitamin D deficiency. Renal failure is associated with hypocalcemia because the kidneys are unable to excrete phosphate and metabolize vitamin D.

Binding of Ca^{++} within the body occurs in pancreatitis. Hemoperfusion or dialysis with citrate may also bind Ca^{++} and lead to hypocalcemia. In addition, rhabdomyolysis can cause hypocalcemia by the precipitation of Ca^{++} in muscles. When the rhabdomyolysis ceases and the Ca^{++} is released, rebound hypercalcemia may occur.

Hypoparathyroidism causes hypocalcemia by decreasing bone resorption. It is associated with low levels of active vitamin D. Hypoparathyroidism may occur after parathyroid surgery, including the inadvertent removal of parathyroid tissue during thyroidectomy. Medical causes of hypoparathroidism other than congenital hypoparathyroidism are uncommon. High phosphate and low serum parathyroid levels are found in hypoparathyroid patients, in addition to hypocalcemia. Low parathyroid hormone (PTH) and Ca^{++} levels also occur in hypomagnesemia, a common problem in poorly nourished patients (including alcoholics) because their low magnesium levels inhibit parathyroid hormone secretion.

The major cause of hypocalcemia due to increased bone formation is the "hungry bone syndrome." This is seen primarily in patients following subtotal parathyroidectomy. The syndrome has also been reported in patients with renal osteodystrophy who are treated with calcitriol.

316

Viral infections and the toxic shock syndrome may cause hypocalcemia by unknown mechanisms. Drugs that may cause hypocalcemia include EDTA, phosphates, diphosphonates, fluoride, calcitonin, mithramycin, and WR-2721.

DIAGNOSIS

Hypocalcemic patients may manifest musculoskeletal symptoms. Their reflexes become hyperactive, and eventually tetany may be seen. Carpopedal spasm is noted when a blood pressure cuff is used to elevate the venous pressure. Chvostek's sign (muscle spasms in face when facial nerve is tapped) is also seen. In addition, seizures may occur. Cardiac dysrhythmias are seen in severe cases. If hypocalcemia is prolonged, bone disease such as osteomalacia will develop.

Even in the presence of symptoms, the diagnosis of hypocalcemia may require laboratory tests. Remember that decreases in serum protein must be accounted for in determining the ionized Ca^{++} concentration. Thus, add 0.8 mg/dl to the serum Ca^{++} to correct for each 1-g/dl decrease in the serum albumin below 4 g/dl. If possible, ionized Ca^{++} should be measured directly.

MANAGEMENT

The treatment of hypocalcemia depends on its underlying cause. If the patient has acute renal failure caused by rhabdomyolysis, Ca^{++} should be given only to prevent symptoms. In cases accompanied by hyperphosphatemia, Ca^{++} should be given with great caution lest these two minerals deposit in the tissues. If hypomagnesemia or vitamin D deficiency are present, treatment is aimed at replacement. The usual daily requirements of Ca^{++} are 800–1000 mg elemental Ca^{++} orally, of which about 200 mg/day are absorbed. Thus, parenteral solutions should contain 200 mg (5 mM) of Ca^{++}; extra may be added as indicated. In cases of tetany or seizures from low Ca^{++}, 10 ml of 10 percent calcium gluconate (which contains 100 mg, 2.5 mM, or 5 mEq Ca^{++}) may be given over 10–20 minutes. More rapid rates may cause hypotension or cardiac arrhythmias.

OUTCOME

Hypocalcemia is easily treated in most critically ill patients who merely have poor intake or hypomagnesemia. Hypocalcemia due to other disorders may be less amenable to therapy.

RECOMMENDED READING

Zaloga GP, Chernow B: Hypocalcemia in critical illness. JAMA 256:1924, 1986.

49. Hypermagnesemia

Susan M. Ott

DEFINITION

Hypermagnesemia is diagnosed when the serum magnesium (Mg^{++}) concentration exceeds the normal range of 1.5–2.5 mg/dl.

PATHOPHYSIOLOGY

Because excess Mg^{++} is readily excreted by the kidneys, hypermagnesemia rarely occurs except in renal failure. Mg^{++} is a small ion and is easily dialyzed, so in patients with renal failure on dialysis, the serum Mg^{++} concentration reflects the levels added to the dialysate and are not elevated unless there has been excessive intake. Mg^{++}- containing antacids can cause hypermagnesemia in a patient with decreased creatinine clearance. Magnesium sulfate is used to treat toxemia of pregnancy; if too much is given patients may become hypermagnesemic.

DIAGNOSIS

No clinical signs or symptoms are seen when the serum Mg^{++} is less than about 4 mEq/L, even though normally the serum levels are less than 2 mEq/L. At higher levels, musculoskeletal symptoms are seen, with weakness and eventually paralysis. The respiratory muscles may become weakened to a point of interfering with ventilation. The patients have hyporeflexia. Complete heart block occurs at levels above 15 mEq/L.

MANAGEMENT

In mild to moderate cases, stopping the Mg^{++} load is sufficient. Rarely, dialysis may be needed to remove the Mg^{++}. Calcium gluconate may be used as a physiologic antagonist if there is respiratory depression.

318

OUTCOME

Hypermagnesemia usually responds to therapy.

RECOMMENDED READING

Dirks JH: The kidney and magnesium regulation. Kidney Int 23:771, 1983.
Rude RK, Singer FR: Magnesium deficiency and excess. Annu Rev Med 32:245, 1981.

50. Hypomagnesemia

Susan M. Ott

DEFINITION

Hypomagnesemia is diagnosed when the serum magnesium (Mg^{++}) concentration is less than the normal range of 1.5–2.5 mg/dl.

PATHOPHYSIOLOGY

Critically ill patients often have low Mg^{++} levels that are overlooked because this "forgotten ion" is not usually included on chemical screening panels. Malnourished patients, including alcoholics, are at particularly high risk. Mg^{++} can also be lost from the gastrointestinal tract, and hypomagnesemia and hypocalcemia occur in pancreatitis, probably owing to deposition in necrotic tissues.

Renal Mg^{++} wasting is seen in several conditions. For example, alcoholism acts to enhance the renal excretion of Mg^{++}. Hyperaldosteronism also contributes to renal Mg^{++} losses, as do diabetic ketoacidosis and other osmotic diuretic states. Several drugs that act on the early distal nephron will cause Mg^{++} wasting; these include furosemide, aminoglycosides, platinum, amphotericin, and digitalis.

DIAGNOSIS

Hypomagnesemia is usually associated with hypocalcemia; hypokalemia may also occur. This may be due to the action of Mg^{++} on the parathyroid gland; hypomagnesemia inhibits parathyroid hormone secretion, which will lower serum calcium. Dysphagia and other musculoskeletal symptoms may occur, which closely resemble hypocalcemia. These symptoms may indeed be due to the hypocalcemia, but in certain experimental situations, the calcium is maintained at a normal level, and the symptoms persist until the Mg^{++} deficiency is corrected.

Management

Parenteral Mg^{++} may be given at about 4 g of magnesium sulfate (32 mEq $MgSO_4$) daily. In more severe cases, up to 100 mEq/day may be infused. Treatment should be carried out for at least 5 days to allow equilibration with intracellular stores. Mg^{++} is a relatively safe ion to administer; if it is given in large amounts (such as are used in the treatment of toxemia), hypotension or hyporeflexia may occur. The serum Mg^{++} concentration may not reflect the degree of total body Mg^{++} depletion; it may rise to low-normal levels even when a significant amount of Mg^{++} depletion still exists intracellularly. One way to check this is to administer a dose of Mg^{++} and then to measure the 24-hour urine excretion. If less than 80 percent of the Mg^{++} is excreted, then Mg^{++} depletion still exists. Unfortunately, when the hypomagnesemia is caused by renal wasting, the urine Mg^{++} will not be helpful, and patients must be treated empirically.

Outcome

Hypomagnesemia should respond to therapy.

RECOMMENDED READING

Dirks JH: The kidney and magnesium regulation. Kidney Int 23:771, 1983.
Kingston ME, AI-Sibà I, MB, Skooge WC: Clinical manifestations of hypomagnesemia. Crit Care Med 14:950, 1986.
Rude RK, Singer FR: Magnesium deficiency and excess. Annu Rev Med 32:245, 1981.

51. Hyperphosphatemia

Susan M. Ott

DEFINITION

Hyperphosphatemia is diagnosed when the serum phosphate (PO_4^{--}) concentration exceeds the normal range of 2.5–4.5 mg/dl.

PATHOPHYSIOLOGY

Hyperphosphatemia occurs most commonly in patients with renal failure who cannot excrete a PO_4^{--} load. This is especially true if rhabdomyolysis is also present. Hypoparathyroidism can also cause hyperphosphatemia, as can rapid lysis of tumors such as Burkitt's lymphoma.

DIAGNOSIS

High PO_4^{--} levels are usually not associated with symptoms. However, they will cause metastatic calcifications if the calcium concentration is normal or high. The calcifications may occur in vessels, leading to ischemic necrosis of the digits. Calcifications in the lungs may occur, but pulmonary function is usually not impaired.

MANAGEMENT

Intestinal absorption of PO_4^{--} can be inhibited by aluminum, which binds the PO_4^{--} in the gut. High doses of calcium carbonate may also be used, especially in young children or in other patients at risk for aluminum intoxication. Dialysis is partially effective in lowering PO_4^{--}, but it will not normalize the levels.

OUTCOME

Hyperphosphatemia is a chronic problem in patients with renal failure, in whom it is difficult to control. In acute renal failure, the hyperphosphatemia usually resolves as the kidneys improve.

RECOMMENDED READING

Maxwell MH, Kleeman CR (eds): Clinical Disorders of Fluid and Electrolyte Metabolism. 3rd edition. New York, McGraw-Hill, Inc., 1980.

52. Hypophosphatemia

Susan M. Ott

DEFINITION

Hypophosphatemia is diagnosed when the serum phosphate(PO_4^{--}) concentration is below the normal range of 2.5–4.5 mg/dl.

PATHOPHYSIOLOGY

Hypophosphatemia is caused by inadequate intake or excessive loss of PO_4^{--} or by a shift of PO_4^{--} into cells. Patients with alcoholism and malnutrition are most likely to have inadequate PO_4^{--} intake. PO_4^{--} can be lost through the gastrointestinal tract or the kidneys; the latter occurs in patients with hyperparathyroidism because parathyroid hormone (PTH) controls the maximum amont of PO_4^{--} that is resorbed. Proximal renal tubular acidosis (Fanconi's syndrome) is associated with PO_4^{--} loss because the damaged proximal tubules cannot resorb the PO_4^{--}. Rare mesenchymal and connective tissue tumors also secrete a factor that causes hypophosphatemia. Osmotic diuresis such as seen in diabetes also leads to renal PO_4^{--} loss. PO_4^{--} can be lost from the gastrointestinal tract during diarrhea. Aluminum-containing antacids will lower PO_4^{--} both by inhibiting absorption and by "trapping" the phosphate, which passively enters the gut.

One of the most common causes of hypophosphatemia in the intensive care unit (ICU) is the use of parenteral nutrition solutions containing glucose that causes PO_4^{--} to enter cells. Alkalosis and refeeding after starvation may also lead to hypophosphatemia by this mechanism. Treatment of folic acid deficiency with folate shifts PO_4^{--} into marrow cells.

DIAGNOSIS

There is a long list of signs and symptoms that can be associated with hypophosphatemia; none is specific, and most are seen when serum levels are below 1.5 mg/dl. These include muscle weakness, rhabdomyolysis, and hemolysis. Chronic low levels of PO_4^{--} that do not cause acute symptoms will lead to bone disease, particularly osteomalacia. Ventilatory failure may be caused by acute or chronic hypophosphatemia, as recent studies have shown.

MANAGEMENT

PO_4^{--} is easily absorbed, and patients without lactose deficiency who can tolerate oral feedings may be given milk as a source of PO_4^{--}. In ICU patients who are receiving intravenous solutions, PO_4^{--} may be given as potassium phosphate. Usually 2.5–5 mg/kg/day ($=0.08$–0.16 mM/kg) will be adequate. Since PO_4^{--} is largely intracellular, serum levels may not reflect the total body status, and daily PO_4^{--} levels should be measured until they are normal and stable.

OUTCOME

Hypophosphatemia should respond to replacement therapy.

RECOMMENDED READING

Aubier M, Murciano D, Lecocguic Y, Viires N, Jacquens Y, Squara P, Pariente R: Effect of hypophosphatemia on diaphragmatic contractility in patients with acute respiratory failure. N Engl J Med 313:420, 1985.
Biberstein M, Packer BA: Enema-induced hypophosphatemia. Am J Med 79:645, 1985.
Knochel JP: The clinical status of hypophosphatemia: an update. 313:447, 1985.
Lentz RD, Brown DM, Kjellstrand CM: Treatment of severe hypophosphatemia. Ann Intern Med 89:941, 1978.
Ritz E: Acute hypophosphatemia. Kidney Int 22:84, 1982.

53. Dialysis

Wendell P. Fleet
David J. Pierson

Introduction

When noninvasive means of controlling acute or chronic renal failure are insufficient, dialysis may be used as a temporary or long-term replacement for normal kidney function. Hemodialysis consists of diverting blood out of the body and past a semi-permeable membrane, on the other side of which is a specially prepared dialysate, into and out of which water, solutes, and other substances move according to its composition. In peritoneal dialysis, a specially prepared dialysate is instilled into the patient's peritoneal cavity and subsequently removed along with excess fluid, metabolic wastes, and other substances as necessary. In recent years, these techniques have been supplemented, in the management of acute renal failure and in certain intoxications, by the introduction of continuous arteriovenous hemofiltration (CAVH), charcoal or resin hemoperfusion, and other techniques.

This chapter summarizes the indications and clinical uses of hemodialysis, peritoneal dialysis, and hemoperfusion in the management of acute renal failure, massive drug overdose, and other intoxications.

Indications

Table 53–1 summarizes the indications for dialysis in acute renal failure. In general, dialysis is indicated for severe, symptomatic uremia or volume overload unresponsive to other measures. Traditionally, it is begun when the blood urea nitrogen (BUN) rises above about 120 mg/dl, although in many centers, a more aggressive approach is used, and dialysis is commenced and repeated frequently to prevent the BUN from exceeding approximately 80 mg/dl. The latter approach permits more liberal fluid and nutritional management and, according to the results of several studies, also lowers morbidity and mortality. In the absence of the specific abnormalities listed in Table 53–1, the best general monitor of the need for and effectiveness of dialysis is the BUN.

Whether hemodialysis or peritoneal dialysis should be used in a given

TABLE 53–1. INDICATIONS FOR DIALYSIS IN ACUTE RENAL FAILURE

Azotemia
  Conservative approach: Prevent BUN from rising above 120–140 mg/dl
  Aggressive (prophylactic) approach: prevent BUN from rising above 80–100 mg/dl
Severe fluid overload (e.g., pulmonary edema)
Severe hyperkalemia (refractory to medical management)
Severe metabolic acidosis (refractory to medical management)
Clinical manifestations of uremia
  Uremic pericarditis
  Severe encephalopathy (confusion, coma, asterixis, muscle twitching, intractable nausea
    and vomiting)
  Seizures
  Overt bleeding due to platelet dysfunction

patient with acute renal failure depends upon the general considerations listed in Table 53–2. Although there are some specific drawbacks for each method, either can be used with equal overall effectiveness. Hemodialysis is more efficient and should thus be used in hypercatabolic patients or in those with immediately life-threatening conditions; peritoneal dialysis should be used in patients who cannot tolerate rapid fluid or electrolyte shifts.

CAVH provides a means of controlling fluid balance, sodium, and acidosis that is simpler than conventional hemodialysis and may thus be used in patients who are more seriously ill and less hemodynamically stable. It also permits more aggressive nutritional support and its attendant high fluid intake. In some centers, CAVH is usually used in patients with acute renal failure, and conventional hemodialysis is reserved for cases of severe hyperkalemia and azotemia. However, because of the relatively small surface area employed, CAVH does not remove uremic toxins in the quantities achieved by hemodialysis, and it must therefore be started earlier.

The addition of an adsorbant such as microencapsulated charcoal to a dialysis or hemoperfusion system permits removal of drugs and exogenous toxins as well as endogenous substances. Although unnecessary in most drug overdoses and intoxications, hemoperfusion can be an effective adjunct to aggressive medical management in severe, life-threatening cases (Table 53–3). However, its use in the conditions listed in the table is controversial, and only for ethylene glycol and theophylline intoxications do clinicians generally agree on its necessity.

CONTRAINDICATIONS

There are no contraindications to dialysis in the usual sense. However, hemodialysis is technically difficult and usually inefficient in patients who are hypotensive or have marked cardiovascular instability or when

TABLE 53–2. RELATIVE ADVANTAGES AND DISADVANTAGES OF HEMODIALYSIS AND PERITONEAL DIALYSIS IN ACUTE RENAL FAILURE

HEMODIALYSIS	PERITONEAL DIALYSIS
Advantages	*Advantages*
Can correct metabolic and fluid abnormalities quickly	Metabolic and fluid changes are gradual
Effective in catabolic patient	Less likelihood of precipitating hypotension because of rapid fluid shifts
Can be done emergently via subclavian catheter	Method of choice for hemodynamically unstable patients
Method of choice in patients with undiagnosed intraabdominal disease or recent abdominal or retroperitoneal surgery	Does not require as much technical expertise and apparatus
Less risk of infection	No need for anticoagulation
	Avoids problems of vascular access
	Drugs can be given intraperitoneally
Disadvantages	*Disadvantages*
Requires 200–300 ml/min blood flow into dialyzer	Slower correction of metabolic abnormalities
Cannot be used in patients with hypotension, cardiovascular instability, or recent cerebrovascular accident	Inadequate in highly catabolic patients
Can cause hypotension and other problems due to rapid fluid shifts	Cannot be used in patients with recent abdominal or retroperitoneal surgery, severe abdominal distention, peritonitis, or reduced peritoneal surface area
Requires anticoagulation	Must be used cautiously in patients with prior abdominal surgery or diabetes mellitus
Requires more specialized expertise and apparatus	Impairs diaphragm function; must be used cautiously in patients with respiratory disease who are not on mechanical ventilation
Must be used cautiously in patients with heart failure or advanced age	

TABLE 53–3. INDICATIONS FOR HEMOPERFUSION IN DRUG OVERDOSE OR INTOXICATION*

Ingestion and probable absorption of a potentially lethal dose
A blood level in the potentially fatal range (e.g., theophylline†)
Massive ingestion of an agent that is metabolized to other, more toxic substances (e.g., methanol, ethylene glycol)
Ingestion of an agent with delayed toxicity (e.g., paraquat; *Amanita phalloides*)
Severe impairment in normal route of excretion, metabolism, or clearance (e.g., severe hepatic or renal insufficiency)
Progressive clinical deterioration despite maximal medical therapy (e.g., progressive hypotension requiring pressor agents)

*Assuming the agent involved is known to be cleared effectively by hemoperfusion.
†Recent reports suggest that oral activated charcoal may be as effective as hemoperfusion.

anticoagulation cannot be tolerated (e.g., active gastrointestinal bleeding, acute cerebrovascular accident). It should also be used cautiously in the elderly and in patients with overt heart failure.

Peritoneal dialysis is ineffective when the peritoneal diffusion surface has been reduced by 50 percent or more, as by fibrosis or resection. It is contraindicated in patients with diaphragmatic defects, massive abdominal distention, undiagnosed acute intraabdominal disease, or active peritonitis. In addition, most clinicians consider peritoneal dialysis relatively contraindicated in the early period following abdominal or retroperitoneal surgery and in patients with colostomy or nephrostomy. Individuals with diverticulosis, hepatitis, and severe obesity have higher complication rates than those without these conditions.

Peritoneal dialysis should be done cautiously in patients with diabetes because glucose (commonly 1.5 or 4.25 percent) is usually the main osmotic agent used in the dialysate. Because rapid instillation of 1–2 liters of intraperitoneal fluid causes ventilatory restriction and can precipitate acute respiratory failure, peritoneal dialysis should be performed with great caution in patients with respiratory disease unless they are being mechanically ventilated.

TECHNICAL ASPECTS

Although most technical aspects of dialysis are beyond the scope of this book, several points should be made. Hemodialysis can be accomplished via percutaneous catheter, external arteriovenous shunt, internal shunt, or artificial or native-vein fistula. The last of these is the preferred method of vascular access for long-term hemodialysis, since it has the greatest durability and lowest complication rate. Percutaneous cannulation via subclavian, internal jugular, or femoral vein provides immediate vascular access and preserves peripheral sites for later long-term dialysis but is generally appropriate only for short-term, interval use.

Peritoneal dialysis can be accomplished either by repeated insertion of a traditional stylet catheter or via a permanently implanted catheter of which there are several types. Surgical insertion of an indwelling catheter is performed in many centers whenever peritoneal dialysis is undertaken in acute renal failure, with stylet catheters reserved for situations, such as certain drug overdoses, in which only a single dialysis will be needed.

COMPLICATIONS

Hemodialysis is associated with numerous alterations in organ-system function. These include abnormalities in lipid, carbohydrate, protein, and vitamin metabolism and changes in cardiovascular, endocrine, gastrointestinal, and hematologic function. A specific type of dementia is also associated with long-term hemodialysis. Dialysis disequilibrium, a syndrome characterized by nausea, vomiting, and headache and sometimes progressing to confusion, psychosis, and seizures, may occur during or immediately following hemodialysis. It is more common in patients who have had high levels of uremic toxins for a prolonged period, as occurs in chronic renal failure. It can be minimized by making alterations in fluid and electrolyte balance more gradual.

The incidence of complications of hemodialysis is increased in patients with serious coexisting medical disease or advanced age. Hypotension and other forms of acute circulatory instability may occur, especially during rapid dialysis, and may precipitate angina, seizures, or cerebrovascular accidents. Hemodynamic instability has been reduced by the substitution of bicarbonate for acetate in the dialysate. Hypoxemia and other respiratory alterations may be seen, possibly due to sensitization of leukocytes by contact with the dialysis surface and subsequent agglutination in the pulmonary vessels; use of newer dialysis membrane materials has reduced this problem. Muscle cramps are common.

Complications may also be related to the hemodialysis apparatus (leakage of dialysate into the patient's circulation; clotting; air embolism [see Chapter 96]), to anticoagulation (bleeding from gastrointestinal tract or elsewhere), or to vascular access (bleeding; clotting; infection; heart failure from the left-to-right peripheral shunt).

The main complication of peritoneal dialysis is peritonitis, the initial clinical manifestations of which may be minimal. Potential cardiorespiratory complications include acute volume overload, dysrhythmias, hypoxemia, respiratory distress, acute ventilatory failure, atelectasis, and sudden massive hydrothorax.

Initial placement of a peritoneal dialysis catheter may be associated with perforation of bowel or bladder; major hemorrhage may rarely occur, although minor bleeding is common, particularly during the first few dialysis passes. Later, the catheter may become displaced or wrapped in omentum, preventing dialysate return. The catheter may work itself partway out of the abdominal wall, exposing the cuff or drainage perforations, in which case it must be removed. Removal of the catheter also becomes necessary if its tunnel tract becomes infected, if a superficial exit site infection fails to respond to initial treatment, if bacterial peritonitis persists despite administration of appropriate antibiotics or recurs with the same infecting organism, or if it clogs and cannot be cleared.

RECOMMENDED READING

Blye E, Lorch J, Cortell S: Extracorporeal therapy in the treatment of intoxication. Am J Kidney Dis 3:321, 1984

Brezis B, Rosen S, Epstein FH: Acute renal failure. In Brenner BM, Rector FC Jr (eds): The Kidney. 3rd edition. Philadelphia, W.B. Saunders Co., 1986, p. 735.

Carpenter CB, Lazarus JM: Dialysis and transplantation in the treatment of renal failure. In Braunwald E, et al (eds): Harrison's Principles of Internal Medicine. 11th edition. New York, McGraw-Hill, Inc., 1987, p. 1162.

Eiser AR: Pulmonary gas exchange during hemodialysis and peritoneal dialysis: interaction between respiration and metabolism. Am J Kidney Dis 6:131, 1985

Golper TA: Continuous arteriovenous hemofiltration in acute renal failure: a review. Am J Kidney Dis 6:373, 1985

Hakim RM, Lazarus JM: Medical aspects of hemodialysis. In Brenner BM, Rector FC Jr (eds): The Kidney. 3rd edition. Philadelphia, W.B. Saunders Co., 1986, p. 1791.

Henrich WL: Hemodynamic instability during hemodialysis. Kidney Int 30:605, 1986.

Hughes R, et al: Clinical experience with charcoal and resin hemoperfusion. Semin Liver Dis 6:164, 1986.

Lazarus JM: Complications in hemodialysis: an overview. Kidney Int 18:783, 1980.

Nolph KD: Peritoneal dialysis. In Brenner BM, Rector FC Jr (eds): The Kidney. 3rd edition. Philadelphia, W.B. Saunders Co., 1986, p. 1847.

Endocrinologic and Metabolic Disorders

54. Adrenal Insufficiency

D. Scott Weigle

DEFINITION

In humans, sudden and total failure of the adrenal glands can be fatal within 7 to 10 days. Although complete adrenal destruction is relatively uncommon, adrenal insufficiency may be associated with a variety of critical systemic illnesses and may contribute importantly to mortality in such conditions.

PATHOPHYSIOLOGY

The adrenal cortex is divided into three anatomic zones. The zona glomerulosa, which is supported largely by the renin-angiotensin system, secretes the mineralocorticoid aldosterone. The zona fasciculata and zona reticularis, both of which are supported by adrenocorticotropic hormone (ACTH) from the pituitary, secrete cortisol and adrenal androgens. In primary adrenal insufficiency, or Addison's disease, all three zones of the cortex are destroyed, leading to both mineralocorticoid and glucocorticoid deficiency. In secondary adrenal insufficiency due to loss of pituitary ACTH secretion, the zona glomerulosa is preserved, leading to selective glucocorticoid deficiency.

Roughly 80 percent of cases of primary adrenal failure are due to autoimmune destruction of either the adrenal glands alone or the adrenal glands along with other endocrine tissues as part of a polyglandular autoimmune syndrome. Tuberculosis is the second leading cause of primary adrenal failure, followed by a variety of other infections, including meningococcal infection (Waterhouse-Friderichsen syndrome), gram-negative sepsis, and systemic fungal disease. Hemorrhagic destruction of the adrenal glands can occur with anticoagulant use, and a variety of tumors can metastasize to the adrenal glands, leading to their destruction. Adrenal failure in connection with the acquired immunodeficiency syndrome has recently been recognized.

The leading cause of secondary adrenal failure is suppression of the hypothalamic-pituitary-adrenal axis, owing to exogenous steroids. The duration of suppression after discontinuation of steroid therapy is related to both the dose and the duration of steroid therapy. Impaired glucocorticoid secretion has been noted for up to 9 months following the discontinuation of long-term steroid therapy. Secondary adrenal failure is caused less commonly by pituitary destruction due to neoplastic, infiltrative, or ischemic disease. Finally, hypothalamic lesions leading to loss of corticotropin-releasing hormone and consequent loss of ACTH secretion can lead to secondary adrenal failure.

There are several important consequences of pure glucocorticoid deficiency. Hypotension occurs, owing to volume depletion, a decreased pressor response to catecholamines, and decreased cardiac contractility. Impaired hepatic glucose production leads to hypoglycemia in approximately one third of cases. High antidiuretic hormone (ADH) levels associated with glucocorticoid deficiency lead to impaired free-water clearance and dilutional hyponatremia. When mineralocorticoid deficiency occurs along with glucocorticoid deficiency, sodium wasting and hypovolemia are worse, and frank azotemia may develop. Impaired exchange of potassium and hydrogen ion for sodium in the distal nephron may lead to marked hyperkalemia or hyperchloremic acidosis.

DIAGNOSIS

In acute adrenal failure, the patient may present in a state of hypovolemic shock with prominant nausea, vomiting, and abdominal pain. Fever, either with or without underlying infection, may be present, and hypoglycemia may occur. This state of adrenal crisis is usually precipitated by an intercurrent illness leading to an increased demand for adrenal hormones that cannot be met by the failing glands. Historical points suggesting primary adrenal failure include progressive weakness, lethargy, weight loss, anorexia, salt craving, or orthostatic light-headedness. A history of predisposing systemic infection, use of anticoagulants, or a family history of autoimmune glandular failure may suggest the etiology of the patient's condition. Historical points suggesting secondary adrenal failure include any use of exogenous steroids for periods in excess of 1 to 2 weeks within the past 6 months. Pituitary dysfunction may be suggested by headache, visual disturbance, decreased libido, loss of body hair, amenorrhea, symptoms of hypothyroidism, or recent pregnancy (Sheehan's syndrome).

Physical examination may reveal evidence of hypovolemia and resting or postural hypotension. A fever may be present. In primary adrenal failure, there is characteristic hyperpigmentation of exposed areas, palmar creases, and the buccal mucosa owing to overproduction of ACTH and, possibly, other cleavage products of the pro-opiomelanocortin molecule. Galactorrhea, myxedematous skin changes, or objective visual field

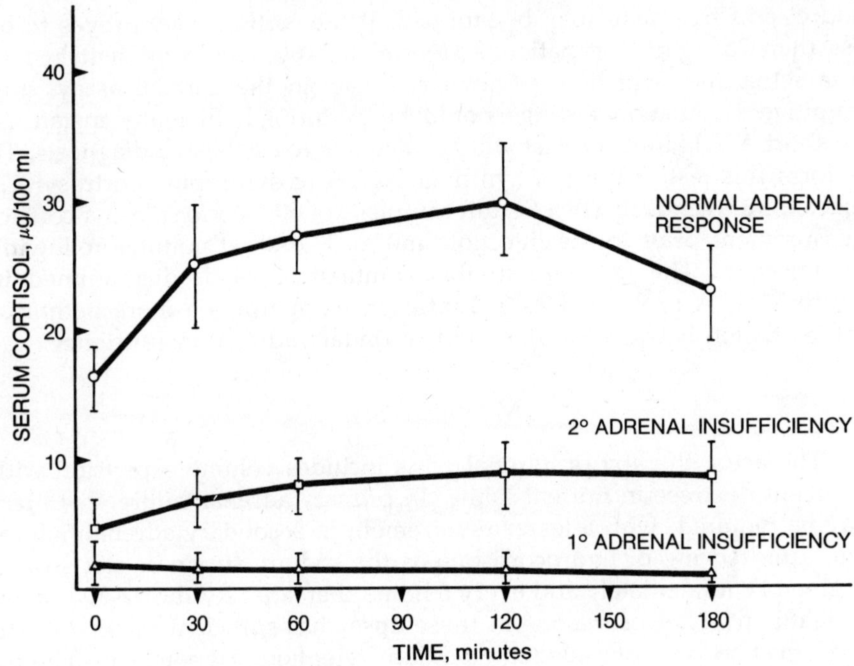

Figure 54–1. Serum cortisol response to 0.25 mg of cosyntropin (Cortrosyn) in normal subjects (n = 9), hypopituitarism (n = 8), and Addison's disease (n = 7). (Adapted, with permission, from Speckart PF, Nicoloff JT, Bethune JE: Screening for adrenocortical insufficiency with cosyntropin (synthetic ACTH). Arch Intern Med 128:761–763, 1971.)

changes may suggest pituitary insufficiency. Features of glucocorticoid excess could point toward previous excessive use of exogenous steroids. Finally, evidence of any predisposing underlying infection should be sought.

The characteristic electrolyte pattern seen in primary adrenal failure includes a decreased serum sodium concentration, increased potassium, and decreased bicarbonate, with a mild hyperchloremic acidosis and azotemia. Eosinophilia is often present, owing to a decreased rate of eosinophil lysis. Neutropenia occurs, owing to increased sequestration of neutrophils in the marginal pool. Anemia and lymphocytosis may occur. Hypoglycemia may be minimal or marked, particularly if there is complete pituitary failure. The electrocardiogram may show low voltage and T-wave flattening.

Definitive diagnosis of adrenal insufficiency requires the demonstration of an impaired glucocorticoid response to provocative stimulation. In emergency situations, a serum sample should be obtained for measurement of cortisol, and treatment should be rendered immediately. A presenting cortisol level in excess of 25 µg/dl essentially excludes adrenal failure, and treatment may be stopped. If the cortisol level proves to be less than 25 μg/dl, the patient's steroid therapy should be switched to dexamethasone, which does not cross-react in the cortisol assay, and definitive stimulation testing should be performed. In many instances, the short ACTH infusion test will be adequate to establish a diagnosis. To perform this test, 250 μg of synthetic ACTH (cosyntropin, Cortrosyn) is injected intravenously (IV). Serum samples are otained for plasma cortisol measurement prior to the injection and at 30 and 60 minutes following the injection. The response to this stimulation test is diagrammed in Figure 54–1. A prolonged ACTH infusion test permits a more definitive differentiation between primary and secondary adrenal insufficiency.

MANAGEMENT

The acute therapy of adrenal crisis includes volume expansion with 5 percent dextrose in normal saline. In primary adrenal failure, 2–4 liters may be required, with a lesser requirement in secondary adrenal failure. One hundred mg of hydrocortisone as the sodium succinate salt should be given IV immediately and every 6 hours thereafter for the first 24 hours of treatment. Hydrocortisone in these doses has sufficient mineralocorticoid effect to promote adequate sodium retention. Hypotension should be corrected by these measures within 3 to 4 hours unless an associated condition such as sepsis is present. After 24 hours, the hydrocortisone dose may generally be reduced to 50 mg IV every 6 hours, with institution of oral maintenance therapy by day 4 of treatment. Treatment of any associated infection or critical illness should be instituted immediately.

The chronic therapy of adrenal insufficiency usually includes cortisol at a dose of 20 mg in the morning and 10 mg between 4 and 6 PM or cortisone acetate at a dose of 25 mg in the morning and 12.5 mg between 4 and 6 PM. This scheme mimics to some extent the diurnal secretory rhythm of cortisol. An equivalent dosage of a longer-acting glucocorticoid preparation such as prednisolone or dexamethasone may be given once daily in the morning as an alternative to the above regimen. In primary adrenal faiure, patients usually require mineralocorticoid replacement as well to control the potassium level and blood pressure. This may be provided in the form of 9-α-fluorocortisol (Florinef) 0.05–0.1 mg daily. Patients should always be cautioned to increase their steroid dose and call a physician during periods of increased stress or intercurrent illness. A medical identification bracelet or wallet card noting the patient's diagnosis is advisable.

OUTCOME

With patient education and appropriate increases in steroid dose during periods of stress, patient survival in primary autoimmune adrenal failure approaches that of the normal population. Acute adrenal failure associated with systemic infection, hemorrhage or neoplastic disease has a less favorable prognosis. Patients with secondary adrenal failure have less risk of developing adrenal crisis, and their prognosis is excellent, provided that the underlying hypothalamic or pituitary disease can be controlled.

RECOMMENDED READING

Bayliss RIS: Adrenal cortex. Clin Endocrinol Metab 9:477, 1980.
Burke CW: Adrenocortical insufficiency. Clin Endocrinol Metab 14:947, 1985.
Byyny RL: Withdrawal from glucocorticoid therapy. N Engl J Med 295:30, 1976.
Fraser R: Disorders of the adrenal cortex: their effects on electrolyte metabolism. Clin Endocrinol Metab 13:413, 1984.
Glasgow BJ, Steinsapir KD, Anders K, et al: Adrenal pathology in the acquired immune deficiency syndrome. Am J Clin Pathol 84:594, 1985.
Greene LW, Cole W, Greene JB, et al: Adrenal insufficiency as a complication of the acquired immunodeficiency syndrome. Ann Int Med 101:497, 1984.
Jordan RM: Endocrine emergencies. Med Clin North Am 67:1193, 1983.
Leshin M: Polyglandular autoimmune syndromes. Am J Med Sci 290:77, 1985.
Nelson AM, Conn DL: Glucocorticoids in rheumatic disease. Mayo Clin Proc 55:758, 1980.
Speckart PF, Nicoloff JT, Bethune JE: Screening for adrenocortical insufficiency with cosyntropin (synthetic ACTH). Arch Int Med 128:761, 1971.

55. Diabetic Ketoacidosis and Hyperosmolar Nonketotic Diabetic Coma

D. Scott Weigle

DEFINITION

Similarities in the pathophysiology and therapy of diabetic ketoacidosis (DKA) and hyperosmolar nonketotic diabetic coma (HNDC) make it reasonable to consider these two disorders together. DKA is the most severe clinical manifestation of marked insulin deficiency in the Type I (juvenile onset) or severely stressed Type II (maturity onset) diabetic patient. This condition is characterized by hyperglycemia, dehydration, and acidosis of the elevated anion gap variety. HNDC is an equally serious condition, typically affecting the elderly patient with either Type II or previously unrecognized diabetes mellitus. This condition differs from DKA in that acidosis is either absent or, if present, is due to lactate accumulation coincident with circulatory failure. Hyperglycemia, hyperosmolarity, and dehydration tend to be worse in HNDC than in DKA.

PATHOPHYSIOLOGY

The altered hormonal milieu responsible for the development of DKA includes an absent or severely decreased insulin level, an increased glucagon level, and increased levels of the counterregulatory hormones epinephrine, cortisol, and growth hormone. The latter three hormones become progressively more elevated as the stress of dehydration and acidosis worsens. The lack of insulin leads to impaired glucose disposal, unrestrained hepatic glucose production, and unrestrained mobilization of fatty acids from the adipose tissue stores. The increased glucagon level enhances hepatic glucose production and ketogenesis from the elevated ambient free fatty acids. The increased levels of all small fuel molecules in the blood lead to a marked osmotic diuresis with consequent dehydration. Fluid loss averages 5–8 liters in DKA. Since glucose is itself cleared to some extent by the diuresis, the elevation of the blood glucose level is

338

variable. Glucose levels above 250 mg/dl imply a falling glomerular filtration rate. DKA with minimal or no glucose elevation has been described. The acidosis is due to titration of free base by acetoacetic and β-hydroxybutyric acids. Whole-body electrolyte depletion is due to increased renal tubular flow and luminal electronegativity created by ketone anions. The patient is in a state of markedly negative potassium, phosphorus, calcium, and nitrogen balance as a result of this process. DKA develops as rapidly as 4–6 hours after complete insulin withdrawal in the Type I diabetic patient. If untreated, the derangements of DKA lead to progressive mental obtundation and death due to circulatory collapse.

The chief difference between HNDC and DKA is that in the former condition, the basal insulin level remains just high enough to restrain lipolysis, thereby limiting the available substrate for ketogenesis. Thus, the insulin deficiency is relative rather than absolute—a situation that often occurs with the stress of intercurrent illness in a patient with Type II diabetes. At first, the patient with HNDC tends to be less acutely ill, owing to the absence of acidosis. This generally results in a more protracted course, so that by the time the patient comes to medical attention, dehydration has progressed to a much more severe degree than in typical DKA. Fluid losses amounting to 20 percent of the body weight have been seen in HNDC, with an average fluid loss of 8–15 liters. The glucose level and serum osmolarity are extremely high, owing to a grossly decreased glomerular filtration rate. If volume depletion has progressed to the point of circulatory collapse, a lactic acidosis may occur because of tissue hypoxia. Extreme volume loss and fluid shifts owing to hyperosmolarity generally result in severe obtundation, often mistaken for a primary neurologic event. Death in HNDC is generally due to circulatory collapse, renal failure, or the intercurrent illness that precipitated the process.

DIAGNOSIS

DKA presents as an acute illness with tachycardia, hyperventilation due to the metabolic acidosis, the breath odor of acetone due to the nonenzymatic decarboxylation of acetoacetate, and severe abdominal pain. Patients tend to be agitated rather than obtunded. HNDC, on the other hand, has a less specific presentation with obtundation easily confused with stroke, overmedication, sepsis, or "failure to thrive" in the elderly patient. Unless glucose is checked early, the diagnosis of HNDC may be delayed with a consequent worsening of the prognosis. A history of insulin omission, past episodes of DKA, or intercurrent illness in a Type I diabetic patient may be helpful. Type II or previously undiagnosed

TABLE 55–1. MEAN LABORATORY VALUES IN DIABETIC KETOACIDOSIS (DKA) AND HYPEROSMOLAR NONKETOTIC COMA (HNDC)

	DKA	HNDC
Glucose (mg/dl)	541	1083
Osmolarity (mOsm)	313	389
Sodium (mM)	133	146
Potassium (mM)	5.3	4.7
Bicarbonate (mM)	8	21

Adapted, in part, from Crapo LM, et al: Med Grand Rounds 2:344, 1983; and from Foster DW, et al: N Engl J Med 309:159, 1983.

diabetic patients may occasionally manifest full-blown DKA in the face of recent surgery, myocardial infarction, infection, or other serious illness.

On physical examination, the patient is tachycardic and may have resting or postural hypotension. Kussmaul's respirations are present in DKA. Although fever may occur because of poor cutaneous perfusion and increased thermogenesis, a careful search for evidence of localized infection, including appropriate cultures, should always be done. Evidence of dehydration is present in DKA and often extreme in HNDC. Focal neurologic findings or seizures may occur, particularly in elderly patients with HNDC who often have underlying cerebrovascular disease.

Laboratory evaluation (Table 55–1) reveals marked hyperglycemia and hyperosmolarity in HNDC. Although the glucose is often 400–600 mg/dl in DKA, any degree of hyperglycemia or even occasionally normoglycemia may occur in this condition. The bicarbonate is often less than 6–8 mEq/l, with an increased anion gap in DKA. The bicarbonate may be mildly depressed in HNDC, owing to the accumulation of lactate or other anions in the event of renal failure. Although total body potassium stores are depleted by as much as 300–400 mEq in DKA, the potassium level is elevated on presentation owing to acidosis-induced shift out of the intracellular compartment. Hyperglycemia or hypertriglyceridemia may factitiously lower the serum sodium despite the hypernatremic nature of the dehydration, resulting from the osmotic diuresis. An increased ratio of the blood urea nitrogen to creatinine reflects poor renal perfusion.

MANAGEMENT

The need for frequent (usually hourly) monitoring of both the DKA and the HNDC patient almost always requires admission to an intensive care unit (ICU). It is essential to keep an accurate flow sheet of vital signs, urine output, fluid and insulin therapy, and laboratory determinations. Mistakes commonly made in treating DKA include termination of insulin and fluid therapy too early during the course of treatment and allowing the development of insulin deficiency in the transition from intravenous to subcutaneous insulin therapy. These mistakes will be avoided if it is recognized that intravenous insulin and fluid treatment must continue until the bicarbonate and pH are normalized and that periods of insulin deficiency as short as 4 hours can allow a return of the acidosis.

Intravenous (IV) fluid therapy in both DKA and HNDC should be started immediately at a rate of 1 liter hourly for the first several hours of therapy. As much as 24–36 hours may be required to fully replace fluid losses in the HNDC patient, owing to the more severe fluid loss and to the risk of precipitating congestive heart failure in the elderly patient. It may be necessary to monitor the central venous or pulmonary arterial wedge pressure in order to avoid the latter situation. Most clinicians recommend starting fluid replacement with normal saline, owing to the intravascular volume depletion and to reports of cerebral or pulmonary edema precipitated by hypotonic replacement, particularly in pediatric DKA patients. Switching to half-normal saline after 3–4 liters will replace free water and lessen the tendency toward prolonged hypernatremia and hyperchloremia. In DKA, it is necessary to shift to 5 percent or 10 percent dextrose/saline solutions as the glucose falls below 250 mg/dl in order to permit continued insulin administration and resolution of the acidosis without causing hypoglycemia.

Low-dose IV insulin treatment is preferred for both DKA and HNDC, although hourly intramuscular injection is an acceptable alternative if establishment of venous access is delayed. Subcutaneous insulin should never be used, owing to poor cutaneous perfusion. A 10–20 unit IV bolus of regular insulin should be given immediately, followed by 8–15 units of insulin per hour mixed into the patient's fluids (albumin is not required in the insulin infusion if the tubing is flushed before administration). The presence of insulin resistance in DKA and a tendency to use too little insulin often leads to undertreatment. There is no harm in giving insulin infusions as high as 20–25 units/hr if it will achieve the desired lowering of glucose at a rate of at least 10 percent per hour. Lowering the glucose at rates exceeding 25 percent per hour may increase the risk of development of cerebral edema.

Although the absence of ketonuria leads to less potassium loss per unit volume of urine, the greater diuresis in HNDC leads to a total body potassium depletion comparable to that seen in DKA. Potassium must be included in IV fluids as soon as the potassium reaches the upper normal range and urine output is established. Potassium should be delivered in the IV fluids at a rate of 20–40 mEq/hr, and the potassium level should be checked at least every 2 hours. Although hypophosphatemia develops during insulin treatment, no benefit of including phosphate in intravenous fluids has been conclusively demonstrated. The importance of bicarbonate treatment in DKA has been heavily disputed. Most authors reserve bicarbonate treatment for patients with exceedingly low pH levels on presentation (less than 7.0–7.1) or circulatory failure due to the negative inotropic effect of acidosis.

In HNDC, once the glucose falls to 200–250 mg/dl and electrolyte and fluid replacement have been completed, IV insulin and fluid administration can be discontinued. The search for a precipitating underlying condition (particularly a treatable infection or a silent myocardial infarction) should be continued; appropriate treatment may obviate the need for long-term insulin therapy. In DKA, on the other hand, once the glucose falls to 200-250 mg/dl, it may be necessary to reduce the insulin infusion rate to avoid hypoglycemia even in the face of 5 percent or 10 percent dextrose/saline infusion. Normalization of the serum bicarbonate and resolution of ketonuria may require an additional 12–24 hours. Often, the anion gap falls and a hyperchloremic acidosis supervenes during this phase of treatment. Only when the pH and bicarbonate return completely to normal should the patient be switched to subcutaneous insulin therapy. It is wise to inject a mixture of intermediate- or long-acting insulin along with regular insulin subcutaneously 30 to 60 minutes before the intravenous insulin infusion is discontinued. This procedure will prevent insulin deficiency in the transition from the ICU to the ward setting. Glucose, electrolytes, and urinary ketones should be monitored at 4–6 hour intervals during this transition period. Since DKA can precipitate acute gastroparesis, food should be introduced with caution. Intravenous access should be maintained until recovery is clearly complete.

OUTCOME

In the absence of a life-threatening infection, renal failure, or vascular accident, the prognosis for complete recovery from an episode of DKA is good, with mortality estimated at only 5–15 percent. Mortality is extremely high, however, in the subgroup of pediatric patients who develop cerebral edema perhaps as a result of overly rapid correction of hyperosmolarity.

In contrast, mortality in HNDC may be as high as 60 percent, because patients are generally elderly, and the condition is so frequently associated with a serious underlying illness. Outcome is worsened by delayed recognition of the problem, either by the patient's caretakers or by the physician who fails to perform a blood glucose test on presentation. Renal failure, myocardial infarction, and stroke are frequent complications of HNDC.

RECOMMENDED READING

Arieff AI, Carroll JH: Non-ketotic hyperosmolar coma with hyperglycemia. Medicine 51:73, 1972.

Barrett EJ, DeFronzo RA, Bevilacqua S, et al: Insulin resistance in diabetic ketoacidosis. Diabetes 31:923, 1982.
Brown RH, Rossini AA, Callaway CW, et al: Caveat on fluid replacement in hyperglycemic, hyperosmolar, nonketotic coma. Diabetes Care 1:305, 1978.
Crapo LM, Reaven G: Hyperosmolar nonketotic diabetic coma. Med Grand Rounds 2:344, 1983.
Fein IA, Rackow EC, Sprung CL, et al: Relation of colloid osmotic pressure to arterial hypoxemia and cerebral edema during crystalloid volume loading of patients with diabetic ketoacidosis. Ann Int Med 96:570, 1982.
Foster DW, McGarry JD: The metabolic derangements and treatment of diabetic ketoacidosis. N Engl J Med 309:159, 1983.
Kitabchi AE, Ayyagari V, Guerra SMO, et al: The efficacy of low-dose versus conventional therapy of insulin for treatment of diabetic ketoacidosis. Ann Int Med 84:633, 1976
Kitabchi AE, Matteri R, Murphy MB: Optimal insulin delivery in diabetic ketoacidosis (DKA) and hyperglycemic, hyperosmolar nonketotic coma (HHNC). Diabetes Care 5(Suppl 1):78, 1982.
Malchoff CD, Pohl SL, Kaiser DL, et al: Determinants of glucose and ketoacid concentrations in acutely hyperglycemic diabetic patients. Am J Med 77:275, 1984.
Miles JM, Rizza RA, Haymond MW, et al: Effects of acute insulin deficiency on glucose and ketone body turnover in man: evidence for the primacy of overproduction of glucose and ketone bodies in the genesis of diabetic ketoacidosis. Diabetes 29:926, 1980.
Oh MS, Banerji MA, Carroll HJ: The mechanism of hyperchloremic acidosis during the recovery phase of diabetic ketoacidosis, Diabetes 30:310, 1981.
Schade DS, Eaton RP: Diabetic ketoacidosis—pathogenesis, prevention and therapy. Clin Endocrinol Metab 12:321, 1983.
Sperling MA: Diabetic ketoacidosis. Pediatr Clin North Am 31:591, 1984
Wright AD, Walsh CH, Fitzerald MG, et al: Low-dose insulin treatment of hyperosmolar diabetic coma. Postgrad Med J 57:556, 1981.

56. Hyperthyroidism

D. Scott Weigle

DEFINITION

The accelerated thyrotoxic state that occasionally follows radioiodine therapy, infection, surgery, trauma, or other serious illness in a hyperthyroid patient is referred to as thyrotoxic crisis or thyroid storm. Since no laboratory tests or pathophysiologic characteristics clearly separate this disorder from uncomplicated hyperthyroidism, thyroid storm remains a clinical diagnosis. Prompt and aggressive medical treatment is necessary to prevent a fatal outcome in this condition. Thyroid storm may occasionally be confused with pheochromocytoma or overdose of stimulant drugs such as amphetamines (see Chapter 87).

PATHOPHYSIOLOGY

The clinical features of thyroid storm can be traced to the extreme hypermetabolism induced by the elevated serum free T3 level. Accelerated membrane sodium-potassium ATPase activity and catabolism of visceral protein and energy stores lead to hyperthermia. The cutaneous vasodilation that occurs to dissipate body heat leads to an expansion of plasma volume, a widened pulse pressure, and the demand for increased cardiac output. Increased β-adrenergic receptor expression despite normal catecholamine levels causes an increased heart rate, contractility, and tendency toward dysrhythmias. Many of the features of thyroid storm in fact resemble chronic β-adrenergic agonist overload. If untreated, the patient usually succumbs to circulatory collapse due either to pump failure or to dysrhythmia.

DIAGNOSIS

Fever and altered mental status, both of which are essential diagnostic features of thyroid storm, usually develop abruptly following the precipitating illness. Since the fever, which marks the transition from compensated hyperthyroidism to thyrotoxic crisis, may be due in part to under-

344

lying infection, a careful search for a source of infection is always necessary. Abnormal mentation may range from anxiety and restlessness through frank psychosis to terminal apathy and coma. A history, if obtainable, may reveal recent radioiodine therapy, nausea, vomiting, abdominal pain, or typical symptoms of hyperthyroidism during the preceding months. Although symptoms may be blunted in the elderly, physical examination generally reveals the patient to be agitated, diaphoretic, and tremulous, with a high fever and tachycardia. The finding of a goiter or exophthalmos in this setting strongly suggests the diagnosis. Evidence of pulmonary edema or congestive heart failure, often with marked hepatic dysfunction due to passive congestion, may be present. Rhabdomyolysis may occur in thyroid storm. Laboratory evaluation should include toxicology screening and appropriate microbiologic cultures. Since total T4 and T3 levels are comparable to those seen in compensated hyperthyroidism, these tests do not establish the diagnosis of thyroid storm. One report found the dialyzable fraction of thyroxine in six cases of thyroid storm to be about twice that seen in compensated hyperthyroidism.

MANAGEMENT

The goals of medical therapy in thyroid storm are to reduce the production of active thyroid hormone (T3), to reverse the hyperadrenergic state, and to treat the precipitating condition as quickly as possible. Toward the first end, the patient should be given propylthiouracil (PTU) at a dose of 250 mg orally or per nasogastric tube every 6 hours. It is important to stress that, for an optimal outcome, treatment must be started immediately after the diagnosis of thyroid storm is suspected. Of the two available thionamide preparations, PTU is preferable to methimazole, since it blocks the peripheral conversion of T4 and T3, in addition to inhibiting thyroidal hormone synthesis. Unfortunately, neither PTU nor methimazole can be given intravenously (IV). In patients with unreliable gastrointestinal absorption, methimazole tablets may be crushed, placed in aqueous solution, and administered rectally at a dose of 40 mg every 6 hr. PTU may not be administered by this route, owing to its poor aqueous solubility. One to 2 hours after starting PTU or methimazole therapy, the patient should be started on 5 drops of saturated solution of potassium iodide (SSKI) orally every 6 hr. Iodide immediately blocks the release of thyroid hormones, and if given after thionamide blockade of thyroidal iodide uptake is established, the administered iodide cannot fuel further hormone synthesis. Iodide may also be administered IV as a sodium iodide at a dose of 1 g every 24 hr.

The hyperadrenergic state is treated by β-blocker therapy. Usually, propranolol at a starting dose of 40–60 mg orally every 6 hr or 0.5–1 mg/min intravenously for a total dose of 2–10 mg is given. If the intravenous route is chosen, the patient should be monitored electrocardiographically. Owing to rapid drug metabolism, it may be necessary to increase the propranolol dose over the course of the first several administrations. In addition to quickly reducing β-adrenergic tone, propranolol has the beneficial effect of inhibiting peripheral T4 to T3 conversion. A selective β-blocker may be used in patients with bronchospasm.

Glucocorticoid administration constitutes the final therapeutic modality generally recommended for thyroid storm. Glucocorticoids block thyroid hormone release and peripheral T4 to T3 conversion. Additionally, any tendency toward hypocortisolism due to accelerated steroid metabolism in the thyrotoxic state is reversed by glucocorticoid administration. Dexamethasone at a dose of 2 mg every 6 hr or hydrocortisone at a dose of 50–100 mg every 6 hr is recommended. Several reports suggest that the radiographic contrast agent sodium ipodate, a powerful blocker of T4 to T3 conversion, produces a greater fall in free T3 levels than is obtained with propranolol and PTU alone. This agent, given at a dose of 1 g orally each day, is useful in the treatment of thyroid storm, although anaphylaxis and renal toxicity are potential side effects. Although plasma exchange therapy has been successfully employed in the treatment of thyroid storm, most patients should respond to the therapeutic measures described above.

Other measures important in the care of thyrotoxic crisis include fluid, electrolyte, and glucose support, external cooling by sponge baths or cooling blankets, and treatment of congestive heart failure with digoxin, oxygen, and, possibly, diuretics. In the setting of severe congestive heart failure or in the elderly patient, β-blocker therapy must be used with caution. It should be remembered that hyperthyroidism accelerates the clearance of digoxin, so that higher doses than usual may be required. Salicylates should be avoided, since they may displace thyroid hormone from binding proteins, thereby increasing free hormone levels. Perhaps most importantly, the infection or other illness precipitating the episode of thyroid storm must be identified and treated.

OUTCOME

The mortality of thyroid storm is estimated to be between 20 and 50 per cent, with serious underlying illness contributing strongly to adverse outcomes. In favorable cases, the patient usually responds to therapy within 24–48 hours, and glucocorticoid and iodide therapy may be slowly discontinued over 6–8 days.

RECOMMENDED READING

Bennett WR, Huston DP: Rhabdomyolysis in thyroid storn. Am J Med 77:733, 1984.

Brooks MH, Waldstein SS: Free thyroxine concentration in thyroid storm. Ann Intern Med 93:694, 1980.

Davis PJ, Davis FB: Hyperthyroidism in patients over the age of 60 years: clinical features in 85 patients. Medicine 53:161, 1974.

Feely J, Forrest A, Gunn A, et al: Propranolol dosage in thyrotoxicosis. J Clin Endocrinol Metab 51:658, 1980.

Gilliland PF: Endocrine emergencies. Adrenal crisis, myxedema coma, and thyroid storm. Postgrad Med 74:215, 225, 1983.

McDermott MT, Kidd GS, Dodson LE Jr, et al: Radioiodine-induced thyroid storm. Case report and literature review. Am J Med 75:353, 1983.

Nicoloff JT: Thyroid storm and myxedema coma. Med Clin North Am 69:1005, 1985.

Sharp B, Reed AW, Tamagna EI, et al: Treatment of hyperthyroidism with sodium ipodate (Oragrafin) in addition to propylthiouracil and propranolol. J Clin Endocrinol Metab 53:622, 1981.

Tajiri J, Katsuya H, Kiyokawa T, et al: Successful treatment of thyrotoxic crisis with plasma exchange. Crit Care Med 12:536, 1984.

57. Hypothyroidism

D. Scott Weigle

DEFINITION

The end-stage presentation of chronic hypothyroidism in the elderly patient is referred to as myxedema crisis or coma. This condition, which is associated with a high mortality, may often result from unrecognized antecedent hypothyroidism. Myxedema coma may be mimicked by a variety of other critical illnesses associated with depressed consciousness and hypothermia. Since serious illness of any cause may be associated with hypothyroxinemia (euthyroid hypothyroxinemia or "sick low T4 syndrome"), accurate diagnosis may be difficult. It is often necessary to treat presumed myxedema coma before definitive laboratory confirmation is available, since rapid therapy may be life-saving in this condition.

PATHOPHYSIOLOGY

Any of the various etiologies of thyroid failure outlined in Table 57–1 may lead to progressive unrecognized hypothyroidism. In the setting of advanced hypothyroidism, the occurrence of infection, trauma, cold exposure, overmedication, or other serious illness may then trigger myxedema coma. The administration of iodide-containing expectorants is an often unsuspected trigger of myxedema coma as well.

Several factors contribute to the morbidity and high mortality of myxedema coma. First, alveolar hypoventilation with carbon dioxide narcosis occurs. This situation is due to reduced hypoxic and hypercarbic respiratory drives, weak respiratory muscles and, occasionally, a concurrent pneumonia. Cardiac output is reduced, owing to decreased heart rate, decreased contractility, and impaired responsiveness to catecholamines. The combination of ventilatory impairment and decreased cardiac output leads to impaired cerebral oxygen delivery and obtundation. The mental status is further impaired by hypothermia and hyponatremia due to impaired free-water clearance. Generalized or focal seizures may occur. Finally, impaired clearance of drugs such as digoxin, anesthetic agents, or sedatives may further complicate the picture. Drugs must be used with extreme caution in myxedematous patients.

348

TABLE 57–1. ETIOLOGIES OF HYPOTHYROIDISM

PRIMARY HYPOTHYROIDISM (95 percent of cases)
  Autoimmune thyroiditis (Hashimoto's disease)
  Postsurgical or ^{131}I therapy for thyrotoxicosis
  Drug-induced
    Lithium
    Amiodarone
  Iodine deficiency (endemic goiter)
  Iodine administration with underlying thyroid disease
  Infiltrative disease
SECONDARY HYPOTHYROIDISM (5 percent of cases)
  Pituitary dysfunction
    Tumor
    Ischemia
    Infiltration
  Hypothalamic dysfunction
    Tumor
    Ischemia
    Infiltration

DIAGNOSIS

Altered mental status is a hallmark of myxedema coma. A classic presentation of this condition would include coma and severe hypothermia in an elderly patient in the winter or after a viral or bacterial infection. It is important to recognize, however, that hypothermia is not totally specific and may accompany a variety of other conditions associated with impaired thermogenesis (Table 57–2). A history obtained from friends or relatives may be helpful in identifying antecedent symptoms of hypothyroidism, such as progressively increasing somnolence, hoarseness, hearing impairment, or characteristic periorbital puffiness. Of particular help is a history of prior neck surgery, radioiodine treatment, or use of thyroid medication. A recently prescribed sedative drug or narcotic analgesic could be the proximate cause of the patient's deterioration.

Physical examination characteristically reveals hypothermia, with a body temperature often less than 30° C. Bradycardia, hypotension, and hypopnea are often present. Skin changes include hyperkeratosis, dryness, and coolness. The skin is usually pale or yellowish in color, owing

TABLE 57–2. ETIOLOGIES OF HYPOTHERMIA

Cold exposure	Endocrine disease
Congestive heart failure	Hypoglycemia
Drug-related	Hypopituitarism
Barbiturates	Hypothyroidism
Alcohol	Hypothalamic disease
Phenothiazines	Sepsis
Anesthetics	Starvation
	Uremia

to anemia, peripheral vasoconstriction, and impaired clearance of carotene pigments. The hair is coarse, and the face is puffy with periorbital edema. The often-mentioned loss of lateral eyebrow hair is a nonspecific finding in the elderly. Neck examination may reveal a goiter or scar from previous thyroid surgery. The tongue is enlarged and, in extreme cases, may cause upper airway obstruction. Delayed relaxation of the deep tendon reflexes or total areflexia may occur. There may be focal neurologic findings or seizures, owing to segmental cerebrovascular disease that frequently exists in this age group. Alternatively, a stroke may have precipitated the deterioration into myxedema coma. In addition to the above findings, evidence for a precipitating infection, abdominal crisis, trauma, or other serious illness should be sought on physical examination.

Nonspecific laboratory findings in myxedema coma include hyponatremia, hypoglycemia, respiratory acidosis, elevated creatinine phosphokinase, and anemia. The total T4 level and free thyroxine index are invariably depressed, and the thyroid-stimulating hormone (TSH) level is elevated unless thyroid failure is due to hypothalamic or pituitary failure. The latter conditions, which ordinarily account for less than 5 percent of cases of hypothyroidism, should be suspected if there has been a history of head trauma, pituitary surgery, or an abnormal sella on skull roentgenogram. It should also be remembered that dopamine infused as a pressor agent can block the TSH elevation normally seen in primary thyroid failure. Electrocardiographic (ECG) changes include sinus bradycardia, prolongation of the P-R interval, low voltage, and flattened or inverted T waves. These changes may be due in part to pericardial effusion.

MANAGEMENT

The decision to treat in suspected myxedema coma must be made on clinical grounds, since any delay in therapy markedly worsens the already poor prognosis of this condition. Definitive laboratory confirmation may take several days, particularly if one is trying to distinguish true hypothyroidism from the "euthyroid sick syndrome" frequently seen in critically ill patients. In the latter condition, the free thyroxine index computed from the total T4 level and the T3 resin uptake may be low despite a euthyroid status and failure to respond to thyroid hormone therapy. These patients maybe distinguished from truly hypothyroid patients by the findings of a normal free T4 level by equilibrium dialysis, a normal TSH level, and an elevated reverse T3 level.

When the clinical suspicion of myxedema coma is high, blood should be drawn for measurement of the total T4, T3 resin uptake, TSH, and baseline cortisol level. Serum should be saved for the possible later determination of reverse T3 level and free T4 level by equilibrium dialysis.

Therapy should then be started immediately, even though thyroid hormone replacement carries some risk in patients with coronary artery disease. Owing to the likelihood of impaired gastrointestinal absorption, thyroid hormone should be administered intravenously as a single 500 μg dose of levothyroxine. This dose is adequate to saturate thyroid hormone binding sites and to quickly restore free hormone levels. Intravenous levothyroxine at a dose of 50–100 μg should be administered daily until the patient is able to reliably take oral medications. At this point oral levothyroxine at a dose of 100–150 μg may be substituted.

Patients should generally have continuous ECG monitoring during the early phase of thyroid hormone replacement owing to the possibility of inducing dysrhythmias during this phase of treatment. Because of the relative cortisol deficiency that accompanies myxedema coma as the metabolic rate increases in response to thyroid hormone replacement, hydrocortisone at a dose of 100 mg every 6 hr should be administered for the first 2–3 days of treatment. Steroid treatment may generally be discontinued at this point, although full recovery of the pituitary-adrenal axis may take 1–2 weeks. Since autoimmune thyroid and adrenal failure occasionally occur together (Schmidt's syndrome), it may be necessary to evaluate the patient more fully for adrenal insufficiency if recovery appears to be delayed (see Chapter 54).

In most cases, an increase in the body temperature, a fall in the TSH, and some improvement in mental status should be seen within the first 24 hours of therapy. It is important during this period to avoid inducing water intoxication or congestive heart failure due to the administration of excessive volumes of hypotonic intravenous fluids. Hypoglycemia should be corrected by intravenous glucose administration. Support of tissue oxygenation is critical and often requires the use of controlled oxygen administration or mechanical ventilation. External rewarming should be avoided, owing to the possibility of inducing circulatory collapse secondary to peripheral vasodilation. Pressor agents should be avoided if possible, since they may exacerbate the tendency to develop dysrhythmias. Efforts should be made to diagnose any underlying infection, trauma, or vascular accident. Finally, routine measures to prevent aspiration, urinary retention, or the development of decubitus ulcers should be undertaken, as in any comatose patient.

OUTCOME

Earlier series placed the mortality rate of myxedema coma as high as 70–80 percent. Despite the use of parenteral thyroxine and steroids, mortality still remains as high as 50 percent. The combination of an elderly patient population and frequently severe associated illness contributes to this unfavorable prognosis.

RECOMMENDED READING

Bastenie PA, Bonnyns M, Vanhaelst L: Natural history of primary myxedema. Am J Med 79:91, 1985.

Gilliland PF: Endocrine emergencies. Adrenal crisis, myxedema coma, and thyroid storm. Postgrad Med 74:215, 1983.

Hamburger S, Collier RE: Myxedema coma (clinical conference). Ann Emerg Med 11:156, 1982.

Hoffenberg R: Thyroid emergencies. Clin Endocrinol Metab 9:503, 1980.

Hylander B, Rosenqvist U: Treatment of myxoedema coma—factors associated with fatal outcome. Acta Endocrinol (Copenh) 108:65, 1985.

Jordan RM: Endocrine emergencies. Med Clin North Am 67:1193, 1983.

Mazonson PD, Williams ML, Cantley LK, et al: Myxedema coma during long-term amiodarone therapy. Am J Med 77:751, 1984.

Nicoloff JT: Thyroid storm and myxedema coma. Med Clin North Am 69:1005, 1985.

Zwillich CW, Pierson DJ, Hofeldt FD, et al: Ventilatory control in myxedema and hypothyroidism. N Engl J Med 292:662, 1975.

Nutrition

58. Nutritional Assessment

Michael S. Hickey
Kristin Weaver

INTRODUCTION

Today, clinicians clearly recognize the role that nutrition plays in the successful management of critically ill patients. Nutritional studies have revealed that nearly 50 percent of all hospitalized surgical and medical patients would benefit from some form of nutritional supplementation. A normal, well-balanced diet provides 1 gram (g) of protein per kilogram (kg) of body weight daily. The daily intake of 10 g of nitrogen, equivalent to 62.5 g of protein, will promote positive nitrogen balance and prevent protein malnutrition in most individuals. The body can assimilate a maximum of 10 g/kg of protein daily. This amounts to nearly 700 g of protein or more than 100 g of nitrogen in the average adult. Daily caloric requirements vary, depending upon the clinical situation and the therapeutic goal. Most individuals require 30–35 kilocalories (kcal)/kg to maintain weight and 35–40 kcal/kg to gain weight.

MALNUTRITION

Patients with inadequate nutritional intake may become malnourished. There are basically two types of malnutrition: Protein malnutrition (kwashiorkor syndrome) occurs when the diet is deficient in protein. Protein-calorie malnutrition (marasmus syndrome) occurs as a consequence of general starvation and the inadequate intake of both protein and calories.

Protein malnutrition, or kwashiorkor syndrome, causes muscle atrophy, delayed wound healing, prolonged ventilatory dependence, impaired immunocompetence, delayed bone callus formation, and abnormal red cell function. It may occur as a result of chronic diarrhea, renal dysfunction, infection, hemorrhage, trauma, or burns. Protein malnutrition is characterized by reduced serum albumin and transferrin levels, decreased serum iron-binding capacity, and delayed cellular immunity. Weight loss is inconsistent and may not be recognized because of fluid retention.

The protein losses that occur during critical illness are primarily the result of protein tissue catabolism. These losses are determined by measuring the 24-hour urinary urea nitrogen excretion. Most body proteins contain 16 percent nitrogen. By dividing 16 into 100, a constant (6.25) is derived. By multiplying 6.25 times the total urinary nitrogen loss, one can calculate the total protein loss. To determine the equivalent amount of catabolized lean wet tissue such as muscle, it is necessary to multiply 6.25 times 5 because muscle protein is bound to 4 volumes of water by weight. Thus, 1 g of urinary nitrogen represents the catabolism of approximately 30 g of muscle tissue. A more precise determination of the degree of skeletal muscle catabolism can be made by measuring the 24-hour urinary excretion of 3-methyl histidine, a nonreducible product of skeletal muscle degradation.

In addition to protein catabolism, patients may have direct losses of intact protein. Whole blood contains 3 g of nitrogen or 19 g of protein/100 ml. Consequently, hemorrhage may result in major plasma protein losses. Pneumonia and empyema induce intrathoracic plasma protein losses. Intestinal obstruction and peritonitis result in losses of plasma protein into the bowel wall and the peritoneal space. Crush injuries and thermal injuries give rise to soft tissue and burn wound protein losses.

Protein-calorie malnutrition, or marasmus syndrome, occurs as a result of general starvation. This form of malnutrition is characterized by weight loss, bradycardia, hypothermia, reduced basal metabolism, depletion of subcutaneous fat and tissue turgor, and the development of wrinkled skin. Patients with protein-calorie malnutrition consistently lose weight and require intense nutritional therapy.

The body's ability to avoid malnutrition during periods of metabolic stress is dependent upon (1) the endogenous energy stores and the availability of biochemically active substrates, (2) the assimilation of exogenous calories and proteins, and (3) the mobilization and utilization of energy stores.

The body has three potential energy sources: carbohydrate (glycogen), protein, and fat (triglycerides). Glycogen is combined with water and is stored in both the muscle (120–130 g) and the liver (60–70 g). Glycogen metabolism yields only 1 or 2 kcal/g in contrast to the 4 kcal/g from the metabolism of dry carbohydrate. The body's entire glycogen reserve is consumed within 18–24 hours of complete starvation. Protein is combined with water and is stored primarily in muscle. The metabolism of muscle protein yields 1 kcal/g whereas the metabolism of exogenous animal protein yields nearly 4 kcal/g. Body proteins are not designed as a primary fuel source. Instead, they function as organic catalysts (enzymes), cellular binding blocks, antibodies, and hormones. Protein that is not utilized to replenish body stores is metabolized, and the nitrogen excreted as urea. The excess calories from this protein metabolism are stored as fat. Fat is essentially water free and yields approximately 9 kcal/g. Fat catabolism

TABLE 58–1. BODY COMPOSITION OF A NORMAL (70-kg) ADULT MALE

WEIGHT (kg)	COMPONENTS	CALORIE EQUIVALENT
48.7	Water and minerals	0
15.0	Fat (adipose triglyceride)	141,000
6.0	Protein (mainly muscle)	24,000
	Glycogen	
0.150	Muscle	600
0.075	Liver	300
69.925	*Subtotal*	165,900
0.020	Glucose (extracellular fluid)	80
0.0003	Free fatty acids (plasma)	3
0.003	Triglycerides (plasma)	30
69.9483	*Total*	166,013

Adapted from Cahill GF, by permission of The New England Journal of Medicine (282:669, 1970).

provides 87 percent of the caloric requirements during metabolic stress and starvation.

Studies have demonstrated that the following metabolic events occur if a 70-kg man who consumes approximately 1800 kcal daily is subjected to a 24-hour period of starvation: (1) The body catabolizes 75 g of protein (primarily from muscle) and 160 g of triglyceride from adipose tissue; (2) the body excretes 12–15 g of urinary nitrogen, primarily in the form of urea; (3) the total body weight decreases approximately 500 g; (4) body glycogen stores yield approximately 180 g of endogenous glucose for ongoing metabolism; (5) the body derives 87 percent of its caloric requirements from fat metabolism and 13 percent from protein tissue catabolism.

The body composition of a normal 70 kg male and the calories derived from each potential fuel source are listed in Table 58–1.

NUTRITIONAL ASSESSMENT

A nutritional assessment examines specific clinical and laboratory parameters and provides an estimate of the patient's general nutritional status. It evaluates the somatic (skeletal) protein store, the visceral protein store, and the fat reserve. The somatic protein store is determined by anthropometric measurement of the midarm circumference and by calculation of the creatinine height index. The visceral protein store is determined from the serum albumin and transferrin levels, total lymphocyte count, and anergy skin testing. The fat reserve is determined by anthropometric measurement of the triceps skin fold. Table 58–2 lists the specific clinical and laboratory parameters evaluated in a nutritional assessment.

If the nutritional assessment indicates that the patient is malnourished, a dietary regimen must be designed that will correct the nutritional

TABLE 58–2. THE SAN FRANCISCO GENERAL HOSPITAL NUTRITIONAL SUPPORT SERVICE NUTRITIONAL ASSESSMENT

CLINICAL/LABORATORY PARAMETERS	EXTENT OF MALNUTRITION		
	Mild	*Moderate*	*Severe*
Albumin (g/dl)	2.8–3.2	2.1–2.7	<2.1
Transferrin (mg/dl)	150–200	100–150	<100
Total lymphocyte count (cells/mm^3)	1200–2000	800–1200	<800
Creatinine/height index (percent) (actual/ideal × 100)	60–80	40–60	<40
Ideal body weight (percent)	80–90	70–80	<70
Usual body weight (percent)	85–95	75–85	<75
Skin tests (number reactive/ number placed)	4/4 (Normal)	1–2/4 (Weak)	0/4 (Anergic)
Weight loss/unit of time	<5 percent/ month <7.5 percent/ 3 months <10 percent/ 6 months	<2 percent/ week >5 percent/ month >7.5 percent/ 3 months >10 percent/ 6 months	>2 percent/ week
Normal anthropometric measurements		*Male*	*Female*
Triceps skin fold (mm)		12.5	16.5
Mid-arm circumference (cm)		29.3	28.5

Adapted, with permission, from Dudrick, SJ, O'Donnell JJ, Weinmann-Winkler S, et al. In Deitel M (ed): Nutrition in Clinical Surgery. 2nd Edition. © The Williams & Wilkins Co., Baltimore. 1985.

TABLE 58–3. THE SAN FRANCISCO GENERAL HOSPITAL NUTRITIONAL SUPPORT SERVICE METHOD FOR CALCULATING THE ADULT (NON-BURN) PATIENT'S TOTAL ENERGY EXPENDITURE (TEE)

CALORIC REQUIREMENT

Male = [66.5 + (13.7 × weight in kg) + (5.0 × height in cm) + (6.7 × age in years)] × AF × IF + 500 kcal

Female = [665.1 + (9.6 × weight in kg) + (1.8 × height in cm) + (4.6 × age in years)] × AF × IF + 500 kcal

PROTEIN REQUIREMENT

Male/Female = total kcal × $\dfrac{\text{g nitrogen}}{150\ \text{kcal}}$ × 6.24

*Activity factor (AF): confined to bed = 1.2; ambulatory = 1.3; fever factor = 1.13/°C

†Injury factor (IF): surgery = 1.1–1.2; infection = 1.2–1.6; trauma = 1.14–1.8; sepsis = 1.4–1.8

Adapted, with permission, from Harris JA, Benedict FG. Carnegie Institute of Washington, Publication No. 279, 1919.

TABLE 58–4. THE SAN FRANCISCO GENERAL HOSPITAL NUTRITIONAL SUPPORT SERVICE TABLE UTILIZED FOR DETERMINING THE PEDIATRIC (NON-BURN) PATIENT'S TOTAL ENERGY EXPENDITURE (TEE)

AGE	KILOCALORIES/KG	PROTEIN (g/kg)
Newborn (term)	117	1.8*
Newborn (premature)	130	1.8*
3 days (term)	130	2.2
10 days	130	2.2
3 months	100–130	3.5–4.0
5 months	100–130	3.5–4.0
9 months	100–130	3.5
1–3 years	90–100	2.5
4–6 years	80–90	2.2
7–9 years	70–80	2.2
10–12 years	60–70	1.8
13–15 years	50–60	1.7
15+ years	40–50	1.4

*g/100 kcal

Adapted, with permission, from Pfeifer JA. Pediatric nutrition. In Kennedy-Caldwell, C. (ed): Nutrition Support Nursing—Core curriculum. 1988 ASPEN Clinical Conference. Published by ASPEN, Suite 500, 8605 Cameron Street, Silver Spring, Maryland 20910.

deficiency and subsequently enhance the overall response to medical therapy. Enteral and parenteral feedings must provide 75–200 (average, 150) nonprotein carbohydrate kcal for each gram of nitrogen administered. This ratio allows the maximum utilization of protein and carbohydrate.

The daily adult (non-burn) total energy expenditure (TEE) is derived from the product of the Harris-Benedict equation and the activity factor (AF) and the injury factor (IF) (Table 58–3). The TEE represents the estimated caloric and protein requirements of an individual at rest.

The daily adult (non-burn) maintenance protein requirement ranges from 0.8–1.5 g/kg of body weight. The protein requirement may increase 30–75 percent in traumatized, critically ill, or metabolically stressed pa-

TABLE 58–5. THE SAN FRANCISCO GENERAL HOSPITAL NUTRITIONAL SUPPORT SERVICE METHOD FOR CALCULATING THE ADULT (BURN) PATIENT'S TOTAL ENERGY EXPENDITURE (TEE)

CALORIC REQUIREMENT

Male = (25 kcal × preburn weight in kg × BMR* age factor) = (40 kcal × percent TBSA† burn)

Female = (22 kcal × preburn weight in kg × BMR* age factor) + (40 kcal × percent TBSA† burn)

PROTEIN REQUIREMENT (>20 percent TBSA†)

Male/Female = (1 g protein × preinjury weight in kg) + (3 g protein × percent TBSA† burn)

*BMR = basal metabolic rate

†TBSA = total body surface area

Adapted, with permission, from Curreri PW, Richmond B, Marvin J, et al. J Am Diet Assoc, 65:415, 1974.

TABLE 58–6. THE SAN FRANCISCO GENERAL HOSPITAL NUTRITIONAL
SUPPORT SERVICE METHOD FOR CALCULATING THE PEDIATRIC (BURN)
PATIENT'S TOTAL ENERGY EXPENDITURE (TEE)

CALORIC REQUIREMENT
(30 − 100 kcal/kg*) + (40 kcal/percent TBSA† burn)

PROTEIN REQUIREMENT
(1.8 − 3.0 g protein/kg*) + (1.5 g protein/percent TBSA† burn)

*Age- and weight-dependent (see Table 58–4)
†TBSA = total body surface area
Adapted, with permission, from Curreri PW, Richmond, B, Marvin, J, et al. J Am Diet
Assoc, 65:415, 1974.

tients. To determine the daily protein requirements in these patients, a
24-hour urinary urea nitrogen collection is performed and the actual
nitrogen losses calculated.

The daily pediatric (non-burn) TEE is age- and weight-dependent.
Pediatric enteral and parenteral feedings are formulated to meet the
specific age-weight and calorie-protein requirements (Table 58–4).

Pediatric patients 15 years of age and older have the same daily TEE
and protein requirements as (non-burn) adults.

The daily adult (burn) TEE is calculated using a modified version of
the Curreri formula (Table 58–5).

The daily pediatric (burn) TEE is also calculated from a modified
version of the Curreri formula (Table 58–6).

Enteral and parenteral diets should provide the daily caloric protein,
fat, electrolyte, mineral, vitamin, and trace element requirements. The
volume of feeding solution infused must *not* exceed the patient's estimated
daily fluid requirement. Several factors such as the maintenance fluid
requirement, fistulae and nasogastric drainage, temperature, cardiovascular function, and so forth, must be considered when the daily fluid
requirement is being estimated. The adult maintenance fluid requirement
for a 70 kg male ranges from 2000–2500 ml daily. The daily pediatric
maintenance fluid requirement is weight-dependent. Table 58–7 provides
a method for estimating the daily pediatric maintenance fluid requirements. The daily pediatric maintenance requirements for electrolytes,
minerals, trace elements, and vitamins are available in any standard
pediatric textbook. The daily adult maintenance requirements for electrolytes, trace elements, vitamins, and minerals are listed in Table 58–8.

TABLE 58–7. DAILY PEDIATRIC MAINTENANCE FLUID REQUIREMENTS

WEIGHT IN KG	FLUIDS
0–10	100 ml/kg
10–20	1000 ml + 50 ml/kg for every kg >10 *but* <20
20–30	1500 ml + 20 ml/kg for every kg >20 *but* <30
>30	2000–2500 ml

TABLE 58–8. DAILY ELECTROLYTE, TRACE ELEMENT, VITAMIN, AND MINERAL REQUIREMENTS

COMPONENTS	DOSAGES	
Electrolytes	*Enteral*	*Parenteral*
Sodium	—	90–150 mEq
Potassium	—	60–90 mEq
Trace Elements		
Chromium*§	5–200 μg	10–15 μg
Copper*§	2–3 mg	0.5–0.15 mg
Manganese*§	2.5–5.0 mg	0.15–0.8 mg
Zinc*	15 mg	2.5–4.0 mg
Iron	10 mg	2.5 mg
Iodine	150 μg	2.5 mg
Fluoride§	1.5–4.0 mg	—
Selenium§	0.50–0.20 mg	20–40 μg
Molybdenum§	0.15–0.50 mg	20–120 μg
Tin‖	—	—
Vanadium‖	—	—
Nickel‖	—	—
Arsenic‖	—	—
Silicon‖	—	—
Vitamins		
Ascorbic acid (C)†	60 mg	100 mg
Retinol (A)†	1000 μg	3300 IU
Vitamin D†	5.0 μg	200 IU
Thiamine (B$_1$)	1.4 mg	3.0 mg
Riboflavin (B$_2$)†	1.7 mg	3.6 mg
Pyridoxine (B$_6$)†	2.2 mg	4.0 mg
Niacin†	19 mg	40 mg
Pantothenic acid†	4–7 mg	15 mg
Vitamin E†	10.0 mg	10 IU
Biotin†§	100–200 μg	60 μg
Folic acid†	400 μg	400 μg
Cobalamin (B$_{12}$)†	3.0 μg	5.0 μg
Vitamin K‡	70–140 μg	10 mg
Minerals		
Calcium	800 mg	0.20–0.30 mEq/kg
Phosphorus	800 mg	300–400 mg/kg
Magnesium	350 mg	0.34–0.45 mEq/kg
Sulfur	2–3 g	—

*Multitrace 5 ml provides the daily requirement
†MVI–12 10 ml provides the daily requirement
‡Weekly requirement
§Estimated safe and adequate dose
‖No data available regarding human requirements

Reproduced, with permission, from Kennedy-Caldwell C. Substrate metabolism: vitamins; Jeffers S. Substrate metabolism: minerals; and Moore MC. Substrate metabolism: Trace elements. In Kennedy-Caldwell C (ed): Nutrition Support Nursing—Core Curriculum. Published by ASPEN, Suite 500, 8605 Cameron Street, Silver Spring, Maryland, 20910.

TABLE 58–9. COMPOSITION OF GASTROINTESTINAL SECRETIONS

SITE	Na^+ (mEq/L)	K^+ (mEq/L)	Cl^- (mEq/L)	HCO_3^- (mEq/L)
Stomach	60	10	130	—
Duodenum	140	5	80	—
Ileum	140	5	104	30
Colon	60	30	40	—
Pancreas	140	5	75	115
Liver (bile)	145	5	100	35

Na^+ = sodium; K^+ = potassium; Cl^- = chloride; HCO_3^- = bicarbonate
Reproduced, with permission, from Shires TG, Canizaro PC. In Schwartz SI (ed): Principles of Surgery. 3rd edition. New York, McGraw-Hill, Inc., 1979, p. 76.

Patients with high nasogastric output or enterocutaneous or colocutaneous fistulae may have significant fluctuations in their serum electrolytes and acid-base balance. Enteral and parenteral diets should replace the electrolyte and bicarbonate losses from the gastrointestinal tract. The electrolyte and bicarbonate contents of specific gastrointestinal secretions are listed in Table 58–9.

RECOMMENDED READING

Askanazi J, et al: Respiratory changes induced by large glucose loads of total parenteral nutrition. JAMA 243:1444, 1980.

Blackburn GL: Hyperalimentation in the critically ill patient. Heart Lung 8:67, 1979.

Copeland EM III, et al: Intravenous hyperalimentation in inflammatory bowel disease, pancreatitis and cancer. Ann Surg 12:83, 1980.

Daly JM, et al: Parenteral nutrition in esophageal cancer patients. Ann Surg 196:203, 1981.

Dudrick SJ, Copeland EM: Nutritional support of the cancer patient. In Miller TA, Dudrick SJ (eds): The Management of Difficult Surgical Problems. Austin, University of Texas Press, 1981, pp. 93–122.

Dudrick SJ, Jackson D: The short bowel syndrome and total parenteral nutrition. Heart Lung 12:195, 1983.

Dudrick SJ, Long JM III: Applications and hazards of intravenous hyperalimentation. Annu Rev Med 28:517, 1977.

Dudrick SJ, et al: Long-term total parenteral nutrition with growth, development, and positive nitrogen balance. Surgery 64:134, 1968.

Dudrick SJ, et al: Parenteral hyperalimentation: Metabolic problems and solutions. Ann Surg 176:259, 1972.

Gregory JA, Schiller WR: Subclavian catheter changes every third day in high-risk patients. Am Surg 51:534, 1985.

Hardin TC, Page CP, Schwesinger WH: Rapid replacement and maintenance of serum albumin in patients receiving total parenteral nutrition. Surg Gynecol Obstet 163:359, 1986.

Miller JJ, et al: Comparison of the sterility of long-term central venous catheterization using single lumen, triple lumen, and pulmonary artery catheters. Crit Care Med 12:634, 1984.

Silberman H, et al: The safety and efficacy of a lipid-based system of parenteral nutrition in acute pancreatitis. Gastroenterology 77:494, 1982.

59. Enteral Nutrition

Michael S. Hickey
Kristin Weaver

INTRODUCTION

Enteral diets are the primary means of nutritional supplementation in malnourished patients with either a functional or a semifunctional gastrointestinal tract. They are simple to administer, require minimal medical management, and are far less expensive than parenteral diets. The disadvantages and potential complications associated with these diets include nausea, vomiting, diarrhea, abdominal distention, hypertonic-nonketotic coma, hyperglycemia, glycosuria, aspiration, peritonitis, hypernatremia, and hyperkalemia.

ENTERAL DIETS

There are several types of enteral diets. Each varies in its source of protein, fat, and carbohydrate; each also varies in the electrolyte, vitamin, mineral, and trace element content; the osmolality; and the caloric content per ml of feeding solution. Most standard, full-strength enteral diets provide 1.0–1.5 kilocalories (kcal)/ml and deliver 75–200 nonprotein carbohydrate kcal/g of nitrogen. They frequently fail to provide the trace elements—selenium, chromium, and molybdenum. They generally contain 0.034–0.064 g of protein per ml, 0.033–0.051 g of fat per ml, 0.152–0.217 g of carbohydrate/ml, and varying amounts of vitamins A, D, E, K, C, B_{12}, folic acid, thiamine, riboflavin, niacin, biotin, pathothenic acid, calcium, phosphorus, iron, magnesium, copper, zinc, and manganese. Except for the special trauma enteral diets and the hepatic, renal, and pulmonary failure enteral diets, most standard enteral diets have a sodium content that ranges from 0.027–0.040 mEq/ml, a potassium content from 0.030–0.040 mEq/ml, and a chloride content from 0.020–0.045 mEq/ml.

The trauma enteral diets and the hepatic, pulmonary, and renal failure enteral diets are formulated to meet the specific nutritional requirements of these disease entities. Enteral diets are categorized into five major groups based upon their protein, fat, carbohydrate, lactose, and caloric content per milliliter, their nonprotein carbohydrate calorie to gram

TABLE 59–1. INTACT PROTEIN AND LACTOSE-FREE ENTERAL DIETS

PRODUCT/ UPDATED	(kcal/ ml)	PROTEIN (source)	(g/dl)	FAT (source)	(g/dl)
Nutri-Aid (Am McGaw) 1/83	1	Sodium and calcium caseinates	3.9	Corn oil	3.7
Renu (Biosearch) 12/80	1	Sodium and calcium caseinates	3.5	Soy oil	4.0
Isotein HN (Doyle) 8/82 powder	1.2	Delactosed lactalbumin, sodium caseinate	8	Soy oil, MCT	4.0
Precision HN (Doyle) 8/82 powder	1.05	Egg albumin	3.7	MCT, soy oil	0.1
Precision Isotonic (Doyle) 8/82 powder	1	Egg albumin, sodium caseinate	3.0	Soy oil	3.1
Precision LR (Doyle) 8/82 powder	1.1	Egg albumin	2.2	MCT, soy oil	0.1
Isocal (Mead Johnson) 1/82	1.06	Calcium and sodium caseinates, soy protein	3.4	Soy oil, MCT (20 percent)	4.4
Sustacal (Mead Johnson) 1/82	1	Calcium caseinate, soy protein, sodium caseinate	6.1	Soy oil	2.3
Enrich (with fiber) (Ross) 12/83	1.1	Sodium and calcium caseinates	4.0	Corn oil	3.7
Ensure (Ross) 5/82	1.06	Sodium and calcium caseinates, soy protein	3.7	Corn oil, soy oil	3.7
Ensure HN (Ross) 6/83	1.06	Sodium and calcium caseinates	4.4	Corn oil	3.5
Osmolite (Ross) 5/82	1	Sodium and calcium caseinates, soy protein	3.7	Corn oil, soy oil, MCT (50 percent)	3.9
Osmolite HN (Ross) 11/82	1.06	Sodium and calcium caseinates, soy protein isolate	4.4	MCT (50 percent), corn oil, soy oil, soy lecithin	3.7
Travasorb (Travenol) 12/80	1	Sodium caseinate, soy protein	3.7	Corn oil, soy oil	3.7
Travasorb MCT (Travenol) 1/84	1.5	Casein, lactalbumin, potassium caseinate	7.4	Sunflower oil MCT (80 percent), mono- and diglycerides	5.0

TABLE 59–1. INTACT PROTEIN AND LACTOSE-FREE ENTERAL DIETS *Continued*

CARBOHYDRATE (source)	(g/dl)	Na⁺ (mEq/dl)	K⁺ (mEq/dl)	PHOSPHORUS (mg/dl)	CALCIUM (mg/dl)	OSMOLALITY (mOsm/L)	VOLUME TO MEET RDA
Corn syrup solids	14.0	3.3	3.2	54	54	290	2000
Maltodextrin sucrose	12.5	2.2	3.2	50	50	300	2000
Fructose maltodextrin	18.4	3.5	2.6	68	68	300	1500
Maltodextrin, sucrose	18.2	3.6	2.0	29	29	525	3400
Glucose oligosaccharides, sucrose, maltodextrin	15.0	3.5	2.6	68	68	300	1500
Maltodextrin, sucrose	20.9	2.6	2.6	49	49	510	2040
Maltodextrin	13.2	2.2	3.2	50	60	300	2000
Sucrose, corn syrup	14.0	4.0	5.3	92	100	625	1080
Hydrolyzed cornstarch, sucrose, soy polysaccharides	16.0	3.6	4.0	70.1	70.1	480	1530
Hydrolyzed cornstarch, sucrose	14.5	3.7	4.9	100	100	450	2000
Hydrolyzed cornstarch, sucrose	13.9	4.0	4.0	75	75	470	1400
Glucose polymers	14.5	2.4	2.6	50	50	300	2000
Hydrolyzed cornstarch, carrageenan	14.1	4.0	4.0	76	76	310	1400
Sucrose, corn syrup solids	14.3	3.1	3.1	53	53	450	2000
Maltodextrin	18.5	2.3	3.7	74	74	420	2000

TABLE 59–2. INTACT PROTEIN, LACTOSE-FREE HIGH-DENSITY
ENTERAL DIETS

PRODUCT/ UPDATED	(kcal/ ml)	PROTEIN (source)	(g/dl)	FAT (source)	(g/dl)
Magnacal (Biosearch) 7/82	2	Sodium and calcium caseinates	7.0	Soy oil	8.0
Isocal HCN (Mead Johnson) 1/82	2	Sodium and calcium caseinates	7.5	Soy oil, MCT (30 percent)	9.1
Sustacal HC (Mead Johnson) 1/82	1.5	Sodium and calcium caseinates	6.1	Soy oil	5.8
Ensure Plus (Ross) 5/82	1.5	Sodium and calcium caseinates, soy protein	5.5	Corn oil, soy oil	5.3
Ensure Plus HN (Ross) 6/83	1.5	Sodium and calcium caseinates	6.3	Corn oil	4.9

Reproduced, with permission, from the Sandoz Nutrition Corporation. Enteral Formula Chart. Sandoz Clinical Products Division, 1987.

nitrogen ratio, and their osmolality. Each group is briefly discussed below. A complete description of each enteral diet is available in the *Physicians' Desk Reference.*

Intact protein and lactose-free enteral diets utilize combinations of sodium and calcium caseinate, soy protein, lactalbumin, and egg albumin as their protein source. The fat source is either corn oil, soy oil, or 20–50 percent medium-chain triglycerides. Maltodextrin, sucrose, corn syrup, and hydrolyzed corn starch provide the carbohydrate source. These diets are lactose free, provide 1.0–1.5 kcal/ml, have nonprotein carbohydrate kcal/g nitrogen ratios of 125:1 to 160:1, and osmolalities that range from 300–625 mOsm/L. They are administered either orally or by feeding tube and are designed to provide complete nutritional maintenance for patients with inadequate lactose concentrations or with lactose intolerance secondary to gastric or intestinal resection, radiation therapy, or chronic disease. Table 59–1 summarizes several key facts regarding intact protein and lactose-free enteral diets.

Intact protein, lactose-free high-density enteral diets have essentially the same protein, fat, and carbohydrate sources as the previous group of enteral feedings; however, the individual concentrations of each are higher. These solutions provide 1.5–2.0 kcal/ml, have nonprotein carbohydrate kcal/g nitrogen ratios of 125:1–154:1, and have higher osmolalities (590–690 mOsm/L). These feedings are administered either orally or by feeding tube. Table 59–2 summarizes several key facts regarding intact protein, lactose-free, high-density enteral diets.

TABLE 59–2. INTACT PROTEIN, LACTOSE-FREE HIGH-DENSITY
ENTERAL DIETS *Continued*

CARBOHYDRATE (source)	(g/dl)	NA$^+$ (mEq/dl)	K$^+$ (mEq/dl)	PHOSPHORUS (mg/dl)	CALCIUM (mg/dl)	OSMOLALITY (mOsm/L)	VOLUME TO MEET RDA
Maltodextrin, sucrose	25.0	4.3	3.2	100	100	590	2000
Corn syrup	22.5	3.5	3.6	67	67	690	1500
Corn syrup solids, sugar	19.0	3.6	3.8	84	84	650	1800
Hydrolyzed cornstarch, sucrose	20.0	4.0	6.0	63	63	600	2000
Hydrolyzed cornstarch, sucrose	19.7	5.1	4.6	104	104	650	1420

Elemental and peptide enteral diets are significantly different from the previous two groups of feedings because they are virtually fiber free, semisynthetic formulations that utilize either essential or nonessential amino acids (30–50 percent branched-chain amino acids), hydrolyzed casein, or hydrolyzed lactalbumin as their protein source; safflower oil, sunflower oil, or medium-chain triglycerides as the fat source; and either glucose, oligosaccharides, maltodextrin, modified starch, or hydrolyzed corn starch as the carbohydrate source. These diets provide approximately one kcal/ml, have nonprotein carbohydrate kcal/g nitrogen ratios of 97:1–281:1; and have osmolalities that range from 310–910 mOsm/L. Elemental diets are utilized for those patients with minimal digestive capacity and are administered as either complete diets or as supplements to another nutritional regimen. Frequently, these diets are unpalatable because of their high nitrogen content and must be administered via feeding tube. The indications for elemental and peptide enteral diets are (1) management of patients with gastrointestinal disease in which the lower digestive tract must be placed at rest (e.g., gastrointestinal fistula, active inflammatory bowel disease, pancreatitis, and radiation enteritis), (2) prevention and correction of negative nitrogen balance, (3) provision of total oral nutrition with minimal residue prior to bowel surgery, and (4) malabsorption states. Table 59–3 summarizes several key facts regarding elemental and peptide enteral diets.

Blenderized meat-based enteral diets utilize beef in combination with sodium and calcium caseinate, vegetables, and cereal as their protein source. Soy oil, mono- and diglycerides, or beef fat provide the fat. Maltodextrin, vegetables, fruit, lactose, or sucrose provide the carbohy-

TABLE 59–3. ELEMENTAL AND PEPTIDE ENTERAL DIETS

PRODUCT/ UPDATED	(kcal/ ml)	PROTEIN (source)	(g/dl)	FAT (source)	(g/dl)
Vivonex (Norwich Eaton) powder	1	Amino acids	2.1	Safflower oil	0.1
Vivonex HN (Norwich Eaton) powder	1	Amino acids	4.4	Safflower oil	0.1
Vivonex T.E.N. (Norwich Eaton) powder	1	Amino acids (33 percent BCAA)	3.8	Safflower oil	0.3
Criticare HN (Mead Johnson) 1/82	1.06	Hydrolyzed casein, amino acids	3.8	Safflower oil	0.3
Vital HN (Ross) 6/80 powder	1	Hydrolyzed whey, soy and meat protein, amino acids	4.2	MCT (45 percent), safflower oil	1.1
Travasorb HN (Travenol) 12/80	1	Hydrolyzed lactalbumin	5.2	MCT, sunflower oil	1.6
Travasorb STD (Travenol) 12/80	1	Hydrolyzed lactalbumin	3.5	MCT, sunflower oil	1.6

Reproduced, with permission, from the Sandoz Nutrition Corporation. Enteral Formulas Chart. Sandoz Clinical Products Division, 1987.

TABLE 59–4. BLENDERIZED MEAT-BASED ENTERAL DIETS

PRODUCT/ UPDATED	(kcal/ ml)	PROTEIN (source)	(g/dl)	FAT (source)	(g/dl)
Vitaneed (Biosearch) 2/83	1	Beef, sodium and calcium caseinates	3.5	Soy oil, mono- and diglycerides	4.0
Compleat B (Doyle) 10/82	1.06	Beef, skim milk, vegetables	4.3	Corn oil, beef fat, mono- and diglycerides	4.3
Compleat B Modified (Doyle) 10/82	1.06	Cereal, beef, calcium caseinate	4.3	Corn oil, mono- and diglycerides	3.7

Reproduced, with permission, from the Sandoz Nutrition Corporation. Enteral Formulas Chart. Sandoz Clinical Products Division, 1987.

TABLE 59–3. ELEMENTAL AND PEPTIDE ENTERAL DIETS *Continued*

CARBOHYDRATE (source)	(g/dl)	Na^+ (mEq/dl)	K^+ (mEq/dl)	PHOSPHORUS (mg/dl)	CALCIUM (mg/dl)	OSMOLALITY (mOsm/L)	VOLUME TO MEET RDA
Glucose oligosaccharides	23.1	2.0	3.0	55.6	55.6	550	1800
Glucose oligosaccharides	21.0	2.3	3.0	55.6	55.6	810	3000
Maltodextrin, modified starch	20.6	2.0	2.0	50	50	630	2000
Maltodextrin, modified cornstarch	22.2	2.7	3.4	53.0	53.0	650	2000
Hydrolyzed cornstarch, sucrose	18.5	1.7	3.0	66.7	66.7	460	1500
Glucose oligo-saccharides	20.0	4.7	3.5	58.5	58.5	450	2000
Glucose oligosaccharides	22.0	4.7	3.5	58.5	58.5	450	2000

TABLE 59–4. BLENDERIZED MEAT-BASED ENTERAL DIETS *Continued*

CARBOHYDRATE (source)	(g/dl)	Na^+ (mEq/dl)	K^+ (mEq/dl)	PHOSPHORUS (mg/dl)	CALCIUM (mg/dl)	OSMOLALITY (mOsm/L)	VOLUME TO MEET RDA
Maltodextrin, vegetables, fruit	12.5	2.2	3.2	50	50	310	2000
Cereal, vegetables, fruit, maltodextrin, lactose, sucrose	13.0	5.6	3.6	133	68	405	1500
Cereal, vegetables, fruit	14.0	3.0	3.6	92	68	300	1500

drate source. These enteral diets provide 1 kcal/ml, have nonprotein carbohydrate kcal/g nitrogen ratios of 131:1–154:1, and have osmolalities that range from 300–405 mOsm/L. They are well tolerated by the gastrointestinal tract because of their natural source of protein and their low osmolality.

Table 59–4 summarizes several key facts regarding blenderized meat-based enteral diets.

The *special enteral diets* are specifically formulated to fulfill the metabolic requirements associated with traumatic injuries and hepatic, pulmonary, and renal failure. In general, these feedings contain protein as free amino acids (30–50 percent branched-chain amino acids), sodium and calcium caseinates, or hydrolyzed lactalbumin; fat as safflower oil, corn oil, soybean oil, sunflower oil, or 12–30 percent medium-chain triglycerides; and carbohydrate as maltodextrin, sucrose, glucose oligosaccharides, corn syrup, or hydrolyzed corn starch. The specific protein, fat, and carbohydrate contents, the kcal/ml, the nonprotein carbohydrate kcal/g nitrogen ratio, and the osmolality of each special enteral diet are discussed below.

Trauma enteral diets such as TraumaCal, Traum-Aid HBC, Criticare HN, Travasorb HN, Magnacal, Vivonex T.E.N., and Stresstein are formulated to provide nutrition for hypermetabolic, stressed trauma patients. They contain high concentrations of protein (0.38–0.083 g/ml), provide 1.2–2.0 kcal/ml, have a lower nonprotein carbohydrate kcal/g nitrogen ratio (97:1–154:1), and have osmolalities ranging from 460–910 mOsm/L.

Hepatic failure enteral diets such as Travasorb Hepatic and Hepatic-Aid II provide nutrition for patients with hepatic failure. Their protein content is lower than that of the other standard enteral diets, ranging from 0.029–0.044 g/ml, and is provided primarily in the form of branched-chain amino acids. Medium-chain triglycerides, sunflower oil, and partially hydrogenated soybean oil furnish the fat needed. The fat content ranges from 0.014–0.036 g/ml. Maltodextrin, sucrose, or glucose oligosaccharides provide the carbohydrate source. The carbohydrate content ranges from 0.169–0.209 g/ml. These feedings provide 1.1–1.6 kcal/ml and have a nonprotein carbohydrate kcal/g nitrogen ratio ranging from 148:1–218:1. They also contain decreased concentrations of sodium, potassium, and phosphorus.

Pulmonary failure enteral diets such as Pulmocare are formulated to provide nutrition for patients with chronic obstructive pulmonary disease (COPD) and high serum carbon dioxide (CO_2) levels. They are unique in that their primary source of calories is the metabolism of fat rather than glucose; this takes advantage of the lower respiratory quotient and decreased CO_2 production associated with fat metabolism. These diets have a protein content of 0.063 g/ml, a fat content of 0.092 g/ml, and a glucose content of 0.106 g/ml. They provide 1.5 kcal/ml and have a nonprotein carbohydrate kcal/g nitrogen ratio of 125:1.

Renal failure enteral diets such as Travasorb Renal and Amin-Aid contain primarily free essential amino acids. Compared to the other enteral diets, these solutions have a low protein content (0.019–0.023 g/ml), a high concentration of glucose (0.271–0.366 g/ml), a high ratio of nonprotein carbohydrate kcal/g nitrogen (363:1–830:1); and a negligible concentration of sodium, potassium, phosphorus, and calcium. Their fat content is 0.018 g/ml and is furnished by medium-chain triglycerides, sunflower oil, or partially hydrogenated soybean oil. Their carbohydrate source is glucose oligosaccharides, sucrose, or maltodextrin. Renal failure feedings supply 1.3–2.0 kcal/ml and have osmolalities that range from 590–1095 mOsm/L.

Enteral diets may be administered either orally or by nasogastric, nasointestinal, gastrostomy, or jejunostomy tube. The position of the feeding tube must be confirmed roentgenographically before infusing the feeding solution. Recommended nasogastric and nasointestinal infusion schedules for isosmolar and hyperosmolar enteral feedings are listed in Table 59–5.

Enteral feedings are infused continuously. The advantages of continuous infusion over bolus therapy are that it (1) is better tolerated, (2) is associated with smaller residual volumes, (3) presents decreased risk of pulmonary aspiration, and (4) requires less supervision, especially when an infusion pump is used.

Routine enteral feeding orders should include the following:

1. Administer tube feeding continuously via pump at the predetermined rate via a nasointestinal feeding tube.

2. Weigh daily and record the weight in kilograms on the vital signs sheet.

3. Record the input and the output every 8 hours and total the input and output every 24 hours.

4. Check the urine for sugar and acetone every 8 hours. If the urine sugar is 4+, request a STAT serum glucose to be drawn. If the serum glucose is *greater* than 160 mg/dl, contact the physician and request treatment orders. If the serum glucose is *less* than 160 mg/dl, no treatment is necessary.

5. Perform routine laboratory tests.

Sunday AM: CBC, copper, zinc, magnesium, total protein, albumin, SGOT, SGPT, alkaline phosphatase, total bilirubin, calcium, phosphorus, globulin, transferrin, triglyceride, electrolytes, blood urea nitrogen, creatinine, glucose, and cholesterol.

Thursday AM: CBC, total protein, albumin, SGOT, SGPT, alkaline phosphatase, total bilirubin, phosphorus, globulin,

TABLE 59–5. RECOMMENDED INFUSION SCHEDULES FOR ISOSMOLAR AND HYPEROSMOLAR ENTERAL FEEDINGS

		HOURS	CONCENTRATION	CONTINUOUS INFUSION (ml/hr via pump*)
Isosmolar	Nasogastric feedings†			
		8	Full strength	20
		12	Full strength	40
		12	Full strength	80
		Final	Full strength	100–125‡
	Nasointestinal feedings			
		8	Full strength	40
		12	Full strength	80
		Final	Full strength	80–125‡
Hyperosmolar	Nasogastric feedings†			
		8	1/4	20
		12	1/2	40
		18	3/4	40
		12	Full strength	40
		12	Full strength	80
		Final	Full strength	100–125‡
	Nasointestinal feedings			
		12	1/4	40
		12	1/2	40
		18	3/4	40
		12	Full strength	40
		12	Full strength	80
		Final	Full strength	100–125‡

*Liquid diets should be administered via controlled volumetric pump.
†Nasogastric feedings should be avoided. Nasointestinal feedings are preferable.
‡The final infusion rate is dependent upon the patient's calculated total energy expenditure (TEE) and overall cardiovascular status.

calcium, sodium, potassium, CO_2, blood urea nitrogen, creatinine, and glucose.

6. Record the daily oral calorie and protein intake.

7. Notify the physician for feeding residuals greater than 100 ml, increasing abdominal distention, nausea, vomiting, or persistent diarrhea.

8. Flush the feeding tube with 10 ml of water every 8 hours.

The basic principles for the administration of enteral tube feeding are as follows:

1. Remember the mnemonic "S-A-F-E":

S = Slowly increase the concentration of a hyperosmolar feeding solution to full strength over 36–48 hours before increasing the infusion rate.

A = Aspirate every 6 hours to determine the amount of residual solution.

F = Flush the feeding tube with 10 ml of water every 6 hours and after administering medication.

E = Elevate the head of the bed at least 30 degrees while the feeding is being infused.

2. Stop the tube feeding for 2 hours if the aspirate is greater than 100 ml, then restart.

3. If the residual remains significant, reduce the infusion rate.

4. If there is abdominal cramping or nausea, the infusion rate should be reduced.

5. Examine the patient daily for evidence of obstruction or the possibility of fecal impaction. If diarrhea occurs, the osmolality of the feeding solution should be reduced or an antidiarrheal agent such as Lomotil, Imodium, or tincture of opium may be added directly to the feeding solution.

6. A serum glucose greater than 160 mg/dl requires treatment with subcutaneous or intramuscular regular insulin.

7. The feeding solution should be continuously administered via a volumetric pump through a nasointestinal tube positioned in the small bowel. Hang no more than a 4-hour supply of feeding solution at any one time.

RECOMMENDED READING

Blackburn GL: Branched chain amino acid administration and metabolism during starvation, injury, and infection. Surgery 86:307, 1979.

Cobb JM, Cartmill AM, Gilsdorf RB: Early postoperative nutritional support using the serosal tunnel jejunostomy. JPEN 5:397, 1981.

Curreri WP: Nutritional replacement modalities. J Trauma 19:906, 1979.

Hiebert JM, et al: Comparison of continuous vs intermittent tube feedings in adult burn patients. JPEN 5:73, 1980.

Kay RM, et al: Elemental and liquid diets in surgery. In Deitel M (ed): Nutrition in Clinical Surgery. Baltimore, Williams & Wilkins, 1980, p. 29.

Larkin JM, Maylan JA: Complete enteral support of thermally injured patients. Am J Surg 131:722, 1976.

Mecray PM, Barden RP, Ravdin IS: Nutritional edema: its effect on the gastric emptying time before and after gastric operations. Surgery 1:53, 1937.

Moss G: Plasma albumin and postoperative ileus. Surg Forum 18:333, 1967.

Moss G: Postoperative metabolism: the role of plasma albumin in the enteral absorption of water and electrolytes. Pac Med Surg 75:355, 1967.

Muggla M, et al: Postoperative enteral versus parenteral nutritional support in gastrointestinal surgery. Surgery 149:106, 1985.

Page CP, et al: Safe, cost-effective postoperative nutrition; defined formula diet via needle-catheter jejunostomy. Am J Surg 138:939, 1979.

Randall HT, et al: Efficacy, feasibility, safety, and cost comparisons of enteral and parenteral elemental nutrition. Contemp Surg 28:4, 1986.

Wilmore DW: Nutrition and metabolism following thermal injury.Clin Plast Surg 1:603, 1974.

60. Parenteral Nutrition

Michael S. Hickey
Kristin Weaver

INTRODUCTION

Intravenous hyperalimentation or total parenteral nutrition (TPN) may be utilized as either a primary source of nutrition for patients with nonfunctional gastrointestinal tracts or as a nutritional supplement when enteral feedings are inadequate.

TPN therapy is expensive. A standard 1000 ml bag of TPN solution costs approximately \$110–150. The average malnourished patient requires approximately 2000–2500 ml of TPN daily. Patients with severe hypoproteinemia may require albumin supplements in addition to the standard TPN solution. The addition of 12.5 g or 25.0 g of albumin to 1000 ml of TPN solution increases the cost \$75–\$125. The high cost of TPN therapy forces physicians to be more alert for errors in the formulation of TPN solutions and to more carefully monitor the patient's therapeutic response.

TPN therapy involves the infusion of hypertonic dextrose, amino acids, electrolytes, vitamins, minerals, and trace elements by means of a catheter in a large, high-flow vein such as the internal jugular vein, the subclavian vein, the superior vena cava, or the inferior vena cava. TPN solutions should provide 75–200 nonprotein carbohydrate kilocalories (kcal)/g of nitrogen in order to achieve maximum utilization of both carbohydrate and protein and to avoid hepatic dysfunction. If the ratio exceeds 200:1, the patient may experience increased glycogen deposition within the liver and, subsequently, the "fatty liver syndrome."

TPN SOLUTIONS

Routine central TPN solutions contain 500 ml of 50 percent dextrose in water (D50W) and 500 ml of 8.5 percent amino acids. D50W contains 50 g of glucose per 100 ml. The metabolism of 1 g of glucose yields appoximately 4 kcal. Therefore, 500 ml of D50W provides 250 g of glucose or approximately 1000 kcal. An 8.5 percent amino acid solution contains 8.5 g of protein/100 ml. The 500 ml of 8.5 percent amino acid contains approximately 42.5 g of protein. One g of nitrogen is equal to approximately 6.25 g of protein. Therefore, 42.5 g of protein are equivalent to approximately 6.8 g of nitrogen. The mixture of D50W, 500 ml, and amino acids 8.5 percent, 500 ml, results in a final dextrose concentration of 25 percent and a final amino acid concentration of 4.25 percent. The nonprotein carbohydrate kcal/g nitrogen ratio is approximately 147:1. This ratio allows the maximum utilization of glucose and protein by the body. If this ratio is exceeded, the fatty liver syndrome may occur as a result of glycogen deposition within the liver. The above TPN formula provides approximately 1.0 kcal/ml, 6.8 g nitrogen/1000 ml, a nonprotein carbohydrate kcal/g nitrogen ratio of 147:1, a final dextrose concentration of 25 percent, and a final amino acid concentration of 4.25 percent.

The dextrose and amino acid content of a TPN solution may be increased (e.g., 60 percent dextrose in water [D60W], 500 ml, plus 10 percent amino acids, 500 ml) if the patient's cardiovascular status requires fluid restriction. The TPN formula, however, *must* maintain a nonprotein carbohydrate cal/g nitrogen ratio of 75–200:1 (average, 150:1).

In addition to the TPN therapy, patients should receive supplements of intravenous fat emulsion. Fat metabolism results in a greater caloric production and a lower respiratory quotient (R) as compared with carbohydrate metabolism. The metabolism of 1 g of glucose yields approximately 4 kcal and has an R of 1.0. The metabolism of 1 g of fat yields 9 kcal and has an R of 0.7. The lower R for fat metabolism increases the value of fat as a caloric source for patients with pulmonary disease and elevated carbon dioxide (CO_2) levels.

Fats should provide 4–6 percent of the daily caloric intake to avoid fatty acid deficiency. However, fats may be utilized to provide as much as 40–60 percent of the daily caloric requirements. There are several commercially available fat emulsions in concentrations of 10 percent (1 kcal/ml) or 20 percent (2 kcal/ml). TPN patients should routinely receive 250 ml or 500 ml of either 10 percent or 20 percent fat emulsion intravenously 3–4 times each week to avoid fatty acid deficiency. Patients with pulmonary disease and elevated CO_2 levels should receive a higher percentage of their caloric requirements as intravenous fat and less as glucose in order to maximize the caloric and R advantages of fat metabolism. Table 60–1 lists several commercially available amino acid solutions.

Amino acid solutions vary in their protein content; thus, 8.5 percent amino acid provides 8.5 g of protein/100 ml, whereas 11.0 percent amino acid provides 11.0 g of protein/100 ml.

Special Amino Acid Solutions

In addition to the standard amino acid solutions, special amino acid solutions have been formulated to meet the nutritional requirements of

TABLE 60–1. AMINO ACID SOLUTIONS WITHOUT ELECTROLYTES

BRAND NAME	AMINO ACID CONCENTRATION (percent)	NITROGEN (mg/100 ml)	OSMOLALITY (mOsm/L)
Aminosyn 3.5%	3.5	0.55	357
Aminosyn 5.0%	5.0	0.79	500
Travasol 5.5%	5.5	0.92	575
Aminosyn 7.0%	7.0	1.10	700
Aminosyn 8.5%	8.5	1.34	850
Novamine 8.5%	8.5	1.35	785
Travasol 8.5%	8.5	1.42	890
FreAmine III 8.5%	8.5	1.30	810
Aminosyn 10%	10.0	1.57	1000
Travasol 10%	10.0	1.65	1000
FreAmine III 10%	10.0	1.53	950
Novamine 11%	11.4	1.80	1049

patients with specific disease entities. Renal failure amino acid solutions such as RenAmin and NephrAmine provide a concentrated source of essential amino acids. Renal failure amino acid solutions provide all the daily essential amino acids in approximately 250 ml of solution. In addition, these solutions provide the basic nonessential amino acids, including histidine and arginine in quantities sufficient to meet the daily requirements of renal failure patients.

Hepatic failure amino acid solutions such as HepatAmine and Branch Amin provide a mixture of essential and nonessential amino acids with a high concentration of methionine and the aromatic amino acids—phenylalanine and tryptophan. Their amino acid composition is specifically formulated to provide a well-tolerated nitrogen source for patients with liver disease and hepatic encephalopathy.

Central TPN solutions (final dextrose concentration greater than 10 percent) must be infused via a high-flow vein such as the internal jugular vein–superior vena cava or the subclavian vein–superior vena cava, in order to avoid thrombotic and phlebitic sequelae. In children 6 years of age and older and in adults, TPN catheters are inserted percutaneously via a mid-third infraclavicular approach into the subclavian vein–superior vena cava or via the neck into the internal jugular vein–superior vena cava. Rarely, TPN catheters are inserted percutaneously into the femoral vein–inferior vena cava.

TPN CATHETERS

There are several types of TPN catheters. The most commonly used temporary percutaneous catheters include the Deseret Intracath (a 16-gauge, 8-inch radiopaque "catheter-through-needle") and the Centrasil catheter (a 16-gauge, 7-inch radiopaque silicone elastomer "catheter-over-wire"). The permanent TPN catheters include the Hickman catheter (a single-lumen, radiopaque rubber 90-cm catheter with a polyester felt cuff and an internal diameter of 1.6 mm), the Broviac catheter (a single-lumen, barium-impregnated silicon rubber 90-cm catheter with a Dacron felt cuff and an internal diameter of 1.0 mm), and the Groshong catheter (a single-lumen, radiopaque, silicon rubber 35–65-cm catheter with a Dacron cuff and a 2-way slit valve adjacent to a rounded, closed tip). The Hickman, Broviac, and Groshong catheters are usually inserted when long-term TPN therapy is necessary.

TPN Bags

TPN solutions are routinely ordered in volumes of 1000 ml. Each TPN bag or bottle is numbered "1," "2," or "3." TPN bag number 1 is infused *each* day, since it contains the amino acids, dextrose, electrolytes, and minerals, plus the trace elements and vitamins. The trace elements (Multitrace 5 ml) and multivitamins (M.V.I.-12 10 ml) are administered daily but *only* in TPN bag number 1. The routine components of TPN bag number 1 are listed in Table 60–2.

Special Problems

The concentrations of specific TPN components frequently require minor adjustment based upon the serum CO_2, sodium, potassium, phosphate, glucose, and prothrombin values. A serum CO_2 of less than 25 mEq/L is treated by administering a portion of the sodium or potassium components as either sodium acetate or potassium acetate. Acetate is converted by the liver to bicarbonate. The additional bicarbonate increases the serum CO_2 level and assists in correcting the metabolic acidosis. A serum CO_2 greater than 25 mEq/L is treated by administering the sodium and potassium components as either sodium chloride or potassium chloride.

The treatment of hyponatremia is dependent upon the clinical situation. Dilutional hyponatremia is corrected by restricting total fluid intake. Hyponatremia secondary to total body sodium depletion is corrected by increasing the TPN sodium content. The total sodium content should *not*, however, exceed 154 mEq/L.

Specific treatment of hypernatremia is also dependent upon the clinical situation. Hypernatremia secondary to dehydration is corrected by the administration of free water. Hypernatremia that occurs in conjunction with normal fluid balance is treated by decreasing the TPN sodium content

TABLE 60–2. STANDARD COMPONENTS AND ROUTINE/OPTIONAL ADDITIVES PER 1000 ML OF CENTRAL TPN SOLUTION

DEXTROSE	
D50W	500 ml
AMINO ACID	
8.5 percent	500 ml
ROUTINE ADDITIVES	
NaCl or Na acetate*	0–145 mEq
KCl or K acetate*	0–40 mEq
KPO_4*	0–20 mM
$MgSO_4$*	10–12 mEq
Ca gluceptate*	4.5 or 9.0 mEq
MVI-12[R]†	10 ml
Multitrace[R]†	5 ml
OPTIONAL ADDITIVES	
$NaPO_4$	0–20 mM
Cimetidine	0–600 mg
Regular insulin‡	0–40 units
Albumin§	12.5 or 25.0 g
Vitamin K‖	10 mg
Imferon¶	0.5–1.0 ml

*Standard components in every 1000 ml volume of central TPN
†Administered once daily in TPN bag number 1
‡Added to each 1000 ml volume of central TPN *if* the serum glucose >160 mg percent
§Added to each 1000 ml volume of central TPN *if* the serum albumin <2.5 g percent
‖Added to TPN bag number 1 on Monday and Thursday *only*
¶A *maximum* of 1 ml is added to TPN bag number 1 daily

or by deleting sodium from the TPN solution until the serum sodium returns to normal.

Hypokalemia is treated by increasing the TPN potassium content. The potassium content should *not*, however, exceed 40 mEq/L. If additional doses of potassium are necessary to correct the deficit, it is much safer and more economical to administer the potassium in a crystalloid medium as either a continuous peripheral infusion or as a series of intravenous interrupts. Hyperkalemia is treated by immediately replacing the potassium-containing TPN infusion with a 10 percent dextrose in water (D10W) infusion at the same infusion rate. Potassium is then deleted from the TPN solution until the serum potassium returns to normal.

Phosphate is added to every bag of TPN solution unless the patient has hyperphosphatemia. Phosphate may be administered as either sodium phosphate or potassium phosphate. Prior to selecting the exact form in which the phosphate will be added, the serum sodium and potassium levels must be determined. Normally, phosphate is administered as potassium phosphate. However, in the event of hyperkalemia or hyponatremia, the phosphate may be administered as sodium phosphate.

Hyperglycemia may occur during TPN therapy. Patients with hyperglycemia complain of polyuria and polydipsia. Clinically, they have marked glycosuria and serum glucose values greater than 160 mg/dl. Hyperglycemia in a patient without fever and with a normal white blood cell count usually represents a mild to moderate intolerance of the hypertonic dextrose infusion. The sudden development of hyperglycemia associated with fever and leukocytosis usually represents infection. Hyperglycemia may result in an osmotic diuresis and, if untreated, hyperosmolar nonketotic coma.

The initial treatment of glycosuria and hyperglycemia greater than 160 mg/dl requires the intravenous administration of regular insulin. A single dose of intravenous regular insulin should *not* exceed 15 units. A serum glucose determination is repeated 30 minutes following the administration of insulin. Additional doses of regular insulin may be necessary if the serum glucose level remains greater than 160 mg/dl. Refractory hyperglycemia is treated by adding regular insulin to the TPN solution. The dosage of regular insulin should not exceed 50 units per 1000 ml of TPN solution (final dextrose concentration of 25 percent). If the addition of regular insulin (maximum, 50 units per bag) fails to correct the hyperglycemia, the TPN dextrose concentration should be reduced. If this fails, the TPN infusion rate must be decreased.

Hypoglycemia may occur if a TPN infusion is suddenly discontinued and the patient has an inadequate caloric intake. To treat this clinical situation, D10W is immediately infused either centrally or peripherally at the previous TPN rate. The D10W infusion will prevent the hypoglycemic "rebound phenomenon" and will allow time for the reinstitution of the TPN therapy.

The inadequate oral intake of vitamin K or failure to provide vitamin K supplements during TPN therapy may result in the prolongation of the prothrombin time. Vitamin K 10 mg is routinely added to TPN bag number 1 every Monday and Thursday to avoid this problem. Additional vitamin K may be required in specific clinical situations.

The addition of 25 percent albumin to TPN solutions is very controversial. Albumin *may* be added to the TPN solution (1) to correct preoperative hypoalbuminemia (less than 3 g/dl) in patients who are scheduled to undergo bowel resection and anastomosis, (2) to provide the temporary oncotic benefits of normal serum albumin (greater than 3 g/dl) until nutritional supplements can permanently maintain a normal serum albumin level, and (3) to increase the serum albumin level (to greater than 3 g/dl) in an effort to enhance gut absorption and decrease diarrhea in patients receiving simultaneous enteral diets or in patients being converted to enteral diets exclusively. Albumin dosages should *not* exceed 25 g/L of TPN solution, and the course of albumin therapy should not exceed 72 hours without the serum albumin level being reevaluated.

Routine TPN orders should include the following:

1. STAT upright expirational portable chest roentgenogram to check the position of the subclavian catheter and to rule out a pneumothorax.

2. Infuse 5 percent dextrose in ½ normal saline at 40 ml/hr by subclavian catheter via pump until the catheter position is confirmed prior to starting the TPN solution.

3. Strict input and output measurement every 8 hours. Total the input and output every 24 hours.

4. Record the daily weight in kg on the vital signs sheet.

5. Check the urine for sugar and acetone every 8 hours. If the urine sugar is 4+, request a STAT serum glucose. If the serum glucose is greater than 160 mg/dl, contact the physician and request treatment orders. If the serum glucose is less than 160 mg/dl, no treatment is necessary.

6. Notify the physician if the oral temperature is greater than 38 °C.

7. Routine TPN laboratory samples are to be drawn at the times specified below. They should include:

Sunday AM:	CBC, copper, zinc, magnesium, total protein, albumin, SGOT, SGPT, alkaline phosphatase, globulin, calcium, sodium, potassium, chloride, CO_2, total bilirubin, phosphorus, transferrin, triglyceride, cholesterol, blood urea nitrogen, creatinine, and glucose.
Tuesday AM:	CBC, sodium, potassium, chloride, CO_2, blood urea nitrogen, creatinine, and glucose.
Thursday AM:	CBC, total protein, albumin, SGOT, SGPT, alkaline phosphatase, total bilirubin, phosphorus, globulin, calcium, sodium, potassium, chloride, CO_2, blood urea nitrogen, creatinine, and glucose.

8. Begin a 24-hour urinary urea nitrogen collection at 6 AM every Monday and Thursday to determine nitrogen balance.

9. Change the TPN subclavian catheter dressings every 48 hours. TPN intravenous tubing and filters should be changed every 24 hours.

TPN infusion rates depend upon the patient's age, TEE, nutritional requirements, cardiovascular status, and the specific disease process. Routine infusion rates for adults are listed in the following table.

ADULT TPN INFUSION RATES

DAY	RATE (ml/hr via pump)
1	40
2	80
3	100–125

Successful TPN therapy requires close adherence to certain basic principles. These principles are listed below:

1. The portable chest roentgenogram must show that the subclavian catheter tip is in the superior vena cava prior to starting of TPN infusion.

2. The initial TPN infusion is started at 40 ml/hr via pump. The TPN infusion rate is increased to 80 ml/hr on day 2 of therapy and to 100–125 ml/hr by day 3 of therapy. The final infusion rate is dependent upon the patient's cardiovascular status, TEE, underlying disease, and general fluid requirement.

3. TPN laboratory samples must be drawn at specific times to eliminate delays in changing TPN components.

4. TPN catheter sepsis is associated with a persistent temperature elevation (greater than 38° C) for several hours or days and *not* with an isolated temperature spike. If catheter sepsis is suspected, blood samples are sterilely aspirated via the catheter for aerobic, anaerobic, and fungal cultures. If a temporary TPN catheter is in place, the catheter is changed over a guide wire. If there is defervescence, *no* further therapy is necessary. However, if the fever persists, the catheter must be removed and a new catheter inserted on the contralateral side. If a permanent catheter is in place, the patient should be started on appropriate gram-negative and gram-positive antibiotic coverage for 72 hours. If the patient remains afebrile during and after antibiotic therapy, no further therapy is necessary. If the fever persists or recurs following antibiotic therapy, the catheter must be removed and a new catheter placed on the contralateral side.

5. The distal port of a triple-lumen catheter may be utilized for the infusion of TPN solution *only* if there is no other central venous access or if a coagulopathy is present that prohibits the safe insertion of a new central catheter. A single-lumen TPN catheter is preferable.

6. Ten percent dextrose in water (D10W) must be infused centrally or peripherally if the TPN infusion is suddenly interrupted (except for patients with adequate caloric intake) to avoid rebound hypoglycemia.

7. A subclavian catheter is *not* to be utilized for the infusion of TPN solution if the catheter has previously been used for central venous pressure monitoring or for the prolonged administration of crystalloid solution or blood products.

8. Blood samples are *not* to be drawn from a single-lumen TPN catheter (except for cultures). Medications and blood components are *not* to be infused through TPN catheters.

9. TPN therapy may result in hyperchloremic metabolic acidosis. This metabolic abnormality is treated by removing the chloride components in the TPN solution and administering the sodium and potassium in their acetate form.

RECOMMENDED READING

Askanazi J, et al: Nutrition and the respiratory system. Crit Care Med 10:163, 1982.

Askanazi J, et al: Nutrition for the patient with respiratory failure: glucose vs fat. Anesthesiology 54:373, 1981.

Bartlett RH, Dechert RE, Mault JR, et al: Measurement of metabolism in multiple organ failure. Surgery 92:771, 1982.

Bassili RH: Nutritional support in long term intensive care with special reference to ventilator patients: a review. Can Anaesth Soc J 28:17, 1981.

Bell SJ, Wyatt J: Nutrition guidelines for burned patients. J Am Diet Assoc 86:648, 1986.

Clowes GHA, et al: Energy metabolism and proteolysis in traumatized and septic man. Surg Clin North Am 56:1169, 1976.

Curreri WP: Metabolic response to thermal injury and its nutritional support. Cutis 22:501, 1978.

Dudrick SJ, et al: The effects of protein calorie malnutrition on immune competence of the surgical patient. Surg Gynecol Obstet 139:257, 1974.

Elwyn DH: Nutritional requirements of adult surgical patients. Crit Care Med 8:9, 1980.

Fischer JF: Amino acid derangements in patients with sepsis: treatment with branched chain amino acid rich solutions. Ann Surg 188:423, 1978.

Kinney JM, et al: Influence of nutrients on ventilation. Rev Clin Nutr 54:921, 1984.

Long CL, Schaffel N, Geiger JW: Metabolic response to injury and illness: estimation of energy and protein needs from indirect calorimetry and nitrogen balance. J Parenter Ent Nutr 3:452, 1979.

Paauw JD, et al: Assessment of caloric needs of stressed patients. (Abstr.) Proceedings of the 23rd annual meeting, American College of Nutrition, Arlington, VA, Oct 4, 1982.

Wilmore DW: The Metabolic Management of the Critically Ill. Plenum Publishing Corp., New York, 1977.

Gastrointestinal and Hepatic Disorders

61. Upper Gastrointestinal Bleeding

James H. Grendell

DEFINITION

Upper gastrointestinal bleeding refers to bleeding from a lesion in the gastrointestinal tract proximal to the ligament of Treitz (esophagus, stomach, duodenum). This clinical problem is responsible for about 150,000 hospital admissions yearly in the United States.

PATHOPHYSIOLOGY

Three types of processes are responsible for upper gastrointestinal bleeding in about 90 percent of patients: (1) acid peptic disease (duodenal and gastric ulcers, esophagitis, gastritis, duodenitis), (2) esophageal varices, and (3) Mallory-Weiss tears of the gastroesophageal junction. Thus, in about one third of patients, the source of gastrointestinal bleeding is at or near the gastroesophageal junction (esophageal varices, Mallory-Weiss mucosal tears, erosive esophagitis); in another third, the source is in the stomach (gastric ulcer, gastritis); and in the last third, it is in the pylorus or duodenum (duodenal or pyloric channel ulcer, duodenitis).

Acid peptic disease and Mallory-Weiss mucosal tears of the gastroesophageal junction produce bleeding by disruption of the mucosal lining of the upper gastrointestinal tract with exposure of and damage to underlying blood vessels. Esophageal varices are submucosal veins that have become dilated and then expand into the lumen and rupture, owing to portal hypertension, usually from cirrhosis, but at times caused by extrahepatic vascular disease. Abnormalities in the coagulation system and thrombocytopenia may contribute to the severity of gastrointestinal bleeding, as is frequently seen in patients with cirrhosis.

Less commonly, upper gastrointestinal bleeding may result from a variety of causes; e.g., gastric cancer, acute duodenal fistula, coagulation abnormalities, vascular malformations, hemobilia (bleeding from the liver or pancreas into the gastrointestinal tract via the biliary tree).

DIAGNOSIS

Patients with upper gastrointestinal bleeding usually present with hematemesis (vomiting of red blood or a dark brown "coffee-ground"–like material) and/or melena (passage of black, tarry stools). When bleeding is massive and rapid, hematochezia (passage of bright red blood through the rectum) may be observed. Patients may also present with evidence of hypovolemia (postural changes in pulse or blood pressure, tachycardia, hypotension, syncope).

On the physical examination, one should look for evidence of chronic liver disease, abdominal surgical scars, coagulopathy, or skin lesions associated with gastrointestinal bleeding (e.g., in hereditary hemorrhagic telangiectasia). A nasogastric tube should be placed as part of the initial evaluation and gastric contents aspirated. If hematemesis has occurred or if blood is present in the nasogastric aspirate, then the source of bleeding is almost certainly proximal to the ligament of Treitz. However, the absence of blood in the nasogastric aspirate does *not* exclude an upper gastrointestinal source of bleeding because blood may not reflux through the pylorus in a patient with an actively bleeding duodenal lesion, or a previously bleeding upper gastrointestinal lesion may have stopped bleeding prior to passage of the nasogastric tube.

Upper gastrointestinal endoscopy is the diagnostic procedure of choice and should be performed in the actively bleeding patient once adequate resuscitation with intravenous fluids and blood has been accomplished. Endoscopy permits the rapid, definitive diagnosis of the site of upper gastrointestinal bleeding in 90–95 percent of patients. In the actively bleeding patient in whom endoscopy is not diagnostic, technetium-labeled red blood cell radionuclide scans or selective mesenteric angiography may identify the location of bleeding. Upper gastrointestinal contrast (barium) roentgenogram studies identify only one to two thirds of lesions causing upper gastrointestinal bleeding, and the presence of barium in the gastrointestinal tract may make endoscopy, angiography, or radionuclide scans difficult or impossible. Contrast roentgenographic studies should be obtained only in patients with "minor" upper gastrointestinal bleeding (absence of postural signs, hematocrit >30) and should be followed up with endoscopy if results are normal or equivocal.

MANAGEMENT

The first objective is to evaluate the degree of volume loss and begin resuscitation. An orthostatic pulse rise of >20/min or blood pressure fall of >10 mm Hg indicates a blood loss >1000 ml. A supine resting pulse

>100/min or systolic BP <100 mm Hg suggests blood loss >1200–1500 ml. Early in the patient's course, the hematocrit may lead one to severely underestimate the degree of blood loss. However, following adequate blood resuscitation, it is a useful indicator of the subsequent severity of bleeding. In patients with evidence of a substantial volume deficit, volume replacement should be initiated with 1–2 liters of 0.9 percent NaCl through a large-bore (14–18 gauge) peripheral intravenous line. Blood loss should be replaced (to a hematocrit of 25–30) as soon as possible by whole blood (if available) or packed red blood cells. Transfusion of fresh frozen plasma or platelets should be restricted to patients with laboratory evidence of a significant coagulopathy. Vital signs and urine output should be closely monitored. Some patients may require placement of an arterial line to monitor blood pressure and a pulmonary artery catheter to guide volume replacement.

Patients found to be bleeding at endoscopy from esophageal varices should undergo endoscopic sclerotherapy to try to stop the bleeding. If this is not successful, balloon tamponade or intravenous vasopressin (0.1–0.5 units/min) may be employed, with emergency portacaval shunt surgery reserved for better risk (Child A and B) patients who continue to bleed despite all these measures. In general, patients with continued nonvariceal active upper gastrointestinal bleeding should be considered for surgery once they have required 6–8 units of blood. Other treatment modalities currently under investigation include angiographic embolization and endoscopic treatment through use of lasers, multipolar electrocautery (Bicap), and thermal cautery (heater probe). The use of antacids and/or histamine-2 (H_2) antagonists have not been shown to alter the course of acute upper gastrointestinal bleeding.

OUTCOME

About 80 percent of patients with upper gastrointestinal bleeding will stop bleeding spontaneously. Patients found at endoscopy to have a "visible vessel" in an ulcer crater or, in some series, other related endoscopic findings (e.g., adherent clot with oozing of blood) have an approximately 50 percent incidence of rebleeding during the same hospitalization, compared with about 5 percent risk if these findings are absent. The overall mortality of upper gastrointestinal bleeding is about 8 percent, with increased mortality in older patients (>55–60 years old) with other significant medical problems, patients with variceal hemorrhage, and patients presenting in shock.

RECOMMENDED READING

Cello JP, Crass RA, Grendell JH, et al: Management of the patient with hemorrhaging esophageal varices. JAMA 256:1480, 1986.

Fleischer D: Endoscopic therapy of upper gastrointestinal bleeding in humans. Gastroenterology 90:217, 1986.

Fleischer D: Etiology and prevalence of severe persistent upper gastrointestinal bleeding. Gastroenterology 87:538, 1983.

Kerlan RK Jr, Pogany AC, Burke DR, et al: Angiographic management of upper gastrointestinal hemorrhage. Am J Roentgenol 147:1185, 1986.

Larson DE, Farnell MB: Upper gastrointestinal hemorrhage. Mayo Clin Proc 58:371, 1983.

Steer ML, Silen W: Diagnostic procedures in gastrointestinal hemorrhage. N Engl J Med 309:646, 1983.

Zuckerman G, Welch R, Douglas A, et al: Controlled trial of medical therapy for active upper gastrointestinal bleeding and prevention of rebleeding. Am J Med 76:361, 1984.

62. Lower Gastrointestinal Bleeding

James H. Grendell

DEFINITION

Lower gastrointestinal bleeding refers to bleeding from a lesion in the gastrointestinal tract distal to the ligament of Treitz (jejunum, ileum, colon, anorectal region). However, the great majority of patients with lower gastrointestinal hemorrhage have a bleeding site in the colon or anorectal region. If one considers lower gastrointestinal bleeding of all degrees of severity, the cause will be found in the anorectal region in almost half of all patients.

PATHOPHYSIOLOGY

Lower gastrointestinal bleeding can result from a large number of causes. Intermittent low-grade bleeding with bowel movements is usually due to anorectal diseases, primarily hemorrhoids and fissures. At times, hemorrhoidal bleeding may be massive, requiring hospitalization and transfusion.

Once anorectal processes are excluded, the majority of patients with lower gastrointestinal bleeding will be found to have colonic cancers or polyps (about 15–30 percent), diverticulosis (15–20 percent), vascular ectasias of the colon (10–25 percent), or an acute colitis (e.g., infectious, ischemic, radiation-induced, or due to inflammatory bowel disease) (5–10 percent). Depending on the diagnostic studies employed, no source of bleeding will be found in 15–60 percent of patients.

Hemorrhoids bleed because of rupture of the vessel wall, presumably owing to an increase in venous pressure such as might be produced by a bowel movement. Anal fissures bleed because of disruption of superficial vessels. Bleeding from colonic cancers and polyps in most cases appears to be due to erosion or ulceration of the surface of these lesions. Diverticular bleeding results from disruption of vessels in the walls of diverticula (usually in the absence of clinically overt diverticulitis). Vascular ectasias (also termed angiodysplastic lesions) may be seen in hereditary conditions such as the Osler-Weber-Rendu syndrome but more commonly occur as an age-related degenerative process. They tend to bleed in a chronic, intermittent fashion rather than as a continuous massive hemorrhage. Various forms of colitis produce lower gastrointestinal bleeding, owing to diffuse inflammation and necrosis of the mucosa lining the colon and rectum.

Rarely, lower gastrointestinal bleeding may result from lesions in the small intestine such as tumors, vascular ectasias, or Meckel's diverticula. As with upper gastrointestinal bleeding, coagulation abnormalities and thrombocytopenia may contribute to the severity of bleeding.

DIAGNOSIS

Patients with lower gastrointestinal bleeding usually present with hematochezia (passage of bright red blood through the rectum). However, if the site of bleeding is in the small intestine or the right side of the colon and if the rate of bleeding is not rapid, melena (passage of black tarry stools) may be observed. Depending on the severity of bleeding, patients may also demonstrate evidence of hypovolemia (postural changes in pulse or blood pressure, tachycardia, hypotension, syncope).

Physical examination generally does not provide information concerning the source of bleeding except in patients with skin lesions associated with gastrointestinal bleeding (e.g., hereditary hemorrhagic telangiectasia syndrome, some forms of familial polyposis). In patients with signs of substantial blood loss, upper gastrointestinal sources must be considered. If aspiration of gastric contents shows no evidence of blood, especially if bile is present in the aspirate, an upper source is unlikely.

Anoscopy and either flexible or rigid sigmoidoscopy should be performed as the initial diagnostic procedure because of the high incidence of anorectal causes of lower gastrointestinal bleeding and the ability to reach a large proportion of polyps and cancers by this technique. In addition, many patients with colitis can be diagnosed by this means. If anoscopy and sigmoidoscopy are not diagnostic and bleeding has stopped or slowed markedly, colonoscopy should be performed following cleansing of the colon with 4–6 liters of an electrolyte/polyethylene glycol solution administered orally or through a nasogastric tube. Barium enema is much less sensitive than colonoscopy in identifying causes of lower gastrointestinal bleeding but may occasionally reveal polyps missed by colonoscopy.

Continuous rapid bleeding makes adequate colonoscopy very difficult or impossible. In such situations, either technetium-labeled red blood cell radionuclide scanning or angiography may be useful in determining the site of bleeding. The technetium red blood cell scan is more sensitive, capable of identifying bleeding at a rate of 1 unit of blood every 2–4 hours, compared with a sensitivity of about 1 unit/hour for angiography. If a technetium red blood cell scan is positive, angiography may help further identify the lesion and permits attempts at embolization. If the scan is negative, it is very unlikely that subsequent angiography will identify a source of bleeding.

MANAGEMENT

As described for patients with upper gastrointestinal bleeding, the first objective is to evaluate the degree of volume loss and then begin resuscitation. Most patients will stop bleeding spontaneously. Patients who continue to bleed are managed in a variety of ways, depending on the site of bleeding. Hemorrhoidal bleeding can usually be stopped by surgical treatment through the operative sigmoidoscope. Bleeding colonic cancers or polyps require excision either surgically or endoscopically. Diverticular bleeding requiring transfusion of 6–8 units of blood should be treated surgically following localization of the bleeding site by technetium red blood cell scan or angiography. In patients who are considered to be poor candidates for surgery, angiographic means may be employed in an attempt to control bleeding. Vascular ectasias are best treated by endoscopic means using laser photocoagulation, multipolar electrocoagulation (Bicap), or thermal coagulation (heater probe). Surgery should be reserved for patients with vascular ectasias with massive bleeding not controllable endoscopically or by angiography. Treatment of lower gastrointestinal bleeding due to colitis should be directed at the underlying disease process.

OUTCOME

Causes of lower gastrointestinal bleeding are much less likely to produce severe, exsanguinating hemorrhages than are causes of upper gastrointestinal hemorrhage. Therefore, the prognosis of a patient with lower gastrointestinal bleeding is usually determined by the underlying disease process causing the bleeding and by other concomitant medical conditions.

RECOMMENDED READING

Allison DJ, Hemmingway AP, Cunningham DA: Angiography in gastrointestinal bleeding. Lancet II:30, 1982.

Athanasoulis CA: Therapeutic applications of angiography. N Engl J Med 302:1117, 1980.

Boley SJ, Sammartano R, Adams A, et al: On the nature and etiology of vascular ectasias of the colon. Degenerative lesions of aging. Gastroenterology 72:650, 1977.

Cello JP, Grendell JH: Endoscopic laser treatment for gastrointestinal vascular ectasias. Ann Intern Med 104:352, 1986.

Forde KA: Colonoscopy in acute rectal bleeding. Gastrointest Endosc 27:219, 1981.

Markisz JA, Front D, Royal MD, et al: An evaluation of ^{99m}Tc-labeled red blood cell scintigraphy for the detection and localization of gastrointestinal bleeding sites. Gastroenterology 83:394, 1982.

Richter JM, Hedberg SE, Athanasoulis CA, et al: Angiodysplasia—clinical presentation and colonoscopic diagnosis. Dig Dis Sci 29:481, 1984.

Tedesco FJ, Waye JD, Raskin JB, et al: Colonoscopic evaluation of rectal bleeding. A study of 304 patients. Ann Intern Med 89:907, 1978.

63. Acute Pancreatitis

James H. Grendell

James H. Grendell

DEFINITION

Acute pancreatitis is an inflammatory process of the pancreas of variable severity ranging from a mild, self-limited form with interstitial edema of the gland and peripancreatic fat necrosis to a severe form with extensive hemorrhagic necrosis of the pancreas and both intra- and peripancreatic fat necrosis, which may have a fatal outcome.

PATHOPHYSIOLOGY

A variety of etiologic factors have been associated with the development of acute pancreatitis, but only two of these, chronic alcohol abuse and gallstone disease, are responsible for 75–80 percent of cases in most series. Other less common but recognized causes include abdominal trauma, hyperlipoproteinemias characterized by very high serum triglyceride concentrations, hypercalcemia, drugs (e.g., azathioprine, thiazide diuretics), pregnancy, penetrating duodenal ulcer, vasculitides, cancer of the pancreas, and some viral and parasitic infections. In addition, acute pancreatitis is rarely observed following surgery or endoscopic retrograde pancreatography. In 5–10 percent of patients in most series, the disease is idiopathic.

Acute pancreatitis is believed to be due to "autodigestion" of the gland produced by premature activation of digestive enzymes leading to damage and necrosis of the enzyme-secreting (acinar) cells; this then results in release and activation of more digestive enzymes. If the process extends beyond the pancreas, it can lead to retroperitoneal and peritoneal fat necrosis, hemorrhage, exudation of peritoneal fluid, disturbances of gastric and intestinal motility (ileus), and obstruction of flow in the common bile duct. Activated pancreatic trypsin can also convert kallikrein to bradykinin, plasminogen to plasmin, and activate complement. These (and probably other substances not yet identified) can contribute to both the local inflammatory process in and around the pancreas and to the systemic manifestations such as metabolic abnormalities (e.g., hypocal-

393

cemia, hyperglycemia), coagulopathy, and renal or pulmonary insufficiency.

Although in most patients acute pancreatitis will spontaneously
resolve, death may occur, usually owing to hypovolemic shock, renal or
pulmonary insufficiency, or the formation of a pancreatic abscess and
sepsis.

DIAGNOSIS

About 95 percent of patients with acute pancreatitis present with
abdominal pain, which, in about 50 percent, will be upper abdominal
pain radiating to the back. Nausea and vomiting are present in 60–80
percent of patients. On physical examination, abdominal tenderness and/
or guarding are observed in 80–90 percent of patients, abdominal distention and tympany in 70 percent, and a low-grade fever (<39 °C) in 50–80
percent. The presence of a higher fever should suggest cholecystitis,
cholangitis, peritonitis, or a pancreatic abscess. Other commonly observed
findings are hypotension, mild jaundice, ascites, or pleural effusion.

The clinical diagnosis of acute pancreatitis requires laboratory or
roentgenographic confirmation because the symptoms and signs are
nonspecific (e.g., a perforated ulcer, cholecystitis or cholangitis, and
intestinal ischemia can present in a similar fashion). Measurement of the
concentration of the pancreatic enzyme amylase in serum or urine has
been the most widely used diagnostic study for confirming this diagnosis.
Although the concentration of amylase is elevated in most patients with
acute pancreatitis, it may be normal (falsely negative) if not measured
within 2–7 days of the onset of symptoms or in 10–30 percent of patients
with acute alcoholic pancreatitis. Falsely positive results may occur in
salivary gland disease; perforation of the esophagus, stomach, or intestine;
intestinal ischemia; gynecologic disorders (e.g., ruptured tubal pregnancy
or ovarian cyst); malignant tumors; renal failure; severe burns; diabetic
ketoacidosis; and macroamylasemia. The measurement of the serum
concentrations of pancreatic isoamylase or of other pancreatic enzymes
such as lipase, trypsin, and elastase is being evaluated in the diagnosis of
acute pancreatitis. However, so far none of these other determinations
has been convincingly shown to improve upon the diagnostic accuracy of
measuring serum amylase concentration.

When the diagnosis remains in doubt following clinical assessment
and serum amylase determination, especially in the more severely ill
patient, abdominal sonography and computed tomography are very helpful in confirming the diagnosis of acute pancreatitis and excluding other
intraabdominal catastrophic processes. However, abdominal sonography

cannot be accurately performed in patients with a moderate-to-severe ileus, and computed tomography is the procedure of choice in that setting.

MANAGEMENT

There is no effective specific therapy to treat the underlying disease process in acute pancreatitis. Therefore the therapeutic approach at present is one of supportive care and treatment of complications. The primary goal, initially, is the replacement of volume deficits and electrolyte losses, which can be massive and life-threatening. Correction of hypocalcemia should be cautious because hypocalcemia in the setting of acute pancreatitis is rarely clinically significant. Patients may require substantial amounts of analgesia, usually with meperidine (Demerol). Oral intake should be prohibited until the patient's clinical condition improves, and nasogastric suction should be employed for patients who are vomiting or have significant abdominal distention. The patient's degree of respiratory effort, chest examination, and arterial blood gas values should be monitored closely, especially early in the hospital course, and oxygen and ventilatory support provided if needed.

The use of prophylactic antibiotics, drugs to "put the pancreas at rest," protease (trypsin) inhibitors, and peritoneal lavage has not been shown to be effective in controlled clinical trials. The value of aggressive surgical debridement and drainage of the pancreatic bed in severe acute pancreatitis and of early surgical or endoscopic removal of impacted gallstones from the common bile duct remains unproven.

In patients with severe pain or elevated serum amylase concentration persisting for more than a week, abdominal sonography or computed tomography should be performed, and a pseudocyst (collection of inflammatory debris and pancreatic secretion) should be sought. In general, pseudocysts in the setting of acute pancreatitis should be followed for at least 6 weeks prior to surgical intervention to allow either spontaneous resolution (about 25 percent) or maturation of the pseudocyst wall to permit internal drainage to the stomach or small intestine. More urgent surgical intervention may be required if the pseudocyst ruptures into the peritoneal cavity, becomes infected, erodes into a blood vessel, or produces protracted biliary or intestinal obstruction.

Patients demonstrating a fever >39 °C, white blood count >20,000/mm^3, or clinical deterioration after initial improvement should be promptly evaluated for the presence of a pancreatic abscess by emergency computed tomography; fine-needle aspiration of any suspicious-looking fluid collections should be done for Gram's stain and culture. If computed tomography and Gram's stain suggest the presence of a pancreatic abscess, the patient should be started on broad-spectrum antibiotics (e.g., ampicillin, gentamicin, and metronidazole) and should undergo emergency surgical drainage of the suspected abscess.

Outcome

Most patients have a self-limiting benign course with ultimate spontaneous resolution, and they return to their previous level of pancreatic endocrine and exocrine function. Overall mortality is generally <10 percent and tends to be somewhat higher in patients with gallstone pancreatitis than in alcohol-related disease. The presence of either renal or respiratory failure is associated with a mortality of >50 percent. The mortality of pancreatic abscess not treated with surgical drainage approaches 100 percent. With the use of broad spectrum antibiotics and of computed tomography and fine-needle aspiration to enable earlier surgical drainage, the mortality has been reduced to 20–25 percent.

Recurrence of acute pancreatitis can be prevented in gallstone patients by cholecystectomy and removal of common duct stones; in patients with hyperlipoproteinemias by normalization of serum triglycerides by diet and/or medication; and, in patients with drug-induced pancreatitis, by removing the offending agent. The effect of abstinence from alcohol on the recurrence rate of acute alcoholic pancreatitis has not been clearly established.

RECOMMENDED READING

Crass RA, Meyer AA, Jeffrey RB, et al: Pancreatic abscess: impact of computerized tomography on early diagnosis and surgery. Am J Surg 150:127, 1985.

Moosa AR: Diagnostic tests and procedures in acute pancreatitis. N Engl J Med 311:639, 1984.

Pellegrini CA: The treatment of acute pancreatitis: a continuing challenge. (Editorial.) N Engl J Med 312:436, 1985.

Ranson JHC: Acute pancreatitis: pathogenesis, outcome, and treatment. Clin Gastroenterol 13:843, 1984.

Steinberg WM, Goldstein SS, Davis ND, et al: Diagnostic assays in acute pancreatitis. A study of sensitivity and specificity. Ann Intern Med 102:576, 1985.

Toskes PP, Greenberger NJ: Acute and chronic pancreatitis. Dis Mon 26:1, 1983.

Weaver DW, Busuito MJ, Bowman DL, et al: Interpretation of serum amylase levels in critically ill patients. Crit Care Med 13:532, 1985.

64. Hepatic Failure and Encephalopathy

James H. Grendell

DEFINITION

Liver failure represents a severe, generalized impairment of liver function that carries a high mortality. When it occurs within 8 weeks of the onset of illness in patients without preexisting liver disease, it is called fulminant hepatic failure. Liver failure may also occur as the end stage of chronic liver disease such as cirrhosis of any cause or massive replacement of liver tissue by primary or metastatic tumors.

PATHOPHYSIOLOGY (Table 64–1)

Fulminant hepatic failure most commonly develops following massive necrosis of liver cells, owing to viral hepatitis. Drugs (e.g., acetaminophen, halothane, isoniazid, methyldopa) and toxins (e.g., *Amanita* mushroom poisoning, carbon tetrachloride, yellow phosphorus) are also important etiologic factors. It may also occur following severe ischemic injury to the liver ("shock liver") and is associated with a variety of other disorders (Reye's syndrome, acute fatty liver of pregnancy, acute hepatic vein occlusion).

Liver failure may also develop in chronic diseases of the liver, including cirrhosis, the "acute" form of Wilson's disease, and massive involvement of the liver by tumor.

DIAGNOSIS

Hepatic encephalopathy is the hallmark of liver failure, with some clinicians requiring the presence of Stage III (somnolence) or IV (coma) for the diagnosis of fulminant hepatic failure. Asterixis, which is typically present in the early stages of hepatic encephalopathy (Stage I: mood alterations, restlessness, decreased attention span; Stage II: lethargy, confusion), is frequently absent in Stages III and IV.

TABLE 64–1. ETIOLOGY OF LIVER FAILURE

ACUTE LIVER DISEASE
Viral hepatitis
Drugs (e.g., acetaminophen, halothane, isoniazid, methyldopa)
Toxins (e.g., mushroom poisoning, carbon tetrachloride, yellow phosphorus)
Ischemia
Reye's syndrome
Acute fatty liver of pregnancy
Acute hepatic vein occlusion

CHRONIC LIVER DISEASE
Cirrhosis
Wilson's disease
Primary or metastatic tumors of the liver

Impairment of liver synthetic function is often present, as reflected by an increased prothrombin time and a decreased serum albumin concentration. Although the serum bilirubin concentration is usually elevated in liver failure in the setting of chronic liver disease, it may be low in the early stages of rapidly progressive fulminant hepatic failure. Serum transaminase concentrations (ALT, AST) may be markedly elevated following massive liver necrosis from viral infections, drugs, toxins, or ischemia; however, these concentrations rapidly fall toward normal. Serum transaminase concentrations in chronic liver disease may only be mildly increased or may even be normal.

MANAGEMENT

An attempt should be made to correct any factors that may be contributing to the development of liver dysfunction and hepatic encephalopathy. These factors include excessive dietary protein, constipation, sedative or potentially hepatotoxic drugs, volume depletion and electrolyte abnormalities, renal failure, hypoxemia, and bacterial infection.

Because there is no specific treatment for liver failure short of liver transplantation, the major focus of efforts should be on providing good supportive care and preventing or treating potential complications (Table 64–2); supportive care includes adequate hydration and careful correction of electrolyte abnormalities, especially hypokalemia, which can worsen

TABLE 64–2. COMPLICATIONS OF LIVER FAILURE

Electrolyte abnormalities	Renal failure
Hypoglycemia	Cerebral edema
Gastrointestinal hemorrhage	Seizures
Hepatic encephalopathy	Hypotension
Infection	Lactic acidosis
Hypoxemia	

encephalopathy. Hypoglycemia is common and should be treated when present with intravenous infusion of 10 percent dextrose solutions, with two to three liters or more a day required at times.

Either H_2-receptor antagonists or antacids should be used to maintain the intragastric pH >4.0 to reduce the risk of gastrointestinal bleeding primarily from stress gastritis. Vitamin K (10 mg subcutaneously) should be given daily to patients with an abnormal prothrombin time, although substantial correction of the prothrombin time with vitamin K does not typically occur in this setting. Administration of fresh-frozen plasma or platelets should be reserved for treatment of significant bleeding in the setting of coagulopathy or thrombocytopenia.

Hepatic encephalopathy of mild-to-moderate severity can be treated by restriction of dietary protein to less than 0.5 g/kg/day, although this may interfere with optimal nutrition if maintained for a prolonged period of time. Oral or parenteral administration of branched-chain amino acids has been recommended, based on animal and limited clinical studies; however, this treatment probably has little, if any, benefit in fulminant hepatic failure. The most useful therapy for hepatic encephalopathy at present is lactulose syrup given orally or by nasogastric tube at 50 ml every 2 hours until diarrhea results. The dose can then be titrated to produce two to four soft-formed stools per day (usually requiring 90–120 ml lactulose per day in divided doses). Neomycin (2–6 g/day in divided doses orally or by nasogastric tube) is also effective but may result in auditory or renal toxicity because small amounts of neomycin are absorbed.

Bacterial and fungal infections frequently occur in liver failure. The frequency of these disorders can be reduced by careful maintenance of genitourinary catheters and intravenous lines and by positioning of the patient so as to minimize the risk of pulmonary aspiration and decubitus ulcers. Strongly suspected or documented infections should be treated with antibiotics as indicated by diagnostic studies and results of cultures. However, prophylactic antibiotics should not be used because of the likelihood of superinfection by resistant bacteria or fungi.

Hypoxemia may be observed in liver failure, owing to intrapulmonary shunting of blood or noncardiogenic pulmonary edema. Administration of oxygen, diuresis (if indicated), and, in some patients, mechanical ventilation with positive end-expiratory pressure may be required.

Renal failure may result from the hepatorenal syndrome, acute tubular necrosis, or hypovolemia. Dialysis has not been shown to improve survival in patients with liver failure whose azotemia is not corrected by appropriate volume expansion.

Cerebral edema may be present in half or more of patients dying of liver failure; it is not responsive to corticosteroids, but, in one study, intravenous mannitol was of benefit to some patients. Seizures may also occur and, if frequent or prolonged, may require the therapy outlined in Chapter 65. Hypotension, which is typically refractory to pressors, is frequently a terminal event as is lactic acidosis. The latter can be treated with intravenous bicarbonate, although this approach may not alter prognosis.

Because of the poor prognosis of liver failure and lack of effective, specific therapy, a variety of techniques have been used to provide temporary hepatic support, analogous to renal dialysis. These have included exchange transfusion, plasmapheresis, cross-circulation with a human or animal, hemodialysis, hemoperfusion through an isolated human cadaver or animal liver, and charcoal hemoperfusion. None of these approaches has been demonstrated to clearly improve survival compared with that of good supportive care. Administration of corticosteroids, L-dopa, and hepatitis B immune globulin has been shown to be ineffective.

The development of liver transplantation provides a new option in the treatment of liver failure. However, few patients with fulminant hepatic failure have received transplants so far because of the rapidity of the disease's course, making procurement of a donor liver difficult; it is also difficult to transport these extremely ill patients to transplant centers. With the spread of transplant centers and improvements in the donor organ procurement system, transplantation may play a larger role in the treatment of fulminant hepatic failure. Patients with liver failure due to cirrhosis may be candidates for liver transplantation depending on age, overall condition, and whether they are active alcohol abusers. Results of transplantation in patients with malignant tumors involving the liver have been poor.

Outcome

Survival in fulminant hepatic failure is only about 20 percent, although preliminary data from a small number of selected patients suggest that liver transplantation may improve upon this. Survivors usually recover completely with little or no evidence of liver disease on subsequent biopsy.

The short-term prognosis of patients with liver failure and chronic liver disease depends on the presence of potentially reversible factors such as volume and electrolyte abnormalities, gastrointestinal bleeding, or infection. However, because these patients generally have end-stage irreversible liver disease, the overall prognosis is generally very poor unless they are candidates for liver transplantation.

RECOMMENDED READING

Canalese J, Gimson AE, Davis C, et al: Controlled trial of dexamethasone and mannitol for the cerebral oedema of fulminant hepatic failure. Gut 23:625, 1985.
Payne JA: Fulminant liver failure. Med Clin North Am 70:1067, 1986.
Tygstrup N, Ranek L: Assessment of prognosis in fulminant hepatic failure. Semin Liver Dis 6:129, 1986.
Williams R, Gimson AES: An assessment of orthotopic liver transplantation in acute liver failure. Hepatology 4:22S, 1984.
Williams R, Gimson A: Management of acute liver failure. Clin Gastroenterol 14:93, 1985.

Neurologic and Psychiatric Disorders

65. Status Epilepticus

John M. Luce

DEFINITION

Status epilepticus is defined as a seizure lasting long enough or repeated frequently enough to produce a fixed and enduring epileptic condition. To most investigators, this means a seizure lasting 30 minutes or longer or a series of seizures without return of consciousness or normal neurologic behavior for 30 minutes.

PATHOPHYSIOLOGY

Status epilepticus is currently classified as (1) convulsive status, in which patients do not regain consciousness during or between attacks; (2) nonconvulsive status, in which patients manifest a prolonged "twilight" or absence state; and (3) continuous partial status or epilepsia partialis continuum, in which consciousness is preserved. Convulsive status is the most common of these types; approximately 100,000 Americans, including 1–5 percent of all persons with epilepsy, will have at least one episode.

The etiologic characteristics of status epilepticus depend, in part, on the age of patients involved. In infants and children, status is often the first ictal event, although other seizures may follow. Causes of status in this age group include (1) intracranial infections such as meningitis and encephalitis, (2) metabolic disorders due to electrolyte imbalance or anoxia, (3) vascular abnormalities and brain malformations, and (4) idiopathic causes. Among adults, status often occurs in the setting of previously diagnosed epilepsy and is rarely the initial manifestation of this condition. Indeed, the most common cause of status in adults is noncompliance with anticonvulsant drug regimens. Other causes include withdrawal from alcohol and other drugs, cerebrovascular disease (including acute stroke), cerebral trauma or tumors (especially those involving the frontal lobes), intracranial infections, metabolic disorders, drug overdosage (e.g., aminophylline, lidocaine, tricyclic antidepressants, and isoniazid), or combinations of the above. No specific cause of status is found in 15 percent of adults.

The neurologic consequences of status epilepticus depend on the type

405

and duration of seizures and the amount of muscle activity as reflected in the body temperature. Convulsive status is accompanied by a profound initial increase in blood pressure and cerebral blood flow (CBF) that results from sympathetic nervous stimulation, increased peripheral vascular resistance, augmented venous return to the central circulation, and cerebral vasodilation. Intracranial pressure may increase in the process, especially among patients whose intracranial compliance is abnormal, owing to cerebral swelling or mass lesions. These events are paralleled by a two- to fivefold increase in the cerebral metabolism of oxygen, glucose, and other substrates.

Hypercapnia is seen in many patients with status and is attributable to diminished ventilatory efforts, to mechanical impairment of breathing by muscle spasms, or to upper airway obstruction. Hypoxemia also is common; its causes include hypoventilation, ventilation-perfusion abnormalities related to increased tracheobronchial secretions, and, possibly, intrapulmonary shunting due to neurogenic pulmonary edema. The last condition most likely results from increased filtration of fluid in the lungs secondary to increased hydrostatic pressures in the pulmonary circulation and increased microvascular permeability, both of which occur during the initial phase of sympathetic overactivity.

Patients in status frequently manifest a peripheral leukocytosis due to demargination of white blood cells. A pleocytosis may also be present in the cerebrospinal fluid; although this may result from status alone, infection must often be ruled out. In addition, the early phase of status is often characterized by hyperglycemia due to catecholamine release and hyperkalemia due to muscle breakdown. Lactic acidosis may increase as seizures progress; so does the core temperature, which may exceed 40°C. Eventually, hypoglycemia results from body as well as brain glucose consumption, and rhabdomyolysis may follow continued muscle breakdown. The blood pressure falls in the presence of acidosis and hypoxemia, and patients may suffer cardiovascular collapse.

DIAGNOSIS

Early diagnosis is essential because status epilepticus is a medical emergency and because anticonvulsant drugs have different effects depending on the type of seizures involved. Status epilepticus should be obvious in unconscious patients with unremitting muscle activity. However, the diagnosis of other types of status may be made only by electroencephalography. Although a full evaluation of the cause of status should not interfere unduly with measures to stop seizures, serum levels of glucose and electrolytes and renal and liver function tests should be obtained in all patients if possible. Blood should be saved for toxicology screens if indicated (consider especially tricyclic antidepressant overdosage, as discussed in Chapter 88). A lumbar puncture should be performed whenever infection is suspected, and computerized tomography should be considered in trauma patients.

MANAGEMENT

Several drugs are available to treat status and all have advantages and disadvantages. For example, diazepam and other benzodiazapines given intravenously should eliminate convulsive status in 90 percent of patients (excluding those with rapidly growing mass lesions), but these agents have only a 15 minute half-life when given intravenously and may cause drowsiness and respiratory depression. Intravenous phenytoin is equally effective in suppressing seizures, is less depressing on the nervous system, and has the additional benefit of being the drug many patients will take after their status is broken. However, phenytoin has a slower onset of action than diazepam and should not be given in doses over 50 mg/min, owing to its own dysrhythmogenic properties and the hypotensive effects of its diluent, propylene glycol. Intravenous or intramuscular phenobarbital, which may also be useful, depresses ventilation and causes peripheral venous pooling that may limit the cardiac output. Other barbiturates have the same properties.

Given these facts and the need to treat status quickly, the following protocol seems advisable. First, protect the airway by positioning patients on their sides and inserting a nasal airway if possible. Place an intravenous catheter, obtain serum for the studies suggested earlier, and give 50 ml of a 50 percent dextrose solution if hypoglycemia is known or strongly suspected. Also give thiamine 50 mg if alcoholism and malnutrition are possible. Then give diazepam 0.3–0.5 mg/kg (adult dose) intravenously over 1–2 minutes. Regardless of the effect of diazepam, load patients with intravenous phenytoin, 15–20 mg/kg (1000–1500 mg) at a rate of 50 mg/ min; phenytoin should be given with saline because it will precipitate in dextrose-containing solutions. During this period, arterial blood gases should be drawn if possible to assess the adequacy of ventilation and oxygenation, and supplemental oxygen should be given. Intubation and mechanical ventilation may be called for, especially if ventilation is depressed by the anticonvulsant drugs.

If seizures persist at this point, several options are available. Some clinicians continue to give intravenous diazepam (100 mg diazepam in 500 ml of D5W at 40 ml/hr) until a total dose of 1 mg/kg/day is reached; this should only be done in intubated patients because apnea is certain. Others proceed to intravenous phenobarbital, giving 15–20 mg/kg (1000–1500 mg) slowly and monitoring ventilation carefully. If these, too, are ineffective, general anesthesia using barbiturates (with or without muscle paralysis) is required. Barbiturate protocols include pentobarbital 5 mg/kg given slowly intravenously, then 1–5 mg/kg/hr; or thiopental 100–250 mg slowly, followed by 80–120 mg/hr.

It must be stressed that this general protocol should be amended in certain circumstances. For example, large doses of diazepam or barbiturates are undesirable in patients with severe cardiopulmonary dysfunction or in patients whose level of consciousness should not be depressed. Intravenous phenytoin is the drug of choice in such patients and in those with partial motor status. At the same time, because most anticonvulsants cross the placenta, obstetricians may prefer to treat status in pregnant women with magnesium sulfate.

OUTCOME

Death was once reported in up to 50 percent of patients with status epilepticus but now occurs in approximately 10 percent. Permanent neurologic damage is uncommon if status is aborted in 1 hour or less but common if it lasts longer. Although neurologic sequelae have been attributed to factors such as hypoxemia, status itself can cause neuroanatomic lesions in experimental animals whose arterial blood gases are normal. Status may follow mild head trauma in children and does not carry a bad prognosis, whereas the prognosis is poor for adults whose status follows head trauma. The likelihood of chronic epilepsy in children following fibrile seizures depends primarily on the presence or absence of preexisting brain disease.

RECOMMENDED READING

Aicardi J, Chevrie JJ: Convulsive status epilepticus in infants and children. Epilepsia 11:187, 1970.

Aminoff MJ, Simon RP: Status epilepticus: causes, clinical features and consequences in 98 patients. Am J Med 69:6576, 1980.

Brown AS, Horton JM: Status epilepticus treated by intravenous infusions of thiopentone sodium. Br Med J 1:27, 1967.

Celesia GG: Modern concepts of status epilepticus. JAMA 235:1571, 1976.

Delgado-Escueta AV, Wasterlain C, Treiman DM, Porter RJ: Management of status epilepticus. N Engl J Med 307:1337, 1982.

Grand W: The significance of post-traumatic status epilepticus in childhood. J Neurosurg 37:178, 1974.

Lockman LA, Kriel R, Zaske D, et al: Phenobarbital dosage for control of neonatal seizures. Neurology 29:1445, 1979.

Meldrum BS, Brierley JB: Prolonged epilepticus seizures in primates: ischemic cell change and its relation to ictal physiological events. Arch Neurol 28:10, 1973.

Meldrum BS, Horton RW: Physiology of status epilepticus in primates. Arch Neurol 28:1, 1973.

Nelson KB, Ellenberg J: Predictors of epilepsy in children who have experienced febrile seizures. N Engl J Med 295:1029, 1976.

Oxbury JM, Whitty CWM: Causes and consequences of status epilepticus in adults. Brain 94:733, 1971.

Prensky AL, Raff MC, Moore MJ, et al: Intravenous diazepam in the treatment of prolonged seizure activity. N Engl J Med 276:779, 1967.

Pritchard JA, Pritchard SA: Standardized treatment of 154 consecutive cases of eclampsia. Am J Obstet Gynecol 101:543, 1975.

Simon RP, Bayne LL, Tranbaugh RF, et al: Elevated pulmonary lymph flow and protein content during status epilepticus in sheep. J Appl Physiol 52:91, 1982.

Wallis W, Kutt H, McDowell F: Intravenous diphenylhydantoin in treatment of acute repetitive seizures. Neurology 18:513, 1968.

66. Delirium and Insomnia

John M. Luce

DEFINITION

Delirium is defined as a wakeful state of metabolic encephalopathy that is often associated with tremulous agitation, hallucinations, and loss of contact with the environment. This condition is also referred to as a toxic psychosis or an acute confusional state. Because sleeplessness frequently accompanies delirium and may be part of its pathogenesis, it also is discussed in this chapter.

PATHOPHYSIOLOGY

Delirium represents a diffuse disturbance of cerebral metabolism that involves the cerebral hemispheres and the brainstem, including the reticular activating system. The hallmark of delirium is an altered state of awareness and activity. Although some patients with delirium due to hypoxia and ischemia or hepatic failure may become quiet or even comatose, most delirious patients are agitated, irritable, distractible, and emotionally labile. They also manifest disturbances of cognition, memory, and judgment, are disoriented, and may hallucinate.

Delirium may result from any or all of the insults outlined in Table 66–1. In critically ill patients, the most common of these abnormalities are hypoxia and ischemia, electrolyte disturbance, liver and renal disease, drug intoxication and withdrawal, and infection. Generally, stimulants cause delirium during their ingestion, whereas sedative-hypnotic agents cause delirium during their withdrawal. The intensive care unit (ICU) setting, which subjects the patient to anxiety, pain, physical discomfort, invasive procedures, and many intrusions upon privacy, has also been implicated in the pathogenesis of delirium; hence, the term "ICU psychosis," which is applied indiscriminately in many cases.

Sleeplessness may be an important contribution to delirium in the critical care environment. Sleep occurs when the arousal activity of the reticular system, which is normally maintained by inputs from higher brain centers as well as the peripheral and autonomic nervous systems, is overwhelmed by stimuli from other areas. The sources of these stimuli

410

TABLE 66–1. COMMON CAUSES OF DELIRIUM IN THE CRITICAL CARE ENVIRONMENT

Hypoxemia
Ischemia
Hypoglycemia
Hyponatremia
Hypomagnesemia
Thiamine deficiency (Wernicke's encephalopathy)
Hepatic failure
Renal failure
Thyrotoxicosis
Drug intoxication or withdrawal (especially alcohol, barbiturates,
    amphetamines, anticholinergics, corticosteroids)
Infections (e.g., meningitis)
Head trauma (e.g., cerebral contusion)
"ICU psychosis" (? sleep deprivation)

include the hypothalamus, which normally imparts a circadian rhythm to sleep and wakefulness in response to light and time cues; and the pons, which contains adrenergic and cholinergic nuclei, whose interactions create 90–100 minute cycles of sleep, usually during the night. These cycles are made up phases 1–4 of nonrapid eye movement (NREM) sleep, which are characterized by depression of the electroencephalograph (EEG), muscle tone, respiratory rate, and blood pressure; and the rapid eye movement (REM) phase, in which there is autonomic hyperactivity and, paradoxically, a paralysis of all but the extraocular muscles. Normally, sleep cycles are repeated throughout the night, with REM phases becoming progressively longer in the early morning hours.

Sleep may be disrupted by several mechanisms: loss of the circadian rhythm, which might occur because of an alteration in external cues or disease of the hypothalamus, or conditions that either increase adrenergic or decrease cholinergic activity in the brainstem. Adrenergic activity is increased by pain, physical activity, and drugs such as caffeine. Cholinergic activity is decreased by anticholinergic agents, including atropine. Because healthy people vary so much in their sleep requirements, sleep deprivation is difficult to define. Nevertheless, loss of one or more nights of sleep is known to increase fatigue and disorientation and to decrease mental acuity. Sleeplessness may also predispose to delirium or potentiate it. In support of this theory is the fact that delirium is usually accompanied by insomnia and may end with a period of prolonged, deep sleep (containing stage 4 NREM as well as REM sleep) from which patients awake with a normal mental status. Drugs such as alcohol and other sedatives suppress REM sleep, and high levels of REM are seen in wakeful patients during the delirium that accompanies withdrawal from these drugs. Nevertheless, "REM rebound" is not observed in all delirious patients, and the relationship between delirium and sleep remains obscure.

DIAGNOSIS

Delirium most commonly occurs in patients over 60 years of age who have a previous history of neuropsychiatric disease and/or alcohol or drug abuse. It is extremely common in the postoperative period and has been reported in as many as 40 percent of patients after open heart surgery. Postoperative delirium generally occurs 2–5 days after surgery and is preceded by a lucid phase. Physical findings suggestive of delirium include hypertension and tachycardia, tremor, asterixis (a sign of metabolic encephalopathy in general, not just hepatic disease), and myoclonus. The pupils should be equal and reactive in delirious patients, except those with drug intoxication due to glutethimide (midposition, fixed pupils) and adrenergic or anticholinergic agents (dilated, fixed pupils).

The cause or causes of delirium may be more difficult to identify. Patient histories may be revealing, especially regarding previous psychosis or drug use. Some diseases such as meningitis, hepatic failure, and thyrotoxicosis may be suggested by the physical examination. Appropriate laboratory tests in delirious patients include complete blood count; electrolytes; blood glucose; liver, renal, and thyroid function tests; cerebrospinal fluid analysis; and toxicology screens. Computerized tomography of the brain is indicated in selected individuals.

MANAGEMENT

The treatment of specific causes of delirium, including drug intoxication and withdrawal, is covered in other chapters. The general management of the disorder involves providing orientation and sleep. Patient orientation can be improved by regular contact with family, friends, nurses, and physicians, who remind the patients of who and where they are. ICU rooms should have windows, clocks, calendars, and televisions or radios. Ideally, the rooms should be quiet and dark at night and patients should be disturbed as little as possible during the nighttime hours. Drugs that cloud the sensorium should generally be avoided, but pain should be treated aggressively, as described in Chapter 79.

If these and other measures fail, sedative-hypnotic drugs may be tried. The benzodiazepine diazepam is an effective anxiolytic and sedative-hypnotic agent that may improve sleep during the first days or nights of its administration. This drug is usually given in 5–10 mg doses; the schedule for treating alcohol withdrawal involves 5 mg doses given every 5–15 min until patients are calm, as discussed in Chapter 84. Unfortunately, diazepam also suppresses REM sleep and is associated with sleep disturbance during its withdrawal. This drug also depresses ventilation and may cause hypotension if given in large doses. Diazepam is absorbed poorly from intramuscular depots and must be given orally or intravenously. In the latter form, its elimination half-life is 24–48 hours; active metabolites of diazepam have their own elimination half-lives as well. The hepatic metabolism of diazepam is attenuated by liver disease and by drugs such as cimetidine. For these reasons, diazepam has a prolonged action in most critically ill patients; this has prompted the development of benzodiazepines with shorter half-lives that do not suppress REM sleep so profoundly. Such agents include lorazepam (12 hour half-life; usual intravenous dose 2–4 mg) and triazolam (1–2 hour half-life; usual intravenous dose 0.25–0.5 mg).

The limitations of diazepam and the similarity between delirium and true psychosis has led many clinicians to use antipsychotic drugs in delirious patients. These agents are not actually sedatives or hypnotics, but their calming effect is often profound. Chlorpromazine should probably be avoided, owing to its α-adrenergic antagonistic and anticholinergic properties. The preferred drug is haloperidol, administered in 5–10 mg intramuscular or intravenous doses until the patient is no longer agitated. Haloperidol does not depress ventilation or suppress REM sleep. Its elimination half-life is approximately 12 hours.

OUTCOME

Depending on its cause, delirium may be either a mild and transient disorder or a medical crisis that culminates in death. However, most patients should survive this condition if it is treated appropriately and if their underlying problems are attended to.

RECOMMENDED READING

Hobson JA: Sleep: order and disorder. Behav Bio Med Monogr 1:1, 1983.
Johns MW, Large AA, Masterton JP, et al: Sleep and delirium after open heart surgery. Br J Surg 61:377, 1974.
Klotz U, Reimann I: Delayed clearance of diazepam due to cimetidine. N Engl J Med 302:1012, 1980.
Moore DP: Rapid treatment of delirium in critically ill patients. Am J Psychiatry 134:1431, 1977.
Ochs JR, Greenblatt DJ, Lauven PM, et al: Kinetics of high-dose IV diazepam. Br J Anaesth 54:849, 1982.
Orr WC, Stahl ML: Sleep disturbances after open heart surgery. Am J Cardiol 39:196, 1977.
Plum F, Posner JB: Diagnosis of Stupor and Coma. 3rd edition. Philadelphia, F. A. Davis Co., 1982.
Sellers EM, Kalant H: Alcohol intoxication and withdrawal. N Engl J Med 294:757, 1976.

67. Coma

John M. Luce

DEFINITION

Coma is a sleeplike state from which patients cannot be aroused. Among other entities, it represents the final stage before brain death along the continuum of depressed mental status. Coma differs from brain death, which is discussed in Chapter 68, in that comatose patients may retain certain reflex responses, such as decerebrate and decorticate posturing, that are absent in brain-dead individuals. Coma also differs from the persistent vegetative state, in which patients may open their eyes but cannot communicate; such patients are said to be awake but unaware.

PATHOPHYSIOLOGY

Normal consciousness is made possible by the coordinated functioning of the brain stem reticular activating system, which is located in the central cone of the brainstem from the midpons to the diencephalon, and the two cerebral hemispheres. Coma occurs when the reticular activating system or both cerebral hemispheres or all three areas are injured. Such injury may be structural, in that specific tissues are damaged by infarction, hemorrhage, infection, or edema; or metabolic, involving diffuse dysfunction of the central nervous system. The causes of structural and metabolic coma are legion; some conditions commonly causing coma are discussed later in this chapter.

DIAGNOSIS

The initial step in evaluating apparently unconscious patients is to determine whether they truly are comatose. This can be accomplished by stimulating them verbally and with noxious physical maneuvers such as pressing on the fingernail beds, the sternum, or the supraorbital ridge. Eye opening, verbal response, and motor response to these maneuvers can be quantitated with the Glasgow Coma Scale (GCS) in patients with

TABLE 67–1. GLASGOW COMA SCALE

EYE OPENING	
Spontaneous	4
To speech	3
To pain	2
Nil	1
MOTOR RESPONSE	
Obeys commands	6
Localizes	5
Withdraws	4
Abnormal flexion	3
Extends	2
Nil	1
VERBAL RESPONSE	
Oriented	5
Confused conversation	4
Inappropriate words	3
Incomprehensible sounds	2
Nil	1

head trauma and other structural lesions but is not so useful in patients with metabolic coma (Table 67–1).

Once the diagnosis of coma is established, clinicians should assure delivery of blood, oxygen, and glucose to the brain. Breathing patterns and pulses should be sought, and cardiopulmonary resuscitation should be administered if vital signs are absent. Arterial blood gases should be obtained, and endotracheal intubation and mechanical ventilation should be initiated if necessary. Blood should be drawn for rapid determination of glucose and electrolyte values, hepatic and renal function, and osmolality, as well as for complete blood count and toxicology screens. Dextrose (50 g) should be given intravenously if hypoglycemia is confirmed or strongly suspected. Thiamine (100 mg) should precede dextrose to prevent the precipitation of Wernicke's encephalopathy in malnourished patients. Naloxone administration (0.4 mg or more) is indicated in all comatose patients who may have taken narcotics. Intravenous antibiotics (2 million units of aqueous penicillin G in adults or cefuroxime in children) should be given as soon as possible if bacterial meningitis is suspected (see Chapter 74).

The cause of coma can frequently be determined by history-taking and physical examination. The history may strongly suggest that the coma is due to hypothermia, diabetes, epilepsy, alcohol or drug overdosage, liver or kidney failure, head trauma, or intracerebral hemorrhage associated with hypertension. The underlying abnormality may also be indicated by physical signs such as fever and nuchal rigidity in patients with meningitis or subarachnoid hemorrhage.

Close attention should be paid to the eyes of comatose patients. The pupils should not be dilated with cycloplegic agents, but the optic fundi should be observed for blurring of the disc margins and for other signs of elevated intracranial pressure; for subhyaloid hemorrhages, which may be seen in subarachnoid bleeding; and for the chronic vascular changes of hypertension and diabetes. The intactness of cranial nerves II (afferent) and III (efferent) is established in patients by noting pupils of equal size and reactivity. Pinpoint, fixed pupils may be seen in pontine hemorrhage or narcotic overdose. Midposition, fixed pupils are suggestive of midbrain lesions or glutethimide overdose. Dilated, unreactive pupils may occur with atropine or sympathomimetic intoxication and occasionally with structural brainstem injury. Unilateral fixed pupils are indicative of third nerve dysfunction, usually caused by herniation of the uncus of the temporal lobe. Ocular immobility or involuntary eye movements are seen in a variety of structural and metabolic processes. The intactness of cranial nerve V (afferent) and VII (efferent) is established by the presence of the corneal reflex.

Oculocephalic and oculovestibular testing are used to determine the intactness of cranial nerves VIII (afferent) and III and VI (efferent) and of the median longitudinal fasciculus. These tests are based on the fact that the vestibular nuclei symmetrically stimulate the oculomotor system and that vestibular tone is affected by the semicircular canals and by proprioceptive inputs. The eyes tend to deviate toward the nucleus with a relative decrease in tone when this symmetry is interrupted. In oculocephalic testing ("doll's eyes" testing), the head is rolled from side to side; as vestibular tone is increased on the side to which the head is turned, the eyes normally deviate in the opposite direction. In oculovestibular testing (caloric testing), cold or ice water (30–50 ml) is instilled against the tympanic membrane with the head at a 30-degree angle from the horizontal; as vestibular tone is decreased by the cold, the eyes normally will deviate toward the side injected. Tonic deviation of the eyes is opposed by saccadic movements if input from above the vestibular nuclei is present. If supranuclear input is lost, the eyes deviate tonically. If the nuclei of cranial nerves III, VI, and VIII are damaged in the pons, the eyes will not deviate. If the median longitudinal fasciculus is damaged for either structural or metabolic reasons, the eyes will not cross the midline.

The motor system examination should focus on involuntary movements suggestive of status epilepticus or myoclonus, which is commonly seen after ischemic-hypoxic events. Decorticate posturing involves flexion of the arms, wrists, and fingers, with extension and internal rotation of the legs, spontaneously or in response to noxious stimuli. This posturing generally indicates that structures below the diencephalon are intact but that damage exists above. Decerebrate posturing, which involves extension and internal rotation of the upper as well as the lower extremities, may indicate dysfunction of the pons and midbrain. These postures,

TABLE 67–2. PROGRESSION OF NEUROLOGIC SIGNS IN CENTRAL TRANSTENTORIAL HERNIATION

Level of Neurologic Deficit	Level of Arousal	Pupillary Response	Oculocephalic/ Oculovestibular Reflex	Respiratory Pattern	Motor Function
Diencephalon	Lethargy, stupor	Small, reactive	Present	Sighs, yawns, Cheyne-Stokes	Semipurposeful, decorticate
Mesencephalon (midbrain)	Coma	Midposition, fixed	Decreased, absent	Tachypneic, hyperpneic	Decerebrate
Pons	Coma	Midposition, fixed	Absent	Eupneic	Decerebrate, flaccid
Myelencephalon (medulla oblongata)	Coma	Midposition, fixed	Absent	Ataxic	Flaccid

together with pupillary responses, oculocephalic or oculovestibular reflexes, and respiratory patterns, have been combined by Plum and Posner (see Recommended Reading) in a diagnostic scheme that allows determination of the progress of central transtentorial herniation (Table 67–2).

Ideally, history-taking and physical examination should help clinicians distinguish structural from metabolic coma and point toward its cause. Blood studies may also help; for example, an elevated osmolality may suggest alcohol intoxication, while other poisonings may be detected on toxicology screens. However, the single most important diagnostic tool is computerized tomography (CT), which can define structural lesions with great precision. Lumbar puncture should not be performed before CT in most patients; concern over the possibility of meningitis may be assuaged by the early empiric use of antibiotics, as discussed in Chapter 74.

MANAGEMENT

Definitive therapy for specific causes of coma cannot be covered here but is discussed in many of the following chapters. The emergency treatment of intracranial hypertension with or without uncal or transtentorial herniation involves the use of hyperventilation, hyperosmolar agents such as mannitol, corticosteroids, and other measures. These are discussed at length in Chapter 77.

OUTCOME

Outcome of coma depends on whether it is structural or metabolic in origin. In general, prognosis in traumatic coma due to diffuse brain disease or focal lesions relates to the patient's age and initial neurologic deficit as quantitated by the GCS. Thus, the majority of elderly patients who present with unreactive pupils within the first 24 hours die or survive in a persistent vegetative state, whereas neurologic improvement can be expected in most younger individuals. The prognosis of metabolic coma is more difficult to establish, owing to the heterogeneity of diseases involved. Patients with drug overdose usually do well, whereas those with ischemic-hypoxic insults do poorly. In general, a survival rate of less than 10 percent is associated with the absence of pupillary, corneal, oculocephalic or oculovestibular, and motor responses to stimulation within the first 24 hours.

RECOMMENDED READING

Caplan LR, Scheiner D: Dysconjugate gaze in hepatic coma. Ann Neurol 8:328, 1980.

Caronna JJ, Finklestein S: Neurological syndromes after cardiac arrest. Stroke 9:517, 1978.

Conomy JP, Swash M: Reversible decerebrate and decorticate postures in hepatic coma. N Engl J Med 278:876, 1968.

Jennett B, Teasdale G, Braakman R, et al: Predicting outcome in individual patients after severe head injury. Lancet 1:1031, 1976.

Keane JR: Ocular skew deviation: analysis of 100 cases. Arch Neurol 32:185, 1975.

Levy DE, Bates D, Caronna JJ, et al: Prognosis in nontraumatic coma. Ann Intern Med 94:293, 1981.

Levy DE, Knill-Jones RP, Plum F: The vegetative state and its prognosis following nontraumatic coma. Ann NY Acad Sci 315:293, 1978.

Newcomer J, Haire W: Coma and thyrotoxicosis. Ann Neurol 14:689, 1983.

Overgaard J, Huid-Hansen O, Land AM, et al: Prognosis after head injury based on early clinical examination. Lancet 2:631, 1973.

Plum F, Posner JE: The Diagnosis of Stupor and Coma. 3rd edition. Philadelphia, F. A. Davis Co., 1980.

Sigsbee B, Plum F: The unresponsive patient: diagnosis and early management. Med Clin North Am 63:813, 1979.

Teasdale G, Jennett B: Assessment of coma and impaired consciousness: a practical scale. Lancet 2:81, 1974.

68. Brain Death

John M. Luce

DEFINITION

Death has traditionally been defined as the end of cardiac and pulmonary function. Although many patients may be dead by these criteria, the development of life-support systems and the feasibility of transplanting organs (including the heart and lungs) has led to the concept that death may also be synonymous with brain death. This term implies the complete and irreversible cessation of all brain functions, including those of the brainstem.

PATHOPHYSIOLOGY

Brain death is due to an absence of flow of oxygenated blood to the brain. It may result from prolonged cerebral ischemia, prolonged cerebral hypoxia, or both mechanisms. One of the most common causes of brain death is cardiopulmonary arrest, which permanently eliminates cerebral blood flow (CBF) unless cardiopulmonary resuscitation is successful.

Brain-dead patients are by definition comatose, that is, unaware of themselves and their environment and unable to respond to external stimuli. Nevertheless, not all comatose patients are brain dead if they manifest CBF. Similarly, although they lack higher cortical functions, patients who are in a chronic vegetative state are not brain dead because their brainstems still function.

The concept of brain death as representing a loss of function of the entire brain, including the brainstem, has been promulgated by the President's Commission for the Study of Ethical Problems in Medicine and Biomedical and Behavioral Research. Its implementation has been endorsed by many medical groups, and approximately 40 states, including California and New York, have adopted brain death statutes. Courts in these and other states have established the ethical legitimacy of monitoring life-support equipment of brain-dead patients. Although it is not legally necessary to establish brain death before removing such equipment from patients who are not likely to benefit medically from further support, many physicians prefer to prove brain death before doing so. Such proof is definitely necessary before organ transplantation.

DIAGNOSIS

A number of criteria for brain death have been devised. Included among them are the Harvard criteria, which require the demonstration of electrocerebral silence on electroencephalograms (EEGs) performed 24 hours apart. Today, the most widely accepted criteria are those of the President's Commission, published in 1981, which require demonstration of the complete and irreversible cessation of brain function. To prove complete cessation, patients must be unresponsive to verbal and painful stimuli (spinal cord reflexes may be present) and must lack pupillary, corneal, oropharyngeal, oculocephalic or oculovestibular, and respiratory reflexes. Moreover, the cause of the patient's coma must be known and be adequate to explain the clinical picture, and drug intoxication, hypothermia (temperature below 32 °C), neuromuscular blockade, and shock must be ruled out. To prove irreversibility, these criteria must be present for an appropriate length of time: 6 hours with a confirmatory isoelectric EEG, 12 hours without an EEG, and 24 hours for brain injury following cardiopulmonary arrest.

Demonstration of absent respiratory reflexes requires apnea testing. The rationale for this test is that in the absence of respiratory depressants, elevation of the arterial carbon dioxide tension ($PaCO_2$) should induce breathing if the brain stem is intact. The average change in $PaCO_2$ in apneic patients whose $PaCO_2$ is normal to begin with (35–45 mm Hg) is 3–6 mm Hg/min. However, the fall in the arterial oxygen tension (PaO_2) is minimal if patients are preoxygenated with 100 percent oxygen (O_2) and are given supplemental O_2 by diffusion during the test.

Prior to apnea testing, a given patient should be shown to not be hypothermic or under the influence of depressant drugs. The patient's family should be told that brain death is likely, that their loved one will be disconnected from the ventilator during the test, and that the patient will not be reattached if apnea is confirmed unless organ transplantation is anticipated. Preoxygenation is then provided for 7 minutes or more, and a PaO_2 greater than 100 mm Hg is demonstrated. Continuous electrocardiographic monitoring is provided. Assuming that the $PaCO_2$ is between 35–45 mm Hg, the patient is disconnected from the ventilator and maintained with a T piece connected to an Ayers bag. The chest and abdomen are exposed, ventilatory efforts are looked for there and with the bag, and arterial blood gases are drawn at least every 5 minutes. The $PaCO_2$ is allowed to reach 70 mm Hg, at which point one of four things happens: (1) the patient displays ventilatory efforts, in which case the ventilator is reattached; (2) the patient displays no ventilatory efforts but develops dysrhythmias or a PaO_2 of less than 60 mm Hg, in which case the ventilator is reattached; (3) the patient displays no ventilatory efforts and is not put back on the ventilator; or (4) the patient displays no ventilatory efforts but is put back on the ventilator pending organ transplantation.

OUTCOME

As noted earlier, brain death is synonymous with death.

RECOMMENDED READING

Eger EI, Severinghaus JW: The rate of rise of $PaCO_2$ in the apneic anesthetized patient. Anesthesiology 22:419, 1961.

Grenvik A, Powner DJ, Snyder JV, et al: Cessation of therapy in terminal illness and brain death. Crit Care Med 6:284, 1978.

Pitts LH, Kaktis J, Caronna J, et al: Brain death, apneic diffusion oxygenation, and organ transplantation. J Trauma 18:180, 1978.

President's Commission for the Study of Ethical Problems in Medical and Biochemical and Behavioral Research. Guidelines for the determination of death. JAMA 246:2184, 1981.

Ropper AH, Kennedy SK, Russell L: Apnea testing in the diagnosis of brain death. Clinical and physiological observations. J Neurosurg 55:942, 1981.

Schafer JA, Caronna JJ: Duration of apnea needed to confirm brain death. Neurology 28:661, 1976.

69. Cerebral Infarction

John M. Luce

John M. Luce

DEFINITION

The term cerebral infarction refers to the death of brain tissue owing to arterial obstruction. Cerebral infarction is therefore differentiated from intracerebral hemorrhage and subarachnoid hemorrhage, the subjects of subsequent chapters. Cerebral infarction accounts for approximately 80 percent of strokes in the United States and, despite the overall decline in cerebrovascular accidents since 1950 in this country, remains a common cause of morbidity and mortality.

PATHOPHYSIOLOGY

Patients with nonhemorrhagic cerebrovascular disease may be divided into four categories that relate to the temporal profile of their symptoms. These categories include: (1) transient ischemic attacks (TIAs)—focal episodes of neurologic dysfunction occurring on a vascular basis that last under 24 hours; (2) reversible ischemic neurologic deficits (RINDs)—focal events that last longer than 24 hours but are resolved within 3 weeks; (3) progressive strokes or strokes-in-evolution—neurovascular events that worsen over time; and (4) completed strokes—fixed neurologic deficits such as cerebral infarction. Progressive strokes may evolve over several hours in the distribution of the carotid artery and over 72 hours in the distribution of the vertebral and basilar arteries. Similarly, completed strokes are defined as those that last for at least 24 hours in the area of the brain supplied by the carotid artery and for 72 hours in the area supplied by the vertebral-basilar system.

In addition to their temporal profile and anatomic features, nonhemorrhagic cerebrovascular events may also be subdivided according to their pathogenesis, as shown in Figure 69–1. Most of these events are thrombotic in nature. The thrombi usually originate in the large neck vessels and may extend into the intracerebral arteries. They consist of platelets, fibrin, and red blood cells that collect on atherosclerotic plaques, often in patients who are hypertensive. Emboli dislodge from these plaques in certain instances, but gradual thrombotic vascular occlusion

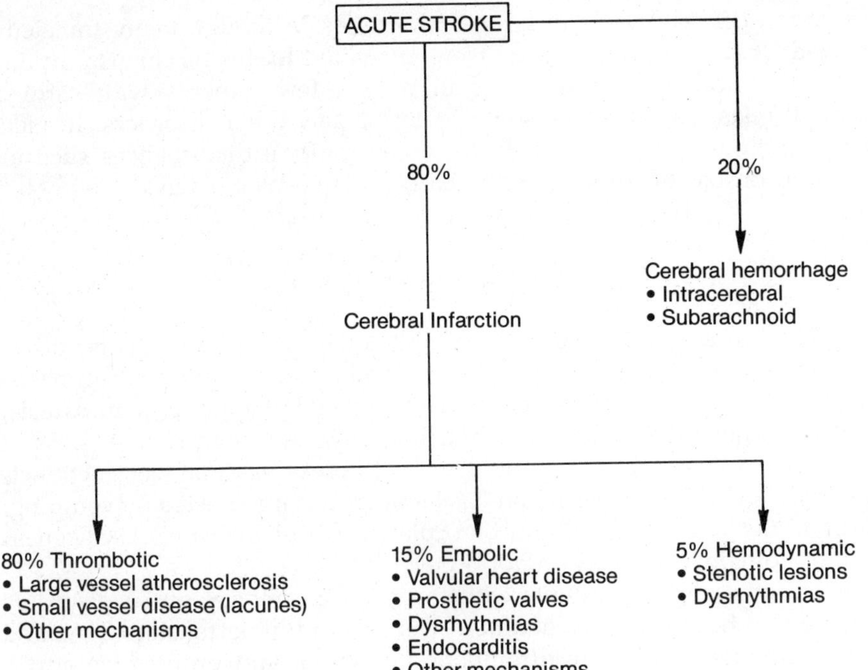

FIGURE 69–1. Subdivision of cerebrovascular events according to pathogenesis. (Adapted, with permission, from Sherman DG, Dyken ML, Fisher M, et al: Cerebral embolism. Chest 89:825, 1986.)

occurs more commonly. Instead of or in addition to large-vessel involvement, some patients suffer small intracerebral vascular occlusions that are called lacunes. Although atherosclerosis and hypertension are important in the pathogenesis of most large and small vessel occlusions, increased coagulability, polycythemia, and vasculitis due either to infection (e.g., syphilis) or to idiopathic causes (e.g., *periarteritis nodosa*) may play a role in certain individuals.

Intracerebral emboli from thrombi in the neck vessels might be considered a form of embolism rather than thrombotic cerebrovascular disease. Nevertheless, the term embolic is generally used to describe clots that emanate from the heart and other extracranial sources. Patients with rheumatic valvular disease, mitral valve prolapse, prosthetic cardiac valves, endocarditis, and myocardial infarction with or without dysrhythmias (especially atrial fibrillation) are the most likely candidates for this condition. Systemic embolism of venous clots or other substances that pass through patent right-to-left intracardiac shunts may also occur.

The third and least common cause of nonhemorrhagic cerebrovascular disease is hemodynamic compromise in patients with stenotic lesions of the large neck vessels or intracerebral arteries. Although many transient or fixed focal neurologic deficits were attributed to this mechanism in the past, it is now known to occur in only a few patients with cardiac dysrhythmias, severe aortic stenosis, and a few other disorders. In fact, such conditions are more likely to cause nonfocal disturbances such as dizziness or loss of consciousness than focal neurologic deficits.

DIAGNOSIS

The clinical manifestations of nonhemorrhagic cerebrovascular disorders relate to their temporal profile, anatomic features, and pathogenesis. Disease of the carotid circulation is characterized by mono- or hemiparesis, aphasia, monocular visual loss, and homonymous hemianopia. Loss of consciousness is rare with carotid events unless vascular obstruction is massive. Disease of the vertebral-basilar system is manifested by vomiting, vertigo, ataxia, dysarthria, and binocular visual disturbance. Drowsiness and loss of consciousness do not occur.

As noted earlier, patients with thrombotic cerebrovascular disorders are likely to have a history of atherosclerosis and hypertension. TIAs and RINDs frequently precede thrombotic infarction, and progressive stroke is also common in this group of patients. In contrast, cerebral embolism usually occurs in patients without atherosclerosis or hypertension but with cardiac disease. TIAs and RINDs are less common in such patients, and stroke is more often sudden than progressive, frequently affecting the distribution of the middle cerebral artery. Finally, hemodynamic compromise from stenotic lesions should be suspected in only a few individuals.

The lumbar puncture is generally normal in patients with cerebral infarction except in cases of infection (e.g., bacterial endocarditis) or vasculitis (e.g., syphilis), in which the pleocytosis and positive VDRL of spinal fluid are diagnostic of infection. Lumbar puncture should therefore be reserved for patients in whom infection or vasculitis is expected and for those in whom intracerebral and subarachnoid hemorrhage have been ruled out. Hemorrhage and ischemic infarction can be differentiated by computerized tomography (CT), which should reveal bland infarction within hours or a few days of an acute nonhemorrhagic event, whereas intracerebral blood should be demonstrated following hemorrhage; CT may be unrevealing in lacunar infarction, however. Cerebral angiography may also be negative in lacunar infarction but should reveal extra- or intracerebral vascular occlusion or stenosis in patients with large-vessel disease. Because CT is so useful, angiography should be used primarily in situations in which it will facilitate the diagnosis (as in vasculitis) or therapy (prior to carotid endarterectomy, for example). Echocardiography should be used to search for an embolic source when cerebral embolism is suspected.

MANAGEMENT

Therapy for cerebral infarction is largely supportive because neurologic deficits, by definition, have already occurred. Such support includes (1) early intubation for patients who cannot protect their airway, (2) administration of oral or intravenous fluids to avoid hyperviscosity, (3) enteral or parenteral nutrition, (4) loading (1 g) and maintenance (300 mg/day) with phenytoin if seizures are present (some clinicians give this drug prophylactically), (5) prevention of deep venous thrombosis and pulmonary embolism with minidose heparin (5000 units subcutaneously BID), (6) treatment of cardiac dysrhythmias if present, and (7) physical therapy to limit contractures. Although severe hypertension probably should be treated, aggressive therapy of mild to moderate hypertension should be avoided to prevent further cerebral ischemia or infarction from occurring.

Full-dose heparin (5000 unit bolus followed by approximately 1000 units/hour to achieve an activated partial thromboplastin time of 2–2½ times control) followed by 3–6 months of Coumadin (dose sufficient to achieve a prothrombin time of 1½–2 times control) has been recommended for patients who have progressive stroke or nonhemorrhagic embolic strokes. However, a recent double-blind trial demonstrated no benefit from anticoagulation in this group, and it can no longer be recommended. Anticoagulation is not effective in thrombotic cerebral infarction and has not been shown to be effective in TIAs or RINDs, although it is often employed in the last two situations. More commonly, patients with TIAs, RINDs, or completed strokes are given oral aspirin, which was first proved to be of benefit in doses of 1300 mg/day. Smaller doses (325 mg) have recently been shown to be equally effective. Some clinicians also add dipyridamole (50 mg or more TID); the benefit of this combination over aspirin alone is uncertain.

A few patients with hemispheric infarction manifest intracranial hypertension and may be candidates for cerebral perfusion pressure monitoring and manipulation, as described in Chapter 77. Nevertheless, hyperventilation with mechanical ventilators, hyperosmolar agents such as mannitol, furosemide and other diuretics, corticosteroids, and barbiturates cannot be routinely recommended. The same is true of systemic vasopressors and cerebral vasodilators.

Carotid endarterectomy has no place in patients with complete cerebral infarctions and may cause perioperative neurologic complications in those with progressive stroke. This procedure may be performed in persons with TIAs and RINDs, although it has not been demonstrated to be superior to medical management in randomized trials. Endarterectomy cannot be easily accomplished in patients with vertebral-basilar disease. Surgical anastomosis of superficial temporal artery and the middle cerebral artery was recently shown not to be beneficial in a large randomized trial.

OUTCOME

The overall mortality from cerebral infarction involving either the carotid or the vertebral-basilar distribution is above 20 percent. The prognosis is worse for patients who present with coma, altered consciousness, or dense hemiplegia with conjugate eye deviation. The prognosis for incomplete nonhemorrhagic cerebrovascular events is less certain. Recent studies suggest that 40 percent of patients with TIAs will suffer a cerebral infarction within 5 years of their first event; the risk is greatest in the first year.

RECOMMENDED READING

Bauer RB, Tellez H: Dexamethasone as treatment in cerebrovascular disease. 2. A controlled study in acute cerebral infarction. Stroke 4:547, 1973.

Buonanno F, Toole JF: Management of patients with established ("completed") cerebral infarction. Stroke 12:7, 1981.

The Canadian Cooperative Study Group: A randomized trial of aspirin and sulfinpyrazone in threatened stroke. N Engl J Med 299:53, 1978.

Christensen MS, Paulson OB, Alexander SC, et al: Cerebral apoplexy (stroke) treated with or without prolonged artificial hyperventilation. 1. Cerebral circulation, clinical course, and cause of death. Stroke 4:568, 1973.

Duke RJ, Bloch RF, Turpie AGG, et al: Intravenous heparin for the prevention of stroke progression in acute partial stable stroke: a randomized controlled trial. Ann Intern Med 105:825, 1986.

The EC/IC Bypass Study Group: Failure of extracranial-intracranial arterial bypass to reduce the risk of ischemic stroke. N Engl J Med 313:1191, 1985.

Fisher CM: Lacunar strokes and infarcts: a review. Neurology 32:871, 1982.

Garraway WM, Whisnant JP, Furlan AJ, et al: The declining incidence of stroke. N Eng J Med 300:449, 1979.

Genton E, Barnett HJM, Fields WS, et al: XIV. Cerebral ischemia: the role of thrombosis and of antithrombotic therapy. Stroke 8:150, 1977.

Jones HR, Millikan CH: Temporal profile (clinical course) of acute carotid system cerebral infarction. Stroke 7:64, 1976.

Jones HR, Millikan CH, Sandok BA: Temporal profile (clinical course) of acute vertebrobasilar system cerebral infarction. Stroke 11:173, 1980.

Sandok BA, Furlan AJ, Whisnant JP, et al: Guidelines for the management of transient ischemic attacks. Mayo Clinic Proc 53:665, 1978.

Sherman DG, Dyken ML, Fisher M, et al: Cerebral embolism. Chest 89:825, 1986.

Smith AL, Hoff JT, Nielsen SL, et al: Barbiturate protection in acute focal cerebral ischemia. Stroke 5:1, 1974.

Yatsu FM: Current concepts of cerebrovascular disease—stroke. Acute medical therapy of stroke. Stroke 13:524, 1982.

70. Intracerebral Hemorrhage

John M. Luce

DEFINITION

Bleeding into the brain parenchyma may be associated with head trauma, intracranial aneurysms, arteriovenous malformations, primary or metastatic brain tumors, cerebral vasculitis, clotting disorders, and anticoagulant therapy. However, the most common underlying cause of spontaneous intracerebral hemorrhage is systemic hypertension. Intracranial hemorrhage accounts for approximately 10 percent of all strokes and is responsible for a high morbidity and mortality.

PATHOPHYSIOLOGY

Intracranial hemorrhage secondary to hypertension happens most frequently in four specific sites: the putamen, the thalamus, the cerebellum, and the pons. Lobar hemorrhage into the subcortical white matter may also occur in hypertensive patients, although the majority of patients with this disorder have a normal blood pressure. In all but lobar bleeding, the most commonly affected vessels are small penetrating arteries at the base of the brain and branches of the basilar artery. Traditional theory has held that microaneurysms in these vessels rupture when exposed to high pressure; an alternate explanation is that fibrinoid necrosis in the vessel walls predisposes to rupture with or without microaneurysm formation.

Once rupture does occur, blood expelled at high pressure damages surrounding brain structure and then tracks along adjacent tissue planes. Over 90 percent of hypertensive hemorrhages enter into the ventricles; rupture into the subarachnoid space is unusual. The physiologic consequence of intracerebral hemorrhage is a loss of cerebral autoregulation that makes cerebral blood flow (CBF) linearly dependent upon cerebral perfusion pressure (CPP), which is the difference between mean arterial pressure (MAP) and intracranial pressure (ICP). Both global and regional CBF may be reduced if MAP is reduced or if ICP becomes elevated,

TABLE 70–1. MANIFESTATIONS OF INTRACEREBRAL HEMORRHAGE

SITE	EYE MOVEMENTS	PUPILS	MOTOR/SENSORY
Putamen	Deviation to side of lesion	Normal	Hemiplegia
Thalamus	Deviation to tip of nose	Small	Hemisensory deficit
Cerebellum	Abnormal conjugate movements	Small	Inability to stand or walk
Pons	Impaired lateral movements	Pinpoint	Quadriplegia

leading to further ischemic tissue damage. Rebleeding is rare; intracranial hematomas are usually resorbed over the subsequent months if the initial rupture is not fatal.

DIAGNOSIS

Like subarachnoid hemorrhage, intracerebral hemorrhage is most often reported in middle-aged persons, especially during activity. Early warning signs of subclinical bleeding do not usually occur, however. Headache may follow intracerebral hemorrhage but may also be absent. Sudden vomiting more often accompanies intracerebral hemorrhage than it does cerebral infarction but is not a universal finding. Of greater importance is the fact that intracerebral hemorrhage more often leads rapidly to coma than does thrombotic or embolic stroke.

The neurologic consequences of intracerebral hemorrhage relate to the site of bleeding (Table 70–1). Putamenal hemorrhage is characterized by progressive hemiplegia with or without sensory loss, accompanied by conjugate deviation of the eyes to the side of the lesion. Classic features of thalamic hemorrhage include hemisensory loss with downward eye deviation. Patients with cerebellar bleeding may manifest eye findings as well as sudden dizziness and inability to stand or walk. Pontine hemorrhage is characterized by coma, quadriplegia, decerebrate rigidity, and pinpoint pupils.

Computerized tomography (CT) is indicated in all patients with suspected intracerebral hemorrhage. This procedure should obviate the need for lumbar puncture, which may cause herniation of brain tissue. If performed, lumbar puncture usually reveals bloody cerebrospinal fluid, although the fluid may be clear. Angiography is usually reserved for patients who are not hypertensive, who have lobar hemorrhage, or who are suspected of having tumors or arteriovenous malformations. Clotting parameters, including the prothrombin time and the activated partial thromboplastic time, should be checked in most patients and are obligatory for those with clotting disorders or for those receiving anticoagulants.

Management

Because intracerebral hemorrhages rarely recur, rigorous "aneurysm precautions" and antifibrinolytic agents such as ε-aminocaproic acid are not indicated in patients with this disorder. They should receive prophylactic anticonvulsants, however, and their CPP should be brought into the normal range or be slightly elevated if it was elevated before hemorrhage occurred. Systemic hypotension should be avoided in patients with intracerebral hemorrhage, and ICP should be reduced by the measures cited in Chapter 77. Such measures include hyperventilation, mannitol, furosemide, and cerebrospinal fluid drainage. Corticosteroids have not been shown to improve the outcome from intracerebral hemorrhage and are not recommended. Vitamin K and fresh frozen plasma should be given if clotting parameters are abnormal, and the platelet count should be kept above 50,000 mm^3.

The place of surgery in managing intracerebral hemorrhage depends largely on the site of bleeding. Many hemorrhages at the base of the brain are too deep to reach, even with microsurgical techniques, and pontine bleeding is rarely approachable. Nevertheless, neurosurgeons may attempt evacuation in patients with lobar and putamenal hemorrhage, especially in those who deteriorate despite medical management. Surgical evacuation may be life saving in patients with large cerebellar hemorrhages that result in significant compression of the brainstem.

Outcome

The prognosis for patients with intracerebral hemorrhage relates to their state of consciousness on admission and the size and accessibility of their lesions. Overall, intracerebral hemorrhage is fatal in some 50 percent of patients. Fortunately, the incidence of this condition has declined in recent years. This decline presumably relates to better identification and control of hypertension in the general population and to the more judicious use of anticoagulants.

RECOMMENDED READING

Brennan RW, Bergland RM: Acute cerebellar hemorrhage: analysis of clinical findings and outcome in 12 cases. Neurology 27:527, 1977.
Cuneo RA, Caronna JJ: The neurologic complications of hypertension. Med Clin North Am 61:565, 1977.
Furlan AJ, Whisnant JP, Elveback LR: The decreasing incidence of primary intracerebral hemorrhage: a population study. Ann Neurol 5:367, 1979.
Herbstein DJ, Schaumburg HH: Hypertensive intracerebral hematoma: an investigation of

the initial hemorrhage and rebleeding using chromium Cr 51-labeled erythrocytes. Arch Neurol 30:412, 1974.

Hier DB, Davis KR, Richardson EP, et al: Hypertensive putamenal hemorrhage. Ann Neurol 1:152, 1977.

Kase CS, Williams JP, Wyatt DA, et al: Lobar intracerebral hematomas: clinical and CT analysis of 22 cases. Neurology 32:1146, 1982.

McCormick WF, Rosenfield DB: Massive brain hemorrhage: a review of 144 cases and an examination of their causes. Stroke 4:946, 1973.

McKinsock W, Richardson A, Taylor J: Primary intracerebral hemorrhage: a controlled trial of surgical and conservative treatment in 180 unselected cases. Lancet 2:221, 1961.

Ojemann RG, Heros RC: Spontaneous brain hemorrhage. Stroke 14:468, 1983.

Ott KH, Kase CS, Ojemann RG, et al: Cerebellar hemorrhage: diagnosis and treatment: a review of 56 cases. Arch Neurol 31:160, 1974.

Paillas JE, Alliez B: Surgical treatment of spontaneous intracerebral hemorrhage: immediate and long-term results in 250 cases. J Neurosurg 39:145, 1973.

Russell RWR: Observations on intracerebral aneurysms. Brain 86:425, 1963.

Silverstein A: Neurological complications of anticoagulation therapy: a neurologist's review. Arch Intern Med 139:217, 1979.

Tellez H, Bauer RB: Dexamethasone as treatment in cerebrovascular disease. 1. A controlled study in intracerebral hemorrhage. Stroke 4:541, 1979.

Walshe TM, Davis KR, Fisher CM: Thalamic hemorrhage: a computed tomographic-clinical correlation. Neurology 27:217, 1977.

71. Subarachnoid Hemorrhage

John M. Luce

John M. Luce

DEFINITION

Blood may enter the subarachnoid space after intracerebral hemorrhage, bleeding from arteriovenous malformations or tumors of the brain or spinal cord, or head trauma. Nevertheless, the most common cause of subarachnoid hemorrhage is rupture of an aneurysm originating from a blood vessel in the subarachnoid space. Subarachnoid hemorrhages account for 10 percent of all cases of stroke; there are approximately 25,000 new cases of subarachnoid hemorrhage in the United States each year.

PATHOPHYSIOLOGY

Intracranial aneurysms may be traumatic, mycotic, or, most commonly, developmental in origin. A developmental etiology is suggested by these facts: (1) aneurysms are found most often among persons, especially women, in the sixth decade of life; (2) aneurysms may occur in association with coarctation of the aorta and polycystic kidney disease; and (3) aneurysms often lack a muscular media and may have a fragmented elastic lamina that indicates degeneration of the vessel wall. Hypertension, which could contribute to developmental changes within aneurysms, is not more prevalent among patients with aneurysms than it is in the general population, although it adversely affects prognosis if it is present.

Aneurysms arise, for the most part, from bifurcations of the major proximal intracranial arteries, especially the internal carotid artery and the anterior communicating arteries. Multiple aneurysms occur in some 20 percent of patients. Aneurysms less than 1 cm in size rarely rupture, whereas those larger than 1 cm are likely to do so eventually. In a minority of patients, rupture leads to massive hemorrhage and swift death. In the majority, bleeding is stopped by surrounding tissue pressure and the formation of a fibrin plug. A number of complications may then ensue.

Perhaps the most feared complication is rebleeding due to fibrinolysis,

TABLE 71–1. CLINICAL GRADING SCALE FOR SUBARACHNOID HEMORRHAGE

GRADE	CRITERIA
I	Asymptomatic or minimal headache and nuchal rigidity
II	Moderate to severe headache; nuchal rigidity; no neurologic deficit other than cranial nerve palsy
III	Drowsy, confused; mild focal deficit
IV	Stuporous; moderate to severe hemiparesis; early decerebrate rigidity
V	Comatose; decerebrate rigidity; moribund appearance

Adapted, with permission, from Hunt WE, Hess RM: J Neurosurg 28:14, 1968.

which occurs in from 25 to 50 percent of patients, most commonly within the first 48 hours after the initial bleed. Equally common and no less potentially catastrophic is cerebral vasospasm, which occurs most often within 7 to 14 days. Vasospasm probably relates to the initial deposition of blood in the subarachnoid space around the circle of Willis and to the release of vasoactive mediators that constrict the proximal intracerebral vessels. Autoregulation of cerebral blood flow (CBF) then is lost, and both global and regional CBF is decreased, causing ischemia and infarction.

Other complications of subarachnoid hemorrhage include cerebral edema and intracranial hypertension, which may retard bleeding but may also displace tissue and reduce CBF. Intracerebral hematoma with tissue bleeding is reported in a few patients with subarachnoid hemorrhage, as are seizures. Irritation of the hypothalmus by blood may lead either to diabetes insipidus or to antidiuretic hormone release. Communicating hydrocephalus may result from the presence of blood in the subarachnoid space, which blocks cerebrospinal fluid absorption by the arachnoid villi.

DIAGNOSIS

Premonitory symptoms such as mild headache may occur before major rupture in many patients with intracranial aneurysms. However, few patients seek medical attention for these symptoms and instead present with acute manifestations of subarachnoid hemorrhage: headache that is classically described as the worst ever experienced, neck and back pain, nausea and vomiting, third nerve palsy (due to compression of this nerve by internal carotid-posterior communicating artery aneurysms), drowsiness, confusion, or coma. Physical examination may reveal nuchal rigidity and focal neurologic deficits; these findings and the presenting symptoms can be combined into a clinical grading scale outlined in Table 71–1. Computerized tomography (CT) should reveal subarachnoid blood and obviate the need for a lumbar puncture. Cerebral angiography is necessary to visualize the presence of single or multiple aneurysms.

Neurologic deterioration that occurs after the diagnosis of subarachnoid hemorrhage may be due to extension of the initial insult, rebleeding, vasospasm, or other problems. Timing of the deterioration may help in differentiating these processes, in that rebleeding is most common shortly after initial hemorrhage, and spasm usually takes several days. Furthermore, intracerebral hemorrhage and vasospasm often cause focal defects, whereas the effects of rebleeding and intracranial hypertension are more generalized. Nevertheless, repeat CT and/or angiography are frequently required to determine the exact cause—or causes—of deterioration.

MANAGEMENT

Traditional management of patients with subarachnoid hemorrhage who survive until hospitalization has centered on "aneurysm precautions" to reduce the risk of rebleeding. These precautions include residence in a dark, quiet room; limitation of such stimuli as visitors or television; the administration of sedatives and antihypertensive agents such as propranolol or hydralazine; and the use of prophylactic phenytoin (1000 mg oral loading dose; thereafter, 300 mg/day) to prevent seizures. Many clinicians also give antifibrinolytic agents such as ϵ-aminocaproic acid in doses of 1.5–2.0 g/hr for 48 hours or longer. The reduction in rebleeding achieved with this drug must be balanced against the increased risk of deep venous thrombosis, pulmonary embolism, cerebral ischemia, and hydrocephalus.

The prevention and treatment of cerebral vasospasm involve maintaining normal and even increased CBF by raising cerebral perfusion pressure (CPP) and reducing cerebrovascular resistance. Mean arterial pressure (MAP) and intracranial pressure (ICP), the two components of CPP, should be monitored and manipulated by the techniques described in Chapter 77. Many clinicians raise MAP by infusing crystalloid, colloid, or volume expanders to maintain a central venous pressure in the range of 15 mm Hg. ICP can be reduced by hyperventilation, by intravenous mannitol and furosemide, or by drainage of cerebrospinal fluid through a ventriculostomy that is also used for monitoring ICP. Such drainage is also recommended for hydrocephalus, which usually resolves within a few days to a week after bleeding. Corticosteroids are of no proven value in this condition.

The most popular approach to reducing cerebrovascular resistance involves the intravenous administration of isoproterenol (1.5 mg/kg/hr), a β-adrenergic agent that dilates vascular smooth muscle by increasing adenyl cyclase and cyclic AMP levels; and aminophylline (1 mg/kg/hr), which elevates cyclic AMP by phosphodiesterase inhibition. Calcium channel blockers such as nimodipine (0.35–0.7 mg/kg q 4 h) may also be useful, although experience is limited with these agents.

The definitive therapy of intracranial aneurysms is clipping or surgical obliteration, which usually is attempted in patients in Grades I–III (Table 71–1). Surgery was formerly delayed for 7–14 days for patients in these groups, owing to unacceptable preoperative morbidity and mortality rates that were attributed to poor surgical technique and cerebral vasospasm. However, with the advent of microsurgery technology and better understanding of vasospasm, many clinicians today advocate early surgery. This approach has the advantage of limiting recurrent hemorrhage and allowing the patients to tolerate the increased CBF that is thought to prevent vasospasm.

Outcome

The outcome of patients with subarachnoid hemorrhage who reach the hospital alive depends on their clinical grade (Table 71–1). If surgery is delayed, approximately 10 percent will die before it is performed. Surgical mortality is approximately 5 percent; immediate complications relate primarily to the size and location of the aneurysm. Another 25–35 percent of patients will die or fail to improve in the next 6 months, often owing to vasospasm. Despite refinements in the management of subarachnoid hemorrhage, the overall prognosis of patients with this condition has not significantly changed.

RECOMMENDED READING

Adams HP, Kassell NF, Torner JC, et al: Early management of aneurysmal subarachnoid hemorrhage: a report of the Cooperative Aneurysm Study. J Neurosurg 54:141, 1981.

Allen GS, Ahn HS, Preziosi TJ, et al: Cerebral arterial spasm—a controlled trial of nimodipine in patients with subarachnoid hemorrhage. N Engl J Med 308:619, 1983.

Artiola I, Fortuny L, Prieto-Valiente L: Long-term prognosis in surgically treated intracranial aneurysms. Part 1: Mortality. J Neurosurg 54:26, 1981.

Artiola I, Fortuny L, Prieto-Valiente L: Long-term prognosis in surgically treated intracranial aneurysms. Part 2: Morbidity. J Neurosurg 54:35, 1981.

Crowell RM, Zervas NT: Management of intracranial aneurysm. Med Clin North Am 63:695, 1979.

Fleischer AS, Tindall GT: Cerebral vasospasm following aneurysm rupture: a protocol for therapy and prophylaxis. J Neurosurg 52:149, 1980.

Heros RC, Zervas NT: Subarachnoid hemorrhage. Annu Rev Med 34:367, 1983.

Hunt WE, Hess RM: Surgical risk related to time of intervention in the repair of intracranial aneurysms. J Neurosurg 28:14, 1968.

Kassell NF, Torner JC, Adams HP: Antifibrinolytic therapy in the acute period following aneurysmal subarachnoid hemorrhage: preliminary observations from the Cooperative Aneurysm Study. J Neurosurg 61:225, 1984.

McCormick WF, Noefzinger JD: Saccular intracranial aneurysms: an autopsy study. J Neurosurg 22:155, 1977.

Stehbens WE: Ultrastructure of aneurysms. Arch Neurol 32:798, 1975.

Sundt TM, Whisnant JP: Subarachnoid hemorrhage from intracranial aneurysms: surgical management and history of disease. N Engl J Med 299:116, 1978.

Whisnant JP, Phillips LH, Sundt TM: Aneurysmal subarachnoid hemorrhage: timing of surgery and mortality. Mayo Clin Proc 57:471, 1982.

Wiebers DO, Whisnant JP, O'Fallon WM: The natural history of unruptured intracranial aneurysms. N Engl J Med 304:696, 1981.

72. Spinal Cord Injury

John M. Luce

Definition

Spinal cord injuries are of two types: (1) traumatic injury, which usually results from motor vehicle accidents, falls, and sports-related trauma; and (2) nontraumatic cord compression, which is caused most often by metastatic tumors, protruding intervertebral discs, epidural abscesses, or hematomas. Traumatic injury is much more common, rendering approximately 12,000 Americans acutely quadriplegic or paraplegic each year.

Pathophysiology

In general, the dura and arachnoid that invest the cord and the anterior and posterior spinal arteries that nourish it remain intact after spinal cord trauma unless transection occurs. However, even with minor cord injury, the small intramedullary vessels may be damaged, leading to hyperemia and hemorrhage in the central gray matter of the cord. As the hemorrhages coalesce, platelet thrombi accumulate in the injured vessels, and water and protein extravasate from them. Norepinephrine and other vasoactive mediators may accumulate in the spinal cord during this period and produce ischemia. Microangiopathic studies of experimental cord injury reveal necrosis of the central gray matter within 4 hours of trauma; vasogenic edema then spreads into the surrounding white matter, whose microvasculature remains normal, although neuronal and axonal degeneration become manifested by 8 hours. Neurologic recovery cannot be expected once necrosis has occurred.

Nontraumatic spinal cord compression is caused by tumors and other processes that originate in the extradural or epidural space. Extradural metastases from primary neoplasms of the lung, breast, and lymphatic tissue usually invade the vertebral bodies first and then push against the dura in the spinal canal. Epidural metastases from these and other primary tumors may grow directly into the spinal cord. Unlike spinal cord trauma, which frequently involves the cervical cord, metastatic tumors most often compromise the thoracic cord. Cord involvement may be the initial

436

manifestation of the primary lesion and can progress rapidly, causing permanent disability in a matter of hours.

The respiratory complications of spinal cord injury depend on the initial level of cord involvement, the completeness of the lesion, and the degree of recovery over time. Severe damage to cord segments C3 to C5 involves the phrenic nerve nuclei and causes partial or complete bilateral hemidiaphragmatic paralysis. Intercostal and abdominal muscle functions also cease, and patients inspire only with their accessory muscles (Fig. 72–1). As a result, acute high cervical quadriplegics are unable to generate an adequate vital capacity during inspiration. They therefore manifest ventilatory failure with a high arterial carbon dioxide tension ($PaCO_2$) and a low arterial oxygen tension (PaO_2) shortly after injury. Hypercapnia and hypoxemia frequently worsen when these patients breathe spontaneously in the supine position, because their abdominal contents force their flaccid hemidiaphragms cephalad.

Low quadriplegic patients whose phrenic nerve nuclei are completely or partially intact can contract their hemidiaphragms to a greater or lesser extent. Nevertheless, they usually lack the intercostal muscle activity necessary to stabilize the rib cage so that the hemidiaphragms can function properly. Furthermore, because they lack abdominal muscle tone, their hemidiaphragms do not contract from the steeply domed position in which their fiber length–tension relationship is optimized (Fig. 72–2); thus, vital capacity will be diminished. This diminution is usually most pronounced when the patient sits up and the hemidiaphragm is not supported by the abdominal contents; it is minimized when the patient is supine.

Paraplegic patients generally maintain hemidiaphragmatic function and also have intact intercostal muscles above the level of their spinal cord injury. However, they may manifest the same lack of abdominal muscle activity as quadriplegics if they have thoracic lesions. Depending on the extent of abdominal muscle involvement, paraplegics may exhibit impaired hemidiaphragmatic performance and a reduced vital capacity and ability to increase minute ventilation. Their lack of abdominal muscle activity, especially when coupled with intercostal muscle dysfunction, prevents paraplegic patients and those with higher lesions from developing the positive airway pressures necessary to expel mucus. Their inadequate cough is responsible in turn for retained secretions and recurrent respiratory infections.

Experimental studies suggest that the immediate cardiovascular response to acute spinal cord trauma is a transient period of hypertension related to sympathetic discharge. This discharge may be sufficient to cause neurogenic pulmonary edema by increasing intravascular hydrostatic pressure, forcing blood into the central circulation, and increasing pulmonary microvascular permeability. Although hypertension may occur

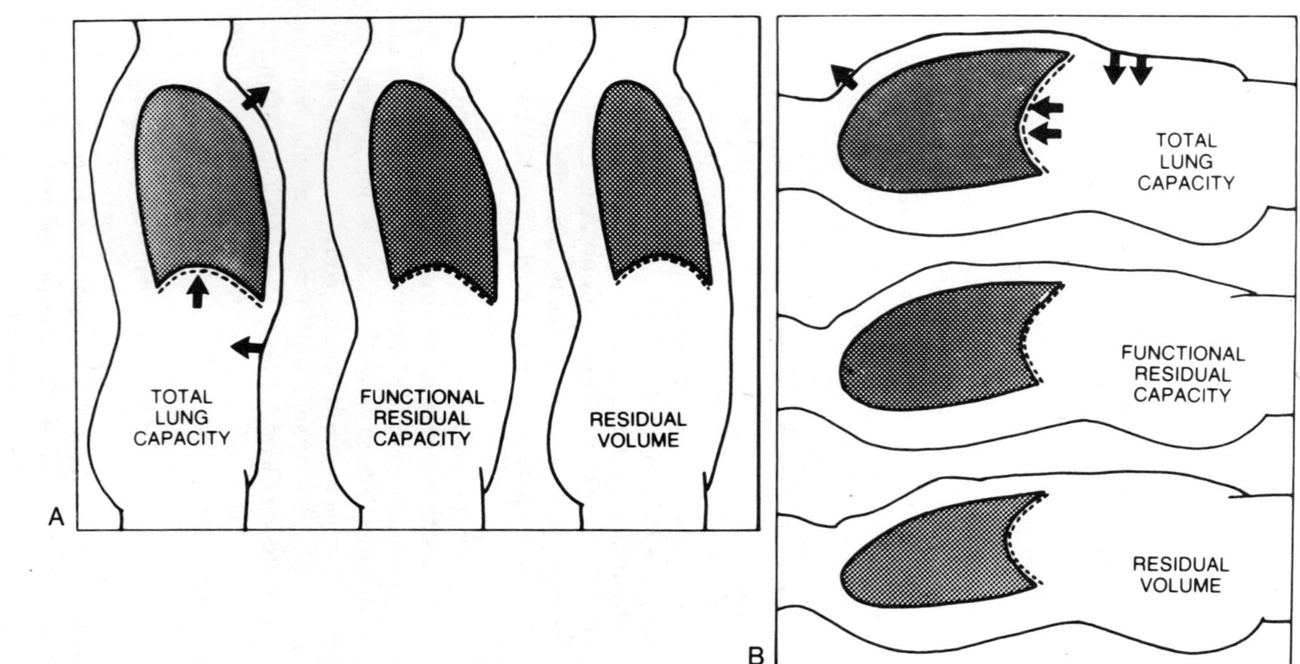

FIGURE 72–1. Breathing patterns in the upright (A) and supine (B) positions in patients with high cervical cord lesions. Because the phrenic and intercostal nerves do not function, patients inspire from functional residual capacity only with their accessory respiratory muscles, and only their upper rib cage moves outward (arrow). This produces a reduced total lung capacity. The situation is worsened in the supine position. Because the abdominal nerves do not function, active expiration is limited, and the patients have a high residual volume. (Adapted, with permission, from Luce JM, Tyler ML, Pierson DJ: Intensive Respiratory Care. Philadelphia, W. B. Saunders Co., 1984, p. 69.)

438

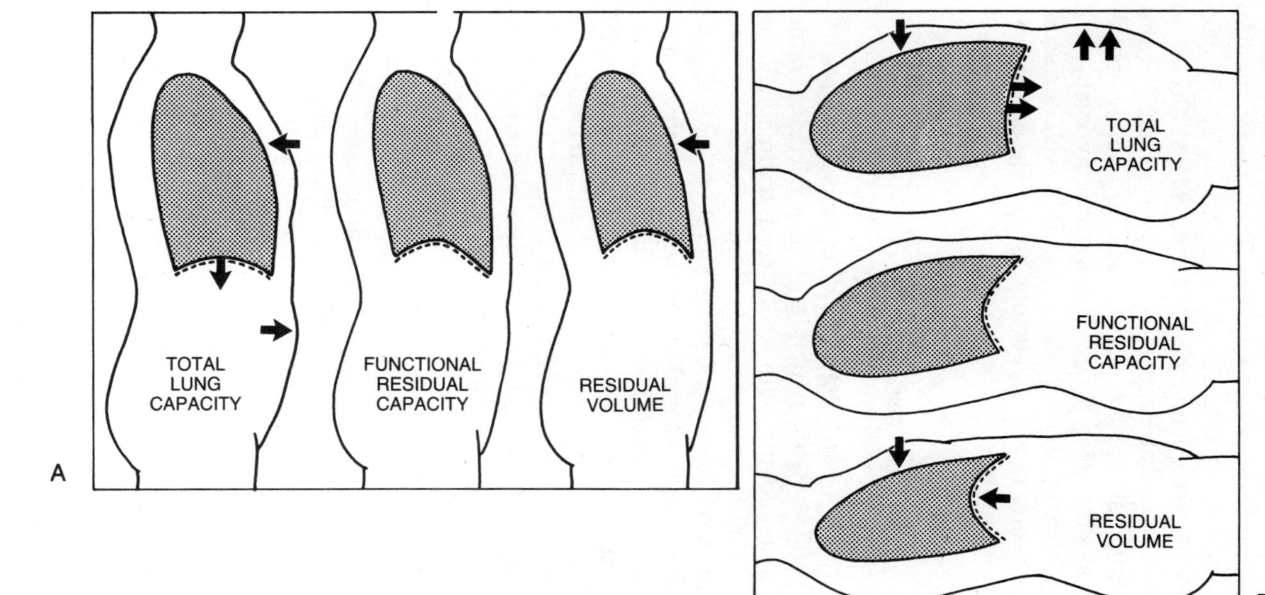

FIGURE 72–2. Breathing patterns in the upright (A) and supine (B) positions with low cervical cord lesions. Because the phrenic nerve functions, patients inspire reasonably well from functional residual capacity. They therefore achieve a total lung capacity that is near normal and is limited only by a lack of abdominal and internal muscle contraction. Inspiration is aided in the supine position, when the abdominal contents force the hemidiaphragms into a domed position from which they contract more effectively. Expiration to residual volume is limited by the lack of abdominal muscles. (Reproduced, with permission, from Luce JM, Tyler ML, Pierson DJ: Intensive Respiratory Care. Philadelphia, W. B. Saunders Co., 1984, p. 67.)

immediately after spinal cord trauma, most patients have hypotension due to increased venous capacitance by the time they reeive medical assistance. Bradycardia progressing occasionally to heart block and poikilothermy (in patients with complete lesions above T1) sufficient to reduce the core temperature several degrees centigrade are part of this picture, which is called spinal shock. Because of their autonomic insufficiency, patients with spinal shock may become profoundly hypotensive if positioned upright. When supine, they appear warm and well perfused, and their systolic blood pressure rarely falls below 70 mm Hg unless they are bleeding from concurrent injuries.

Diagnosis

Spinal cord trauma should be suspected in all unconscious patients, including head-injured patients who exhibit muscular flaccidity rather than reflex posturing. Most patients with acute cord trauma who are conscious can testify to numbness and paralysis. When these symptoms are present or patients are unconscious, the spine should be immobilized as the physical examination and diagnostic studies are performed. A complete physical examination is mandatory in all patients with known or suspected spinal cord trauma, because associated injuries occur in 25–60 percent of such individuals. Diagnostic studies should include plain cervical spine roentgenograms with a lateral vertical view with the shoulder pulled down. Computerized tomography (CT) adds additional information and should be performed if available. Sensory-evoked potentials, discussed in Chapter 75, may also be used to determine the extent and location of nervous system injury.

Patients with nontraumatic spinal cord compression usually present with progressive pain, weakness, sensory loss, and autonomic dysfunction, in that order. The pain frequently increases when these patients are recumbent. Unfortunately, because of the fact that autonomic dysfunction occurs last, a majority of patients with metastatic cord involvement are diagnosed only when their bladder or bowel function is impaired. Roentgenograms of the spine may reveal bony lesions in such patients. Conventional myelography or CT with metrizamide may demonstrate impaired or absent flow of subarachnoid contrast material.

Management

Although immobilization must be maintained, patients with spinal cord trauma may require an artificial airway if they are not ventilating, cannot manage their secretions, or are comatose. Most patients can be intubated by the blind nasotracheal method or by direct laryngoscopy without unduly extending the neck. Alternatively, intubation may be accomplished by advancing the endotracheal tube over a fiberoptic laryngoscope or bronchoscope. Emergency tracheostomy is rarely required and may interfere with anterior spinal fusion. Unless such fusion is anticipated, however, early tracheostomy should be considered in patients who are likely to need prolonged mechanical support. Tracheostomy facilitates eating, talking (through devices that direct airflow cephalad through the vocal cords) and tracheopulmonary toilet, and increases patient comfort.

Intubated patients who can maintain normal ventilation should probably receive supplemental oxygen with or without small amounts of continuous positive airway pressure, in order to prevent microatelectasis. Patients whose $PaCO_2$ is elevated during spontaneous breathing are candidates for intermittent positive-pressure ventilation with or without positive end-expiratory pressure. There is no indication that any particular ventilatory mode (e.g., intermittent mechanical [mandatory] ventilation) is inherently superior for such patients. Nevertheless, patients whose ventilatory reserve is severely limited should probably not receive intermittent mechanical ventilation at a low ventilatory rate. This provision is especially applicable at night, when hypoventilation may worsen.

Patients with high cord injuries usually need assistance in clearing secretions. Quad coughing, in which one pushes forcefully on the abdomen, is useful in generating the positive airway pressure necessary to expel mucus. Intubated patients may be helped to cough in this fashion or can be suctioned gently through the endotracheal tube after the intravenous administration of atropine, if necessary, to prevent severe bradycardia or heart block. The sputum obtained by suctioning should be Gram-stained and examined under the microscope to determine changes in bacterial flora. Antibiotics should be administered promptly on the basis of Gram-stain results in the presence of fever, leukocytosis, and infiltrates on the chest roentgenogram. Prophylactic antibiotics should be avoided to prevent the emergence of more resistant microorganisms. Full-dose heparin is indicated for deep venous thrombosis and pulmonary embolism; some authors recommend low-dose heparin to prevent these conditions.

The autonomic lability of patients with spinal cord injury dictates that vasoactive drugs and those affecting the heart be used sparingly. This provision applies equally to anesthetic agents. Sympathetic deficiency or excess should be treated with the infusion of direct-acting vasoconstrictors such as Neo-Synephrine, vasodilators such as nitroprusside, cardiac stimulants such as isoproterenol, and depressants such as propranolol, rather than adrenergic agonists or antagonists that might indirectly alter catechol concentrations. Succinylcholine and other depolarizing agents should not be used during the first 6 months after spinal cord injury, to avoid hyperkalemic crises.

Although opinions vary, most investigators agree that fluid and blood replacement should be limited in patients with spinal shock, to avoid potentiation of pulmonary edema. The sensitivity of patients with spinal cord injury to fluids, drugs, and the stress of hospitalization suggests the desirability of close hemodynamic monitoring. Such monitoring may be limited to frequent checking of vital signs in some patients, but others require systemic and pulmonary artery catheters. Pulmonary artery catheters should be inserted as soon as possible in unstable patients. Intracranial pressure monitoring is indicated in patients with concurrent head injury. The high incidence of significant poikilothermy in patients with spinal cord injury above T1 underscores the importance of temperature support and monitoring. A nasogastric tube should be passed as soon as possible after trauma and should be maintained in place until gastrointestinal atony is resolved. The urinary bladder should be catheterized, and urine output should be followed.

A variety of drugs and procedures, including spinal cord cooling, have been used to maintain the cord microcirculation after spinal cord trauma, but none of these has been proven effective. This is not the case with metastatic lesions, which generally respond to corticosteroids (10–50 mg dexamethasone initially, followed by lesser doses on a QID schedule) and perhaps to mannitol. Decompressive laminectomy and other kinds of surgery are rarely performed on patients with spinal cord trauma unless the cord is impinged upon by bony fragments, and a return of neurologic function is anticipated following their removal. Radiation therapy is also preferred to surgery in patients with nontraumatic cord compression by known primary malignancies. However, surgical decompression may be chosen if the primary lesion is not known, if patients have not responded to irradiation, or if another process such as epidural abscess or hematoma is suspected.

OUTCOME

Unfortunately, irreversible neurologic damage has frequently occurred before the diagnosis of traumatic or nontraumatic spinal cord injury is made. By that time, patients with permanent deficits are usually suffering from infections of the lungs or urinary bladder, depending on the level and nature of their lesions. Meticulous respiratory care and intermittent, rather than continuous, bladder catheterization can help keep these complications to a minimum.

RECOMMENDED READING

Bosch A, Stauffer ES, Nickel VL: Incomplete traumatic quadriplegia: a ten-year review. JAMA 216:473, 1971.

DeTroyer A, Heilporn A: Respiratory mechanics in quadriplegia: the respiratory function of the intercostal muscles. Am Rev Respir Dis 122:591, 1980.

Eidelberg EE: Cardiovascular response to experimental spinal cord compression. J Neurosurg 38:326, 1973.

Fairholm DJ, Turnbull IM: Microangiographic study of experimental spinal cord injuries. J Neurosurg 35:277, 1971.

Feuer H: Management of acute spine and spinal cord injuries. Arch Surg 3:638, 1976.

Gilbert H: Neoplastic epidural spinal cord compression: a current prospective. JAMA 241:2771, 1978.

Ledsome JR, Sharp JM: Pulmonary function in acute cervical cord injury. Am Rev Respir Dis 124:41, 1981.

Livingston KE, Perrin RG: The neurosurgical management of spinal metasteses causing cord and *cauda equina* compression. J Neurosurg 49:339, 1978.

Luce JM: Medical management of spinal cord injury. Crit Care Med 13:126, 1985.

McKinley AC, Auchincloss KH, Gilbert R, et al: Pulmonary function, ventilatory control, and respiratory complications in quadriplegic subjects. Am Rev Respir Dis 100:526, 1969.

Mullins GM, Flynn SPG, El-Mahde AN, et al: Malignant lymphoma of the spinal epidural space. Ann Intern Med 74:416, 1971.

Perot PL: The clinical use of somatosensory-evoked potentials in acute spinal cord injury. Clin Neurosurg 20:367, 1973.

Silver JR, Gibbon NOK: Prognosis in tetraplegia. Br Med J 4:79, 1968.

Silver JR, Moulton A: Prophylactic anticoagulant therapy against pulmonary emboli in acute paraplegia. Br Med J 2:338, 1973.

73. Head Trauma

John M. Luce

Definition

Head trauma is of two types: closed head injury, in which the cranial vault remains intact; and open head injury, in which the brain is exposed. Of the two, closed head injury is much more common owing to the strength of the skull. Although closed head injury may produce little more than a transient loss of consciousness, more severe insults are the most common cause of disability and death among trauma patients, particularly those under 50 years of age.

Pathophysiology

Two kinds of damage result from head injury: primary damage, attributable to the trauma itself, and secondary damage, related to expanding mass lesions and brain swelling, displacement of brain tissue caused by increased intracranial pressure (ICP), and concomitant or late ischemic, hypoxic, metabolic, and infectious abnormalities. The basic mechanism of primary brain damage is believed to be cerebral concussion, in which rotational shear forces following abrupt acceleration or deceleration disrupt axons and myelin sheaths. The shear forces are maximal at the brain surface, minimal at its center, and intensified where the brain is exposed to bony or dural protrusions such as those at the frontal and temporal tips. The forces therefore cause a centripetal pattern of nerve fiber injury that affects subcortical structures only after the cortex is involved.

Focal injuries may occur alone or in concert with concussion. Such injuries include cerebral contusion, which is characterized by subpial and intracerebral extravasation of blood, and cerebral laceration, in which the pia mater is torn. Contusion and laceration may occur under areas of extreme impact and most often involve the frontal and temporal poles. However, they may also accompany penetrating injuries such as stab, puncture, or missile wounds that damage deeper brain structures.

Brain swelling is a common secondary consequence of diffuse brain injury. In adults, the swelling is usually attributed to vasogenic edema,

444

which presumably results from increased permeability of the cerebral microvasculature caused by a brief increase of blood flow to the brain immediately following injury. Cerebral blood flow (CBF) usually decreases in adults following the initial surge of blood, in part owing to cerebral vasospasm. In children and adolescents, however, CBF usually remains elevated following severe head trauma and accounts for much, if not all, of the brain swelling.

Secondary brain injury may involve expanding mass lesions in addition to generalized swelling of the brain. Epidural hematomas most often arise from temporal skull fractures that are associated with lacerations of the middle meningeal artery. By contrast, subdural bleeding usually emanates from small cerebral veins bridging the cortex and the superior sagittal sinus, especially in the frontal region. Intracerebral hematomas may result from penetrating injuries or other conditions in which great force is applied to a small area of the brain. Abscesses and empyema also may follow penetrating injuries or depressed skull fractures.

As is the case with brain swelling, expanding mass lesions injure the brain largely by increasing ICP. Shortly after hospital admission, ICP is increased above the normal level of 10 mm Hg in more than 80 percent of patients with severe head trauma, and it is almost invariably elevated in those with rapidly expanding mass lesions. ICP increases when the volume of one or more of the intracranial components (water, blood, solids, or cerebrospinal fluid [CSF]) increase without a commensurate decrease in another component. When new lesions are not present, ICP generally reaches its zenith some 2 to 3 days after head trauma, a point at which cerebral swelling is most severe.

Intracranial hypertension damages the brain by compressing, distorting, and displacing tissue. The latter effect is seen most dramatically during transtentorial herniation, when ICP rises on the cephalad side of the tentorial notch and forces brain structures caudad because pressure is lower on that side. During the descent, compression of the brainstem and the third nerve by the temporal lobe is responsible for a combination of ipsilateral oculomotor nerve paresis, contralateral hemiparesis progressing to decerebrate rigidity, and altered level of consciousness. Ventilatory irregularities that culminate in apnea and marked hypertension with or without bradycardia (called the hypertensive or Cushing response) result from increased pressure in the posterior fossa with medullary dysfunction.

Another important consequence of intracranial hypertension is a global reduction in CBF. CBF is directly proportional to the cerebral perfusion pressure (CPP) and inversely proportional to the cerebral vascular resistance (CVR). When autoregulation is impaired, owing to brain injury, and CVR does not vary, CBF is dependent entirely upon CPP. The cerebral perfusion pressure is equal to mean arterial pressure (MAP), the inflow pressure, minus ICP, which resembles pressure in the cerebral veins and therefore can be used as the effective outflow pressure. Studies have demonstrated that CBF decreases significantly when ICP exceeds 40 mm Hg under experimental circumstances; assuming a normal MAP of 90 mm Hg, this ICP rise would produce a CPP of 50 mm Hg. A poor outcome from head trauma is associated with a CPP of 60 mm Hg or less.

Intracranial hypertension may be associated with hypoxemia in some patients. This is rarely due to hypoventilation, because most patients without medullary depression manifest a normal or reduced $PaCO_2$. Occasionally, hypoxemia correlates with ICP and can be attributed to neurologic pulmonary edema, which probably results from transient increases in pulmonary blood flow and microvascular permeability related to the Cushing response. Nevertheless, neurogenic pulmonary edema should usually be considered a diagnosis of exclusion, and other causes of hypoxemia such as pneumonia, gastric aspiration, and overly vigorous fluid resuscitation should be ruled out.

Diagnosis

The initial evaluation of head-injured patients is essential in determining the extent of damage to the brain and to other vital organs, in directing treatment, and in estimating prognosis. However, thorough history-taking and physical examination should not be performed until the cervical spine is immobilized, the airway is protected, bleeding is controlled, seizures are treated, arterial blood gases are drawn, a naso-gastric tube and bladder catheter are passed, and ventilation is supported if necessary.

The examination of head-injured patients should focus on their level of consciousness, pupillary size and reaction to light, corneal reflexes, oculomotor function (usually determined by oculovestibular rather than oculocephalic testing, owing to the possibility of spinal cord damage), condition of retinal vessels, gag reflex, cough reflex, rectal tone, and pattern of ventilation. In addition to noting these variables, it may be helpful to categorize patients by means of the Glascow Coma Scale (GCS), which is based on their best level of eye opening and verbal and motor responses.

Patients with signs of tentorial herniation may be candidates for exploratory bur holes at this stage in their evaluation. However, if time permits and proper facilities are available, diagnostic roentgenographic studies should be performed. These should usually include cervical spinal views and a chest roentgenogram. Plain skull roentgenograms were once taken routinely in trauma patients, but computerized tomography (CT) can visualize brain structures in addition to the skull. Angiography may be used if CT is not available or if additional information is required.

MANAGEMENT

The surgical management of head trauma is directed toward recognition and removal of mass lesions responsible for increasing ICP. Such lesions are found in up to 40 percent of severely head-injured patients and are specially likely to be present if ICP is markedly elevated. Although evacuation of mass lesions may restore the ICP to normal levels, a large number of patients continue to maintain or develop intracranial hypertension. Thus, in many patients, the ICP must be reduced by medical means.

Specific measures to monitor and manipulate ICP are covered in Chapter 77. Beyond these measures, the medical management of head injury is intended to insure systemic and cerebral homeostatis. From a cardiovascular standpoint, this means that MAP should be maintained in the normal range so that CPP does not fall near the critical level of 50–60 mm Hg or rise to such an extent that CBF is greatly increased. Fluids or vasopressors may be used to support MAP if necessary. Alternatively, MAP may be lowered by vasodilators in the occasional hypertensive patient. MAP should be lowered with extreme caution, however, because an elevated MAP may reflect chronic hypertension or the hypertensive response to brainstem ischemia.

From a respiratory standpoint, airway protection is the first priority. Mechanical ventilation should also be instituted in hypercapneic patients because the elevated $PaCO_2$ may dilate cerebral vessels and increase CBF. Hypoxemia should be corrected by supplemental O_2 with the addition of positive end-expiratory pressure (PEEP) if necessary to avoid O_2 toxicity, despite the fact that PEEP may compromise venous return. The ideal PaO_2 is uncertain in head-injury patients, but, generally, it should exceed 100 mm Hg to avoid cerebral tissue hypoxia during hyperventilation therapy.

Measures to insure cerebral homeostatis include the administration of metabolic substrates and the normalization or reduction of cerebral metabolic needs. All patients in coma should receive 100 mm Hg of thiamine and 0.4 mg of naloxone as soon as possible; dextrose should be added if hypoglycemia is demonstrated. Adequate nutrition is essential thereafter; caloric intake should be greater than the basal needs of 25 cal/kg/day to offset the stress of injury. Cerebral metabolic needs can be normalized by the therapeutic or prophylactic administration of phenytoin (loading, 1 g; maintenance, 300 mg/day) to abolish seizures, the administration of antipyretics and appropriate antibiotics to treat fever, and the use of sedatives and muscle relaxants to reduce agitation. The latter agents are discussed in Chapter 78.

Outcome

Two important questions related to the issue of outcome from head trauma are (1) How can outcome be predicted? and (2) Is it altered by medical intervention? Regarding the first question, studies have demonstrated that the initial clinical evaluation focusing on level of consciousness, motor behavior, and pupillary reflexes is most predictive of recovery from blunt head trauma. The GCS was introduced, in part, to facilitate prognostication on the basis of early physical examination, and it is accurate in 80 percent of patients. Other clinical aspects, such as decerebrate rigidity, are also important indicators of outcome. Age appears to be most important, however, in that children and adolescents frequently recover from severe head trauma despite decerebrate rigidity. Indeed, the death rate from head trauma in an unselected pediatric population should be as low as 33 percent or less.

That initial clinical evaluation alone is highly predictive of outcome following head trauma suggests that morbidity and mortality cannot be greatly influenced by therapy. This conclusion is supported by the uniform death rate of 50 percent among head-injured patients, most of them adults, in three countries with different care systems and management details. In marked contrast, some American investigators have claimed that aggressive head injury management has lowered mortality to 30 percent. An intermediate viewpoint would be that clinical outcome depends on both the degree of initial damage and recognition and management of treatable injuries.

RECOMMENDED READING

Becker DP, Miller JD, Ward JD, et al: The outcome from severe head injury with early diagnosis and intensive management. J Neurosurg 47:491, 1977.

Berger MS, Pitts LH, Lovely M, et al: Outcome from severe head injury in children and adolescents. J Neurosurg 62:194, 1985.

Bruce DA, Alavi A, Bilaniuk L, et al: Diffuse cerebral swelling following head injuries in children: the syndrome of "malignant brain edema." J Neurosurg 54:170, 1981.

Bruce DA, Gennarelli TA, Langfitt TW: Resuscitation from coma due to head injury. Crit Care Med 6:254, 1978.

Bruce DA, Langfitt TW, Miller JD, et al: Regional blood flow, intracranial pressure, and brain metabolism in comatose patients. J Neurosurg 38:131, 1973.

Bruce DA, Schut L, Bruno LA, et al: Outcome following severe head injuries in children. J Neurosurg 48:679, 1978.

Jennett B, Teasdale G, Galbraith S, et al: Severe head injuries in three countries. J Neurol Neurosurg Psychiatry 40:291, 1977.

Kety SS, Shenkin HA, Schmidt CF: The effects of increased intracranial pressure on cerebral circulatory functions in man. J Clin Invest 27:493, 1948.

Mackersie RC, Christensen JM, Pitts LH, et al: Pulmonary extravascular fluid accumulation following intracranial injury. J Trauma 23:968, 1983.

Miller JD, Becker DP, Ward JD, et al: Significance of intracranial hypertension in severe head inury. J Neurosurg 47:503, 1977.

Ommaya AK, Gennarelli TA. Cerebral concussion and traumatic unconsciousness: correlation of experimental and clinical observations on blunt head injuries. Brain 97:633, 1974.

Overgaard J, Hvid-Hansen O, Land AM, et al: Prognosis after head injury based on early clinical examination. Lancet 2:631, 1973.

Pitts LH, Martin N: Head injuries. Surg Clin North Am 62:47, 1982.

Teasdale G, Jennett B: Assessment of coma and impaired consciousness. Lancet 12 July:81, 1974.

74. Infectious Meningitis

John M. Luce

DEFINITION

Meningitis is an inflammation of the meninges that is caused by a variety of infectious and noninfectious agents. Bacterial meningitis, which occurs in over 25,000 Americans each year, is perhaps the most potentially treatable of neurologic emergencies.

PATHOPHYSIOLOGY

Approximately 70 percent of patients with bacterial meningitis are children less than 12 years of age. *Escherichia coli*, other gram-negative organisms, and group B streptococci are the most common causes of meningitis in neonates. After the first month of life and into adulthood, most cases of bacterial meningitis are due to *Haemophilus influenzae* and *Neisseria meningitidis*; the latter organism may cause epidemics among military recruits and other groups of young people. *Streptococcus pneumoniae* becomes an increasingly common cause of meningitis as adulthood progresses. *Staphylococcus aureus* may be responsible for this disease in patients with endocarditis or following neurosurgical procedures. Gram-negative meningitis also occurs in the latter group and in immunosuppressed patients, as does meningitis due to *Listeria monocytogenes*. Fungal meningitis caused by organisms such as *Cryptococcus neoformans* also occurs most often in the immunocompromised.

The meninges may be seeded through hematogenous spread of organisms or by extension of contiguous infection. The former route is the most common, with organisms originating either at a distant site, such as the heart or lung, or from the colonized nasopharynx. Most individuals develop antibodies against nasopharyngeal bacteria that can prevent the spread of infection. However, when immunologic defenses break down, meningitis may occur. The importance of such defenses is underscored by the increased incidence of meningitis in patients with hypogammaglobulinemia, sickle cell disease, complement deficiency, hyposplenism, and the acquired immunodeficiency syndrome (AIDS).

Meningeal infection can also occur by direct extension from a nasopharyngeal site if the dura is disrupted in areas such as the cribriform plate and the paranasal or ethmoid sinuses. Such disruption may result from a distant or recent episode of head trauma. Meningitis may also be seen in patients with parameningeal infections such as otitis media, mastoiditis, brain abscess, or subdural empyema. Similarly patients with congenital defects, including myelomeningocele and dermal sinus tracts, are candidates for meningitis, as are persons who have undergone neurosurgical procedures and those who have indwelling intracranial pressure monitors, especially ventriculostomies.

Once bacterial organisms reach the cerebrospinal fluid (CSF), host defenses are usually incapable of halting their rapid growth. Purulent exudate accumulates quickly and causes cranial nerve dysfunction as it pools in the basilar cisterns. The inflammatory reaction may also cover the cerebral convexities, produce cerebral edema, and lead to thrombosis in the penetrating cerebral vessels. Ventriculitis may also occur. Patients who were not bacteremic to begin with may become so, owing to absorption of organisms into the arachnoid villi, and hydrocephalus may result when this absorptive mechanism is eventually disrupted by the inflammatory response.

DIAGNOSIS

Patients with acute bacterial meningitis most often experience the sudden onset of fever, headache, vomiting, and neck stiffness. Myalgias, weakness, and mental status changes also occur. Cranial nerve involvement may be evident, and seizures or strokes may occur, owing to vascular thrombosis. These symptoms may be all but absent in very young or old patients, however, and patients with meningitis following neurosurgical procedures may have a more indolent course characterized by the gradual onset of obtundation.

In most acutely ill patients, evidence of meningeal irritation, including neck stiffness and Kernig's and Brudzinski's signs, will be apparent on physical examination. Hypotension may also exist in septic patients. Signs of primary or parameningeal involvement may be elicited on examination. The presence of a petechial, purpuric, or ecchymotic rash suggests infection with *N. meningitidis*, although such abnormalities are not specific for this organism. Although cranial nerve dysfunction, focal neurologic deficits, and mental status changes may be found, evidence of elevated intracranial pressure, including papilledema and decerebrate or decorticate posturing, are usually not present.

The definitive diagnosis of infectious meningitis requires lumbar puncture and CSF analysis. Lumbar puncture should be performed in *all* patients before roentgenographic procedures unless an intracerebral mass lesion is strongly suspected. If it is, penicillin G can be administered empirically to adults or cefuroxime to children while other diagnostic studies are being performed, without significant impact on subsequent CSF cultures. When lumbar puncture is accomplished, the opening pressure is usually elevated, owing to cerebral edema. The CSF white blood count (neutrophils) should exceed 100 cells/mm^3; more than 50,000 cells/mm^3 suggests ventricular rupture of an intracerebral abscess. The CSF glucose should be less than 40 mg/dl (or less than 50–60 percent of the simultaneous blood level) in patients with infectious meningitis, owing to alteration of glucose transport across the blood-brain barrier and not to increased utilization by white blood cells. The CSF protein should also exceed 100 mg/dl. Gram's stain of the spun sediment is often helpful in identifying bacteria prior to culture; alternatively, the organisms may be detected using special stains, such as India ink for *Cryptococcus*, or specific antigens. Roentgenograms of the chest and facial structures may be useful in determining the initial site of infection, as may computerized tomography.

MANAGEMENT

The surgical therapy for meningitis involves debridement of infected parameningeal foci and repair of dural defects if necessary. The antibiotic therapy is of two types: empiric and specific; that is, directed by culture results. Empiric therapy for neonates should cover gram-negative organisms and might include either chloramphenicol and gentamicin or a third-generation cephalosporin such as moxalactam or cefotaxime. Empiric therapy in children is aimed primarily at *H. influenzae* and should include either cefuroxime or chloramphenicol; ampicillin should not be used routinely, owing to the increasingly high resistance of the organisms to this antibiotic. Penicillin G constitutes empiric therapy in adults because it is active against both pneumococci and meningococci. Cefuroxime is also good empiric therapy. Nafcillin or vancomycin should be added for *S. aureus* coverage as well as a third-generation cephalosporin or chloramphenicol and gentamicin when gram negative coverage is required. The specific therapy of commonly identified pathogens is outlined in Table 74–1. In general, treatment should last for 1–2 weeks for *N. meningitidis* and *H. influenzae*, 2 weeks for *S. pneumoniae*, and 3 weeks for gram-negative organisms.

In patients with meningitis who are comatose or who show signs of elevated intracranial pressure, cerebral perfusion pressure monitoring and manipulation, which are discussed in Chapter 77, may be applied. The most theoretically beneficial of these modalities are high-dose corticosteroids given to reduce the inflammatory response, although this approach

TABLE 74–1. ANTIBIOTIC THERAPY FOR BACTERIAL MENINGITIS IN ADULTS

| | 1ST CHOICE | | 2ND CHOICE | |
ORGANISM	Drug	24-Hr IV Dose	Drug	24-Hr IV Dose
GRAM-POSITIVE				
Streptococcus pneumoniae	Penicillin G	20 million units	Cefuroxime	6 g
Staphylococcus aureus	Nafcillin*	12 g	Vancomycin	2 g
Listeria monocytogenes	Ampicillin	2 g	Chloramphenicol	4 g
GRAM-NEGATIVE				
Neisseria meningitidis	Penicillin G	20 million units	Chloramphenicol	4 g
Haemophilus influenzae	Cefuroxime	6 g	Chloramphenicol	4 g
Escherichia coli	Cefotaxime	12 g	Gentamicin	400 mg
FUNGAL				
Cryptococcus neoformans	Amphotericin	25–50 mg		

*If susceptible

has not been tested in humans. Hyperosmolar agents, hyperventilation therapy, and other techniques may also be useful, although, again, data are lacking.

OUTCOME

The prognosis of patients with bacterial meningitis has improved greatly since the advent of antibiotics, and the mortality rate for patients with disease due to *H. influenzae*, *N. meningitidis*, and *S. pneumoniae* should be less than 5, 10, and 30 percent, respectively. The relatively high mortality rate resulting from the pneumococcus reflects the presence in many patients of factors such as advanced age, coexistent illnesses, coma, delay in instituting therapy, and bacteremia that contribute to the poor prognosis with this disease.

RECOMMENDED READING

Berk SL, McCabe WR: Meningitis caused by gram-negative bacilli. Ann Intern Med 93:253, 1980.
Buckwold FJ, Hand R, Hansebout RR: Hospital-acquired bacterial meningitis in neurosurgical patients. J Neurosurg 46:494, 1977.
Carpenter RR, Petersdorf RG: The clinical spectrum of bacterial meningitis. Am J Med 33:262, 1962.
Ernst JD, Decazes JM, Sande MA: Experimental pneumococcal meningitis: role of leukocytes in pathogenesis. Infect Immun 41:275, 1983.
Feigin RD, Shackelford PG: Value of repeat lumbar puncture in the differential diagnosis of meningitis. N Engl J Med 289:571, 1973.
Kaplan SL, Mason EO, Garcia H, et al: Pharmacokinetics and cerebrospinal fluid penetration of moxalactam in children with bacterial meningitis. J Pediatr 98:152, 1981.

Sande MA, Tierney LM: Meningitis. West J Med 140:433, 1984.

Swartz MN, Philip RD: Bacterial meningitis—a review of selected aspects. I. General clinical features, special problems and unusual meningeal reactions mimicking bacterial meningitis. N Engl J Med 272:725, 779, 842, 898, 1965.

Täuber MG, Doroshow CA, Hackbarth CJ, et al: Antibacterial activity of β-lactam antibiotics in experimental meningitis due to *Streptococcus pneumoniae*. J Infect Dis 149:568, 1984.

75. Neurologic Monitoring

John M. Luce

Introduction

Like the monitoring of other organ systems, neurologic monitoring refers to the repeated or continuous assessment of the patients and their physiologic function either by direct observation or by specific procedures. Such monitoring is used most often in patients whose neurologic status is expected to change frequently or suddenly and has the goal of identifying abnormalities and of directing appropriate therapy.

Serial Measurements of Vital Signs and Repeated Physical Examinations

Initial and subsequent recording of vital signs and repeated physical examination remain the basis of neurologic monitoring, even in technologically sophisticated institutions. Blood pressure, pulse, respiratory rate, and temperature are measured serially in most intensive care units (ICUs). The neurologic physical examination focuses on mental status and responsiveness; cranial nerve integrity; the optic discs; spinal reflexes; and motor, sensory, and cerebellar function. Pupillary response to light and the corneal, oculocephalic, and oculovestibular reflexes are particularly important in comatose patients, as discussed in Chapter 67. The Glasgow Coma Scale, also discussed in Chapter 67, may be used to quantitate the severity of coma and to follow changes in patients with structural lesions. Also discussed in Chapter 67 is a scheme to document the progression of neurologic signs in transtentorial herniation.

Assessment of Central Nervous System Anatomy

Routine roentgenograms of the skull, spine, and other structures may be essential in the evaluation of patients with neurologic disease. These studies can also be performed sequentially; for example, cervical spine roentgenograms may be obtained in a patient with neck injury before and after traction is applied. In addition, cerebral angiography is useful in evaluating and following patients with such conditions as intracranial aneurysms. Radionuclide brain scans have been used to diagnose abscesses, tumors, and other processes that disrupt the blood-brain barrier. One-dimensional ultrasound may detect shifts in the cerebral ventricles. Two-dimensional cranial ultrasonography, in which sound waves are directed through the anterior fontanel to provide a dynamic view of movement of the cerebral arteries, has been employed to identify irreversible brain injury in infants and neonates.

To date, the most precise, readily available images of structures in the central nervous system have been provided by computerized tomography (CT). The addition of iodinated contrast media to routine CT scanning allows further visualization of vascular structures, whereas metrizamide can be used to delineate the anatomy of the spinal and intracranial cerebrospinal spaces. CT is repeated so often in the evaluation of neurologic patients that it almost constitutes a monitoring rather than a diagnostic technique at some centers. The same may prove to be true of magnetic resonance imaging, which provides an even clearer picture of central nervous system anatomy.

ELECTROENCEPHALOGRAPHY

The standard electroencephalogram (EEG) records at the skin surface the electrical activity of multiple cortical neurons. During states of alertness or mental activity, the EEG shows a desynchronized pattern, with no obvious dominant frequency. During mental inactivity, sedation, or anesthesia, the EEG becomes synchronized, with characteristic waves (alpha, beta, theta, and delta) of varying frequencies and amplitude. Alterations in EEG frequencies and their relative amplitudes may reflect improvement or decline in cortical function. For example, characteristic changes are seen following reductions in cerebral blood flow to the ischemic threshold, which is 15–20 ml/min/100 g tissue (Table 75–1). The EEG can also be used to detect seizure activity.

TABLE 75–1. NORMAL VALUES FOR CEREBRAL PRESSURES, BLOOD FLOW, AND METABOLIC RATES

Mean arterial pressure (MAP)	90 mm Hg
Intracranial pressure (ICP)	10 mm Hg
Cerebral blood flow (CBF)	50 ml/min/100 g tissue
Ischemic threshold for CBF	15–20 ml/min/100 g tissue
Cerebral tissue oxygen tension	10 mm Hg
Cerebral metabolic rate for oxygen ($CMRO_2$)	3 ml/min/100 g tissue
Minimal $CMRO_2$ for aerobic metabolism	0.2 ml/min/100 g tissue
Cerebral metabolic rate for glucose (CMRG)	4.5 mg/min/100 g tissue

Evoked Potentials

In addition to assessing spontaneous neuronal activity, electrophysiologic studies can also be used to measure the body's response to sensory or motor stimulation. For example, stimulating a peripheral nerve (usually the ulnar nerve at the wrist or elbow) and visually observing contraction of the fingers is a common method of detecting the magnitude and type of neuromuscular blockade. A portable electromyograph also allows the twitch response to be recorded continuously on a dial or strip chart without requiring observation of the fingers.

Just as muscle potentials produced by motor nerve stimulation can monitor neuromuscular blockade, so potentials elicited by sensory stimulation can assess sensory receptors and pathways. These potentials also serve as general indicators of function in adjacent structures. Sensory-evoked potentials are usually recorded on the scalp following visual, auditory, or peripheral nervous stimulation. They may be used to determine the extent and location of nervous system injury in patients with such conditions as spinal cord compression and head trauma. Sensory-evoked potentials also can be employed to determine the depth of anesthesia.

Evaluation of Arterial Blood Gas Values

The arterial carbon dioxide tension ($PaCO_2$) and the arterial oxygen tension (PaO_2) have profound effects on cerebral blood flow (CBF). Studies have demonstrated that a 1 mm Hg increase or decrease in $PaCO_2$ within the range of 20 mm Hg to 80 mm Hg results in an increase or decrease in CSF of 1 ml/min/100 g tissue, with cerebral metabolism unchanged. The change in CBF is virtually immediate and is thought to occur secondary to changes in the pH of brain extracellular fluid surrounding arterioles. CBF plateaus as the $PaCO_2$ is increased above 80 mm Hg, presumably because maximum cerebral vasodilatation has been achieved. Minimal blood flow is reached at a $PaCO_2$ of 20 mm Hg because the resultant vasoconstriction causes tissue ischemia and hypoxia (cerebral tissue oxygen tension less than 10 mm Hg), which tends to cause vasodilatation. Vasodilatation and an increase in CBF also follow a fall in the PaO_2 below 60 mm Hg.

The profound impact of $PaCO_2$ and PaO_2 on CBF should prompt frequent measurement of these variables in most neurologic patients. In place of PaO_2, the arterial oxygen saturation may be measured continuously by oximetry techniques. Transcutaneous carbon dioxide tension and oxygen tension may also prove useful, and end-tidal carbon dioxide tensions may be sampled continuously and measured by mass spectro-photometry. The end-tidal carbon dioxide tension and $PaCO_2$ correlate closely in patients with normal lung function. Despite this fact, the $PaCO_2$ should be used for medicolegal purposes to confirm brain death by apnea testing.

ESTIMATION OF CEREBRAL BLOOD FLOW AND METABOLISM

Although CBF and metabolism can be inferred from the cerebral perfusion pressure, direct measurement of flow and metabolic activity would seem to be desirable. This can be achieved by measuring the clearance of radioactive gas tracers following their injection as a bolus into the carotid artery. Assuming that the tracer is almost completely exhaled on passage through the lungs and has minimal recirculation, the change in brain concentration over time, and hence in CBF, can be described by a simple exponential equation. Either radioactive krypton (^{85}Kr) or radioactive xenon (^{133}Xe) is used because each is relatively insoluble and, hence, rapidly excreted by the lungs. As gamma-emitting isotopes, they can also be detected through the skull, with one or more cameras that measure regional as well as hemispheric CBF. The flow itself is resolved into fast (gray matter) and slow (white matter) compartments. Studies of cerebral metabolic rate for oxygen ($CMRO_2$) and cerebral metabolic rate for glucose (CMRG) can also be performed using arterial and venous samples. However, because the technique requires arterial puncture, its use is generally limited to patients requiring carotid arteriography, and it cannot be performed repeatedly. In addition, because isotope is delivered to only part of the brain, global function cannot be evaluated.

CBF can be measured noninvasively by a technique that uses a 2-minute period of ^{133}Xe inhalation followed by a 40–60-minute washout period that allows separation of flow into fast, slow, and slowest compartments, the last of which is assumed to represent extracranial recirculation. Arterial samples can be obtained directly (along with jugular bulb samples to assess metabolic function), or values can be estimated indirectly by sampling end-tidal expired gases. This technique appears to be an ideal clinical tool, in that total and regional CBF over both hemispheres can be measured noninvasively. At the same time, serial studies are limited only by cumulative radiation exposure. Nevertheless, questions remain regarding the accuracy of this method. Its long washout period precludes its steady use, and expired gas samples cannot be substituted for arterial samples in patients with pulmonary disease.

The newest technique for assessing CBF and metabolism is positron emission tomography (PET). This method utilizes isotopes such as $C^{15}O2$, $^{15}O2$, and ^{18}F deoxyglucose. Given intravenously or by inhalation, these isotopes decay into two positrons emitted 180 degrees apart. By using two electronically linked coincidence detectors that record only events seen simultaneously, one can locate the source of the positrons in one dimension. Similarly, a three-dimensional change can be visualized with computer-assisted rotations or stationary isotope detectors. PET potentially offers precise imaging of CBF, $CMRO_2$, and CMRG. However, the technique is expensive and requires short-lived isotopes generated by an on-site cyclotron. Although imaging quality may suffer somewhat, the disadvantages of PET may be overcome by single-positron emission tomography (SPECT), using isotopes such as ^{81}Kr for measuring perfusion and N-isopropyl-p-{^{123}I}-iodoamphetamine (IMP) for metabolic studies.

RECOMMENDED READING

Greenberg RP, Becker DP, Miller JD, et al: Evaluation of brain function in severe human head trauma with multimodality evoked potentials. Part 2: Localization of brain dysfunction and correlation with posttraumatic neurological conditions. J Neurosurg 47:163, 1977.

Greenberg RP, Mayer DJ, Becker DP, et al: Evaluation of brain function in severe human head trauma with multimodality evoked potentials. Part 1: Evoked brain-injury potentials, methods, and analysis. J Neurosurg 47:150, 1977.

Kuhl DE, Barrio JR, Huang SC, et al: Quantifying local cerebral blood flow by N-isopropyl-p-{^{123}I}-iodoamphetamine (IMP) tomography. J Nucl Med 23:196, 1982.

Lassen NA: Control of cerebral circulation in health and disease. Circulation 34:749, 1974.

Lassen NA, Goedt-Rasmaussen K, Sorensen SC, et al: Regional cerebral blood flow in man determined by krypton. Neurology (NY) 13:719, 1963.

Luce JM: Neurologic monitoring. Respir Care 30:471, 1985.

McDowall DG: Monitoring the brain. Anesthesiology 45:117, 1976.

Naidich TP, Moran CJ, Pudlowski RM, et al: Advances in diagnosis: cranial and spinal computed tomography. Med Clin North Am 63:849, 1979.

Obrist WD, Thompson HK, King CH, et al: Determination of regional blood flow by inhalation of 133-xenon. Circ Res 20:124, 1967.

Perot PL Jr: The clinical use of somatosensory evoked potentials in spinal cord injury. Clin Neurosurg 20:367, 1973.

Phelps ME, Mazziotta JC, Kuhl DE, et al: Tomographic mapping of human cerebral perfusion using a single-photon emitter (krypton-81 m) and a rotating gamma camera. J Nucl Med 21:1139, 1980.

Plum F, Posner JB: The diagnosis of stupor and coma. 3rd edition. Philadelphia, F. A. Davis Co., 1980.

Teasdale G, Jannett B: Assessment of coma and impaired consciousness: a practical scale. Lancet 2:81, 1974.

76. Neuromuscular Diseases

John M. Luce

DEFINITION

Neuromuscular diseases affect nerves, muscles, or the myoneural junction. Despite the decline of poliomyelitis, these disorders remain a significant cause of morbidity and mortality. Reviewed in this chapter are the three most common neuromuscular diseases—Guillain Barré syndrome, myasthenia gravis, and botulism—that cause acute weakness and respiratory failure.

PATHOPHYSIOLOGY

The Guillain Barré syndrome, also called acute inflammatory polyradiculoneuropathy, results from an immunologically mediated segmental demyelination of the peripheral and autonomic nervous systems. The demyelination leads to progressive motor weakness, areflexia, sensory changes, and autonomic dysfunction. The Guillain Barré syndrome occurs most frequently after viral or mycoplasmal infections, immunization, surgery, or other presumed immunologic challenges. It is characterized histologically by a perivascular lymphocytic infiltration.

Although also an immunologic disorder, myasthenia gravis differs from the Guillain Barré syndrome in that it results from circulating antibodies directed against the acetylcholine receptors in the neuromuscular junction. In addition to these humoral aspects, cell-mediated immunity involving lymphocytes and the thymus gland also plays a pathogenic role in the disorder. The end result is that potential interactions between acetylcholine and receptor molecules are reduced, leading to low amplitude motor end-plate potentials that may fail to trigger strong muscle contractions. This, in turn, causes muscle weakness and fatigability that resembles that seen in poisoning by curare.

Botulism also affects the myoneural junction. However, this disease is not immunologic but is caused by a sporulating gram-positive anaerobic bacterium, *Clostridium botulinum*. Ubiquitous in nature, this organism produces potent neurotoxins, designated A through G, that bind irreversibly to the myoneural junction and inhibit the release of acetylcholine.

460

Botulism occurs in three forms: (1) food-borne botulism, in which pre-formed toxin is ingested in nonacidic home-canned or factory-canned vegetables or meat; (2) infant botulism, in which the organism and its spores are ingested in honey or other foods; and (3) wound botulism, in which *C. botulinum* and its spores contaminate traumatic or surgical wounds. In patients with these conditions, the neurotoxin produces a paralytic state that initially involves the cranial nerves and progresses downward. It also causes parasympathetic complaints, such as ileus, and small unreactive pupils.

DIAGNOSIS

The differential diagnosis of muscle weakness includes severe hypocalcemia, tick paralysis, organophosphate poisoning, diphtheria, acute intermittent porphyria, and lead neuropathy, in addition to the diseases highlighted in this chapter. Many of these conditions may be ruled out on clinical and epidemiologic grounds, but distinguishing the Guillain Barré syndrome, myasthenia gravis, and botulism from one other may be difficult. An absence of reflexes is the clinical feature most suggestive of the Guillain Barré syndrome. Additional features are the progression and relative symmetry of the muscle weakness, the likelihood of cranial nerve involvement (50 percent in most series), the presence of paresthesias, and autonomic dysfunction. Myasthenia gravis and botulism are characterized by bulbar and especially ocular weakness that precedes limb weakness, a preservation of reflexes, and a lack of sensory involvement or autonomic disturbance. In botulism, weakness is progressive over hours to days, whereas myasthenia gravis becomes symptomatic over months and causes fluctuating symptoms induced by fatigue.

The classic laboratory feature of the Guillain Barré syndrome is an increase in cerebrospinal fluid (CSF) protein in the absence of inflammatory cells or reduced glucose levels. Nerve conduction studies usually reveal decreased conduction velocities and reduced evoked motor responses, owing to conduction block. Myasthenia gravis causes no characteristic CSF or nerve conduction changes but can usually be diagnosed by giving acetylcholinesterase (AChE) inhibiting agents that increase the interaction between acetylcholine and its receptors at the motor end-plate. Thus, transiently increased strength should be achieved within 30 seconds following the intravenous injection of edrophonium chloride (Tensilon). Botulism is best diagnosed by demonstrating toxin in the stool, gastric contents, or serum of affected patients or in specimens of contaminated food they have ingested. This condition is characterized by post-tetanic facilitation of the muscle action potential on electromyography.

MANAGEMENT

The general management of patients with neuromuscular disease focuses on their muscle disturbance, autonomic dysfunction, and immobility. As shown in Table 76–1, these patients often have difficulty in coughing, clearing secretions, avoiding atelectasis and aspiration, and ventilating adequately. They frequently need chest physical therapy, suctioning, and careful enteral or parenteral feeding; the latter approach is preferred if ileus is present. Pulmonary function should be followed closely, and intubation and mechanical ventilation should be provided if the vital capacity is 10–15 ml/kg, the maximum inspiratory force is 20–25 ml/kg, or significant hypoxemia or hypercapnia are present. Tracheostomy may be performed if sustained weakness is anticipated.

Autonomic dysfunction in the Guillain Barré syndrome may take the form of either over- or underactivity of the sympathetic nervous system. Hypertension, diaphoresis, and tachycardia may be treated with α- or β-adrenergic antagonists. Hypertension may be treated with fluids or α-adrenergic agonists, whereas bradycardia is best treated with atropine. Bedridden patients require scrupulous nursing care, physiotherapy, and the use of insulating pads or kinetic beds to prevent compression neuropathies. Subcutaneous heparin (5000 units BID or TID) should be given to prevent deep venous thrombosis and pulmonary embolism.

Beyond these and other general measures, the neuromuscular diseases discussed in this chapter are treated differently. Corticosteroids do not routinely improve patients with Guillain Barré syndrome; plasmapheresis is of proven benefit only in rapidly progressive disease that is treated early. Plasmapheresis may be of considerable benefit in patients with severe myasthenia gravis who have not responded to more conser-

TABLE 76–1. RESPIRATORY COMPROMISE DUE TO NEUROMUSCULAR DISEASES
CAUSING WEAKNESS

FINDING	COMPROMISE
Vital Capacity	
<30 ml/kg	Inability to cough adequately
<20 ml/kg	Inability to sigh or prevent atelectasis
<10 ml/kg	Inability to ventilate adequately
Maximum Ventilatory Forces	
Maximum expiratory force < 40 cm H_2O	Inability to clear secretions
Maximum inspiratory force < 20 cm H_2O	Inability to ventilate adequately
Dysphagia With Bulbar Paralysis	Inability to avoid aspiration
Arterial Blood Gases	
Hypoxemia	Inability to sigh or prevent atelectasis
Hypercapnia	Inability to ventilate adequately

Adapted, with permission, from O'Donohue WJ, Baker JP, Bell G, et al. JAMA 235:733–735, 1976. Copyright 1976, American Medical Association.

vative therapy, which usually includes AChE inhibiting agents (e.g., pyridostigmine bromide [Mestinon] 60 mg/day in 2 hour doses), corticosteroids (e.g., prednisone up to 100 mg/day in a single or BID dose), and thymectomy. Depending on its type, botulism is treated with gastric lavage and enemas to remove unabsorbed toxin, the administration of trivalent antitoxin (against toxin A, B, and E) to neutralize circulating toxin in the serum, the administration of high-dose penicillin (3 million units intravenously q 4 h) to kill *C. botulinum* organisms if present, and surgical debridement of offending wounds.

OUTCOME

Most patients with Guillain Barré syndrome recover completely if they are adequately supported during the active phase of their disease. The course of myasthenia gravis is much more variable; some patients have easily treated extraocular or bulbar symptoms, whereas others suffer repeated acute deteriorations (due either to disease or to overdosage with anticholinesterase medications), and still others have chronic weakness that does not respond to therapy. Food-borne botulism carries a case fatality rate of approximately 15 percent. Mortality in all forms of botulism relates to the rapidity of progression of neurologic symptoms, the degree of respiratory dysfunction, and the quality of patient care.

RECOMMENDED READING

Arnon SS: Infant botulism. Annu Rev Med 31:541, 1980.

Asbury AK, Arnason BG, Adams RD: The inflammatory lesion in idiopathic polyneuritis: its role in pathogenesis. Medicine 48:173, 1969.

Black LE, Hyatt RE: Maximal static respiratory pressures in generalized neuromuscular disease. Am Rev Resp Dis 103:641, 1971.

NINCDS Committee: Criteria for diagnosis of Guillain-Barré syndrome. Ann Neurol 3:565, 1978.

Dau PC, Lindstrom JM, Cassel CK, et al: Plasmapheresis and immunosuppressive drug therapy in myasthenia gravis. N Engl J Med 297:1134, 1977.

De Troyer A, Borenstein S: Acute changes in respiratory mechanics after pyridostigmine injection in patients with myasthenia gravis. Am Rev Resp Dis 121:629, 1980.

Drachman DB: Myasthenia gravis. N Engl J Med 298:136, 186, 1978.

Harrison BDW, Collins JV, Brown KGE, et al: Respiratory failure in neuromuscular diseases. Thorax 26:579, 1971.

Henderson DK, Tillman DB, Webb HH, et al: Infectious disease emergencies: the clostridial syndromes. West J Med 129:101, 1978.

Hughes RAC, Newsom-Davis JM, Perkin GD, et al: Controlled trial of prednisolone in acute polyneuropathy. Lancet 2:750, 1978.

Leventhal SR, Orkin FK, Hirsh RA: Prediction of the need for postoperative mechanical ventilation in myasthenia gravis. Anesthesiology 53:26, 1980.

Nielsen VK, Paulson OB, Rosenkvist J: Rapid improvement of myasthenia gravis after plasma exchange. Ann Neurol 11:160, 1982.

O'Donohue WJ, Baker JP, Bell G, et al: Respiratory failure in neuromuscular disease: management in respiratory intensive care units. JAMA 235:733, 1976.

Schmidt-Nowara WW, Samet JM, Rosario PA: Early and late pulmonary complications of botulism. Arch Intern Med 143:451, 1983.

77. Monitoring and Manipulation of Cerebral Perfusion Pressure

John M. Luce

INTRODUCTION

Cerebral blood flow (CBF) is directly related to the perfusion across the brain, the cerebral perfusion pressure (CPP), and is inversely related to cerebral vascular resistance (CVR). CPP is equal to the cerebral arterial inflow pressure, the mean arterial pressure (MAP), minus the cerebral venous outflow pressure. Pressure in the cerebral veins is difficult to measure in patients, but it closely resembles the pressure of the intracranial cerebrospinal fluid (CSF), which is called the intracranial pressure (ICP). The reason for this is that the brain behaves like a Starling resistor in which the pressure in the cerebral veins is established by the ICP to which they are exposed. CPP therefore equals MAP minus ICP. Given a normal MAP of 90 mm Hg and an ICP of 10 mm Hg or less, CPP should be approximately 80 mm Hg.

Assuming normal cerebral metabolism and arterial blood gas values, the body maintains a constant CBF of 50 ml/min/100 g tissue by adjusting CVR over CPPs that range from 50 to 150 mm Hg; this mechanism is called autoregulation. However, autoregulation is lost in many, if not most, patients with brain injury, in whom CBF varies linearly with CPP. Thus, CBF may fall below 50 ml/min/100 g tissue and reach an ischemic threshold between 15 and 20 ml/min/100 g tissue if CPP falls below 50 mm Hg. CBF may also increase above normal levels if CPP exceeds 50 mm Hg. If the resultant increase in cerebral blood volume is not accomplished by a reciprocal decrease in the other intracranial contents (water, solids, and CSF), ICP will rise. This rise will be especially pronounced if intracranial volume and ICP are increased to begin with, as occurs with many brain diseases, including those that cause cerebral swelling (see Fig. 77–1). CPP falls without a compensatory increase in MAP, and cerebral ischemia ensues.

CPP monitoring is made possible by the simultaneous use of an indwelling systemic arterial catheter to measure MAP and of indwelling

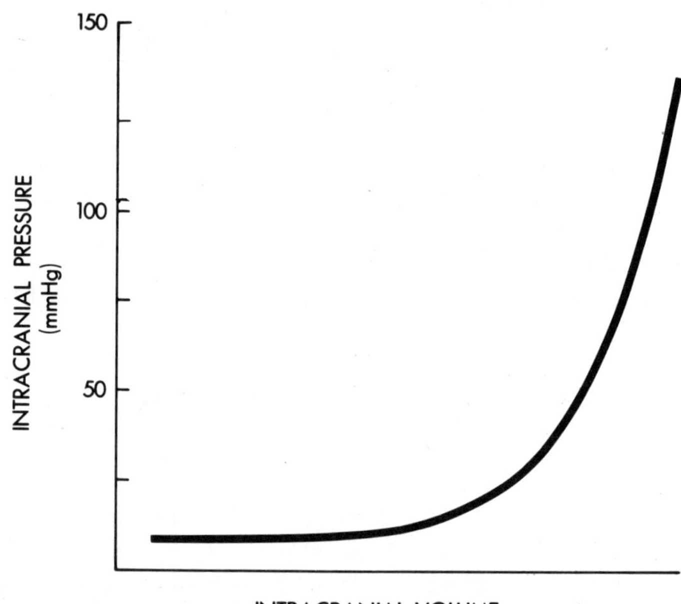

FIGURE 77–1. Intracranial pressure increases markedly if intracranial volume is increased to begin with—and then increases still more. (Reproduced, with permission, from Luce JM: Cerebral resuscitation. In Bone RC (ed): Critical Care: A Comprehensive Approach. Park Ridge, Ill., American College of Chest Physicians, 1984, pp. 403–418.)

devices, which are discussed later, to measure ICP. Once monitoring is available, CPP can be manipulated by altering MAP, ICP, or both. MAP is maintained near-normal levels in most patients, although MAP may be increased on purpose in patients with cerebral vasospasm due, say, to subarachnoid hemorrhage from an intracranial aneurysm. ICP should also be reduced to normal levels by the measures discussed later in this chapter.

ICP monitoring allows assessment of the effects of measures designed to reduce ICP. The impact of positive end-expiratory pressure (PEEP) and other therapies that may elevate ICP by increasing right atrial pressure and by decreasing venous return from the brain can also be assessed. Similarly, one can evaluate the actions of techniques that may affect MAP and ICP simultaneously, such as barbiturate loading for ICP reduction and volume infusion in combination with isoproterenol and aminophylline for cerebral vasospasm. Patients receiving these and other therapies may be candidates for hemodynamic monitoring with right atrial or pulmonary artery catheters as well.

Indications

Despite the physiologic information gained by CPP monitoring and the dramatic immediate effects of therapy in MAP and ICP, the long-term benefits of CPP monitoring and manipulation are unclear. The identification of intracranial hypertension is of prognostic value, and neurologic recovery is less likely in head trauma patients whose ICP is elevated on admission. An improved outcome from severe head injury caused by mass lesions such as subdural hematoma with early diagnosis and treatment has also been demonstrated. Nevertheless, overall improvement has never been demonstrated by a randomized trial. A trial of this sort seems unlikely because clinicians now use ICP monitoring in comatose or potentially unstable patients with head trauma, intracerebral masses, subarachnoid hemorrhage, hydrocephalus, and the metabolic encephalopathy associated with Reye's syndrome. These patients generally have a Glasgow Coma Scale (GCS) rating of 7 or less (see Chapter 66). Monitoring has also been recommended for comatose patients with massive stroke, encephalitis and meningitis, and anoxic encephalopathy following cardiopulmonary arrest, although its usefulness in these situations is unclear.

Contraindications

Because CPP should be monitored only in severely ill patients, there are few, if any, contraindications to the procedure. ICP monitoring devices should not be placed in or through infected spaces, however, and should be removed if infection occurs.

Techniques

Placement of indwelling systemic arterial catheters to measure MAP is discussed in the section on cardiovascular disorders (see Chapter 15). ICP is presently monitored by several methods. Fluid-filled catheters placed directly into the lateral ventricles were the first devices used for this purpose; these catheters can be used to reduce ICP by drawing off CSF and to determine the intracranial compliance or volume-pressure relationship (VPR) by injection of small amounts (usually 1 ml) of saline or mock CSF. Ventriculostomies cannot be readily performed in infants or adult patients with small ventricles. Because of this and of the possibility of insertion-related trauma as well as the fact that a subsequent infection rate of 2–5 percent exists with use of ventricular catheters, clinicians may prefer to measure ICP either with fluid-filled subarachnoid screws that lie

TABLE 77–1. COMPARISON OF THREE METHODS OF
MONITORING INTRACRANIAL PRESSURE

METHOD	EASE OF INSERTION	ACCURACY	INFECTION RATE	VPR AND CSF DRAINAGE?
Ventricular catheter	Problem with small ventricles	Excellent	2–5 percent	Yes
Subarachnoid screw	Little difficulty	Good	1–2 percent	No
Epidural transducer	Little difficulty	Variable	Negligible	No

VPR = volume-pressure relationship; CSF = cerebrospinal fluid

just beneath the dura or with miniature transducers in the epidural space. These two devices are associated with fewer infections but may measure local rather than general ICP changes. In addition, they do not allow assessment of VPR or drainage of CSF. See Table 77–1 for details.

COMPLICATIONS, CARE, AND REMOVAL

As noted earlier, tissue injury and subsequent infection are the most common complications associated with ICP catheters. Infection probably correlates with the condition of the catheter insertion site, the length of time it is in place, and how it is used. Thus, sterile technique must be obeyed during insertion. Catheters should be removed as soon as possible and almost always after 5 days; they may be used for drainage but should only rarely be flushed. Flushing when absolutely necessary with a gentamicin or tobramycin solution (30 mg in 30 ml saline) appears advisable. Clinicians should recall that the pressure measured when a fluid-filled catheter is draining reflects the pressure at the drainage site and not the true ICP.

REDUCING INTRACRANIAL PRESSURE

Intracranial hypertension may occur if cerebral blood volume increases owing to decreased venous drainage. Because this may be caused by kinking of the jugular veins and lowering the brain below the level of the heart, the heads and necks of patients with intracranial hypertension should be kept near the midline position and elevated 30 degrees. These simple measures often serve to blunt the diminution in venous drainage that is caused by coughing, straining, and other activities that increase intrathoracic pressure. If they do not, sedatives and muscle relaxants may be given to limit muscle activity.

Positive pressure ventilation with or without PEEP may also increase

ICP by decreasing cerebral venous return. Studies in animals and humans have demonstrated that PEEP is more likely to increase ICP if intracranial compliance is low or respiratory system compliance is high. This is because PEEP-induced increases in intrathoracic pressure are applied more profoundly to intrathoracic vessels in the latter circumstances. Because PEEP is indicated primarily to treat pulmonary edema, which decreases respiratory system compliance, it should not adversely affect ICP in most circumstances. Nevertheless, both MAP and ICP should be followed closely in patients receiving this therapy.

Hyperventilation may be expected to decrease CBF by causing cerebral vasoconstriction via an increase in the pH of brain extracellular fluid. The reduction in CBF is probably maximal at $PaCO_2$ levels of 20 mm Hg because the vasoconstriction is offset by the vasodilatory effect of cerebral tissue hypoxia. Although cerebral vascular responsiveness to hyperventilation varies even in health, head-injured and other patients manifest at least some reactivity to changes in $PaCO_2$. However, after 8 hours or more of hyperventilation, the pH of brain extracellular fluid may be restored to normal by active transport processes. The $PaCO_2$ should therefore be normalized as soon as possible, providing ICP does not increase.

Hyperosmolar agents reduce ICP—first, by decreasing brain water through the creation of an osmolar gradient between the bloodstream and brain cells and, second, through a reduction in total body water. Most clinicians administer 20 percent mannitol either in high intermittent doses (0.25–0.5 g/kg every 1–2 hours) or by continuous infusion (0.05–0.1 g/kg). A serum osmolality of approximately 325 mOsm/l should not be exceeded because excessive hyperosmolarity may injure neurons. Mannitol depletes the body of sodium and potassium as well as water and must be used cautiously. Also, it should be given sparingly to head-injured children because it may transiently increase intravascular volume, CBF, and ICP.

Diuretics are given to decrease ICP by reducing intravascular volume. Furosemide in doses of 40–80 mg is most commonly employed for this purpose; it has the additional advantage of reducing CSF production by unknown mechanisms. Water intake is usually restricted in patients receiving diuretics, although the efficacy of this approach has yet to be demonstrated.

Acetazolamide is a carbonic anhydrase inhibitor that limits ion exchange across the choroid plexus. This agent is used frequently to reduce CSF production in patients with communicating hydrocephalus. The usual dose of acetazolamide is 250 mg BID or QID. Furosemide may also be used to reduce CSF production, as noted earlier. Although acetazolamide may occasionally be helpful, CSF drainage via a ventriculostomy is usually a more effective method of reducing the contribution of CSF to intracranial hypertension.

Corticosteroids have been assumed to prevent vasogenic brain edema through their stabilizing effects on vascular membranes. This assumption is supported by studies that have demonstrated a reduction in the size of experimental lesions in animals pretreated with dexamethasone. Nevertheless, neither low- (16 mg/day) nor high- (96 mg/day) dose dexamethasone sufficiently affected ICP or outcome in severely head-injured patients in one study. Thus, although corticosteroids are generally effective in reducing peritumor edema in patients with cerebral neoplasms, they need not be routinely given to patients with head trauma, cerebral infarction, or subarachnoid hemorrhage.

Barbiturates may reduce CBF and ICP by decreasing cerebral metabolism or by lowering the effective circulating intravascular volume through peripheral venous dilation and a mild depression of the cardiac output. High-dose pentobarbital therapy (3–5 mg/kg loading dose; 1–5 mg/kg/hr thereafter) normalized ICP and reduced daily mannitol requirements in a majority of severely head-injured patients in one study, although subsequent controlled trials failed to demonstrate any benefit from barbiturates. These agents should only be given as a last resort in patients with refractory intravascular hypertension.

Other therapies to reduce ICP include hypothermia, which reduces CBF as barbiturates do but is logistically difficult to administer; and hyperbaric oxygenation, which causes cerebral vasoconstriction similar to that achieved by hyperventilation but is much more expensive and cumbersome. Dimethyl sulfoxide (DMSO) also reduces ICP in some patients but has not been shown to improve outcome; it therefore cannot be generally recommended.

RECOMMENDED READING

Bruce DA, Langfitt TW, Miller JD, et al: Regional cerebral blood flow, intracranial pressure, and brain metabolism in comatose patients. J Neurosurg 38:131, 1973.

Burchiel KJ, Steege TD, Wyler AR: Intracranial pressure changes in brain-injured patients requiring positive end-expiratory pressure ventilation. Neurosurgery 8:443, 1981.

Jacobson SA, Rothballer AB: Prolonged measurement of experimental intracranial pressure using a subminiature absolute pressure transducer. J Neurosurg 26:603, 1967.

Kindt GW, Waldman J, Kohl S, et al: Intracranial pressure in Reye's syndrome: monitoring and control. JAMA 231:822, 1975.

Luce JM: Neurologic monitoring. Respir Care 30:471, 1985.

Luce JM, Huseby JS, Kirk W, et al: A Starling resistor regulates cerebral venous outflow in dogs. J Appl Physiol 53:1496, 1982.

Lundberg N, Troupp H, Lorin H: Continuous recording of the ventricular-fluid pressure in patients with severe acute traumatic brain injury. J Neurosurg 22:581, 1965.

Miller JD, Becker DP, Ward JD, et al: Significance of intracranial hypertension in severe head injury. J Neurosurg 47:503, 1977.

Teasdale G, Jennett B: Assessment of coma and impaired consciousness: a practical scale. Lancet 2:81, 1974.

Vries JK, Becker DP, Young HF: A subarachnoid screw for monitoring intracranial pressure. J Neurosurg 39:416, 1973.

78. Neuromuscular Blockade

John M. Luce

John M. Luce

INTRODUCTION

Neuromuscular blocking agents relax skeletal muscles by interfering with the transmission of impulses between them and motor nerves. This occurs at the myoneural junction, which consists of the terminal membrane of the nerve axon, the postjunctional membrane of the muscle, and the subneural space or cleft between them (Fig. 78–1). The nerve axon synthesizes acetylcholine (ACh) from choline and acetic acid and stores it within vesicles at its terminus. When the nerve is stimulated, the vesicles release ACh in surplus amounts into the cleft. Receptors in the membrane, which is also termed the motor end-plate, accept ACh and open channels for the passage of calcium and sodium ions, which depolarizes the muscle. Depolarization, in turn, generates an end-plate potential which, if sufficient enough, triggers contraction of muscle myofibrils. The ACh is then broken down into choline and acetic acid by an enzyme, acetylcholinesterase (AChE) in the subneural cleft. These products then diffuse into the nerve axon for resynthesis of ACh, the postjunctional membrane becomes repolarized owing to ion flux, and the muscle returns to its former condition.

Neuromuscular blocking agents are quaternary ammonium compounds that are structurally related to ACh and either inhibit or mimic its effects at the motor-end plate. The nondepolarizing muscle relaxants include D-tubocurarine (DTC), gallamine, pancuronium (Pavulon), metocurine, vecuronium, and atracurium. These agents block the action of ACh by combining with the motor end-plate receptors that normally accept this substance. When a majority of receptors are blocked, the end-plate potential falls short of the threshold levels, and muscle contraction does not occur. Because nondepolarizing agents inhibit ACh competitively, their effect can be overcome by increases in ACh concentration within the subneural cleft. Such increases can be induced by drugs such as edrophonium (Tensilon), neostigmine (Prostigmin), and pyridostigmine (Mestinon) that inhibit AChE. Because nondepolarizing agents do not cause muscle contraction, the neuromuscular blockade they produce is not associated with fasciculation of muscle fibers. Furthermore, the twitch response decreases after repeated single stimuli and also fades after tetanic

"

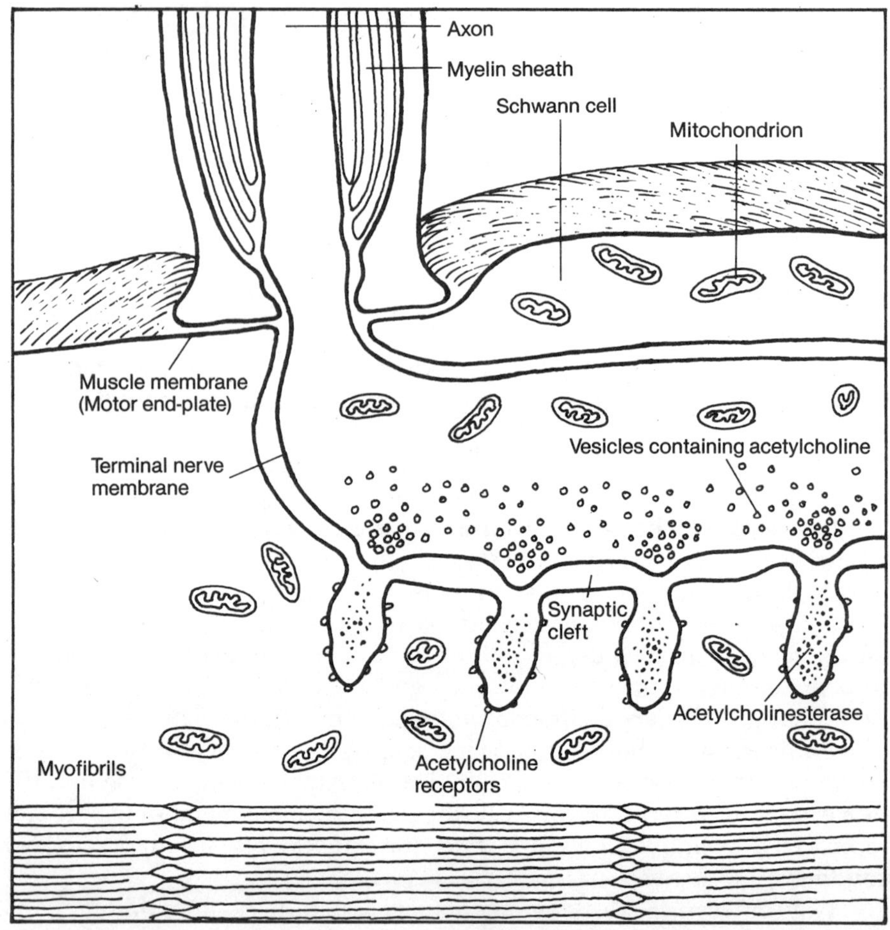

FIGURE 78–1. Diagram of the myoneural junction. See text for explanation.

or rapid rates of stimulation, and when twitch is resumed after tetany, an increase in the response, called post-tetanic facilitation, occurs.

The depolarizing muscle relaxants include succinylcholine (SCh) (Anectine) and decamethonium. Initially, these drugs mimic the effect of ACh on the motor end-plate, producing depolarization of the postjunctional membrane and contraction of the muscle. Because the membrane remains depolarized, it develops resistance to the passage of nerve impulses, and the muscle eventually relaxes. This early phase of depolarization block is characterized by muscle fasciculations, lack of fade with twitch or tetanic stimulation, and absence of post-tetanic facilitation. The postjunctional membrane eventually achieves repolarization in the presence of depolarizing agents, but desensitization to the effects of ACh occurs. This causes a fade with tetanic stimulation and also produces post-tetanic facilitation similar to that seen with nondepolarizing agents.

Neuromuscular blocking agents of both sorts can alter the transmission of nerve impulses at pre- and postganglionic endings in the autonomic nervous system in addition to their action at the myoneural junction. They may also liberate histamine from nerve endings. These actions help explain the cardiovascular effects of the agents that are discussed later in this chapter. It is generally believed that the drugs are not active within the central nervous system.

INDICATIONS

In the critical care setting, neuromuscular blockers are used primarily to provide brief or sustained muscle relaxation to facilitate endotracheal intubation, mechanical ventilation, bronchoscopy, and minor surgical procedures. They are also used to treat status epilepticus (Chapter 65), strychnine poisoning, and tetanus, in which a neurotoxin produced by the spores of a gram-positive anaerobic bacterium, *Clostridium tetani*, blocks inhibitory motor transmission in the spinal cord and thereby produces muscle spasms. In addition, patients with incomplete reversal of neuromuscular blocking agents in the operating room may require intensive care unit (ICU) admission.

CONTRAINDICATIONS

Neuromuscular blocking agents are rarely contraindicated because of their cardiovascular side effects. However, other contraindications should be noted. First, because these drugs paralyze the respiratory muscles, they should not be given without proper observation of the patient and, if necessary, access to endotracheal intubation and mechanical ventilatory support. Second, hyperkalemia to a level associated with cardiac arrest may follow the administration of SCh to patients with burns, traumatic insults, and neuromuscular disease. This complication apparently results from an increased density of ACh receptors in the muscles of these patients in such a way that intense contraction results from depolarization. Although hyperkalemia is most likely in the first 60 days following injury or illness, use of SCh is best avoided at all times in these individuals. Finally, blocking agents should not be given to patients who are not sedated or receiving analgesics because they will feel anxiety and pain but not be able to communicate these sensations while paralyzed.

TECHNIQUES

SCh in intravenous doses of 1 mg/kg has been used for hurried endotracheal intubation, owing to its rapid onset (60 seconds) and short duration of action (5–10 minutes). However, as noted earlier, SCh should not be used in many critically ill patients. Furthermore, when it is used, SCh may cause painful muscle contractions in addition to other side effects that will be discussed. The muscle contractions can be prevented by prior administration of DTC (0.25–0.5 mg/kg) or another nonpolarizing agent.

Intermediate or long-acting nondepolarizing drugs are the agents of choice when sustained paralysis is required. Previously, DTC (paralyzing dose: 0.5 mg/kg; maintenance dose: 5 mg/hr/70 kg) was most often used for this purpose, but pancuronium (paralyzing dose: 0.8–1.0 mg/kg; maintenance dose: 5–10 mg/hr/70 kg) is perhaps more popular today. The effects of these drugs are allowed to disappear gradually in most circumstances. However, if rapid reversal is necessary, patients may be given intravenous edrophonium (0.5–1.0 mg/kg), or neostigmine (2.5–5.0 mg/70 kg). Intravenous atropine (1.0–1.5 mg) should be administered with the latter two agents to prevent miosis, bradycardia, bronchospasm, increased secretions, and other muscarinic effects.

The adequacy of reversal may be ascertained by determining grip strength, maximum inspiratory force, vital capacity, and other indicators of muscle function. More sophisticated techniques include stimulation of a peripheral nerve and evaluation of the twitch or tetanic motor response of a muscle supplied by that nerve. This can be accomplished by stimulation of the ulnar nerve at the wrist and measurement of either the tension developed by or the elctromyographic signal of, the thumb adductor, the adductor pollicis brevis.

COMPLICATIONS

As mentioned earlier, many of the neuromuscular blockers produce cardiovascular and other side effects. In particular, SCh may produce an initial bradycardia and hypotension that may be associated with atrioventricular block via vagal stimulation, followed by tachycardia and hypertension due to autonomic stimulation. The vagal effect is more common in children and in patients taking digitalis, and it can be prevented by atropine. SCh also increases intraocular pressure, probably by extraocular or orbital smooth muscle contraction. In addition, it increases intragastric pressure by contracting the abdominal muscles. Of the nonpolarizing agents, DTC and metocurine tend to decrease pulse and blood pressure, owing to a combination of histamine release and autonomic blockade. On the other hand, pancuronium causes vagal block in the sinus node and is associated with tachycardia.

Clinicians should be aware that both the desired and the undesired effects of neuromuscular blockers may be potentiated in certain patients. In general, the effects of nondepolarizing agents are prolonged by inhaled anesthetics, acidosis, hypothermia, hypokalemia (especially DTC and pancuronium), renal failure (DTC and pancuronium), biliary and hepatic disease (pancuronium and vecuronium), myasthenia gravis, amyotrophic lateral sclerosis, and the Eaton-Lambert syndrome. The undesired effects of depolarizing agents may be potentiated by liver disease, cytotoxic drugs, and AChE inhibitors.

RECOMMENDED READING

Ali HH, Savarese JJ: Monitoring of neuromuscular function. Anesthesiology 45:216, 1976.

Bogetz MS, Katz, JA: Recall of surgery for major trauma. Anesthesiology 61:6, 1984.

Fahey MR, Rupp SM, Fisher DM, et al: The pharmacokinetics and pharmacodynamics of atracurium in patients with and without renal failure. Anesthesiology 61:699, 1984.

Furguson A, Egerszegi P, Bevan DR: Neostigmine, pyridostigmine, and edrophonium as antagonists of pancuronium. Anesthesiology 53:390, 1980.

Gissen AJ, Katz RL: Twitch, tetanus and post-tetanic potentiation as indices of nerve-muscle block in man. Anesthesiology 30:481, 1969.

Gronert GA, Theye RA: Pathophysiology of hyperkalemia induced by succinylcholine. Anesthesiology 43:89, 1975.

Katz RL: Clinical neuromuscular pharmacology of pancuronium. Anesthesiology 34:550, 1971.

Katz RL: Neuromuscular effects of D-tubocurarine, edrophonium, and neostigmine in man. Anesthesiology 28:327, 1967.

Lebrault C, Berger JL, D'Hollander A, et al: Pharmacokinetics and pharmacodynamics of vecuronium (ORG NC 45) in patients with cirrhosis. Anesthesiology 62:601, 1985.

Miller RD, Rupp SM, Fisher DM, et al: Clinical pharmacology of vecuronium and atracurium. Anesthesiology 61:444, 1984.

Miller RD, Savarese JJ: Pharmacology of muscle relaxants and their antagonists. In Miller RD (ed): Anesthesia. 2nd edition. New York, Churchill Livingstone Inc., 1986.

Stoelting RK: The hemodynamic effects of pancuronium and D-tubocurarine in anesthetized patients. Anesthesiology 36:612, 1972.

79. Pain

John M. Luce

Definition

Pain is an unpleasant sensory or emotional experience associated with actual or potential tissue damage. Pain is of two types: acute pain, which usually responds to analgesic agents and has a small psychologic component; and chronic pain, which is harder to treat and has a strong psychologic overlay. Only acute pain is considered in this chapter.

Pathophysiology

The word pain comes from the Greek and Latin words for payment or punishment. Consciously or not, many people still think of pain in terms of punishment. However, from a scientific standpoint, pain is best understood as the result of peripheral sensations and central perceptions. The sensations of pain derive from free nerve endings, called nociceptors, that are activated by mechanical deformation and extremes of temperature. Substances such as histamines and prostaglandins, which are released from injured tissues, may lower the threshold of the nociceptors and thereby contribute to painful sensations. Acetylsalicylic acid, acetaminophen, and nonsteroidal antiinflammatory agents probably relieve pain by inhibiting prostaglandin release peripherally.

The nociceptors are linked with two kinds of peripheral nerve fibers: large, myelinated A fibers, which conduct impulses rapidly and are associated with sharp pain sensations; and small unmyelinated C fibers, which transmit more slowly and are associated with dull pain. The fibers arise from nuclei in the substantia gelatinosa of dorsal root ganglia and ascend the spinal cord in Lissauer's tract, where they synapse with other neurons. These, in turn, cross the thalamus, from which other fibers project to the cerebral cortex and perhaps to the limbic system and to the reticular activating system in the brainstem. Local and regional anesthesia presumably decrease painful secretions by interfering with the conduction of nerve impulses from the peripheral to the central nervous system.

Recent evidence suggests that a neural mechanism in the *substantia gelatinosa* acts like a "gate" that can also decrease the flow of nerve

476

impulses from the periphery. The degree of modulation appears to be determined by the relative amount of transmission in the inhibitory A fibers, the facilitatory C fibers, and the fibers that descend from higher centers. Thus, rubbing the skin or stimulating it with a transcutaneous electrical nerve stimulator may serve to increase transmission in the A fibers, close the "gate," and decrease transmission through the C fibers to the brain.

Although this review stresses the importance of nerve transmission, pain sensation and perception also appear to be modulated by enkephalins or endorphins, natural morphinelike substances that serve as neurotransmitters in what has been called the endorphin-mediated analgesic system. These substances, which are also known as endogenous opioids, are produced by the brain and the pituitary gland and bind to receptors in the limbic system and other sites. Pain intensity is probably determined by body levels of these endogenous opioids and by the availability of enkephalin-binding sites, both of which vary from one person to another. Such variation presumably accounts in part for individual differences in pain perception. Furthermore, the presence of the endorphin-mediated analgesic system probably accounts for the dramatic pain relief achieved with exogenous opioids, such as morphine, that either bind to central sites, in the case of systemically administered agents, or to receptors in the *subtantia gelatinosa*, in the case of narcotics applied directly to the spinal cord. Finally, the prominence played by the limbic and reticular activating systems in pain perception may explain the benefits of anxiolytic and sedative-hypnotic drugs in pain patients; just as pain can cause anxiety and ruin sleep, so can anxiety and sleeplessness amplify pain.

Diagnosis

As an experience, pain as best diagnosed—and described—subjectively. This means that most patients should be taken seriously when they say they are in pain. It also means that pain is not necessarily proportionate to obvious tissue injury; as noted earlier, patients vary in how they perceive pain. From an objective standpoint, most patients with acute pain manifest tachycardia, diaphoresis, pupillary dilation, and other signs of autonomic excess; these signs are absent in chronic pain. That the physiologic manifestations of acute pain are reversed by narcotics underscores the importance of the endorphin-mediated analgesic system in the pain experience.

Management

The major problem in pain management is attitudinal: far too many physicians, nurses, and other health professionals do not understand the pathophysiology of pain. They also underestimate dose regimens when giving narcotic analgesics, overestimate the duration of activity of these agents, and exaggerate the dangers of addiction and side effects. Clinicians may also cling to the concept of pain as punishment and use it to hurt patients unwittingly. One thing is certain: most people who have had painful experiences are more sympathetic toward others in pain.

Once attitudinal obstacles are overcome, pain relief requires a step-by-step approach. The first step usually involves the oral administration of acetylsalicylic acid, acetaminophen, or nonsteroidal antiinflammatory agents. The latter include propionic acid derivatives such as ibuprofen (Motrin) and naproxen (Naprosyn), indolacetic acid derivatives such as indomethacin (Indocin), and nonacetylated salicylates such as diflunisal (Dolobid). All these agents inhibit action of prostaglandin synthetase, although acetaminophen has a somewhat less antiinflammatory effect. The principle adverse side effects of acetylsalicylic acid are gastrointestinal irritation and interference with platelet activity; the drug has also been implicated in the pathogenesis of Reye's syndrome. Acetaminophen causes hepatoxicity only in high doses in normal patients but may be more toxic in alcoholics with preexisting liver disease. The nonsteroidals may be nephrotoxic, especially in patients with volume depletion or preexisting renal disease.

Narcotic agonists relieve pain without causing sleep except in high doses, are reversed by antagonists such as naloxone (Narcan) that presumably block endorphin receptors in the nervous system, and produce tolerance and physical dependence that leads to autonomic hyperactivity during their withdrawal. Narcotics also decrease cough, ventilatory drive, temperature, blood pressure, pupillary size, and propulsion within the gastrointestinal tract and increase histamine release and pressure within the biliary system. Their most common side effects are pruritis, nausea, and constipation.

The analgesic effects of narcotics relate to the individual actions of the drugs, the balance between their agonistic and antagonistic properties, and their route of administration. Because most narcotics are rapidly cleared by the liver (first-pass phenomenon), increased oral doses are required to produce a significant analgesia. As a result, the drugs are best given intramuscularly, intravenously, sublingually, or by the epidural route. Intramuscular administration on a regular basis may be problematic because impaired absorption leads to variations in serum levels that provide unsustained pain relief and reinforce physical dependence (Fig. 79–1). Intramuscular dosing on an irregular PRN schedule is even less effective. Intravenous or epidural administration, ideally done on a continous basis, is therefore preferred.

The commonly prescribed narcotics are outlined in Table 79–1. Morphine is the standard against which all other analgesics must be compared.

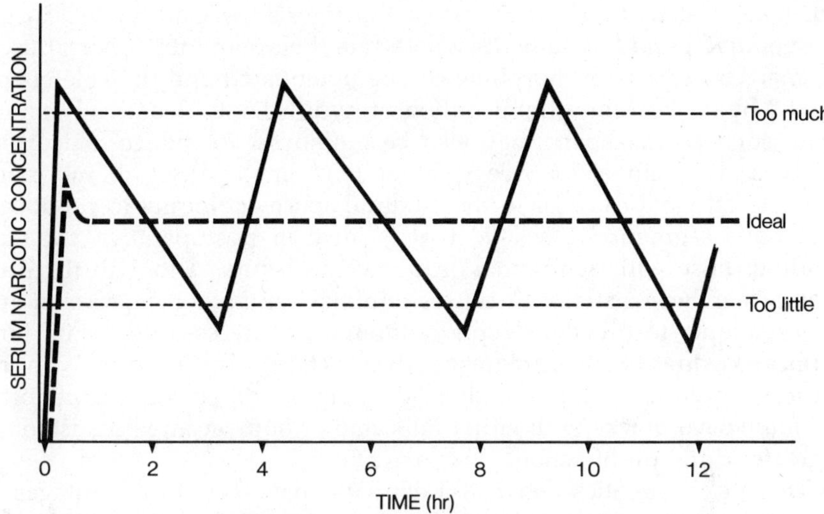

FIGURE 79–1. Intermittent administration of narcotics in intramuscular or other forms produces wide swings in serum levels. Continuous intravenous or epidural administration, which produces steady serum levels, is advised. (Adapted, with permission, from Edwards TW, Burney RG, Kupferberg IM: Management of pain, anxiety, and psychosis in the critically ill. In Rippe JM, Irwin RS, Alpert JE, et al (eds): Intensive Care Medicine. Boston, Little, Brown & Co., Inc., 1985, p. 1015.)

TABLE 79–1. COMMONLY PRESCRIBED NARCOTICS

AGENTS	RELATIVE POTENCY	DURATION OF ACTION (hr)	ORAL DOSE* (mg)	IM DOSE† (mg)	IV DOSE	IV INFUSION DOSE	EPIDURAL DOSE
Morphine	1	4–6	60	10	10 mg	1–5 mg/hr	5–10 mg
Codeine	0.01	4–6	200	NA	130 mg	NA	NA
Heroin	3	4–6	NA	NA	NA	NA	NA
Fentanyl (Sublimaze)	100	1–3	NA	NA	100 mg	10–15 mg/hr	25–50 mg/hr
Meperidine (Demerol)	0.1	2–4	NA	100	100 mg	20 mg/hr	NA
Methadone (Dolophine)	1	12–24	10	10	NA	NA	NA
Hydromorphone (Dilaudid)	4	2–6	NA	1.5	1.5 mg	NA	NA

IM = intramuscular; IV = intravenous; NA = not applicable.
*Oral doses are equivalent to 10 mg of IM morphine.
†IM dose is equivalent to 10 mg of IM morphine.

It is particularly safe to use in a critical care setting because it is easily reversed by naloxone (0.4 mg injections repeated as needed). Recent studies suggest that sufficient and safe analgesia can be achieved in the postoperative period by patients who titrate their own intravenous doses. The analgesic effects of morphine can be potentiated and the side effects reduced by concurrent administration of hydroxyzine. Sedative-hypnotic agents such as diazepam may also be employed to reduce concurrent anxiety and to aid sleep (see Chapter 66). Single doses of morphine administered via a catheter in the epidural space act locally to produce a 12–24 hour segmental blockade that is ideal in postoperative patients, including those with abdominal or thoracic incisions. Although the drug eventually moves rostrally, it causes minimal ventilatory depression and allows patients to breathe deeply (although not necessarily to full lung volumes, owing to diaphragmatic dysfunction). In patients with rib fractures, epidural analgesia is therapeutically and logistically superior to local intercostal blocks with either lidocaine or bupivacaine because of its far greater duration of action.

The other narcotics listed in Table 79–1 have certain advantages or disadvantages compared with those of morphine. Codeine is suitable only in oral form and provides no more analgesia than standard doses of non-narcotic agents such as acetaminophen unless it is given in large amounts. Fentanyl is much more powerful and expensive than morphine and can be given by the epidural or intravenous route; its short half-life may be advantageous in some patients, although it is probably less suitable than morphine in those with lingering pain. Meperidine, the most frequently prescribed narcotic in hospitals, is often not administered frequently enough to overcome its relatively short half-life. Heroin is more powerful than morphine but has no other intrinsic benefits. The long half-life of methadone can be utilized to provide a substrate of analgesia that can be augmented with morphine; it also is useful in withdrawing patients from narcotics, as discussed in Chapter 86. Clonidine, a centrally active α-agonist, has a synergistic inhibitory effect with opiates on central sympathetic overflow and may decrease narcotic requirements. It also is useful in treating narcotic withdrawal.

OUTCOME

As noted earlier, acute pain should be relieved if patients are treated appropriately and adequately.

RECOMMENDED READING

Bailey PW, Smith BE: Continuous epidural infusion of fentanyl for postoperative analgesia. Anesthesia 35:1002, 1980.

Bennett RL, Batenhorst RL, Bivins BA, et al: Patient-controlled analgesia: a new concept of postoperative pain relief. Ann Surg 195:700, 1981.

Bromage PR, Camporesi EM, Durant PA, et al: Rostral spread of epidural morphine. Anesthesiology 56:4316, 1982.

Church JJ: Continuous narcotic infusion for relief of postoperative pain. Br Med J 1:977, 1979.

Ghignone M, Quintin L, Duke PC, et al: Effects of clonidine on narcotic requirements and hemodynamic response during induction of fentanyl anesthesia and endotracheal intubation. Anesthesiology 64:36, 1986.

Gustafsson LL, Friberg-Nielsen S, Garle M, et al: Extradural and parenteral morphine: kinetics and effects in postoperative pain. A controlled clinical study. Br J Anaesth 54:1167, 1982.

Luce JM, Thompson TL, Getto CJ, et al: New concepts of chronic pain and their implications. Hosp Pract 14:113, 1979.

Marks RM, Sachar EJ: Undertreatment of medical inpatients with narcotic analgesia. Ann Intern Med 78:173, 1973.

Melzak R, Wall PD: Pain mechanisms: a new theory. Science 150:971, 1965.

Solomon RA, Viernstein MC, Long DM: Reduction of postoperative pain and narcotic use by transcutaneous electrical nerve stimulation. Surgery 67:142, 1980.

Utting JE, Smith JM: Postoperative analgesia. Anaesthesia 34:320, 1979.

Wang JK, Nauss LA, Thomas JE: Pain relief by intrathecally applied morphine in man. Anaesthesia 30:149, 1979.

Yaksh TL, Rudy TA: Analgesia mediated by a direct spinal action of narcotics. Science 192:1357, 1976.

Hematologic Disorders

80. Hemostatic Failure

Judith A. Luce

DEFINITION

Bleeding resulting from defects in the hemostatic mechanism is a common cause of morbidity in critically ill patients. Fortunately, death due to uncontrollable hemostatic defects is rare. However, clinicians are frequently frustrated by the seeming complexity of coagulation problems and approach them with a random, "shotgun" management plan. This chapter is offered to encourage the systematic evaluation and simplified treatment of bleeding problems.

PATHOPHYSIOLOGY

Blood clotting following interruption of a vessel occurs in a rapid and organized fashion, with three chief physiologic systems taking part. The first, the circulatory system, when interrupted, provides a bare, highly thrombogenic, platelet-adherent surface on which all later events are initiated. The vessel wall must constrict; in addition, a host of substances are released from the vascular endothelium: factors that stimulate clotting, such as kinins and the Fletcher factor; prostaglandins, which may either attract or "repel" platelets, depending on the situation; and substances that initiate fibrinolysis. Vessels with increased fragility, such as those in patients with connective tissue disorders, scurvy, or steroid therapy, are more prone to bleed. The microvascular abnormalities of diabetes and hypertension also predispose to bleeding. The rheology of the blood passing through the vessel is equally important: patients with altered blood viscosity related to hyperglobulinemia or polycythemia are more likely to bleed.

Platelets are the second major system and the cellular component of the blood clotting process. When contact with the subendothelial vessel surface occurs, a platelet undergoes sequential changes in shape, assumes a more adherent surface, and releases adenosine diphosphate (ADP) and thromboxane A_2, which attract other platelets, and serotonin, which has important local vascular effects. A primary plug of adhered platelets forms the first line of defense against further hemorrhage and, in addition,

TABLE 80–1. DRUGS ASSOCIATED WITH BLEEDING DISORDERS

PLATELET DYSFUNCTION
  Aspirin, nonsteroidal antiinflammatory agents
  Dipyridamole
  Dextran
  Ethanol
  β-lactam drugs in high doses: penicillin, semisynthetic penicillins, cephalothin,
    moxalactam, etc.
  Nitrofurantoin
  Clofibrate

THROMBOCYTOPENIA
  Heparin
  Ristocetin
  Quinine, quinidine, and related drugs
  Sulfonamides, sulfonylureas, and related drugs
  Gold salts
  Local and general anesthetics
  Selected antihistamines, tricyclics, phenothiazines
  Ethanol
  Thiazides, α-methyldopa
  Organic arsenicals
  Rifampin, PAS, isoniazid
  Ethchlorvynol
  Penicillins (immune-mediated)
  Digitoxin
  Many classes of cancer chemotherapeutic agents
  Aspirin
  (and more, still rarer—consult the PDR)

COAGULOPATHY
  Heparin
  Protamine
  Warfarin/dicoumarol
  Insect bites, snake bites
  Broad-spectrum antibiotics (vitamin K deficiency)
  Lupus-like syndromes from procainamide, quinidine (inhibitors of coagulation)
  Streptokinase, urokinase
  Tissue plasminogen activator

provides a matrix for fibrin clot formation. Platelets must be present in adequate numbers and must function normally in order for adequate hemostasis to be achieved.

Thrombocytopenia is a commonly acquired problem in the critically ill. Drugs are the chief offenders: a brief list in Table 80–1 describes the wide variety of classes of drugs that may cause poor platelet production or, in some cases, platelet destruction. Because normal body platelet turnover is slow (7–10 days), consumption of platelets may cause thrombocytopenia in a variety of ways. Nonimmune-mediated causes include disseminated intravascular coagulation (DIC) (see Chapter 81), thermal injury, cardiopulmonary bypass, hypersplenism, massive transfusion without adequate replacement, and the hemolytic-uremic syndrome and thrombotic thrombocytopenic purpura (TTP). Immune-mediated platelet destruction occurs in acute and chronic idiopathic thrombocytopenic purpura, following isoimmunization by transfusion or in neonates, following many kinds of infections of viral, rickettsial, and parasitic origin, and after the use of some kinds of drugs.

Disorders of platelet function may be important contributors to bleeding problems, although by themselves are not usually severe enough to cause significant hemorrhage. Aspirin, which irreversibly alters the platelet membrane cyclooxygenase, markedly reduces platelet aggregation *in vitro* and, as measured by the bleeding time, *in vivo*. Its effect on bleeding time is unmeasurable in most normal individuals after 24 hours, but in certain individuals, the effect of aspirin may be more prolonged and more profound. Ethanol has a very mild effect on platelet function, although it heightens the effect of aspirin, and, in addition, when consumed chronically, ethanol produces sometimes severe decreases in platelet production. Nonsteroidal antiinflammatory drugs may produce generally milder and more transient inhibition of platelet aggregation; certain semisynthetic penicillins and other β-lactam drugs may also inhibit platelet function.

The third and final step, the culmination of the coagulation process, the fibrin clot, is formed from a series of rapid, linked enzymatic steps— a "cascade." The extrinsic system, triggered by tissue thromboplastin, is fast, relatively insensitive to circulating anticoagulants, and of key importance in tissue injury such as trauma or surgery. The intrinsic system, triggered by nonendothelial surfaces, is slower and more sensitive to circulating and exogenous anticoagulants. The end product of both of these cascades is fibrin monomer, which polymerizes in the presence of Factor XIII to a stable complex. The entire series is dependent on calcium as a cofactor, platelets to provide a phospholipid-rich surface on which thrombin is activated (Factor II), and vitamin K as a cofactor in the hepatic synthesis of Factors II, VII, IX, and X. Once activated, most of these "serine proteases" have a fairly long half-life, although they may be inhibited by other circulating factors. Factors V and VIII may be consumed during rapid and intense coagulation.

DIAGNOSIS

The first step in the evaluation of a bleeding patient is the assessment of the medical history, drugs, and other illnesses that might predispose to bleeding. A previous surgical history is very important. Blood loss well in excess of that expected for a given procedure is an important indicator of past (perhaps even congenital) coagulation problems. Patients are generally not very accurate at assessing blood loss short of transfusion-requiring levels, however. Obstetrical histories may be misleading, too, as there are many intrapartum causes of massive bleeding in perfectly normal individuals. Dental histories are fairly useful. "Easy bruisability" is also difficult to assess, although large ecchymoses of nonexposed surfaces, mouth, or eyes are more likely to be pathologic. Oozing that occurs during and immediately after a procedure is most suggestive of poor platelet function; bleeding that begins hours after a procedure more strongly suggests a coagulation factor deficiency.

Review of the patient's drug history is extremely important. As previously mentioned, a variety of drugs may cause either platelet numbers or function to decrease. Vitamin K–dependent factor synthesis may be reduced by hepatic and nonhepatic disorders, but broad-spectrum antibiotic therapy, which reduces the enteric production of vitamin K, is by far the most common problem. Combined with inadequate nutrition, this form of coagulopathy may arise rapidly in seriously ill patients. Other potential drug interactions are outlined in Table 80–1.

Other medical problems are extremely important considerations in patients with hemostatic defects. The clinical setting is perhaps the most valuable piece of information when the diagnosis of DIC (Chapter 81) is being made. Uremia is an important cause of platelet dysfunction, which is thought to be mediated by dialyzable molecules interfering with platelet membrane functions. Patients with liver disease may have a host of abnormalities, including soluble factor deficiencies (either synthetic failure or K deficient), enhanced fibrinolysis, thrombocytopenia, platelet dysfunction due to lipid and bilirubin elevations, and persistence of fibrin split products (which act as antithrombins). Myeloproliferative disorders and chronic inflammatory diseases are important risk factors for DIC, acquired inhibitors of clotting, and platelet abnormalities. Cancer is a not infrequent cause of chronic DIC, chronic fibrinolysis, or other coagulopathies.

The physical examination in the critical care setting is centered on assessing the severity of the disorder. Postoperative bleeding from a surgical site only is most often due to wound failure. However, when patients are also bleeding from arterial and venous puncture sites, from endotracheal tubes and enteric tubes, as well as from surgical wounds, reexploration is unlikely to be of benefit to them. Rarely, patients will be found to have the stigmata of specific bleeding disorders, such as mucous membrane telangiectasias, vasculitis or scurvy. Petechiae are a reliable sign of either severe thrombocytopenia or severe hyperglobulinemia.

The basic laboratory screening for a critically ill bleeding patient should test all phases of blood clot formation (Fig. 80–1). A bleeding time, prothrombin time (PT), partial thromboplastin time (PTT), and platelet count should be done in every patient. Blood smear examination and fibrinogen level are strongly recommended. Other tests of specific factor

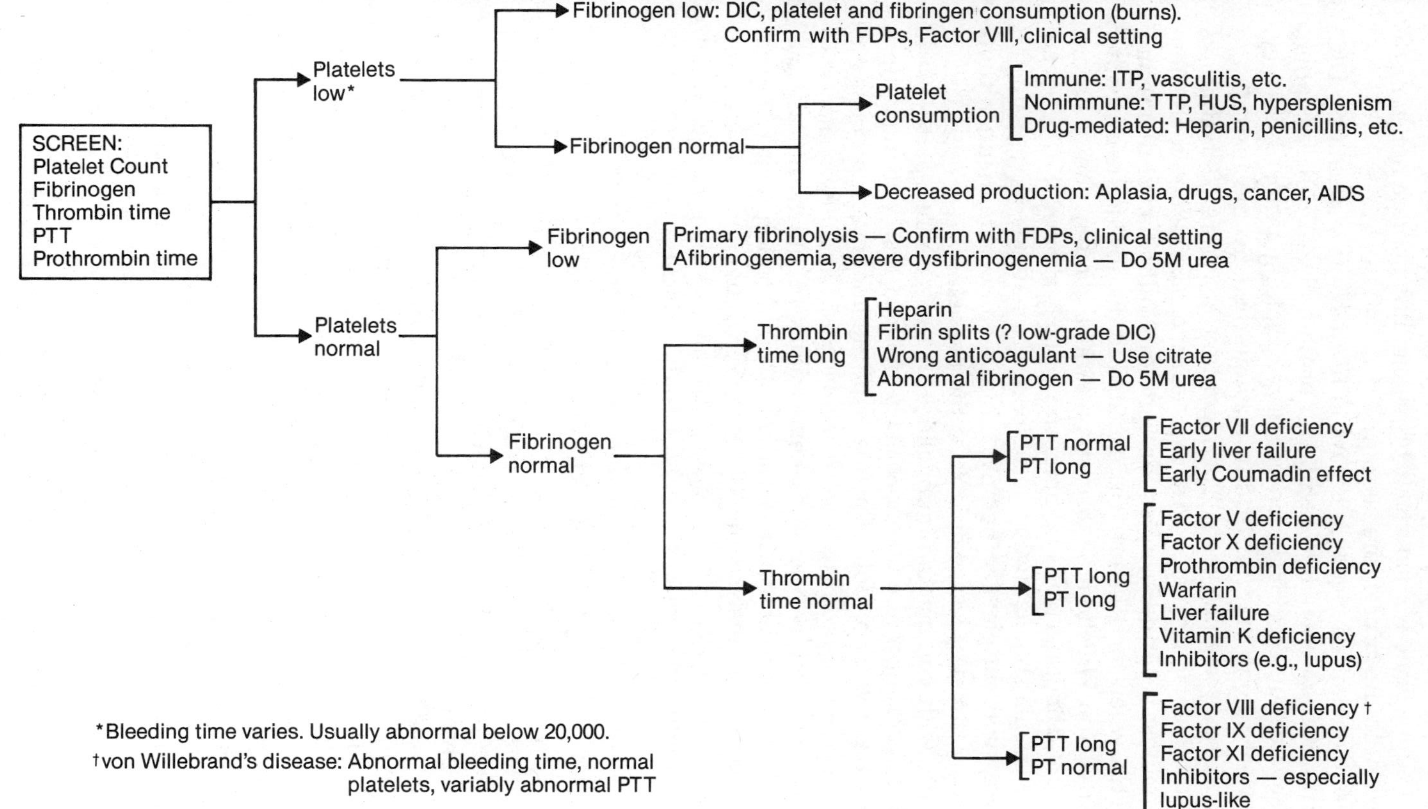

FIGURE 80–1. Algorithm for bleeding disorders. See text for explanation. PTT = partial thromboplastin time; PT = prothrombin time; DIC = disseminated intravascular coagulation; FDPs = fibrin degradation products; HUS = hemolytic-uremic syndrome; AIDS = acquired immuno-deficiency syndrome; 5M urea = test of total fibrinogen, done overnight in 5M urea solution; ITP = idiopathic thrombocytopenic purpura; TTP = thrombotic thrombocytopenic purpura.

489

levels and sophisticated *in vitro* tests of platelet function are not immediately relevant to the critical care setting.

Severe, generalized bleeding occurs in relatively few situations: DIC, severe thrombocytopenia, anticoagulation or fibrinolysis, and, less often, a fairly severe but previously unrecognized clotting factor deficiency. These few situations may be readily distinguished by the history and initial laboratory screening tests. The algorithm in Figure 80–1 attempts to clarify the mental sorting process necessary to narrow down a coagulopathy. Soluble factor deficiencies (or significant inhibitors of them) may be suspected when the PTT or PT is elevated in the absence of any other abnormality. Von Willebrand's disease presents a combination of normal platelet count, abnormal bleeding time, and variably abnormal PTT. Severe thrombocytopenia should always be suspected when massive transfusion has occurred without platelet therapy: transfusion of more than ten units of blood in 12 hours or less should raise the possibility.

Patients with combined abnormalities in two or more parts of the coagulation mechanism are far more likely to bleed than patients with a single abnormality; correction of as many of the underlying problems as possible is needed in order to restore hemostasis. Difficulty in diagnosis may arise from an absence of baseline values or other clinical data; completely empiric treatment is common in this situation. Finally, specimens for coagulation analysis must be properly drawn and collected and bleeding time measurement performed by an experienced technician; improper handling can result in very misleading results.

MANAGEMENT

Treatment depends on the nature of the coagulation problem and may therefore be classified by the system that has failed and by available therapeutic products.

Platelet numbers may be increased by transfusion of banked platelets; usually, one unit of platelets raises the recipient platelet count by approximately $10,000/mm^3$. Goals for adequate hemostasis are $\geq 50,000/mm^3$ for spontaneous bleeding or controlled general surgery and $\geq 100,000/mm^3$ for major vascular or trauma surgery and cardiopulmonary bypass. When platelet dysfunction is occurring, such as in uremia, transfused platelets will be of little efficacy unless the underlying problem is corrected.

In the presence of immune-mediated platelet destruction, platelet transfusions may result in prompt consumption. Occasionally, HLA or single-donor matching may help overcome this problem (see Chapter 82). In such cases, careful attention must also be given to normalizing other coagulation problems, to local measures to attenuate bleeding, and to efforts to remove the underlying cause of platelet consumption. Persistent random donor platelet transfusion should only be considered in the most desperate of emergencies, such as intracerebral bleeding or exsanguination. Recent data suggest that it may be possible to give high doses of intravenous gamma globulin followed by platelet transfusions in these life-threatening situations.

Platelet functional abnormalities are treated by removing the offending drug agent, such as aspirin, in the most common situations. Most patients' bleeding times will revert to normal within 24 hours after aspirin ingestion. Studies of elective abdominal surgery following aspirin ingestion show no increased risk of hemorrhagic complications. Uremic platelet dysfunction may be treated with dialysis. When dialysis is either not available or not tolerable, uremic patients may be treated either with cryoprecipitate infusion (see Chapter 82) or by administration of DDAVP (1-deamino-8-D-arginine-vasopressin), which causes release of Factor VIII-von Willebrand's factor, whose interaction with platelets is affected by uremia.

Cryoprecipitate, whose administration is further covered in Chapter 82, is given in doses of 8–12 bags, with a peak effect on bleeding time in about 4 hours. Its effect in uremia is gone at 24 hours; repeated dosing should occur at 8- to 12-hour intervals, depending on the clinical situation. This is similar to its use in von Willebrand's disease; therapy for patients with hemophilia A is more intense. DDAVP is given intravenously over 15–30 minutes at a dose of 0.3 μg/kg, with effects similar to those of cryoprecipitate, although with a slightly shorter half-life. Repeated doses are usually necessary. Many patients with von Willebrand's disease and some with mild hemophilia A are also responsive to DDAVP infusion. Cryoprecipitate and DDAVP are not useful for other forms of platelet dysfunction.

Coagulation factor deficiencies are treated in a variety of ways. The most common deficiency, that of vitamin K, may be rapidly corrected with 10 mg of parenteral AquaMEPHYTON. Most patients show normalization of PTs in 24–48 hours, although this assumes no other drugs, normal liver function, and some late lag in true correction of all four factor levels, owing to differential rates of production. More rapid reversal can be obtained by administering fresh frozen plasma, although the large volumes required to fully correct some patients may be intolerable to them.

Empiric treatment of assumed coagulation factor deficiency with fresh frozen plasma, when specific factor assays may not be available, is not harmful to patients, but may prove cumbersome (in that large volumes may be required to truly correct an abnormality) and largely ineffective, especially in adults with acquired inhibitors to coagulation. Plasma is frequently overused after transfusion as well. There is poor correlation between circulating factor levels and the number of transfused units of packed red blood cells; a better guide to the need for supplemental plasma in a heavily transfused patient is PT or PTT values. If PT and PTT are starting to rise in a patient receiving a large volume of packed cells, the addition of plasma is reasonable (and omission of platelets unforgivable!).

The clinical use of ε-aminocaproic acid (Amicar) is limited. This drug, a weak inhibitor of fibrinolysis, may be given orally or intravenously and requires a 6-hourly dosing schedule because of its short half-life. It is most often used to augment hemostasis in hemophiliacs undergoing surgery of the oral cavity, where salivary fibrinolytic activity is high. It is weak in its antifibrinolytic activity, however; and although it has been tried for post-streptokinase therapy and in spontaneous fibrinolytic states and DIC, its action does not justify a significant clinical role.

RECOMMENDED READING

Bachmann F: Diagnostic approaches to mild bleeding disorders. Semin Hematol 17:292, 1980.

Baldini MG: ITP and ITP syndrome. Med Clin North Am 56:47, 1972.

Bick RL: Hemostasis defects associated with cardiac surgery, prosthetic devices, and other extracorporeal circuits. Semin Thromb Hemost 11:249, 1985.

Bowie ESW, Owen CA Jr: Hemostatic failure in clinical medicine. Semin Hematol 14:341, 1977.

Counts RB, Haisch C, Simon TL, et al: Hemostasis in massively transfused trauma patients. Ann Surg 190:91, 1979.

Janson PA, Jubelirer SJ, Weinstein MJ, et al: Treatment of the bleeding tendency in uremia with cryoprecipitate. N Engl J Med 303:1318, 1980.

Malpass TW, Hanker LA: Acquired disorders of platelet function. Semin Hematol 17:242, 1980.

Mannucci PM, Remuzzi G, Pusiner F, et al: Deamino-8-D-arginine vasopressin shortens the bleeding time in uremia. N Engl J Med 308:8, 1983.

Miesscher PA: Drug-induced thrombocytopenia. Semin Hematol 10:311, 1973.

Prentice CRM: Acquired coagulation disorders. Clin Haematol 14:313, 1985.

Ridolfi RL, Bell WR: Thrombotic thrombocytopenic purpura. Report of 25 cases and review of the literature. Medicine 60:413, 1981.

Urbaniak SJ, Cash JD: Blood replacement therapy. Br Med Bull 33:273, 1977.

81. Disseminated Intravascular Coagulation

Judith A. Luce

DEFINITION

Disseminated intravascular coagulation (DIC) is one of the most common and often the most ominous acquired disorders of coagulation seen in the critical care setting. Indeed, in one large hospital series, 70 percent of the patients having DIC were already in the intensive care unit (ICU) and 85 percent of them died. For survivors, recovery was complete; DIC clearly complicated the course of nonsurvivors, but was rarely the sole cause of death. For this reason, treatment emphasizes recognition of the cause, anticipation of the situations in which DIC might occur, and early intervention to abort the process by dealing with the underlying pathology.

PATHOPHYSIOLOGY

The understanding of the pathophysiology of DIC rests on an understanding of the normal hemostatic mechanism. Clot formation is the result of the interaction of vascular endothelium, platelets, and soluble circulating factors, resulting in the polymerization of fibrin molecules (see Chapter 80). Fibrinolysis is also initiated by tissue factors and by vascular endothelium, is linked at several steps to the coagulation mechanism, and exists in an equilibrium with it. The DIC state is thought to represent overactivity brought on by extremely potent stimuli that overwhelm the normal checks and balances between the two systems.

Numerous mechanisms of initiation of DIC have been identified and act at various stages in the coagulation and fibrinolytic mechanisms. Vascular endothelial injury, for example, has been shown to cause platelet activation and deposition as well as fibrinolytic and soluble factor activation. Trauma, thermal injury, and other local mechanical stimuli are thought to trigger DIC by nonspecific endothelial damage. Platelet injury, which has been shown to trigger DIC in laboratory models, may act by releasing phospholipid into the circulation, much as an intravascular hemolytic episode does; phospholipids are potent stimuli to coagulation. Direct activation of the extrinsic system (via Factor VII) or intrinsic system (via Factor XII) may occur with tissue injury or be mediated by a variety of substances, including kallikreins and, perhaps, other leukotrienes. There is probably a multistep mechanism that activates coagulation when the release of various substances into the circulation occurs: amniotic fluid, thromboplastinlike substances from red and white blood cells, placenta cells, and unknown substances from tumors. Proteolytic enzymes such as zymosan and the thrombinlike substances from snake venoms are potent activators of the coagulation system; similarly, potent plasmin activators such as urokinase are capable of initiating DIC also. Endotoxin, perhaps the most common mediator, may actually act through some other factors such as interleukin 1 or another lymphokine in order to cause endothelial injury and to activate both coagulation and fibrinolysis.

Once activated, the entire hemostatic system rapidly becomes involved in DIC; evidence of all phases of clotting may be found in the disorder, although at times fibrinolysis may dominate over thrombus formation or vice versa. Consumption of the substrates of clot formation then occurs: platelets and fibrinogen are foremost, but to a lesser extent Factors V, VII, VIII, X, XIII, and sometimes II, as well as antithrombin III, plasminogen, and α_2-antiplasmin disappear from the circulation. Some controversy exists over the degree to which the latter are consumed, and static measurement of these factors fails to tell either how fast they are disappearing or from what level they might have fallen.

In addition to consumption of substrates, the appearance of by-products of the clotting process occurs; these are important both as markers of the process itself and as physiologic factors in the process. Fibrin is metabolized either into polymers (with the aid of Factor XIII) or, in the presence of plasmin activity, into a series of smaller peptides known as fibrin degradation products. In the presence of excess plasmin activity, fibrinogen may also be broken down into smaller peptides. Both fibrin and fibrinogen degradation products may be measured, and both are potent inhibitors of thrombin activity and important in the bleeding diathesis of DIC. Normally cleared in the urine and reticuloendothelial cells, fibrin and fibrinogen degradation products (FDPs) may not be cleared adequately in DIC both because they are being generated too rapidly and because of end-organ dysfunction. Soluble complexes of fibrin monomers appear in greater amounts; similarly, fibrin-fibrinogen complexes can be found. Both may be incorporated into clot, although the fibrinogen-fibrin complexes may not form stable clot.

The net effect of rapid and tumultuous turnover of coagulation is impaired hemostasis due to the combination of depletion of the requisite substrates, circulating inhibitors, and increased clot lysis. Thrombus formation may be seen and may occasionally (especially in the chronic DIC state) dominate the clinical picture. Thrombi may be large and either arterial or venous, or may be microscopic and diffuse. Diffuse microvascular thrombi are thought to complicate DIC by producing dysfunction in a variety of organs, from brain to kidney to liver and heart, organs that may already be compromised by the underlying illness causing DIC. Local effects of vascular thrombi may be seen dramatically in patients with purpura fulminans, in which hemorrhagic necrosis of skin occurs in the setting of gram-negative sepsis. DIC is thought to contribute significantly to the pathophysiology of two important associated conditions, adult respiratory distress syndrome and acute tubular necrosis.

Diagnosis

Making the diagnosis of DIC early in its course largely depends on recognizing a situation in which it might occur; interpretation of the laboratory tests for DIC is based to a large extent on the setting in which it is observed. It is hoped that early recognition and treatment can lead to better management, although the clinical data suggest that this rarely happens. Table 81–1 is a summary of the causes of DIC.

The association of sepsis, particularly with endotoxin-producing organisms, and DIC is well recognized. Endotoxin is a potent initiator of DIC as well as of a host of other manifestations of the septic state and probably acts through a variety of mediators of the inflammatory response. Other infectious diseases cause DIC more rarely, but overwhelming viral and ricksettsial disease and occasionally disseminated mycobacterial infections are associated with DIC.

Shock probably causes DIC through the same mechanisms as endotoxin, although the exact process has yet to be elucidated. Any cause of shock may be associated with DIC, although, clearly, sepsis predominates in the ICU setting. Burns may be associated with DIC or without shock; so also can other thermal injuries such as heat stroke.

Obstetrical causes of DIC are quite diverse but, fortunately, short-lived. *Abruptio placentae*, retained dead fetus, and severe toxemia are the most easily treated, i.e., by delivery of the fetus; vaginal delivery actually places less stress on the hemostatic mechanism than does cesarean section. Amniotic fluid embolism is very dangerous and lethal; it may occur in the setting of induced abortion as well as in term delivery and is accompanied often by severe pulmonary insufficiency and right heart failure as well as DIC. An extremely rare event, acute fatty liver of pregnancy, has a high mortality because of concomitant liver failure and DIC. Obstetric patients display a variety of abnormalities of coagulation that render them vulnerable to clotting and make the diagnosis of DIC more difficult. At term, levels of fibrinogen in the blood are high; levels of Factor VIII and

TABLE 81–1. CONDITIONS THAT MAY TRIGGER DISSEMINATED INTRAVASCULAR COAGULATION (DIC)

OBSTETRIC
  Retained dead fetus
  Abruptio placentae
  Amniotic fluid embolism
  Severe toxemia
  Septic abortion/intrauterine infection
  Hydatidiform mole
  Placenta accreta
  Prolonged shock from obstetrical causes
  Intravascular hemolysis

ACUTE, CRITICAL CARE
  Shock, any etiology
  Sepsis, especially gram-negative or meningococcal
  Anaphylaxis
  Burns
  Heat stroke
  Severe hemolytic transfusion reaction
  Severe viral and rickettsial infections
  Surgery or manipulation of the urinary tract and prostate
  Snake venom

CAUSES USUALLY ASSOCIATED WITH CHRONIC DIC
  Neoplasms, particularly adenocarcinomas, urinary tract, and acute leukemia
  Myeloproliferative diseases
  Autoimmune disorders
  Kasabach-Merritt syndrome
  "Hypercoagulable states," such as thrombophlebitis, use of oral contraceptives, chronic inflammatory disease, postoperative state

antithrombin III are also abnormal. Hepatic and reticuloendothelial clearance of activated factors may be abnormal as well. Patients with preeclampsia may develop low-grade DIC.

Chronic DIC, a less hyperactive version of acute DIC, is known to occur in a host of different settings, but mainly in patients with cancer and chronic inflammatory diseases such as autoimmune disease. DIC in these settings may also be complicated by the presence of other circulating inhibitors of coagulation. It is important to recognize patients with chronic DIC because they are at a much heightened risk of thrombosis and bleeding in the hospital, particularly intra- and postoperatively.

There are several clinical situations occurring in the ICU that may resemble DIC but must be distinguished from it. Much of the older literature includes thrombotic thrombocytopenic purpura and hemolytic-uremic syndrome in the causes of DIC. These conditions may display red cell shearing and hemolysis, thrombocytopenia, and bleeding on that basis. However, fibrinogen turnover is near normal and coagulation parameters should be normal. The treatment for these two disorders is very different than that of DIC, and clinical and laboratory distinctions must be drawn.

Another disorder that may resemble DIC and be difficult to distinguish from it is the coagulopathy of advanced liver disease. Patients with liver failure display many of the same abnormalities as those with DIC: low platelet counts, low fibrinogen levels (although usually very late in their disease), abnormal coagulation tests, elevated levels of FDPs, and abnormalities of fibrinolysis that may arise from either poor hepatic clearance of FDPs and plasmin or from poor hepatic synthesis of α_2-antiplasmin. Signal differences are that the liver-failure patient's coagulopathy is relatively static, in that consumption of substrates is not usually occurring at the same rate as in DIC. Unfortunately, clinicians cannot obtain dynamic measurements for the most part and must try to use available static tests to differentiate DIC. Factor VIII levels are often elevated in patients who have an inflammatory component to their liver disease; therefore, patients with low or merely low-normal levels of this factor may be having DIC. Similarly, Factor V, not made by the liver, may be depressed in DIC. Changes in previously observed levels of platelets, fibrinogen, or FDPs may also be a clue to the development of DIC. Other sophisticated tests, such as fibrinopeptide generation, reptilase clotting times, and other factor levels, have not proven clinically useful.

Laboratory screening for DIC employs tests that are both readily available to clinicians and abnormal in most patients with DIC. These are listed in Table 81–2. The "DIC screen" that is performed by most laboratories consists of prothrombin time (PT), partial thromboplastin time (PTT), FDPs, fibrinogen, and platelet count. The findings of depressed platelet numbers and fibrinogen level, increased FDPs and mild elevations in PT and PTT are typical of DIC.

The thrombin time (TT) measures only the final steps in coagulation, since thrombin is added directly to plasma. It is extremely sensitive to fibrinogen levels and inhibitors of thrombin activity. Thrombin times are always abnormal in patients with DIC, since FDPs are inhibitors of thrombin. Heparin, by binding to antithrombin III, is a potent thrombin inhibitor and also raises the TT markedly. Therefore, TTs may be used when the clinician is uncertain whether near-normal PT or PTTs are significant, when the PTT is much higher than the PT elevation and heparin has been given, and when platelet counts, fibrinogen levels, and FDPs are not particularly diagnostic and heparin has not been given.

The peripheral blood smear may be a useful adjunct to the diagnosis of DIC. In addition to noting a decrease in the number of platelets, one might expect to see red cell morphologic changes suggestive of intravascular red cell destruction: schistocytes, helmet cells, and other red-cell fragments. These are produced by collisions between red cells and fibrin strands formed in small vessels, with mechanical shearing of the red cells.

Factor levels may be useful in evaluating patients with DIC, as long as the results are not needed promptly. As previously mentioned, Factors

TABLE 81–2. LABORATORY DIAGNOSIS OF DISSEMINATED INTRAVASCULAR COAGULATION (DIC)

TEST	NORMAL VALUE	ACUTE DIC	PERCENT OF PATIENTS ABNORMAL	CHRONIC DIC
Platelet count	175,000–400,000/mm³	<150,000 Often very low	50–90	Variable; often low-normal
Fibrin degradation products	<10 µg/ml	>40 µg/ml	75–100	Should be abnormal
Prothrombin time	11–12.5 seconds*	2–5 seconds longer	70–80	Usually normal
Partial thromboplastin time	*	2–20 seconds longer	70–80	Mildly increased; may be shorter
Fibrinogen	185–300 mg/dl	≤100 mg/dl	40–70	May be normal
Thrombin time	<20 seconds*	5–60 seconds longer	60–80	Should be abnormal
Red cell morphology (blood smear)	Normal appearance	Schistocytes	40–70	May be normal
Euglobulin lysis time	Hours*	Variable: long, short, or normal	30	Variable
Factors V and VIII	50–150 percent	Variable	20–80	Variable
Antithrombin III	>50 percent	<50 percent	60–80	May be low or normal

*Based on individual laboratory controls.

V and VIII are consumed stoichiometrically in the coagulation process and may fall during DIC. The use of these levels is complicated, since they may rise in inflammatory states and fall into the normal range with consumption. While other factor levels fall more variably, they are less useful measures of the consumptive process.

When heparin has been given to patients, its presence confounds the diagnosis. FDPs and low fibrinogen levels should not be seen in a patient who has been given heparin, but in case these values are borderline, many laboratories provide biochemical tests for the presence of heparin, including simply serial additions of small amounts of protamine to the plasma.

A variety of tests of fibrinolysis have been devised, but the most widely used is the euglobulin lysis time. This is not a rapid assay and is only useful when a clinician is considering therapy directed at fibrinolysis. Simple whole-blood clotting times and the appearance of clots are not useful tests—they are time-consuming, not very reproducible, and should optimally be done in a 37° C bath, not in the operating room or the ICU.

Finally, if the diagnosis of DIC is uncertain and steps have been taken to treat other potential coagulation problems and hemorrhage continues, repeating the laboratory screening tests is mandatory. Because DIC is a rapid process in most cases, changes in fibrinogen and platelets, and perhaps even elevations in FDP levels, may be seen over a period of only a few hours; this demonstration of ongoing consumption may be all that is necessary to make the diagnosis clear.

MANAGEMENT

The treatment of DIC has long been a source of controversy, primarily because no specific therapy solves the clinical problem. A host of supportive and palliative therapies have been offered, but mortality remains high. Clearly, the patients who survive DIC have two characteristics: mild DIC or rapid resolution of the underlying stimulus. Therefore, the single most important aspect of DIC treatment lies not in treating its symptoms but in discovering and treating its cause.

Therapy of DIC falls into two categories: transfusion support and pharmocologic intervention. The rationale for transfusion therapy is that patients could not recover without support, even if this support risks adding "fuel to the fire" of DIC. Pharmacologic interventions have been directed at various aspects of the process, including fibrinolysis and thrombin activity.

Transfusion with red blood cells to replace hemorrhagic losses is the most important part of DIC therapy, since, obviously, intravascular volume loss will exacerbate the problem. Platelet support is also widely regarded as necessary and important; ideally, maintaining a platelet count at or above 50,000/mm^3 would help hemostasis. Since platelets are rapidly consumed in DIC, this may be nearly impossible to accomplish, but there is no clinical data to suggest that it is harmful.

Plasma and plasma products have been variably used in DIC. Fresh frozen plasma provides all of the missing soluble components, but carries hepatitis and other disease risks, is cumbersome to thaw, and may be required in very high volumes. In addition, it may not be necessary to replace all factors, since the depressions in many are not significant. Cryoprecipitate is preferred by many clinicians, since its volume is low, and it contains three substances known to be diminished in DIC— fibrinogen, Factor VIII, and fibronectin. The last is a plasma substance thought to be important in platelet-endothelial interactions and in opsonization and clearance of debris and bacteria from the circulation. It is unclear that real benefit accrues to patients treated with cryoprecipitate because of fibronectin replacement, but this has been advocated. As with platelets, use of plasma products should be followed by some measurement of their effect. A target of PT and PTT levels below 1½ times normal is not unreasonable, since hemostasis can often be achieved at these levels. Fibrinogen levels over 100 mg/dl are desirable but must be higher if bleeding persists at this level.

Exchange transfusion and pheresis are radical approaches to the patient with DIC and are of unproven benefit. They are probably too cumbersome and destabilizing for the average critically ill patient, and their use could only be undertaken in a patient whose inciting illness had clearly been arrested.

Pharmacologic tactics in the treatment of DIC have had a varied history. Heparin was one of the first agents used. In laboratory models such as snakebite, endotoxic shock, heat stroke, and some obstetric models, heparin is of no demonstrable use. Its clinical application has been in a variety of situations. In acute DIC, it is most likely that the risk of increased bleeding outweighs the clinical benefit: a small minority of patients display improvements in laboratory abnormalities, and a larger fraction sustain increased bleeding. Heparin has been successfully applied in a few limited situations: prophylactic treatment of leukemic patients who either have DIC or are at high risk (especially myelomonocytic leukemia and promyelocytic leukemia), prophylactic treatment of obstetric patients with retained dead fetus prior to the delivery of the fetus, and in some chronic DIC patients with malignancy or inflammatory diseases. The use of warfarin anticoagulation in such patients is of no benefit.

Antiplatelet agents such as aspirin and dipyridamole have a role in the treatment of TTP or hemolytic-uremic syndrome but have no defined role in DIC. Still more obscure is the potential role of antithrombin III and other pharmacologic antithrombins. These drugs may actually exacerbate the coagulopathy and, given the lack of good clinical trials, should only be used in the research setting.

The use of fibrinolytic inhibitors is also controversial. The usual clinical doses of ϵ-aminocaproic acid are capable of inhibiting plasmin activity (see Chapter 80). The risk exists that its use may convert a primarily hemostatic defect into a thrombotic problem, since the clotting cascade remains unchecked. In occasional patients, the laboratory data predominantly suggest fibrinolysis, that is, high levels of FDPs, abnormal euglobulin lysis, and relatively little effect on PT and PTT. In a patient whose condition could lead to mostly fibrinolysis, such as one who has had surgery on the urinary tract or one with a malignancy of the urinary tract, a cautious trial of fibrinolytic agents is indicated.

OUTCOME

The criteria for a response to therapy for DIC are vague but are based on a reduction or cessation of bleeding and some normalization of hemostasis. The half-time of disappearance of FDPs from the circulation is approximately 9 hours, and, in conjunction with the fall in FDPs, the PTT and TT should improve. Removal of fibrin-fibrinogen complexes and fibrin-fibrin degradation complexes may take much longer. Fibrinogen levels may take several days to rise to normal, depending greatly on the state of the patient's nutrition and liver. The platelet count is the slowest to rise and usually requires the most support. Normal platelet turnover is a week to 10 days, and increases in production occur only very slowly. Marrow depression is a frequent occurrence in a serious illness, so that replacement may barely occur at all for many days after the DIC episode resolves. A stationary platelet count is probably an encouraging sign in such a patient.

DIC is associated with a high mortality. As mentioned in the introduction, 85 percent of patients having acute DIC in a large hospital series died. However, more than 70 percent of the entire series had failure of one or more organ systems, and the mortality in the ICU patients was 91 percent. Fewer than 5 percent of patients in the series had hemorrhage or thrombosis as a major cause of death. DIC clearly complicates the care of these ill patients, and acute respiratory failure and acute renal failure were concomitant with DIC in 40 percent of patients. Those patients who survive are less ill at the onset, have fewer severe hematologic abnormalities, and have the most reversible clinical situations.

RECOMMENDED READING

Bone RC, Francis PB, Pierce AK: Intravascular coagulation associated with the adult respiratory distress syndrome. Am J Med 61:585, 1976.

Boulton FE, Letsky E: Obstetric haemorrhage: causes and management. Clin Haematol 14:683, 1985.

Brodin B, Hesselvik F, Blomback M, et al: Fibronectin and other DIC-related variables in patients with moderately severe infections receiving cryoprecipitate. Scand J Clin Lab Invest 45:57, 1985.

Colman RW, Robboy SJ, Minna JD: Disseminated intravascular coagulation (DIC): an approach. Am J Med 52:679, 1972.

Corrigan JJ Jr, Jordan CM: Heparin therapy in septicemia with disseminated intravascular coagulation. N Engl J Med 283:778, 1970.

Deykin D: The clinical challenge of disseminated intravascular coagulation. N Engl J Med 283:636, 1970.

Drapkin RL, Gee TS, Dowling MD, et al: Prophylactic heparin therapy in acute promyelocytic leukemia. Cancer 41:2484, 1978.

Feinstein DI: Diagnosis and management of disseminated intravascular coagulation: the role of heparin therapy. Blood 60:284, 1982.

Mant MJ, King EG: Severe, acute disseminated intravascular coagulation. Am J Med 67:557, 1979.

Sherman LA: Therapeutic problems of disseminated intravascular coagulation. Arch Intern Med 132:446, 1973.

Siegal T, Seligsohn U, Aghai E, et al: Clinical and laboratory aspects of disseminated intravascular coagulation (DIC): a study of 118 cases. Thromb Haemost 39:122, 1978.

Spero JA, Lewis JH, Hasiba U: Disseminated intravascular coagulation: findings in 346 patients. Thromb Haemost 43:28, 1980.

Spicer TE, Rau JM: Purpura fulminans. Am J Med 61:566, 1976.

82. Blood Banking and Blood Products

Judith A. Luce

INTRODUCTION

Safe, sophisticated blood product support has been one of the chief reasons for the development of trauma and burn centers and for the success of major surgical procedures such as cardiac surgery and invasive vascular surgery. Advances in blood banking have also permitted the safer and more sophisticated treatment of medical patients in intensive care units as well as patients with hematologic and immunologic disorders and patients undergoing intensive cancer treatment. This chapter covers the availability, indications, administration, and complications of blood products.

RED BLOOD CELLS

Whole blood is rarely available to clinicians, particularly in the centers that are large enough to support intensive care units. Blood banks increasingly produce either packed red blood cells or, occasionally, a product that has had various plasma components, mainly platelets, removed. This may be called "reconstituted" whole blood or "processed" whole blood. The reasons for this trend are several: First, most locales experience difficulty and great cost in obtaining donors of fresh whole blood in emergent situations. Second, storage at refrigerator temperatures results in the prompt deterioration of platelet function; thus, the value of the platelet component of whole blood is lost. And, finally, increased use of cryoprecipitate for hemophilia treatment has led many centers to remove this plasma fraction early in the storage process as well. Packed red blood cells have become the standard item for support of patients requiring red cell transfusion.

The definition of transfusion requirement and, therefore, the indications for transfusion of red blood cells, are highly variable. Actively bleeding patients have requirements based on blood pressure, volume of blood loss, and ability to tolerate intravascular volume changes; these

502

requirements may fluctuate, and rigid criteria cannot be laid out. Chronically anemic patients may have widely differing requirements for intravascular volume, for oxygen-carrying capacity, and for tissue oxygen delivery. Ultimately, the goal is adequate tissue oxygenation, but arriving at an accurate simple measure of this is difficult. Tissue oxygen extraction (as measured by the arterial-mixed venous oxygen difference $[a - \bar{v}]O_2$) may be measured in most patients in the intensive care unit (ICU), but other factors influencing this value, including metabolic demands and cardiac function, are not readily taken into account. In general, a hemoglobin level of 10 g/dl or greater is compatible with life in virtually all situations. Most surgical literature of untransfused patients with acute bleeding suggests that the survival of patients with hemoglobin levels of 7 g/dl or greater is not influenced by the lack of transfusion. Mortality due to tissue oxygen deprivation begins to occur at hemoglobin values below this level. Several clinical parameters have been proposed as guidelines to inadequate tissue oxygenation in critically ill patients. These include a mixed venous oxygen tension ($P\bar{v}O_2$) of less than 25 mm Hg, oxygen consumption falling to less than 50 percent of the patient's baseline value (assuming that this is known), and an oxygen extraction ratio of more than 50 percent; that is,

$$\frac{\text{oxygen consumed}}{\text{oxygen delivered}} \geq 50 \text{ percent, or } \frac{CaO_2 - C\bar{v}O_2}{CaO_2} \geq 0.5$$

Beyond these simple guidelines, the choice and the amount of red cell transfusions are highly individualized.

Other forms of red cells are increasingly available. Washed, or "leukocyte-poor," red cells are used for patients with repeated intolerance of packed cell transfusions, presumably due to febrile or other reactions to contaminating white blood cells. Red blood cell preparations may also be irradiated to render leukocytes inviable so that inadvertent engraftment in an immunosuppressed recipient does not occur. Of potentially wider use, however, are frozen red cells. Frozen in glycerol, these red blood cells have a longer shelf-life, and although they may not be used routinely, they may be useful in extending the shelf-life of rare donor type units of blood.

Artificial blood substitutes have been devised and are of two general types. The first is denatured hemoglobin, which is a less efficient molecule than the tetramer in the red cell, but by polymerization or conjugation with other carrier molecules, such as dextrans, the developers hope to create a product that is both a more efficient carrier and has a longer circulatory half-life than the free hemoglobin monomers. This product has seen very little clinical testing. On the other hand, the perfluorocarbons are molecules with high solubility for oxygen that have been clinically tested as Fluosol DA. These products are marred by their relatively short circulatory half-life (24 hours) and by the requirement for high inspired oxygen concentrations for efficient loading of the molecules. Recent clinical data suggest little or no clinical benefit of the commercially available product at safe, nontoxic doses.

Transfusion of red blood cells is quite straightforward. Meticulous care must be paid to the identification of the patient, the blood to be transfused, and the verification of the typing data. Half of all hemolytic transfusion reactions are due to clerical or nursing errors. Large-bore catheters or needles (< 20-gauge) are required, both for the speed of flow and to avoid shearing red cells. In-line filters do effectively screen large clumps of adhered or denatured red cells and cellular debris; their use has diminished the incidence of nonspecific reactions. Heating, if necessary, is accomplished with a variety of commercial devices but must be carefully monitored, since red cell hemolysis occurs at temperatures as low as 40 °C. Patient management includes nursing observation for fever, urticaria, and hypotension. Monitoring for intravascular volume overload and response to therapy are important parameters.

White Blood Cells

White blood cells may also be transfused but are of limited usefulness. Leukocytes are harvested from individual donors, using apheresis equipment and often supplemental steroids, hydroxyethyl starch, or other additives to improve yield. Once obtained, leukocytes must be promptly administered, since *in vitro* they adhere to one another and degranulate, and their survival is only a few hours. Their use has been largely confined to neutropenic patients with infection. Clearly, in a neutropenic patient with a documented bacterial infection that is not responding to appropriate antibacterial therapy, leukocyte transfusions may be life-saving. However, the empiric or prophylactic use of white cell transfusions in any febrile neutropenic patient is not supported by the literature. Their prophylactic use in the bone marrow transplant setting may be justified. Leukocyte transfusions carry a heightened risk of transmission of cytomegalovirus, and, theoretically, a heightened risk of HIV-1, and the virus responsible for the acquired immunodeficiency syndrome (AIDS) as well.

Platelets

Platelets are harvested from whole blood by a sedimentation process before it is refrigerated. Together with a small amount of plasma, platelets are stored at room temperature under continuous gentle agitation for 72 hours to a week. Platelet function deteriorates steadily under these conditions, probably owing to random collisions triggering adhesion and degranulation. The platelets from a single unit of blood are sufficient to raise the platelet count of an average-sized recipient by about 10,000/mm^3. Goals for platelet counts for most routine general surgery are $> 50,000/$mm^3. Higher numbers, $\geq 100,000/$mm^3, are required for cardiopulmonary bypass and major trauma surgery. Obviously, numbers are as important as function, and no platelet transfusion should be undertaken without concurrent assessment of platelet function, such as a bleeding time. Spontaneous hemorrhage starts to occur in patients having fewer than 20,000/mm^3 platelets; most clinicians consider this their threshold for "routine" transfusion to prevent potentially lethal spontaneous hemorrhage. However, some patients, particularly those with stable, immune-mediated destruction of platelets, may tolerate platelet levels as low as 5,000/mm^3 before evidence of spontaneous blood loss starts to appear.

Platelets are a very important component of the transfusion therapy of all seriously bleeding patients. Since stored whole blood contains, for practical purposes, *no* viable platelets, and since bone marrow recovery from depletion of circulating platelets may be too slow or slowed by metabolic insults, clinicians must remember to give adequate numbers of platelets when resuscitating a massively bleeding patient. Rapid transfusion of 10 or more units of blood over a few hours (less than 12 hours, as a rule), should automatically require at least checking the patient's platelet count. Empiric usage is difficult to prescribe, since some patients consume platelets extremely rapidly—patients with disseminated intravascular coagulation (DIC), burns, massive crush injury, and sepsis, for example. Their platelet requirements may easily exceed the 10-units-of-red-cells rule of thumb. A general rule is to obtain platelet counts regularly in any bleeding patient. The only situation in which platelets are not always given is in patients with idiopathic thrombocytopenic purpura, in whom the rapid immune destruction of platelets renders them useless, and theoretically, may even aggravate the problem.

PLASMA AND PLASMA FRACTIONS

Plasma may be available to clinicians in several forms: fresh-frozen plasma is exactly what the name implies, although it is devoid of platelets and sometimes of cryoprecipitate also. Plasma expanders (such as Plasmanate) are usually globulin-free, processed products that are less allergenic, free of clotting factors, and therefore useful as volume expanders only. Albumin may be obtained in small quantities and makes an expensive but concentrated form of volume expander. Fresh frozen plasma is a useful product for the clinician who requires volume supplementation in the transfused patient and is concerned about the so-called "washout" syndrome, in which albumin and plasma proteins, including clotting factors, are diluted when massive quantities of red cells and saline are given in transfusion. The difficulty in quantitating the "washout" syndrome is that there is a poor correlation between the number of units of red cells and saline transfused and clotting factor levels measurable in the recipients. Nonetheless, there are patients for whom fresh frozen plasma is important; they can be found by evaluating the prothrombin or partial thromboplastin times in transfused patients.

Fresh frozen plasma is routine treatment for patients who exhibit vitamin K-dependent factor depletion (from any source, including warfarin therapy), who are bleeding and require rapid correction of their coagulopathy. However, since large volumes of plasma may be required to fully correct the clotting abnormality, vitamin K must always be administered concomitantly and intravascular volume monitored. Fresh frozen plasma is a routine source for rare factors such as XIII, XII, and XI; in addition, it may be part of the therapy for thrombotic thrombocytopenic purpura. Fresh frozen plasma is useful for replacement following pheresis. It may be necessary in patients with C1 esterase deficiency who are having life-threatening angioedema. Administration follows immediately after thawing the units in a controlled fashion, to avoid overheating. In-line filters are recommended, as is monitoring for febrile and urticarial reactions.

Cryoprecipitate is formed when fresh plasma is rapidly frozen, then carefully thawed to only 60 °F. Factor VIII precipitates out of the solution, along with roughly one third of the fibrinogen; this precipitate is harvested by centrifugation and is resuspended in a very small volume of saline or dried (in the commercial preparations), pooled, and stored. Cryoprecipitate is a safe, usually inexpensive form of Factor VIII and, in addition, makes a low-volume source of fibrinogen. Aside from its use in the treatment of von Willebrand's disease, for which it supplies the complete Factor VIII–von Willebrand's factor molecule, in hemophilia A and in primary and secondary afibrinogenemia, cryoprecipitate may be a useful adjunct in the treatment of DIC (Chapter 81); it may also have a role in the treatment of uremic platelet dysfunction. Once resuspended, cryoprecipitate should be given promptly, intravenously, with the use of an in-line filter. General dose guidelines are stated in Table 82–1.

Concentrates of Factors VIII and IX are commercially available products used specifically for the treatment of hemophiliacs. The dose and general use are outlined in Table 82–1. The goal of treatment is to raise the patient's plasma factor level to that desired for treatment of spontaneous or surgical bleeding. The frequency with which the factor is given depends on the duration of symptoms or the period of surgical risk. Factor IX preparations are much more difficult to use, in part because the

TABLE 82–1. PROTOCOL FOR FACTOR REPLACEMENT

| | PERCENT OF NORMAL REQUIRED | | | | | PERCENT RECOVERY OF |
FACTOR	Minor Surgery	Major Surgery*	SOURCE	Dose (per kg)	HALF-LIFE (hr)†	TRANSFUSED PATIENTS
I	50–100 mg/dl	>100 mg/dl	Cryoprecipitate	0.3 bag	96–144	50
II	10–15	20–40	Plasma	20 ml	50–80	40–100
V	5–15	15–25	Plasma	10 ml	12–24	50–80
VII	5–10	10–20	Plasma	10 ml	4–6	70–100
VIII	15–20	50	Concentrate Cryoprecipitate	40 units‡ (80–100 U/bag)	6–12	70–80
IX	10–15	50	Concentrate	80 U§	20–30	25–50
X	5–10	15–20	Plasma	10 ml	25–50	50–100
XI	5–15	15–25	Plasma	20 ml	40–84	90
XII	less than 10		None	None	Unknown	
XIII	1	5	Plasma or Cryoprecipitate	5 ml 0.1 bag	150	50–100
VWF	20?	50?	Cryoprecipitate‖	0.6 bag	6–12¶	70–80

*Includes dental extractions.
†Tranfusion interval may vary; does not include consumption states.
‡Dose depends on initial factor level; 1 unit = 100 percent normal activity/ml plasma.
§Factor IX concentrate varies in viability; recovery is so poor that transfusion is impractical, except in emergencies.
‖Do not use factor VIII concentrate to correct platelet dysfunction.
¶Half life of VIII coagulant activity; half life of effect on bleeding time about 4 hrs.
VWF = von Willebrand factor
Adapted, with permission, from Urbaniak SJ, Cash JD: Br Med Bull 33:273, 1977.

bioavailability of the preparation is poor. Particularly difficult to treat are severe hemophiliacs who have acquired antibodies to Factor VIII or IX. An experienced hematologist should guide the management of hemophiliac patients once they are hospitalized.

BLOOD CROSSMATCHING AND COMPATIBILITY

Red blood cells are characterized by a variety of protein antigens associated with their membranes, substances that are genetically determined. ABO is the terminology that describes a densely distributed set of surface antigens derived from the metabolism of a single protein called H. ABO antigens are ubiquitous in the human environment because of their secretion in bodily fluids. Because of their prevalence in the environment, these antigens are recognized by all persons not possessing them; hence, all individuals have circulating IgG antibodies to their "foreign" ABO antigens, even if they have never been transfused or exposed to blood before. No other series of red cell antigens is similar; all others require previous exposure and/or re-exposure for expression of antibodies.

Rh is the most common terminology for another complex locus of linked antigens; the term Rh-negative usually implies the absence of the most potent of these antigens, called D. A host of other antigens are variably distributed within the population, with racial and ethnic distributions reflecting their genetics. These minor antigens are either less densely distributed on red cells or less antigenic, and therefore antibodies to them are much less common.

Immune-mediated destruction of red blood cells may proceed in two ways: most spectacular is the intravascular hemolytic reaction, caused when complement is fixed to red cells and they are lysed within the circulation. Massive intravascular reactions are generally only associated with ABO reactions, but may occur, if slightly more slowly, in strongly immunized individuals; this occurs most commonly with Rh incompatibility and Kell or Duffy antigen incompatibility. Extravascular hemolysis may occur when antibody bound to a red cell does not fix complement but is recognized by the Fc receptor of a fixed tissue macrophage, as in the spleen, and the red cell is engulfed and destroyed. Clearly, it is the goal of the crossmatching process to avoid either of these forms of destruction by identifying compatible units of blood.

Typing is performed by incubation of red cells from the recipient with antisera containing known reactivity. ABO and Rh characteristics are routinely typed; more complicated typing may be made necessary by difficulty finding compatible units of blood. Compatibility testing or crossmatching is done by incubation of donor and recipient sera and red cells and by watching for agglutination reactions in the test tube. It is an exacting process but obviously important. Errors in typing may occur with prolonged storage of donor or recipient red cells (thus the demand for fresh clots when new units of blood are crossmatched after 24 or more hours). Massive transfusion or plasmapheresis may dilute recipient antibodies; circulating immune complexes and agglutinins may interfere with *in vitro* reactions. Weak expression of red cell antigens is seen in the very elderly and in neonates and may also confuse typing. Antibodies present in the recipient may have low affinity for donor cells under laboratory conditions and may not be accurately observed in the crossmatching process.

Platelets are not crossmatched, largely because the ABO antigens are not expressed on their surfaces and because the amount of plasma transmitted with the platelets may not be sufficient to react with the recipient's red cells. In general, most blood banks supply ABO and Rh-specific platelets, but that they are not always able to is not usually clinically significant. However, with repeated exposure to heterologous platelets, virtually all immunocompetent recipients will develop antiplatelet antibodies, and significant immune-mediated platelet destruction will occur. Platelets express HLA antigens and, in addition, express a series of unique platelet antigens. Under certain specific circumstances, blood banks may provide HLA-matched single-donor platelets to avoid the problem of platelet transfusion refractoriness. These platelets are obtained from individual volunteer donors by pheresis and are therefore more expensive and difficult to obtain.

Plasma is also not crossmatched; type-specific plasma rarely causes any specific immune reactions except in recipients who are IgA deficient.

COMPLICATIONS OF BLOOD AND BLOOD-PRODUCT TRANSFUSION

Reactions to the administration of blood and blood products are both common and potentially serious; therefore recognition of the signs and symptoms of transfusion reactions and prompt treatment are important in the critical care setting.

A hemolytic transfusion reaction occurs when sufficient complement-fixing antibody is bound to the red cell to promote intravascular lysis. When ABO incompatibility occurs, the reaction is rapid and massive; when other antigens are involved, the reaction may be slower or delayed in onset until antibody titers reach the critical point to promote a high degree of lysis. The release of the contents of the red cell into the circulation causes the subsequent physiologic changes. Most studies suggest that the red cell membranes, not the freed hemoglobin, are responsible for triggering the reaction.

Rapid, massive intravascular hemolysis results in a host of symptoms: flushing and warmth, first along the course of the vein, then widespread; fever, chills, and sweating; headache, chest pain, and, often, severe back pain in the area of the kidneys. Gross hemoglobinuria may be seen; urticaria is rather unusual. The release of complement, kinins, leuko-trienes, and a host of other mediator substances strongly resembles the effect of endotoxin, with resulting hypotension, triggering of DIC, adult respiratory distress syndrome (ARDS), and acute renal failure. The effect is dose-related, and if the transfusion is stopped quickly enough, mortality is rare. Overall, fewer than 10 percent of patients who receive incompatible blood die from the resulting disease.

Diagnosis of a major hemolytic transfusion reaction is usually straightforward. When the transfusion is stopped, samples of the recipient's blood and urine are assayed for free hemoglobin and haptoglobin and are used to recrossmatch the offending unit of blood. Urine hemoglobin or hemosiderin, plasma bilirubin, LDH, and even complement levels may be used to document red cell destruction under certain circumstances. Approximately one half of such diagnostic work-ups reveal the source of error to be clerical or technical.

Treatment of major hemolytic transfusion reactions begins with prompt cessation of the transfusion. Analgesics are administered where appropriate, and fluid, mannitol, and other blood volume support are given aggressively. Urine output is maintained by the use of volume expansion, vasoactive drugs, and occasionally diuretics when indicated. Other intensive support for disorders such as DIC and ARDS is used as indicated. There is no conclusive clinical data to support the use of steroids, heparin, and other "prophylactic" measures. Fortunately for most patients, the illness induced by transfusion reaction is very self-limited.

Two other common types of transfusion reaction may also occur. The first is a nonspecific reaction to leukocytes in the transfused blood. This reaction is characterized by flushing and warmth followed by fever and chills, often of impressive proportions. Dyspnea, cough, and fleeting pulmonary infiltrates may occur; these are usually only seen as a reaction to transfused granulocyte preparations, as the transfused white blood cells may pool transiently in the pulmonary capillary bed. Rarely, patients may experience ARDS or DIC following a leukocyte reaction. A leukocyte reaction may present as an isolated reaction to a specific unit of blood. However, 15–20 percent of regular recipients of red cell transfusions may repeatedly experience these reactions. Leukocyte-poor preparations may be used in these patients; alternately, pretreatment with antipyretics or steroids may be used to abort these reactions.

A second minor transfusion reaction is not so much minor as it is rare: IgA deficiency, a rare but notable inherited trait, results in urticaria and anaphylaxis when recipients are exposed to IgA-containing blood products. This problem is usually unsuspected, but may be avoided by the use of frozen or rewashed red cells or, in extremely sensitive individuals, by the use of IgA-negative donors. Urticarial, even anaphylactoid, reactions may occur for other, nonspecific reasons during transfusion. These are rarely life-threatening and may be treated with antihistamines or other symptomatic medications. The exact basis of minor urticarial reactions is unknown.

Transfusion of blood and blood products carries a variety of other hazards. The transmission of disease is of major concern to clinicians and patients alike. All types of hepatitis may be transmitted by most whole blood components, although screening of donors has significantly reduced the incidence of hepatitis A and B and will, perhaps, in the near future reduce the acquisition of non-A, non-B hepatitis. Cytomegalovirus may be transmitted to susceptible patients, mainly seronegative or very immunosuppressed patients, via whole blood and granulocyte transfusions; the vector appears to be leukocytes. HIV, the AIDS virus, may also be transmitted in unscreened blood. Factor concentrates, immunoglobulin preparations, processed plasma fractions, and other pooled plasma preparations, including human-origin hepatitis vaccine, are, if properly prepared, considered to be free of the risk of transmission of AIDS virus or hepatitis. The incidence of acquisition of these illnesses varies depending on the source of donor blood and the regional disease prevalence.

The acute transfusion process may be complicated by fluid overload, excessive cooling (especially when transfusion is massive and surgery is being carried out simultaneously) and only very rarely by citrate toxicity. Citrate toxicity seems to occur mainly in situations of hepatic failure and massive transfusion; it results in hypocalcemia and electrolyte abnormalities and may be treated with intravenous calcium chloride. Massive transfusion has been reported to cause a fall in patients' P_{50} (the pressure of oxygen at which hemoglobin is 50 percent saturated), owing to falls in 2,3-DPG levels in stored blood. The clinical significance of this abnormality, which corrects rapidly in the absence of other metabolic problems, is uncertain. When patients require repeated episodes of transfusion over a long period of time, other problems appear: iron overload, progressive sensitization to exogenous blood products, and increasing rates of minor transfusion reactions occur in chronically transfused patients.

RECOMMENDED READING

Aach RD and Kahn: Post-transfusion hepatitis B: current perspectives. Ann Int Med 92:539, 1980.
Counts RB, Haisch C, Simon TL: Hemostasis in massively transfused trauma patients. Ann Surg 190(1):91, 1979.
Daly PA, Schiffer CA, Aisner J, et al: Platelet transfusion therapy. JAMA 243:435, 1980.
Giblett ER: Blood group alloantibodies. Transfusion 17:279, 1977.
Goldfinger D: Hemolytic transfusion reactions—a fresh look at pathogenesis and considerations regarding therapy. Transfusion 17:85, 1977.
Gould SA, Rice CL, Moss GS: The physiologic basis of the use of blood and blood products. Surg Annu 16:13, 1984.
Gould SA, Rosen AL, Sehgal LR, et al: Fluosol DA as a red-cell substitute in acute anemia. N Eng J Med 314:1653, 1986.
Higby DJ, Burnett D: Granulocyte transfusions: current status. Blood 55:2, 1980.
Lostumbo MM, Holland PV, Schmidt PJ: Isoimmunization after multiple transfusions. N Engl J Med 275:141, 1966.
Pineda AA, Taswell HF, Brzica SM: Delayed hemolytic transfusion reactions. Transfusion 18:1, 1978.
Sherman LA: New plasma components. Clin Haematol 13:17, 1984.
Tremper KK, Friedman AE, Levine EM, et al: The preoperative treatment of severely anemic patients with a perfluoro chemical oxygen transport fluid, Fluosol DA. N Engl J Med 307:277, 1982.
Urbaniak SJ, Cash JD: Blood replacement therapy. Br Med Bull 33:273, 1977.
Widmann FK: Untoward effects of blood transfusions. Postgrad Med 69:40, 1981.

83. Anticoagulation and Fibrinolysis

Judith A. Luce

INTRODUCTION

This chapter discusses the use and complications of a diverse group of drugs whose primary effects are to impair the coagulation system and whose clinical use is directed at arresting or reversing the adverse effects of thrombosis.

HEPARIN

Heparins are a heterogeneous group of naturally occurring mucopolysaccharides that are commercially produced from liver, lung, and intestine. Heparins are found in all mast cells and are released from their granules. Heparins are extremely anionic molecules with a high degree of fat solubility. They are neutralized by protamine, a highly cationic molecule with which heparins form a stable salt.

The action of heparin as a potent anticoagulant is based upon its interaction with antithrombin III (AT III), a circulating inhibitor of thrombin. When heparin binds to AT III, the latter's affinity for thrombin is greatly enhanced, and the complex becomes a highly efficient inhibitor. Heparin also acts to inhibit activated Factor X's action on prothrombin and also to inhibit activated Factors IX, XI, and XII.

INDICATIONS

Heparin has become the standard anticoagulation therapy for thrombotic disease, especially venous thrombosis and pulmonary embolism. Its role has not been supplanted by the fibrinolytic agents, even though heparin does not actively promote clot dissolution. Heparin is of more equivocal usefulness when thrombosis has been long-standing. In addition, its use in myocardial infarction (as a sole agent) and in cerebrovascular accident is controversial.

512

Heparin may also be administered in lower doses subcutaneously and in this mode has been used prophylactically to prevent thrombosis in high-risk clinical situations. This usage has been controversial as well, especially in the postoperative setting, and most currently, heparin prophylaxis is not considered routine. Heparin is the drug of choice for thrombosis during pregnancy; it is not indicated for patients suffering from AT III deficiency. Low-dose instillation in in-dwelling catheters has been shown to effectively maintain their patency.

MANAGEMENT

The parenteral route of administration is the only available mode of therapy with heparin; the drug is equally absorbed intravenously and subcutaneously, though the latter route is associated with slower absorption. Available in a wide variety of concentrations and soluble in any intravenous solution, heparin is also very inexpensive. Intramuscular treatment of any kind is contraindicated in a patient on heparin, and subcutaneous injection sites require careful local care to insure that excessive bleeding does not occur.

Heparin has a short half-life when given intravenously, and its half-life is dose-dependent, so that higher boluses will have a longer half-life. A practical dosing frequency is every 4–6 hours, and at this dose interval with average doses, the half-life is roughly 1 hour. All heparin therapy must be initiated with a loading dose to saturate fat stores and the distribution space. The usual loading dose is 100–150 units/kg. All large bolus doses are followed by a period of time, usually about 1 hour, when coagulation function is markedly depressed and clotting times are essentially infinite. In order to avoid this event, continuous infusion therapy for chronic anticoagulation is recommended and is indeed safer with respect to bleeding complications. When continuous infusion therapy is used, coagulation times must be measured 4–6 hours after loading and starting the infusion; repeated smaller loading doses may be necessary if adequate anticoagulation is not achieved with the initial dose. When bolus dosing is used, nadir clotting function must be measured 4–6 hours after the course is begun and frequently remeasured and doses adjusted.

Heparin dosing is based on the effect of the drug on coagulation. Since patients with active thrombosis may have widely differing levels of antithrombin III activity, their heparin requirements to achieve the same level of anticoagulation may vary widely. In addition, heparin requirements generally decrease as active thrombosis slows and clot endothelialization occurs. An average patient may require approximately 25,000–30,000 units of heparin in 24 hours, and this may be given as a continuous infusion or in divided doses administered over 10–30 minutes each or subcutaneously.

Goals of heparin therapy may be measured in several ways in the laboratory. The whole-blood clotting time is the most functionally similar to the *in vivo* process of heparin anticoagulation but is cumbersome because of the longer time it requires and lower reproducibility. A whole-blood clotting time of 2–3 times normal has been shown to be effective anticoagulation. In all laboratory measurements of anticoagulation, the base parameter used is the laboratory normal, not the patients' times, since their starting coagulation tests may be abnormal for a variety of reasons. The partial thromboplastin time (PTT), because of its reproducibility and rapidity, is the most commonly used measure of heparin effect. A PTT of 1½ to 2½ times the normal control value is the empirically correct value. It is important that each laboratory standardize the sensitivity of its PTT to heparin, since times may vary widely depending on the reagents used; some laboratories may report their PTT values in terms of equivalence to heparin concentration in the plasma. Thrombin times are extremely sensitive to heparin effect and are therefore not useful; the prothrombin time does reflect heparin effect but over too narrow a range to be clinically useful.

Heparin therapy is usually maintained for 7–10 days; this is thought to be necessary in order to observe the complete endothelialization of thrombus. Most clinicians feel that, since the highest risk of pulmonary embolus is within the first 48 hours of hospitalization, adequate anticoagulation during this time is extremely important. Use of arbitrary doses of heparin without monitoring PTT has been associated with higher risk of pulmonary embolism and with increased bleeding. Once a patient is adequately orally anticoagulated, heparin may be discontinued (see the following section on warfarin). Long-term subcutaneous treatment with heparin has been shown to be both therapeutic and well tolerated.

Heparin prophylaxis, as previously mentioned, has appeal in a wide variety of clinical situations of high thrombosis risk but is of uncertain benefit to patients at risk. Prophylaxis usually consists of doses of 5,000 units delivered subcutaneously every 8-12 hours. A brief period of abnormal coagulation should follow such doses, but patients' PTTs or whole blood clotting times should be normal most of the time.

COMPLICATIONS

Complications of heparin therapy are fairly common. Bleeding is the major risk and may occur in as many as 20 percent of patients on the drug. Bleeding risk is higher in patients over 60, particularly women, and in patients with gastrointestinal lesions. When intravenous infusion therapy is used and coagulation parameters are carefully monitored, complication rates are markedly decreased: 1–2 percent of patients have major bleeding, and fewer than 20 percent of patients have minor bleeding, one half the rate seen with bolus therapy. Catastrophic bleeding due to heparin may be reversed by the use of protamine, which is also given intravenously. Protamine 1.0 to 1.25 mg will neutralize 100 units of heparin, and using a heparin half-life of 1 hour, most patients' doses may be simply calculated. A PTT may be measured soon after protamine is given, but one must bear in mind that too much protamine may also raise the PTT. Some laboratories have immunologic or biochemical techniques for distinguishing between heparin and protamine effect if this becomes a question.

Heparin also causes thrombocytopenia, and although the incidence of this complication is debated, it is probably less than 10 percent. The thrombocytopenia is immune-mediated and dependent on the presence of the drug in the circulation; it therefore resolves quickly, within the limits of the patient's ability to make new platelets, when the drug is withdrawn. It is not dose-dependent and is not clearly related to previous exposure to heparin. Withdrawal of the drug is the key to treatment; steroids and other modalities used to treat immune-mediated thrombocytopenia should not be necessary. Indeed, once the drug has cleared the plasma, platelets may usually be transfused without immune destruction occurring. Arterial thrombosis may be associated with this syndrome.

Other complications of heparin therapy include alopecia, osteoporosis (usually with chronic administration), *dysesthesia pedis*, and, rarely, skin or fat necrosis of subcutaneous injection sites.

Oral Anticoagulants and Antiplatelet Agents

Warfarin and related drugs, derivatives of the naturally occurring substance coumarin, form another class of potent anticoagulant. This class of drugs competes with vitamin K to inhibit the final step in the hepatic synthesis of Factors II, VII, IX, and X. The effect of the coumarin derivatives is therefore dependent on a host of factors: the amount of vitamin K available in the diet or as a result of intestinal flora production, the rate of hepatic synthetic activity, the half-lives of the factors affected (VII, shortest; II, longest), and the half-life of the drug, which is dependent upon hepatic metabolism. In addition, the drugs are plasma protein–bound, and other drugs that affect this binding may affect anticoagulant properties.

Antiplatelet agents are a variety of drugs that have effects on the prostaglandins in platelets, and hence on their aggregration, after the release of granule contents. The two most potent drugs in this group are aspirin and dipyridamole, and, since these have seen the widest use, they will be the most discussed. Aspirin irreversibly acetylates platelet membrane cyclooxygenase; the effect is mitigated only as platelets are replaced. The action of dipyridamole is primarily on platelet phosphodiesterase, which thus raises intracellular levels of cyclic adenosine monophosphate. It is reversible, and therefore dosing on a 6–8-hour basis is desirable.

INDICATIONS

Oral anticoagulants are the mainstay of therapy for outpatients who have sustained thrombotic disease. The duration of therapy is partly determined empirically, such as the 3-month average following pulmonary embolism, and partly it is a subjective judgment based on the clinical situation of the patient and the duration of risk of thrombosis. Oral anticoagulants are used indefinitely following insertion of mechanical prosthetic heart valves and, generally, following embolic phenomena in patients with paroxysmal atrial fibrillation. Their routine use following myocardial infarction, once discarded, has been revived for use following fibrinolytic therapy.

Antiplatelet drugs have been widely applied in clinical medicine. They have a major role in maintaining the patency of vascular endoprostheses and implants, although their potential role in preventing thrombosis in arterial systems in patients at risk is more controversial. Aspirin and another agent, sulfinpyrazone, have been shown to be effective in preventing myocardial infarction and other complications of coronary artery disease in patients with unstable angina and previous myocardial infarction; dipyridamole has not been shown to be of benefit by itself in this group. Aspirin and dipyridamole have a role in preventing stroke in patients who have sustained previous transient ischemic attack. Aspirin is the drug of choice for patients with thrombocytosis and vascular events. Whether antiplatelet agents have a role in all persons at risk of vascular thrombotic events is unclear; in addition, their effects on women are not well enough studied.

MANAGEMENT

Warfarin is the most commonly used oral anticoagulant; dicoumarol is the second. They are both administered by the oral route and are well absorbed and metabolized by the liver. Oral loading doses of these drugs are not necessary and may be associated with bleeding risk. Their effect is measured by the prothrombin time (PT); this test is most sensitive to the lowering of Factor VII levels—this factor also has the shortest half-life. Therefore, 5–7 days of oral therapy are felt to be required before acceptable reductions in the other factors, especially prothrombin, have been achieved. Most patients who are begun on coumarin drugs are already on heparin, and some caution is required, since heparin does affect the PT and coumadin the PTT. Both drugs may be given in slightly lower doses when used concomitantly, and PT should not be measured immediately after a heparin bolus.

The average daily dose of warfarin is 5 mg on an international normalized scale. The goal of therapy is a PT between 1½ and 2 times the normal value; this usually results in a prothrombin level around 20 percent of normal, which has been empirically found to be within a range of safety and efficacy for these drugs.

The key to oral anticoagulant therapy is extremely careful monitoring of other drug interactions, which are numerous and potentially dangerous. Many, if not most, patients can be maintained on a stable oral dose if no changes are made in any medications; once any new drug is added or the regimen altered, the coumadin dose must be evaluated and altered. An exhaustive list of the drug interactions with warfarin and dicoumarol is not possible in this space, but each and every new drug, especially and including over-the-counter medications, must be checked. Antiplatelet drugs are contraindicated in patients on warfarin. Ingestion of alcohol, particularly in amounts that can significantly impact on liver function, is also contraindicated.

Reversal of the effect of oral anticoagulants can be done with the use of vitamin K, which is available both in oral and parenteral form. Repeated oral dosing may be necessary, but a single parenteral dose (intravenous if the patient has significant bleeding, as hematoma formation may preclude adequate absorption intramuscularly) is usually sufficient. Because patients on warfarin may have high levels of factor precursors, a rebound hypercoagulability may be seen in patients whose oral anticoagulation is rapidly reversed in this manner; however, since the clinical situation usually warrants rapid correction of the coagulopathy, the risk of rebounding is much lower. The time course of changes in the PT following administration of vitamin K is quite variable, but 12–24 hours is sufficient for most patients to normalize. Since synthetic rates vary, complete normalization of all factors may not occur for several days. Treatment with fresh frozen plasma is justified when patients have life-threatening bleeding and when vitamin K has also been administered.

Antiplatelet agents are also orally administered. Aspirin, because it has a long biologic half-life, may be dosed once daily (unless platelet turnover is exceedingly rapid). The precise required dose is unknown, but small amounts of aspirin, below the level detectable in serum, are sufficient for full antiplatelet effect. The doses used in the large drug trials have been 2½ to 5 grains daily or twice daily; minimal toxicity has been associated with these doses. Dipyridamole, with its shorter biologic effect, is usually dosed 2–3 times daily, with an average dose of 150–200 mg/ day.

COMPLICATIONS

As with heparin, the potent anticoagulant effects of coumarin derivatives most often result in bleeding as a complication. Excessive bleeding may be the result of inappropriate dosing or of drug interactions. However, when patients exhibit significant bleeding in the gastrointestinal or genitourinary tracts, most clinicians recommend, and some clinical evidence supports this idea, that a thorough evaluation for an occult source of blood loss be undertaken.

Many patients are at high risk with warfarin therapy. Warfarin is contraindicated in pregnancy because it crosses the placental barrier and may cause fetal hemorrhage; it is also probably teratogenic. Similarly, the drug is contraindicated in individuals with active bleeding sources or recent bleeding in the central nervous system, eye, or other vulnerable sites. It must be used extremely cautiously or reversed in patients in whom minor surgical procedures are contemplated. For major surgery, the drug must be discontinued or reversed; closed biopsies are considered to require reversal also.

Other side effects are less common. Warfarin may cause alopecia and, rarely, urticaria or other dermatitis. Acrocyanosis, nonspecific gastrointestinal symptoms, cutaneous necrosis and hemorrhagic infarction, priapism, and fever have been observed.

The chief side effects of aspirin are gastrointestinal irritation and ulcerogenesis. Whether the doses of aspirin used for their antithrombotic effects have a significant effect in this regard is not known; it is known that serum levels of salicylate are virtually unmeasurable with these doses. Immediate stomach irritation may be avoided with the use of enteric coated tablets. Patients with aspirin hypersensitivity should not use aspirin, even at low doses. Discontinuing aspirin therapy is advised prior to potentially bloody surgery, such as procedures on the urinary tract, cardiothoracic surgery, or major vascular surgery. However, prophylactic doses of aspirin have been shown to pose no additional risk to patients undergoing elective abdominal surgery.

Dipyridamole is a well-tolerated drug. Headache, nausea, dizziness, and flushing have been reported. The drug causes vasodilation in large doses and should be used cautiously in patients with hypotension and cardiac disease.

Fibrinolytic Agents

This group of drugs is enjoying a new and more widespread application in internal medicine and surgery, largely as a result of their wider use in acute myocardial infarction.

Mechanism of Action

The formation of fibrin clots is described in Chapter 80. In parallel and precise coordination, an endogenous mechanism for the lysis of clots by the sequential breakdown of fibrin is initiated. The protein released by endothelial cells in response to clot formation is called tissue plasminogen activator (TPA). This substance has a high affinity for fibrin, and thus *in vivo* is mostly found in association with clot. When bound to fibrin, it enzymatically cleaves another circulating plasma protein, plasminogen. Activated plasmin efficiently cleaves fibrin molecules into a series of smaller fragments dubbed "fibrin degradation products" (see Fig. 83–1).

Plasmin is inhibited by another circulating protein, α_2-antiplasmin, which binds irreversibly to the active site of the protease. α_2-Antiplasmin

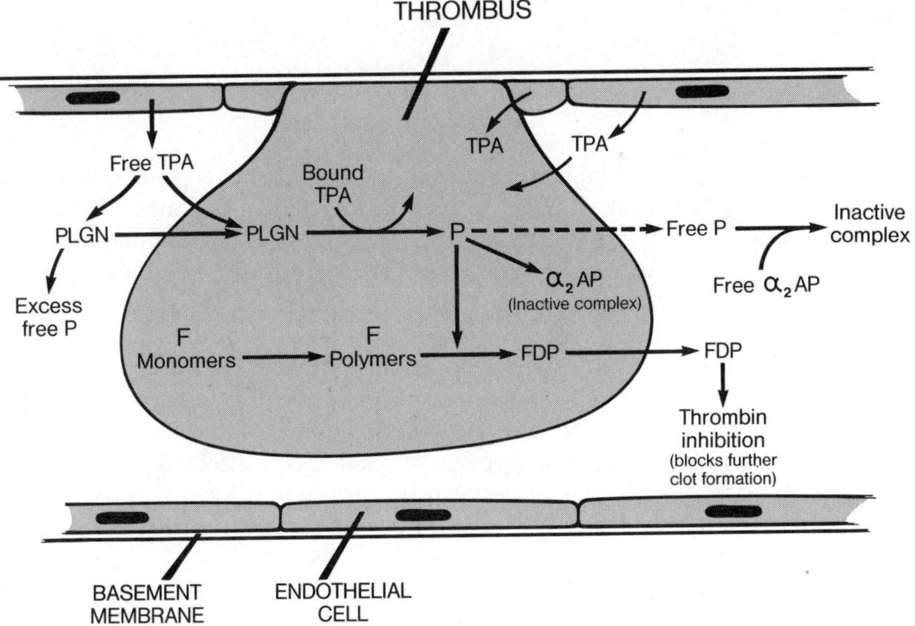

Figure 83–1. Scheme of fibrinolysis. See text for explanation. TPA = tissue plasminogen activator; PLGN = plasminogen; P = plasmin; α_2AP = alpha-2-antiplasmin; F = fibrin; FDP = fibrin degradation products.

binds circulating plasmin better than fibrin-bound plasmin, so it acts as a natural brake on excessive fibrinogen or fibrin lysis.

Clearly, drugs that activate plasminogen in the circulation or suppress α_2-antiplasmin activity can have potent effects on fibrinolysis. One such substance is urokinase, a large protein molecule produced by kidney cells and released into the excretory urinary tract, where it effectively prevents thrombosis. It has little affinity for fibrin, and cleaves plasminogen readily. Streptokinase, a protein product of β-hemolytic streptococci, is also capable of cleaving and activating plasmin. It does so indirectly, by binding to plasmin or plasminogen, and this complex in turn cleaves and activates other plasminogen molecules. Streptokinase also has a low affinity for fibrin, so, like urokinase, it mostly cleaves circulating fibrin and fibrinogen.

The theoretical use of fibrinolytic agents is in dissolving formed clot, and their effectiveness in doing so depends on a variety of factors. Mature clots are less sensitive to plasmin action because α_2-antiplasmin is incorporated in the clot as the fibrin crosslinks are formed. Studies of deep venous thrombosis suggest that clots less than a week old are more likely to respond to fibrinolytic therapy. In addition, the affinity of the fibrinolytic agent for fibrin-bound plasminogen, the perfusion of the clot, and the duration of exposure of the drug to the clot are important variables. The ideal fibrinolytic agent is one that is specific for clots only, is well tolerated by patients, and is effective in achieving measurable clinical benefit.

INDICATIONS

Treatment of deep vein thrombosis has been perhaps the oldest use of fibrinolytic agents, in an effort to prevent morbidity and mortality from pulmonary embolism and to prevent the late complications of postphlebitic syndrome and pulmonary insufficiency. Trials performed to date appear to show efficacy of streptokinase and urokinase in lysis of thrombi, although symptoms may improve in the absence of clot dissolution. Late patency of veins is improved, but no good data exist on the incidence of postphlebitic syndrome in heparin-treated patients; hence, no comparison with fibrinolytic agents may be made. The incidence of and mortality from pulmonary embolism do not appear to have been affected. Toxicity is greater compared with that of heparin therapy when longer infusions of fibrinolytic agents are used but are comparable to heparin toxicity when the agents are used for periods of less than 3 days.

Patients having pulmonary embolism have also been treated in a few comparative studies of heparin versus fibrinolytic agents. The latter are given as a loading dose, followed by intravenous infusions of 24–48 hours' duration; patients are then continued on standard heparin and warfarin therapy. Early lysis of thrombi has been demonstrated angiographically, and the streptokinase- or urokinase-treated patients have a slightly higher rate of lysis as compared with heparinized patients. However, the rates of patency of vessels and appearance of lung scans up to a year after the embolic event are identical in the two groups. Controversy exists as to whether other parameters such as arterial blood gases and pulmonary artery pressures show improvement early or at one year in a significant number of patients treated with fibrinolysins. Mortality and reembolism rates do not differ markedly. Some authors recommend that because of the complications of fibrinolytic therapy, the use of these agents in pulmonary embolism ought to be restricted to high-risk patients who have massive embolism (two or more lobes affected) and other serious signs such as hypotension. Heparin therapy and oral anticoagulation drugs are mandatory following the use of fibrinolytic agents for treating this disease.

Scattered reports of the use of fibrinolytic agents in arterial thrombotic disease suggest a role for this therapy. Dissolution is accomplished by catheter-directed local infusion of the drugs, using relatively low doses and infusion periods of up to 24 hours. Patency rates are impossible to assess, since the reported cases are in selected patients and are not from randomized trials. Because of the lower toxicity of local infusion, fibrinolytic agents may be appropriate therapy for patients with recent arterial occlusion who refuse or are not candidates for surgical therapy.

Following the demonstration that acute thrombosis played a significant role in acute myocardial infarction, intense study of the use of fibrinolytic agents in this disease has ensued. Since myocardial survival depends on prompt reperfusion, most studies have emphasized treatment in the first 6 hours after the onset of symptoms. Intracoronary instillation of streptokinase has resulted in a 60–80 percent rate of reperfusion; restoration of myocardial function has been demonstrated. Some, but not all, studies have shown lowered mortality. Long-term follow-up is somewhat lacking, but vessel patency definitely decreases with time, and clearcut long-term benefit of this procedure *alone* in acute myocardial infarction remains equivocal. Because of the expense and difficulty of angiographic intervention and intracoronary therapy, the use of higher doses of intravenous fibrinolytic agents has been examined. Overall, vessel patency and myocardial restoration rates drop, but approximately 60 percent of patients treated with TPA and 40 percent of patients treated with streptokinase experience vessel patency after the infusion. These patients are also treated with heparin and then oral anticoagulants following fibrinolytic therapy. There is an increasing trend toward definitive surgery or angioplasty following fibrinolytic therapy, and the ultimate place of this type of therapy in the treatment of myocardial infarction is clearly still in evolution.

Fibrinolytic agents have proven useful in other clinical situations. A single instillation of streptokinase in relatively nontoxic doses is a useful maneuver to restore patency in thrombosed arteriovenous shunts and indwelling intravenous catheters. Isolated reports have shown efficacy for these drugs in other acute thrombotic disorders such as priapism, renal artery thrombosis, and the Budd-Chiari syndrome. The use of fibrinolytic agents in cerebrovascular disease, on the other hand, has produced very poor results, and any type of cerebrovascular event is now regarded as a contraindication to the use of these drugs. Fibrinolytic drugs have proven no better than heparin in the treatment of retinal vein thrombosis.

MANAGEMENT

Streptokinase is commercially available for intravenous use in a lyophilized form that is usually given as a loading dose followed by an infusion of variable duration. 250,000 units given intravenously over 30 minutes is a standard loading dose for pulmonary embolism, followed by an infusion of 100,000 units/hr. The half-life of the agent has two phases, the longer phase being roughly 80 minutes. Doses for clot lysis in intravenous cannulae are single doses of up to 250,000 units. Trials of intravenous streptokinase in acute myocardial infarction have used single doses of 500,000 to 1,500,000 units given as a rapid (usually 1 hour or less) intravenous infusion. Clearly, the total dose and duration of therapy are to be considered jointly in assessing toxicity; patients who receive brief exposure to high doses seem to have fewer complications.

Urokinase, similarly available in lyophilized form, is dosed differently, generally based on the patient's weight. This drug is very expensive in the usual clinical doses and therefore has been used much less than streptokinase. Typical intravenous loading doses are 4,000–5,000 units/kg over 10–15 minutes, followed by maintenance infusions of the same dose on an hourly basis. Higher-dose, single-infusion treatments for myocardial infarction have not been reported.

Tissue plasminogen activator is a recombinant DNA product that is highly purified and is currently available for investigational use only. In the Thrombosis in Myocardial Infarction Trial, this drug was employed in escalating doses. Total doses of greater than 80 mg and durations of over 3 hours seemed to be associated with significant systemic fibrinolysis. At this maximum dose, satisfactory levels of thrombolysis were observed. Intravenous half-life is well below 1 hour.

Monitoring of therapeutic efficacy and toxicity of this group of drugs is very simple. There are yet not available reliable measures of plasma levels of any of these drugs, and there is no relationship yet apparent between therapeutic benefit and any parameter of either drug level or coagulation effect. What is done in most trials is a simple demonstration of fibrinolytic effect: an abnormal thrombin time (TT), PTT, euglobulin lysis time, or fibrinogen level, or, alternately, an elevated level of fibrin degradation products. Thrombin times and PTTs are usually used for simplicity and cost-effectiveness. No target coagulation time is sought. Depressions of fibrinogen tend to be smallest with TPA, but depressed levels may persist for 24 hours after cessation of the drugs. Urokinase has the shortest plasma half-life, and hence the most rapid recovery.

For virtually all treatment with fibrinolytic agents, long-term anticoagulation is indicated and is routinely instituted following the termination of fibrinolytic therapy, except in patients with bleeding. Switching to heparin is done by measuring the PTT at the end of the fibrinolytic infusion, then periodically reassessing the PTT and starting a continuous heparin infusion without a loading dose when the PTT falls to the therapeutic range for heparin.

COMPLICATIONS

Bleeding is the notable toxicity of these agents: other side effects are relatively few. The precise incidence of major and minor bleeding events is a source of controversy and a point of contention in the wider use of these drugs. In centers in which patients are stringently screened, mortality from CNS or other severe hemorrhage is less than 1–2 percent; morbid bleeding complications range from IV-site hematomas to gastrointestinal bleeding to larger localized hematomas. These complications have been reported in up to half of patients receiving the drugs.

Because of the bleeding risks, most studies eliminate a large number of patients at risk: persons over 70–75 years of age; anyone with a recent stroke, surgery, or vaginal delivery; anyone having had a recent closed biopsy or cardiac massage; and anyone with either active bleeding or a coagulopathy. Avoidance of invasive procedures and the placement of arterial or central venous catheters is an important part of avoiding bleeding complications. Simultaneous use of aspirin, heparin, and warfarin is to be avoided.

Treatment of hemorrhage during thrombolytic therapy is straightforward. Bleeding sites that can be managed locally must be treated with pressure, and if the blood loss is minor, this is usually sufficient. Any percutaneous vascular puncture sites must be held for 30 minutes. Bleeding of greater magnitude must be treated with the immediate cessation of thrombolytic therapy. Restoration of normal coagulation may be attempted with infusion of fresh frozen plasma or cryoprecipitate. The latter is a low-volume source of fibrinogen and should be available in any institution that undertakes fibrinolytic therapy. It requires no thawing and can be given in large doses of 5–15 bags by rapid infusion intravenously. A PTT or TT may be used to assess the efficacy of transfusions and additional fibrinogen given. Fortunately, the relatively brief duration of the fibrinolytic agents themselves usually makes restoration of normal clotting possible within a few hours. Perhaps of value in suppressing endogenous plasmin activity is ϵ-amino caproic acid (Amicar); its role in the fibrinolytic state induced by these agents is not well established, and its potency is minor compared with that of other drugs, so it is likely to be of less value. Amicar may be given as an oral or intravenous loading dose at 100 mg/kg, followed by either a continuous infusion at the same dose hourly or in divided doses every 6 hours.

Hypersensitivity is the only other risk for the use of streptokinase. No valuable predictive test has been developed, and simply monitoring patients early in therapy for signs and symptoms of hypersensitivity is required; this is not a problem with urokinase or TPA.

RECOMMENDED READING

Chatterjee K: Thrombolysis in acute myocardial infarction. Hosp Pract 21:117, 1986.

Deykin D: Warfarin therapy. N Engl J Med 283:691, 1970.

Genton E, Hirsh J: Observations in anticoagulant and thrombolytic therapy in pulmonary embolism. Prog Cardiovasc Dis 17:335, 1975.

Harker LA: Clinical trials evaluating platelet-modifying drugs in patients with atherosclerotic cardiovascular disease and thrombosis. Circulation 73:206, 1986.

Hull RD, Raskob GE, Hirsh J, et al: Continuous intravenous heparin compared with intermittent subcutaneous heparin in the initial treatment of proximal-vein thrombosis. N Engl J Med 315:1109, 1986.

Jick H, Slone D, Borda IT, Shapiro S: Efficacy and toxicity of heparin in relation to age and sex. N Engl J Med 279:284, 1968.

Koch-Weser J, Sellers EM: Drug interactions with coumarin anticoagulants. N Engl J Med 285:487, 1971.

Marder VJ: The use of thrombolytic agents: choice of patient, drug administration, laboratory monitoring. Ann Intern Med 90:802, 1979.

O'Reilly RA, Aggeler PM: Studies on coumarin anticoagulant drugs: initiation of warfarin therapy without a loading dose. Circulation 38:169, 1968.

Pedersen AK, FitzGerald GA: The human pharmacology of platelet inhibition: pharmacokinetics relevant to drug action. Circulation 72:1164, 1985.

Salzman EW, Deykin D, Shapiro RM, et al: Management of heparin therapy. N Engl J Med 292:1046, 1975.

Sharma GVRK, Cella G, Parisi A, et al: Thrombolytic therapy. N Engl J Med 306:1268, 1982.

Sherry S (Chairman): Thrombolytic therapy in thrombosis: a National Institutes of Health consensus development conference. Ann Intern Med 93:141, 1980.

The TIMI Study Group: The thrombolysis in myocardial infarction (TIMI) trial: Phase I findings. N Engl J Med 312:932, 1985.

Topol EJ, Bell WR, Weisfeldt ML: Coronary thrombolysis with recombinant tissue-type plasminogen activator: a hematologic and pharmacologic study. Ann Intern Med 103:837, 1985.

Drug Overdosage and Withdrawal

84. Alcohol Overdosage and Withdrawal

John M. Luce

Definition

Ethyl alcohol or ethanol is the most commonly used intoxicant—and the most common cause of drug toxicity—in our society. Other aliphatic alcohols, including isopropyl alcohol, methyl alcohol or methanol, and ethylene glycol may also be consumed for their mood-altering qualities. Because these other alcohols are even more acutely toxic than ethanol, they cannot be ingested in large enough quantities or long enough to cause symptoms during their withdrawal.

Pathophysiology

Ethyl alcohol, which is found in concentrations of 5 percent in beer, 12 percent in wine, 20 percent in fortified wine, and 43 percent in distilled spirits (86 proof), is the only commercially available alcoholic intoxicant. Isopropyl alcohol, methyl alcohol, and ethylene glycol are sold either as adulterants or solvents, or as constituents of copy fluids, aftershave lotions, and antifreeze. When ingested by mouth, the aliphatic alcohols are absorbed primarily by the proximal small bowel. The presence of food, especially protein, in the stomach delays gastric emptying and thereby decreases the rate of alcohol absorption and the onset of intoxication.

Once absorbed, alcohol is distributed to tissues with the highest water content. Small amounts of alcohol are excreted by the kidneys and lungs; however, most of the drug—80 percent in the case of ethanol—is metabolized in the liver, primarily by the enzyme alcohol dehydrogenase (ADH). Ethyl alcohol is converted by ADH into acetaldehyde, which is then converted into acetate and acetyl CoA, which enters the Krebs cycle. The oxidation of ethanol involves the reduction of a coenzyme, nicotinamide adenine dinucleotide, that causes a change in the redox potential. This change results, in turn, in an accumulation of lactate and β-hydroxybutyrate; this causes a mild metabolic acidosis, which is known as alcoholic ketoacidosis even though lactate is the more important anion. In a normal

TABLE 84–1. CHARACTERISTICS OF ALCOHOL INTOXICATION

| | TYPE OF ALCOHOL | | | |
CHARACTERISTIC	Ethyl	Isopropyl	Methyl	Ethylene Glycol
PRIMARY TOXIC ENTITY	Metabolites	Parent drug	Parent drug	Metabolites
ONSET	Rapid (30–60 minutes)	Late (24 hours)	Rapid (30–60 minutes) Late (24 hours)	Rapid (30–60 minutes)
METABOLIC ACIDOSIS	Mild (lactate)	Mild (lactate)	Severe (formic acid, lactate)	Severe (oxalate, glyoxalate, lactate)
KETONES	Acetoacetate, hydroxybutyrate	Acetone	Ketobutyric	None
ANION GAP	+ +	+	+ + +	+ + +
SERUM OSMOLALITY	Each 350 mg/dl, add 80 mOsm to calculated	Each 340 mg/dl, add 60 mOsm to calculated	Each 80 mg/dl, add 27 mOsm to calculated	Each 21 mg/dl, add 4 mOsm to calculated
SERUM GLUCOSE	Hypoglycemia	Hypoglycemia	Hyperamylasemia	Hypocalcemia
OTHER CHANGES	Gastritis	Gastritis	Retinal edema	Crystaluria (oxalate)

Adapted, with permission, from Lacouture PG, Wason S, Abrams A, et al.: Am J Med 75:680–686, 1983.

70 kg adult, approximately 7–10 g of ethanol are metabolized each hour. This amounts to approximately 1 oz of distilled spirits or a glass of wine or beer.

Isopropyl alcohol is also metabolized by ADH and other enzymes in the liver, but in this case, the end product is acetone, which causes a very mild metabolic acidosis. Methyl alcohol is initially converted into formaldehyde and then to formic acid, which is ultimately oxidized to carbon dioxide and water by a folate-dependent system. Formic acid and the lactate also resulting from the oxidations of methanol cause a very severe metabolic acidosis, and formate is highly toxic to organs such as the eye. Ethylene glycol is converted by ADH into glycoaldehyde, which is then converted into glycolate, and glyoxalate; along with lactate, these toxic by-products also cause a severe metabolic acidosis (Table 84–1).

Ethanol and the other aliphatic alcohols are classified pharmacologically as sedative-hypnotic agents. As such, they act as central nervous system depressants. This depression usually involves the most cephalad structures first and then moves caudad, affecting the cerebral cortex, limbic system, cerebellum, brain stem reticular activating system, and medullary control centers, in turn. As a result, disinhibition of the higher centers and a feeling of euphoria usually precede ataxia, depression of consciousness, and cardiovascular and respiratory collapse. The effects of alcohol are also dose-related: most light drinkers achieve relaxation at a blood alcohol concentration (BAC) of 50 mg/dl; incoordination occurs at

100 mg/dl, coma at 300 mg/dl, and death at 500 mg/dl. Tolerance is also important, and chronic heavy drinkers may look sober at potentially lethal BACs. In all drinkers, the effects of alcohol are more evident as the BAC is rising, so that one may appear sober at a high but steady BAC.

Alcohols and their metabolites cause toxicity beyond their depressant effects. Ethyl alcohol, for example, is responsible for severe gastritis and upper gastrointestinal hemorrhage in many patients. Chronic drinkers may suffer from a variety of nutritional disorders, including alcoholic hypoglycemia (related both to depleted liver glycogen stores and to impaired glyconeogenesis), hypokalemia, and Wernicke's encephalopathy and other manifestations of thiamine deficiency. Alcoholics also are subject to alcoholic steatosis, hepatitis, and cirrhosis that may culminate in hepatic encephalopathy or coma. Other common causes of coma in alcoholics are head trauma and meningitis.

Isopropyl alcohol causes greater nervous system depression at a low serum concentration that does ethanol. Oral ingestion of isopropyl alcohol may also lead to severe gastritis. Methyl alcohol intoxication is associated with early gastrointestinal side effects and subsequent development of severe metabolic acidosis and ocular injury that may range from blurred vision to blindness. Seizures and cardiovascular collapse occur late in the course of methanol intoxication; the same symptoms may result from even small amounts of ethylene glycol and its metabolites. Ethylene glycol intoxication also causes hypocalcemia due to the chelation of calcium ions by oxalate and late renal failure due to the cytotoxic effects of drug metabolites and, to a lesser degree, the deposition of oxalate crystals in the kidney. Oxalate crystals may also deposit in the central nervous system and contribute to cerebral edema, coma, and death.

In contrast to the depression caused by ongoing ingestion of ethanol, withdrawal from this agent is associated with systemic adrenergic hyperactivity. This hyperactivity is usually manifested shortly following abstinence in previously heavy drinkers, when the BAC is at or near zero. First in sequence, with a peak occurring at 8–12 hours, are tremors, tachycardia, disorientation, and insomnia (Fig. 84–1). These symptoms may be followed by single or multiple seizures, usually grand mal in nature, that relate in part to respiratory alkalosis and hypomagnesemia (status epilepticus rarely occurs during withdrawal and should prompt a search for other causes). After 48 hours, a minority of withdrawing patients experience delirium tremens, a condition characterized by extreme diaphoresis, tachycardia, hypertension, hallucinations, and profound agitation and physical activity. Delirium tremens frequently occurs in patients with concurrent illness such as pneumonia. It may be due, in part, to a rebound of rapid eye movement sleep that affects alcoholics who are sleep-deprived.

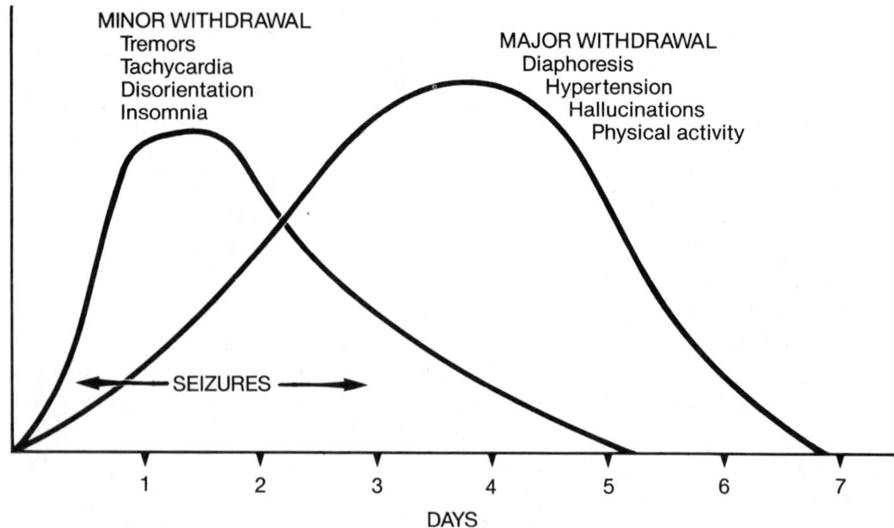

FIGURE 84–1. Major and minor alcohol withdrawal symptoms, with their usual times of onset following abstinence, and their duration. Note that withdrawal seizures may occur at any time within the first 3 days. (Adapted, with permission, from Kalant H, Sellers EM: N Engl J Med 294:757, 1976.)

DIAGNOSIS

Alcohol intoxication should be considered in the differential diagnosis of mental status alterations up to and including coma. Such intoxication may be suggested by patient behavior and habitus, the smell of alcoholic beverages on the breath, and the identification of bottles and containers at a drinking site. Other important clues are the presence of anion and osmolar gaps. As discussed in Chapter 41, a normal difference or gap of 10 mEq/L exists on laboratory electrolyte panels between the major serum cation—sodium—and the major anions—chloride and bicarbonate—because certain organic acids are not routinely measured. Thus, when $Na^+ - (Cl^- + HCO_3^-)$ is greater than 10 mEq/L, it bespeaks the presence of added anions such as lactate, various ketones, or the acidic metabolic byproducts of substances such as methanol or ethylene glycol. A handy mnemonic for these substances is SALAD: *s*alicylates, *a*lcohols, *l*actic acidosis, *a*nuria, and *d*iabetic ketoacidosis.

The calculated serum osmolality is equal to

$$2 \times Na^+ \text{ concentration} + \frac{\text{glucose concentration}}{18} + \frac{\text{blood urea nitrogen}}{2.8 \text{ or } 3}$$

Normally a 10 mOsm/L difference or gap exists between the calculated osmolality and the osmolality actually measured by freezing point depression. If the difference is greater, it indicates the presence of extra osmols from any of the aliphatic alcohols or other substances. Alcohol intoxication is the reason for an increased osmolar gap in most circumstances.

Anion and osmolar gaps should be looked for in all obtunded patients, including those with possible alcohol intoxication. If such gaps exist, the differential diagnosis may be aided by analysis of serum ketones and by the serum levels of various alcohols. If the latter are not available, the concentration of ethanol in mg/dl may be calculated by multiplying the osmolar gap by 5. The presence of hypoglycemia or hypocalcemia may also suggest a specific intoxicant, and crystaluria should be sought on urinalysis. The diagnosis of alcohol withdrawal, as opposed to alcohol intoxication, is usually made on clinical grounds. Certainly other causes of autonomic excess should be considered in all patients.

MANAGEMENT

Supportive care is essential in all forms of intoxication. This should include airway protection, mechanical ventilation for severe respiratory depression, fluids and vasoactive agents for hypotension, and prompt attention to concurrent problems. Gastric lavage should be used to remove residual drug from the stomach (2–3 L lukewarm tap water given via 37–40 F gastric hose following tracheal intubation to protect the airway). However, activated charcoal should not be given to patients with methanol or ethylene glycol poisoning because it does not adsorb these drugs.

Beyond these measures, the treatment of all alcohol ingestions, except those of ethyl and isopropyl alcohol, is to prevent the accumulation of toxic metabolites by administering ethanol to saturate hepatic ADH. Although ethyl alcohol can obviously be given by the mouth, some patients cannot tolerate this route of administration, owing to gastritis; as a result, it is best to give an intravenous solution of ethanol (i.e., 50 g of 50 percent ethanol in 1000 ml D5W) to achieve a BAC of 100–200 mg/dl. Hemodialysis should then be employed to facilitate removal of the toxins and to treat acidosis, to prevent ocular damage, and to ameliorate cardiovascular collapse. Although the indications for this procedure are unclear, many clinicians would dialyze patients with serum methanol levels greater than 50 mg/dl (or formic acid levels greater than 20 mg/dl) and ethylene glycol at all levels. Folic acid, 50 mg intravenously q 4 h, should be given to patients with methanol toxicity.

Alcohol withdrawal may also be treated with oral or intravenous ethanol, but this merely prolongs exposure to the responsible intoxicant. A preferred approach is to substitute another depressant for alcohol and to gradually wean patients from it. Although paraldehyde has been used for this purpose, most clinicians prefer diazepam given in 5 mg intravenous doses every 5–15 minutes until patients are calm, then in 5–15 mg maintenance doses of 6–12 hours for 24–48 hours and thereafter in tapered doses. Atenolol and other β-adrenergic antagonists have also been used to treat the autonomic aspects of withdrawal. Phenytoin should not be given as seizure prophylaxis unless patients are regularly taking this medication for established epilepsy or if they have a history of withdrawal seizures.

Outcome

Although most persons survive acute ethanol and even isopropyl alcohol intoxication, ingestion of methanol or ethylene glycol too frequently ends in death. Alcohol withdrawal is generally well tolerated, but delirium tremens has a 5 percent mortality rate despite aggressive treatment of concurrent illness and the judicious use of benzodiazepines.

RECOMMENDED READING

Becker CE: Acute methanol poisoning—"the blind drunk." West J Med 135:122, 1981.

Benowitz NL, Rosenberg J, Becker CE: Cardiopulmonary catastrophes in drug-overdosed patients. Med Clin North Am 63:267, 1979.

Gabow PA, Clay K, Sullivan JB, et al: Organic acids in ethylene glycol intoxication. Ann Intern Med 105:16, 1986.

Kalant H, Sellers EM: Alcohol intoxication and withdrawal. N Eng J Med 394:757, 1976.

Kraus ML, Gottlieb LD, Horwitz RI, et al: Randomized clinical trial of atenolol in patients with alcohol withdrawal. N Eng J Med 313:905, 1985.

Lacouture PG, Wason S, Abrams A, et al: Acute isopropyl alcohol intoxication. Diagnosis and management. Am J Med 75:680, 1980.

McMartin KE, Ambre JJ, Tephly TR: Methanol poisoning in human subjects: role for formic acid accumulation in the metabolic acidosis. Am J Med 68:414, 1980.

Osterloh JD, Pond SM, Grady S, et al: Serum formate concentrations in methanol intoxication as a criterion for hemodialysis. Ann Intern Med 104:200, 1986.

Parry MF, Wallach R: Ethylene glycol poisoning. Am J Med 57:143, 1974.

Peterson CD, Collins AJ, Himes JM, et al: Ethylene glycol poisoning: pharmacokinetics during therapy with ethanol and hemodialysis. N Engl J Med 304:21, 1981.

Smithline N, Gardner KD: Gaps—anionic and osmolal. JAMA 236:1594, 1976.

Swartz RD, Millman RP, Billi JE, et al: Epidemic methanol poisoning: clinical and biochemical analysis of a recent episode. Medicine 60:373, 1981.

Thompson WL: Management of alcohol withdrawal syndromes. Arch Intern Med 138:278, 1978.

Thompson WL, Johnson AD, Maddrey WL, et al: Diazepam and paraldehyde for treatment of severe delirium tremens: a controlled trial. Ann Intern Med 82:175, 1975.

Wolfe SM, Victor M: The relationship of hypomagnesemia and alkalosis to alcohol withdrawal symptoms. Ann NY Acad Sci 162:973, 1969.

85. Sedative-Hypnotic Drug Overdosage and Withdrawal

John M. Luce

DEFINITION

Sedative-hypnotic agents cause sedation and sleep and have anxiolytic and anticonvulsant properties. These drugs are also used as intoxicants. Among this class of agents are alcohols, barbiturates, benzodiazepines (e.g., diazepam [Valium]), chloral hydrate, ethchlorvynol (Placidyl), glutethimide (Doriden), meprobamate (Miltown), and methaqualone (Quaalude). Ethanol and similar aliphatic alcohols are the subject of Chapter 84; the other sedative-hypnotics, especially barbiturates, are discussed here.

PATHOPHYSIOLOGY

Barbiturates are derived from barbituric acid, and their pharmacologic properties depend largely on the chemical nature of their side chains. In general, barbiturates with long side chains have a short duration of action and a high potency after a single dose and are metabolized by the liver, whereas those with shorter side chains have a longer duration of action and a low potency and are excreted by the kidney. Short-acting barbiturates are active for 2–4 hours after a single dose; they include pentobarbital (Nembutal) and secobarbital (Seconal). Intermediate-acting barbiturates are active from 4–6 hours after a single dose and include amobarbital (Amytal) and butobarbital (Butisol). The major long-acting barbiturate, phenobarbital (Luminal), is active for over 6 hours after a single dose. The nonbarbiturate sedative-hypnotics listed earlier are generally intermediate- to long-acting after a single dose. The duration of action of all sedative-hypnotics is determined by their distribution after multiple doses or overdosage. As a result, their activity is prolonged in the latter situations.

The primary action of barbiturates and other sedative-hypnotics is central nervous system depression. As with alcohol, this depression begins in the cerebral hemispheres and then spreads to the limbic system, cerebellum, brain stem reticular activating system, and medullary cardiovascular and respiratory control centers. The drugs therefore cause disinhibition followed by sedation and coma, nystagmus and gait instability, hypotension, bradycardia, and hypopnea or respiratory arrest. These effects relate to both the dose and the potency of the agents; for example, in normal persons, coma can be expected at plasma levels of 10–15 mg/dl for secobarbital, 20–30 mg/dl for amobarbital, and 50–80 mg/dl for phenobarbital. Tolerance to the drugs also is important, in that people who chronically take barbiturates may manifest few effects at these doses. As a result, drug levels may not be helpful in predicting the effects of barbiturates; such levels are even less helpful with agents such as glutethimide.

Persons who abuse prescription sedative-hypnotics may have few concurrent medical problems. However, these agents are frequently mixed with alcohol or other drugs and are responsible for or reinforce a self-neglecting lifestyle. As a result, nutritional deficiencies, liver disease, and trauma must be anticipated in chronic sedative-hypnotic abusers. Similarly, acute overdosage may be associated with aspiration of gastric contents, increased microvascular permeability, pulmonary edema due either to aspiration or to drug effects upon the lung, orthopedic injury, and either pressure necrosis or rhabdomyolysis due to prolonged unconsciousness while lying in one position.

Tolerance develops to chronic ingestion of sedative-hypnotics largely because their rate of hepatic degradation increases over time. Patients who develop tolerance to one agent, such as glutethimide, will be tolerant of other sedative-hypnotics as well. When they stop taking the drugs, these patients manifest a withdrawal syndrome similar to that seen in alcoholics. The onset of the syndrome usually occurs within 8–12 hours of abstinence from short- and intermediate-acting preparations but may take up to 24 or 48 hours with phenobarbital. Tremulousness, agitation, and tachycardia are the initial manifestations, followed by seizures and, in a minority of patients, a state of extreme autonomic excess similar to delirium tremens. Withdrawal seizures are usually multiple, and status epilepticus is more common during withdrawal from barbiturates than during alcohol withdrawal.

Diagnosis

Sedative-hypnotic overdosage is suggested by such symptoms as slurred speech, nystagmus, and obtundation, especially when a history of drug ingestion is obtained. The possibility of alcohol and other agents contributing to drug intoxication should also be raised. Anion and osmolar gaps do not occur with nonalcoholic sedative-hypnotic overdosage in the absence of concurrent metabolic disturbances or lactic acidosis secondary to shock or hypoperfusion. In many cases, toxicology screens must be relied on for diagnosis.

MANAGEMENT

Specific antidotes are not available for sedative-hypnotics, so therapy is largely supportive. Acute overdosage should be treated with gastric lavage after a cuffed endotracheal tube has been passed in unconscious patients and by the instillation of activated charcoal (1 gm/kg orally or by nasogastric tube in a slurry made with magnesium citrate 4 ml/kg or sorbitol 1 ml/kg). Repeated doses of oral charcoal have been shown to increase the elimination of phenobarbital. Mechanical ventilation should be provided when necessary, as should blood pressure support with fluid and vasoactive agents such as dopamine.

Alkalinization of the urine is indicated for phenobarbital overdosage; forced diuresis should be avoided because it contributes to pulmonary edema. Most sedative-hypnotics are poorly removed from the body by hemoperfusion or hemodialysis; these modalities are usually used only in patients with cardiovascular collapse or the likelihood of prolonged coma due to drugs like phenobarbital. Although some persons take street amphetamines to counter the effects of sedative-hypnotics, medical analeptics have no place in the treatment of sedative-hypnotic overdose.

The management of sedative-hypnotic withdrawal is similar to that of alcohol or narcotic withdrawal: substitution of a long-acting agent for shorter-acting ones. Here the drug of choice is phenobarbital. If the patient's daily sedative-hypnotic dose is not known, 200 mg or repeated doses of phenobarbital may be given orally or intravenously to the point of mild intoxication. If the sedative-hypnotic dose is known, 30 mg of phenobarbital can be substituted for the 100 mg of secobarbital or pentobarbital, 500 mg of chloral hydrate, 250 mg of ethchlorvynol, 400 mg of meprobamate, 300 mg of methaqualone, and 50 mg of diazepam. The total daily phenobarbital requirement should be given in four divided doses. If the patient becomes tremulous or agitated between doses, 100 or 200 mg of phenobarbital can be given immediately. On the other hand, if no symptoms appear between doses, the next dose may be held. In general, the total daily phenobarbital dose should be reduced by 30-60 mg/day; more sudden discontinuation is usually not tolerated, owing to the long half-life of phenobarbital. Phenytoin should not be given in the absence of documented epilepsy because it has little or no prophylactic effect during sedative-hypnotic withdrawal.

OUTCOME

Patients with sedative-hypnotic overdosage who receive supportive care are likely to survive hospitalization unless they suffer from severe concurrent illness. If managed properly, sedative-hypnotic withdrawal also carries a low mortality.

RECOMMENDED READING

Benowitz NL, Rosenberg J, Becker CE: Cardiopulmonary catastrophes in drug-overdosed patients. Med Clin North Am 6:267, 1979.

Berg MJ, Berlinger WG, Goldberg MJ, et al: Acceleration of the body clearance of phenobarbital by oral activated charcoal. N Engl J Med 307:642, 1982.

Busto D, Sellers EM, Naranjo CA, et al: Withdrawal reaction after long-term therapeutic use of benzodiazepines. N Engl J Med 315:854, 1986.

Chazan JA, Garella S: Glutethimide intoxication. A prospective study of 70 patients treated conservatively without hemodialysis. Arch Intern Med 128:215, 1971.

Greenblatt DJ, Shader RI: Drug therapy. Benzodiazepines. N Engl J Med 291:1011, 1239, 1974.

Jay SJ, Johanson WG, Pierce AK: Respiratory complications of overdose with sedative drugs. Am Rev Respir Dis 112:591, 1975.

Lynn RI, Honig CL, Jatlow PI, et al: Resin hemoperfusion for treatment of ethchlorvynol overdose. Ann Intern Med 91:549, 1979.

Robinson RR, Gunnells JC, Clapp JR: Treatment of acute barbiturate intoxication. Mod Treat 8:561, 1971.

Schultz JC, Crowder DG, Medart WS, et al: Excretion studies in ethchlorvynol (Placidyl) intoxication. Arch Intern Med 117:4091, 1966.

Setter JG, Maher JF, Schreiner GE: Barbiturate intoxication. Arch Intern Med 117:224, 1966.

Smith DE, Wesson DR: Phenobarbital technique for treatment of barbiturate dependence. Arch Gen Psychiatry 24:56, 1971.

Teehan BP, Maher JF, Carey JJ, et al: Acute ethchlorvynol (Placidyl) intoxication. Ann Intern Med 72:875, 1970.

Wesson DR, Smith DE: Barbiturates. Their Use, Misuse and Abuse. New York, Human Sciences Press, Inc., 1977.

86. Narcotic Overdosage and Withdrawal

John M. Luce

DEFINITION

Acute overdosage with narcotics is a significant cause of morbidity and mortality, especially among young people. The medical sequelae of chronic narcotic abuse are also frequently encountered among patients receiving intensive care. Narcotic withdrawal may occur in these patients or in other persons receiving narcotics for pain.

PATHOPHYSIOLOGY

Narcotic analgesics reduce pain and produce euphoria at less than hypnotic doses. The prototype narcotic is morphine, the major alkaloid present in opium. Two narcotics are derived from the morphine molecule: codeine, which is methyl morphine, and heroin, which is diacetyl morphine. Commonly used semisynthetic or synthetic narcotics include methadone (Dolophine), oxycodone (Percodan), meperidine (Demerol), fentanyl (Sublimaze), and propoxyphene (Darvon).

Morphine is a weak base that is relatively miscible in gastric acid. It and most other narcotics are rapidly metabolized in the liver (first-pass phenomenon) and hence have little activity when taken by mouth except in high doses, although they may be used in such doses for pain. Given parenterally, morphine has a fast onset of action, achieving peak serum levels within 5 minutes of intravenous injection. Morphine crosses the blood-brain barrier more slowly and therefore causes less of a "high" than heroin, which is more lipid-soluble.

The analgesic effects of morphine and other narcotics stem from their interaction with the body's own endorphin-mediated analgesic system. Endorphin or enkephalins, so-called endogenous opioids, are produced by the brain and the pituitary gland and bind at various receptor sites in the central nervous system and in the *substantia gelatinosa* of the spinal cord, where they alter pain transmission. The variation in pain perception among individuals presumably relates to the number of receptor sites they each possess. Exogenous opioids such as morphine are thought to bind to these sites and thereby to reduce pain.

Narcotics also act upon the oculomotor nerve to cause miosis and upon the brain stem to depress respiration, heart rate, and consciousness. These drugs also cause peripheral vasodilation by relaxing vascular smooth muscle and cause atony through their effects on the gut. The degree of these and other side effects depends on both the dose of a given narcotic and its duration of action; such effects may be brief in the case of short-acting narcotics such as fentanyl but prolonged in the case of methadone.

As might be expected, narcotic overdosage is characterized by pupillary constriction, hypopnea or apnea, slight bradycardia, hypotension, gastric and intestinal atony, and an alteration in mental status ranging from lethargy to profound coma. Hypoxemia is usually caused by hypoventilation; however, the alveolar-to-arterial oxygen tension difference $(P[A-a]O_2)$ may be increased by concurrent pneumonia, gastric aspiration, chronic talcosis of the lung parenchyma due to recurrent intravenous injection of contaminants, or narcotic-induced pulmonary edema. The last entity has been reported with most narcotics and may be present to some degree in all patients who die of overdosage. It probably results from increased pulmonary microvascular permeability caused by some component of narcotic drugs or from neutrophil activation in the lungs caused by unknown factors.

Overdosed patients may also suffer from pressure necrosis and necrotizing fasciitis if they lie for prolonged periods in one position. Severe necrosis may be associated with rhabdomyolysis, hyperkalemia, and renal failure. In addition to these problems, narcotic abusers may suffer from cellulitis, tetanus, hepatitis, bacterial endocarditis, and, with increasing frequency, the acquired immunodeficiency syndrome (AIDS). A diffuse vasculitis similar to *periarteritis nodosa* has been described in heroin addicts; many of these patients manifest the complications of abuse of other drugs, including alcohol.

The abrupt discontinuation of narcotics will precipitate drug withdrawal in chronic narcotic abusers and in patients receiving these drugs; as is the case in withdrawal from alcohol and other sedative-hypnotics, this withdrawal state is characterized by rebound excitability in those organs whose function was previously depressed by the drugs. The severity of withdrawal relates to the level of prior drug usage and the degree of tolerance to narcotics that has developed. Most patients manifest mydriasis, piloerection ("cold turkey"), mild tachycardia, and hypertension, irritability, myalgias, and abdominal cramping and diarrhea.

Diagnosis

Narcotic overdosage is easily diagnosed from physical findings such as miosis, depressed consciousness, hypotension, bradycardia, and gastrointestinal atony. A prompt response to narcotic antagonists, discussed in the next section, aids in the diagnosis. Anion and osmolar gaps should not be present in pure narcotic overdosage unless there is lactic acidosis due to shock; if these gaps are present or if polydrug overdosage is suspected, toxicology screens may be called for.

Management

Narcotic overdosage is treated specifically with naloxone (Narcan), which antagonizes the effects of morphine and other agents by displacing the drugs from endorphin-binding sites in the body. Naloxone is given in 0.4 mg or greater intravenous doses every 10–30 minutes as needed; larger initial doses may be required in patients who have taken large amounts of narcotics (especially propoxyphene), and the doses should be repeated over 4–8 hours in persons using methadone (0.8–1.2 mg/hr). Naloxone may also be given by continuous infusion (4.8 mg naloxone in 1000 ml normal saline, given at 250 ml/hr).

Supportive therapy may also be needed, as with other overdosages. Gastric lavage and charcoal instillation should be performed if polydrug overdosage is suspected, with airway protection as needed to prevent aspiration. Hypotension not responsive to naloxone should be treated with intravenous fluids and vasoactive agents such as dopamine. If present, bradycardia should respond to atropine. Rhabdomyolysis may be prevented in some patients with intravenous infusion of bicarbonate and diuresis aided by mannitol and furosemide. The treatment of rhabdomyolysis is discussed further in Chapter 40.

Patients undergoing severe narcotic withdrawal may benefit from a single small intramuscular dose of a short-acting narcotic such as morphine 10 mg. However, it is better to start with oral methadone, which is usually substituted on a 1-to-3 basis for heroin. If the patient's regular dose of narcotic is not known, one may start with 20-40 mg methadone, watching for signs of sedation or autonomic excess. The methadone is then tapered at the rate of 10 mg/day. Nonnarcotic withdrawal may be accomplished with oral clonidine at a dose of 0.8 mg/day in divided doses. Alternatively, clonidine may be applied in transdermal patches that are active for 7 days or more; this central α-adrenergic agent usually reduces all the objective manifestations of narcotic withdrawal.

Outcome

Narcotic overdosage is rarely fatal if treated appropriately; most deaths occur outside the hospital. Similarly, few patients die from or during narcotic withdrawal.

RECOMMENDED READING

Becker CE: Medical complications of heroin addiction. Calif Med 115:42, 1971.

Benowitz NL, Rosenberg J, Becker CE: Cardiopulmonary catastrophes in drug-overdosed patients. Med Clin North Am 6:267, 1979.

Duberstein JL, Kaufman DM: A clinical study of an epidemic of heroin intoxication and heroin-induced pulmonary edema. Am J Med 51:704, 1971.

Frand UI, Shim CS, Williams MH Jr: Methadone-induced pulmonary edema. Ann Intern Med 76:975, 1972.

Fultz JM, Senay EC: Guidelines for the management of hospitalized narcotic addicts. Ann Intern Med 82:815, 1975.

Gold MS, Pottash AC, Sweeney DR, et al: Opiate withdrawal using clonidine: a safe, effective, and rapid nonopiate treatment. JAMA 243:343, 1980.

Katz S, Aberman A, Frand UI, et al: Heroin pulmonary edema: Evidence for increased pulmonary capillary permeability. Am Rev Respir Dis 106:472, 1972.

Martin WR: Naloxone. Ann Intern Med 85:765, 1976.

Norris JV, Don HF: Prolonged depression of respiratory rate following methadone analgesia. Anesthesiology 45:361, 1976.

Paré JAP, Fraser RG, Hogg JC, et al: Pulmonary "mainline" granulomatosis: talcosis of intravenous methadone abuse. Medicine 58:229, 1979.

Sturner WQ, Garriott JC: Deaths involving propoxyphene. JAMA 223:1125, 1973.

Swartzfarb A, Singh G, Marcus D: Heroin-associated rhabdomyolysis with cardiac involvement. Arch Intern Med 137:1255, 1977.

87. Stimulant Drug Overdosage

John M. Luce

DEFINITION

Stimulants such as amphetamines and cocaine increase the concentration of neurotransmitters within the central and autonomic nervous systems. Many hallucinogenic drugs also have stimulant properties, and some are chemically related to amphetamines. Stimulant drugs are used primarily for their euphoric properties on an illicit basis. If taken in excess, all of these agents can cause serious medical problems.

PATHOPHYSIOLOGY

Amphetamines (including amphetamine sulfate [Benzedrine], dextroamphetamine sulfate [Dexedrine], and methamphetamine), cocaine (benzoylmethylecgonine), and hallucinogens (including lysergic acid diethylamide [LSD] and 3-methoxy-4,5-(methylenedioxy)-amphetamine [MMDA]) either cause the release of endogenous catecholamines such as epinephrine, norepinephrine, dopamine, and serotonin at nerve endings or inhibit their reuptake and chemical degradation. Cocaine is also a local anesthetic and a powerful vasoconstrictor; the latter property is shared by many stimulants. The profound psychic alterations produced by hallucinogens ("psychedelics") are not well understood but may involve agonistic effects on serotonin receptors in the midbrain.

All of these stimulants are readily absorbed from the upper gastrointestinal tract and metabolized by the liver. They are also excreted by the kidneys in a similar fashion, although amphetamines, being weak bases, are eliminated in greater quantities in an acidic urine. The average plasma half-life of stimulants is 6–8 hours; this may be increased in the case of amphetamines when the urine is alkaline and is usually briefer in the case of cocaine.

Stimulants are active within the central nervous system approximately 30 minutes after oral ingestion; their time until onset is reduced when the drugs are ingested intravenously or sniffed or smoked, in the case of cocaine. Tolerance develops to the central and autonomic nervous system effects of the amphetamines in particular, so progressively greater doses may be required to achieve the effects of an initial dose. As a result, uncomfortable or dangerous overdosage most commonly occurs among persons who have not developed tolerance or who are exposed to extremely high concentrations of stimulants. Among the latter group are persons who inject comparatively pure preparations of cocaine (which is usually diluted or "cut" with lidocaine, quinine, or other substances); persons who smoke the cocaine alkaloid ("free base"); and those "body packers" who smuggle cocaine in condoms, foil packages, and other packets that rupture within the gastrointestinal tract.

Stimulant drug overdosage is characterized by initially pleasurable central nervous system effects, such as euphoria, that quickly give way to hyperactivity, anxiety, confusion, combativeness, paranoia, and hallucinations (the last mental status change is most common in hallucinogenic drug overdosage). Patients may ultimately have seizures or become comatose. The autonomic aspects of stimulant overdosage include mydriasis, dry mouth, diaphoresis, hyperpyrexia, hypertension, tachycardia, cardiac dysrhythmias, and cardiovascular collapse. Myocardial infarction due either to coronary artery spasm or to thrombosis has been reported in cocaine users, as have intestinal ischemia and rupture of the ascending aorta. Hypertension may be associated with central nervous system bleeding that is postulated to occur at sites where stimulant drugs or adulterants have caused vasculitis. Alterations of consciousness may also result from intense vasospasm not associated with bleeding.

DIAGNOSIS

Stimulant drug overdosage should be considered in all patients of drug-taking age who manifest signs of central nervous system hyperactivity and autonomic excess. Mydriasis, hypertension, and tachycardia are particularly suggestive physical signs. These signs should be looked for in patients in coma and cardiovascular collapse. In the appropriate clinical setting, "body packing" is suggested by the finding of radiopaque packets on plain radiographs of the abdomen. Specific stimulants and hallucinogens can be identified by toxicologic screens.

MANAGEMENT

Patients who are significantly compromised by the overdosage of oral stimulants or hallucinogens should undergo forced emesis or gastric lavage followed by the instillation of activated charcoal. Condoms and other containers used by "body packers" can be removed in some patients by the use of cathartics; although most require only endoscopy or colonoscopy, surgical removal is necessary if these containers have burst. The renal excretion of amphetamines, which are weak bases, is facilitated by acidification of the urine with ascorbic acid (500–2000 mg orally or intravenously). The intravenous administration of ammonium chloride or dilute hydrochloric acid has also been recommended; however, there is the very real risk of producing a severe metabolic acidosis.

The autonomic excess associated with stimulant drug overdosage is best treated with β-adrenergic antagonists such as propranolol, which may be given in sequential 1 mg intravenous doses up to a total of 8 mg. The possible adverse consequence of this approach is that β-blockade will leave the α-adrenergic effects of the stimulants unopposed and intensify the patient's hypertension. Given this possibility, the combined α- and β-adrenergic blocker labetalol, which can be titrated in 20 mg intravenous doses, may be the best therapy. An alternative approach is to give the relatively short-acting α-adrenergic antagonist phentolamine (Regitine) in 5 mg intravenous doses titrated to produce a normal blood pressure in concert with propranolol.

Outcome

Patients with stimulant drug overdosage can usually be managed effectively if they reach the hospital. However, out-of-hospital deaths due to cocaine, in particular, are increasingly common in our society.

RECOMMENDED READING

Bowen JS, Davis GB, Kearney TE, et al: Diffuse vascular spasm associated with 4-bromo-2,5-dimethoxyamphetamine ingestion. JAMA 249:1477, 1983.
Cregler LL, Mark H: Medical complications of cocaine abuse. N Engl J Med 315:1495, 1986.
Freedman DX: The psychopharmacology of hallucinogenic agents. Ann Rev Med 20:409, 1969.
Hart SB, Wallace J: The adverse effects of amphetamines. Clin Toxicol 8:179, 1975.
Isner JM, Estes NAM, Thompson PD, et al: Acute cardiac events temporally related to cocaine abuse. N Engl J Med 315:1438, 1986.
Jonsson S, O'Meara M, Young JB: Acute cocaine poisoning: importance of treating seizures and acidosis. Am J Med 75:1061, 1983.
Kendrick WC, Hull AR, Knochel JP: Rhabdomyolysis and shock after intravenous amphetamine administration. Ann Intern Med 86:381, 1977.
McCarron MM, Wood JD: The cocaine "body packer" syndrome. JAMA 250:1417, 1983.
Pentel PR, Mikell FL, Zavoral JH: Myocardial injury after phenylpropanolamine ingestion. Br Heart J 47:51, 1982.
Rappolt RT, Gay GR, Soman M: Treatment plan for acute and chronic adrenergic poisoning

crisis utilizing sympatholytic effects of the B1–B2 receptor site blocker propranolol (Inderal) in concert with diazepam and urine acidification. Clin Toxicol 14:55, 1979.
Smith DE: Amphetamine use, misuse, and abuse. Boston, G.K. Hall & Co., 1979.
Wetli CV, Wright RK: Death caused by recreational cocaine use. JAMA 241:2519, 1979.
Wilson DJ, Wallin JD, Vlachakis ND, et al: Intravenous labetalol in the treatment of severe hypertension and hypertensive emergencies. Am J Med 95:95, 1983.

88. Tricyclic Antidepressant Overdosage

John M. Luce

DEFINITION

Tricyclic antidepressants and related drugs are used in treating depression in adult patients. These agents are also prescribed for enuresis, hyperkinesis, and school phobia as well as depression in younger persons. Because depressed persons of all ages are often suicidal and because tricyclics may be prescribed in large amounts, overdosage commonly occurs. In fact, 20 percent of patients admitted to hospitals with self-poisoning have ingested a drug of this group either alone or in combination with other drugs, including alcohol, and tricyclic antidepressants may account for up to 40 percent of poison-related admissions to intensive care units (ICUs).

PATHOPHYSIOLOGY

Tricyclic antidepressants are called tricyclics because they possess a three-ring nucleus; these agents are also called tertiary amines. The prototype tricyclics are imipramine (Tofranil) and amitriptyline (Elavil); their secondary amine metabolites, desipramine and nortriptyline, are pharmacologically active and have been used clinically but are not so popular as the parent compounds. Doxepin (Sinequan) and protriptyline (Vivactyl) differ from the other tricyclics in their ring structure. Tetracyclics such as maprotiline (Ludiomil) have recently become available. The metabolism of the tricyclics involves demethylation of the nitrogen atom in their ring, the generation of active metabolites mentioned earlier, and further hepatic degradation. Hepatic uptake (first-pass phenomenon) results in a limited bioavailability of drugs taken by mouth. Up to 90 percent of the compounds that escape the liver are protein bound; this factor plus their lipid solubility leads to a wide distribution in body tissues. As a result, although the plasma half-life of the tricyclics and their metabolites is relatively short, the drugs may remain in the body for a long time.

545

The antidepressant effects of the tricyclics have been attributed to blockade of the amine pump, a transport system in the presynaptic nerve endings that accepts neurotransmitters such as serotonin and norepinephrine. Blockade presumably increases circulating amounts of these neurotransmitters that may otherwise be reduced in depressed patients. Unfortunately, the amine hypothesis of depression is not universally accepted, and the psychiatric effects of the tricyclics remain largely unknown.

The unwanted side effects of these drugs relate primarily to the sedation they cause; to their anticholinergic properties, which may produce mydriasis, dry mouth, sweating, delayed gastric emptying, constipation, and urinary retention; and to their cardiovascular effects. In part because they are anticholinergic, the tricyclics frequently cause tachycardia. They are also α-adrenergic antagonists and therefore may produce postural hypotension. Because the tricyclics have quinidine-like properties, they may impair myocardial conduction and contraction. By inhibiting neuronal uptake of norepinephrine, they tend to induce dysrhythmias and seizures. A final explanation for their cardiovascular effects is inhibition of sympathetic reflexes within the central nervous system.

One study has suggested that tricyclic overdosage is manifested by the following abnormalities in order of increasing plasma drug levels: abnormal deep tendon reflexes, respiratory depression, heart rate greater than 120 beats/min, QRS prolongation greater than 100 msec, dysrhythmias (including atrial and nodal tachycardia, intraventricular conduction delay, bundle-branch heart block, and sinus and ventricular tachycardia), cardiac arrest, seizures, and death. Seizures are especially problematic because the heat generated by muscle activity cannot be dissipated in patients who are atropinized.

Diagnosis

Tricyclic overdosage should be suspected in patients, especially those who are comatose, who present with signs of anticholinergic excess, seizures, or dysrhythmias. The combination of hypotension, hyperthermia, and a hyperdynamic circulation is also suggestive of tricyclic overdosage. Specific diagnosis may be aided by toxicologic analysis. Severity of overdosage was once thought to correlate with plasma tricyclic concentrations in excess of 1000 ng/ml. However, a recent study suggested that levels are less predictive than once believed, that a QRS duration of 100 msec or longer indicates a high likelihood of seizures and dysrhythmias, and that ventricular dysrhythmias can be expected if the QRS duration is 160 msec or longer.

MANAGEMENT

Treatment of tricyclic overdosage often requires intubation and mechanical ventilation. Conscious patients or unconscious patients who are intubated should receive gastric lavage to remove the drugs and should be given activated charcoal to delay their absorption. Hypotension should be treated with Trendelenburg positioning, intravenous fluids, and pressor drugs such as dopamine if required. Insertion of a pulmonary artery catheter may be helpful in guiding fluid management. The effects of overdosage appear to be worse if the pH becomes acidic; this may be due either to increased intracellular binding of the drug owing to acidosis or to concurrent shifts of potassium. Treatment, therefore, should include the administration of supplemental bicarbonate or hyperventilation to maintain the pH above 7.45.

The therapy of tricyclic-induced seizures is similar to that of status epilepticus, in general, as discussed in Chapter 65. The patient's temperatures should be monitored by deep rectal or esophageal probes, and hyperthermia should be treated with external cooling, volume replacement with cool intravenous fluids, and, perhaps, muscle paralysis. Rhabdomyolysis should be anticipated and treated with intravenous mannitol and bicarbonate.

Beyond attempts to maintain alkalemia, the therapy of dysrhythmias associated with tricyclic overdosage is controversial. Physostigmine, which was once used to treat seizures as well as rhythm disturbances (and which can help diagnose overdosage if anticholinergic and other side effects are readily reversed by therapy) cannot generally be recommended because it may cause severe bradycardia or seizures. Prophylactic phenytoin also has been advocated, but its benefits have never been demonstrated in a prospective trial. The best advice is not to treat tachycardia unless it is hemodynamically compromising, in which case it can be reversed with β-blockers such as propranolol, assuming that these agents are given carefully so as not to further reduce the cardiac output and blood pressure. Patients whose QRS exceeds 100 msec and those with atrioventricular block or bradycardia that is hemodynamically significant should receive temporary transvenous pacemakers (Chapter 16). Ventricular tachycardia and fibrillation should be treated with the drugs discussed in Chapter 3. Quinidine and Pronestyl should be avoided in all patients with overdosage because these drugs augment the effects of the tricyclics.

Hemodialysis should not be useful in tricyclic poisoning, owing to the limited amounts of circulating drug or metabolite that are not protein bound. Nevertheless, dramatic reversal of coma and dysrhythmias have been reported following charcoal or resin hemoperfusion despite the fact that the total amount of tricyclic removed from the body by this method is also small. Most patients can probably be managed without hemoperfusion, but it may be helpful in those who do not respond to routine therapy.

OUTCOME

Tricyclic overdosage remains one of the most common causes of death due to overdosage in hospitalized patients. It is hoped that the introduction of less toxic agents and the reduction in the amount of tricyclics prescribed for depressed patients at any one time will decrease the incidence of fatal overdosage.

RECOMMENDED READING

Benowitz NL, Rosenberg J, Becker CE: Cardiopulmonary catastrophes in drug-overdosed patients. Med Clin North Am 63:267, 1979.

Biggs JT, Spiker DG, Petit JM, et al: Tricyclic antidepressant overdose. JAMA 238:135, 1977.

Boehnert MT, Lovejoy FH Jr: Value of the QRS duration versus the serum drug level in predicting seizures and ventricular arrhythmias after an acute overdose of tricyclic antidepressants. N Engl J Med 313:474, 1985.

Hollister LE: Tricyclic antidepressants. N Engl J Med 299:1168, 1978.

Kingston ME: Hyperventilation in tricyclic antidepressant poisoning. Crit Care Med 7:550, 1979.

Petit JM, Biggs JT: Tricyclic antidepressant overdoses in adolescent patients. Pediatrics 59:283, 1977.

Petit JM, Spiker DG, Ruwitch JF, et al: Tricyclic antidepressant plasma levels and adverse effects after overdose. Clin Pharmacol Ther 21:47, 1976.

Snyder BD, Blonde L, McWhirter WR: Reversal of amitriptyline intoxication by physostigmine. JAMA 230:1433, 1974.

Starkey JR, Lawson AA: Poisoning with tricyclic and related antidepressants—a ten-year review. Q J Med 193:33, 1980.

89. Salicylate Overdosage

John M. Luce

DEFINITION

The major derivatives of salicylic acid include acetylsalicylic acid (aspirin), sodium salicylate, and methylsalicylate. These and other salicylates are used medically for their analgesic, antipyretic, and antiinflammatory effects. Salicylates are also taken intentionally or accidentally in excess, both by young people who acutely overdose and by older persons on a chronic basis; this is one of the commonest overdosages requiring intensive care.

PATHOPHYSIOLOGY

When ingested orally, salicylates are rapidly absorbed by the upper gastrointestinal tract. The drugs are then converted into salicylic acid on their first passage through the liver. Salicylic acid that is not protein bound enters cells, including those of the cerebral nervous system, but not in ionized form. Their uptake is therefore facilitated by acidemia, whereas alkalemia tends to retain ionized salicylic acid in the extracellular space. Salicyclic acid is ultimately metabolized by the liver, and its metabolites are excreted in the urine; renal excretion, again, is pH-dependent, with more drug excreted when the urine is alkaline. Although the plasma half-life of salicylic acid is approximately 4 hours under normal conditions, it may be delayed when toxic concentrations are ingested.

Salicylate overdosage may be characterized by any or all of the following: (1) central nervous system alterations, including coma and seizures, that result both from impaired oxidative phosphorylation and from decreased intracellular glucose concentrations, (2) respiratory alkalosis due to direct stimulation of the brain stem ventilatory control center, (3) ketonemia due to inhibition of enzymes active in the Krebs cycle, (4) metabolic acidosis due to the accumulation of salicylic acid, lactic acid (resulting from the drug-induced block in oxidation phosphorylation), and ketones, (5) nausea and vomiting due to the direct action of the salicylates on gastric mucosa as well as to their central effects, (6) tinnitus, (7) hypothermia related to increased oxygen consumption and heat production, (8) hypovolemia due to vomiting and hyperthermia, (9) hypokalemia that results from vomiting and increased excretion of potassium by the kidneys, (10) direct hepatotoxicity, (11) proteinuria and impaired renal function, (12) bleeding related to inhibition of platelet aggregation as well as elevation of the prothrombin time due to decreased hepatic synthesis of factor VII, and (13) protein-rich pulmonary edema, especially in older patients who chronically use salicylates, that probably results from increased pulmonary microvascular permeability and parallels the leakage of protein into the urine.

DIAGNOSIS

The diagnosis of salicylate overdosage should be suspected in patients with the aforementioned derangements, especially if they have ready access to these drugs. The findings of hypoglycemia, hypokalemia, an elevated prothrombin time, and a mixed respiratory alkalosis and metabolic acidosis (with an anion gap) are especially suggestive of salicylate overdosage. The combination of metabolic acidosis and respiratory acidosis in patients who have taken salicylates usually reflects the concurrent ingestion of narcotics, sedative-hypnotics, or alcohol, which depress ventilation. Although a serum salicylate level in excess of 30 mg/dl is compatible with overdosage, higher concentrations may be well tolerated by chronic salicylate users, and lower levels may be associated with symptoms in persons unfamiliar with the drugs. If salicylate levels are not available, the urine should be tested with Phenistix; conversion of the reagent strips to a purple color suggests a salicylate level of 70 mg/dl or greater.

MANAGEMENT

Therapy of salicylate overdosage includes the induction of vomiting or the use of gastric lavage to reduce absorption of the drugs as well as the instillation of activated charcoal to bind them in the gut and to prevent further absorption. Patients should thus receive intravenous bicarbonate to raise the pH to 7.50 and thereby limit the intracellular accumulation of salicylic acid and hasten its excretion by the kidneys. Although fluids should be given to hypotensive patients, overhydration and especially forced diuresis should be avoided lest they exacerbate pulmonary edema. Supplemental glucose should be given whether or not hypoglycemia is documented in order to raise intracellular glucose concentrations. Potassium should be administered if hypokalemia is present, vitamin K should be used to correct the prothrombin time, and external cooling should be employed to normalize the patient's temperature.

Although this conservative approach should suffice in most patients, some may require hemodialysis or hemoperfusion with charcoal or resin. Refractory coma or seizures, persistent acidosis, inappropriateness of bicarbonate therapy, owing to concurrent hypervolemia or to impaired cardiac function, and salicylate levels above 120 mg/dl are generally accepted indications for these procedures in patients with acute intoxication. Hemodialysis should be considered at salicylate levels in the range of 60 mg/dl in patients with chronic intoxication.

OUTCOME

Salicylate overdosage in young people who are treated expeditiously has, approximately, a 2 percent mortality rate. However, mortality approaches 25 percent in elderly users of salicylates in whom acute to chronic overdosage is not recognized. Because of this, clinicians should maintain a high suspicion of salicylate overdosage in older patients who may take excessive amounts of drugs in treating pain and medical problems.

RECOMMENDED READING

Anderson RJ, Potts DE, Gabow PA, et al: Unrecognized adult salicylate intoxication. Ann Intern Med 85:745, 1976.

Bowers RE, Brigham KL, Owen PJ: Salicylate pulmonary edema: the mechanism in sheep and review of the clinical literature. Am Rev Respir Dis 115:261, 1977.

Davies MG, Vella Briffa D, Greaves MW: Systemic toxicity from topically applied salicylic acid. Br Med J 1:661, 1979.

Gabow DE, Anderson RJ, Potts DE, et al: Acid-base disturbances in the salicylate-intoxicated adult. Arch Intern Med 138:1481, 1978.

Heffner JE, Sahn SA: Salicylate-induced pulmonary edema: clinical features and prognosis. Ann Intern Med 95:405, 1981.

Hormaechea E, Carlson RW, Rogove H, et al: Hypovolemia, pulmonary edema and protein changes in severe salicylate poisoning. Am J Med 66:1046, 1979.

Kimberly RP, Plotz PH: Aspirin-induced depression of renal function. N Engl J Med 296:418, 1977.

Prescott LF, Balali-Mood M, Critchley H, et al: Diuresis or urinary alkalinisation for salicylate poisoning. Br Med J 285:1383, 1982.

Sbarbaro JA, Bennett R: Aspirin hepatotoxicity and disseminated intravascular coagulation. Ann Intern Med 86:183, 1977.

Winchester JF, Gelfand MC, Helliwell M, et al: Extracorporeal treatment of salicylate or acetaminophen poisoning—is there a role? Arch Intern Med 141:370, 1981.

90. Acetaminophen Overdosage

John M. Luce

DEFINITION

Acetaminophen (*N*-acetyl-*p*-aminophenol) is a phenacetin derivative that is used medically for its analgesic and antipyretic actions. This drug has become increasingly popular because it is considered safer than aspirin, which has gastrointestinal toxicity, and phenacetin, which is associated with renal toxicity (analgesic nephropathy). Because of its widespread availability, acetaminophen now is taken acutely or chronically in excess by many persons and has become a common cause of liver toxicity.

PATHOPHYSIOLOGY

Following oral ingestion, acetaminophen is readily absorbed by the upper gastrointestinal tract and distributed in a nonprotein-bound state throughout body fluids. It has a plasma half-life of approximately 3 hours. Most of the drug is conjugated in the liver by glucuronide or sulfate and excreted in the urine. In addition, a small amount is normally converted throughout the cytochrome P_{450} mixed-oxidase enzyme system to a toxic acylated metabolite. This metabolite, in turn, is conjugated with glutathione within hepatocytes and excreted. However, when large amounts of acetaminophen are ingested on either an acute or a chronic basis, hepatic glutathione may become depleted. The acylated metabolite then binds to nucleophilic proteins in hepatocytes and causes necrosis of these cells.

Hepatic toxicity may result from an acute ingestion of as little as 10 g of acetaminophen (30 single-strength or 15 double-strength Tylenol tablets), and 25 g may be fatal. The liver may also be damaged by the chronic ingestion of 5 g of acetaminophen or more each day. The likelihood of hepatic toxicity is increased substantially in alcoholic patients either because the activity of the cytochrome P_{450} system is increased by concurrent metabolism of ethanol or because malnutrition reduces liver stores of glutathione.

Acute acetaminophen overdosage is usually manifested by nausea and vomiting and a depressed mental status (especially if other drugs are taken) that resolve within 12–24 hours. Patients, thereafter, may feel well and may have no delayed hepatotoxicity if their plasma acetaminophen concentrations are less than 150 μg/dl 4 hours after ingestion or less than 50 μg/dl 12 hours after ingestion. However, if their drug levels are higher, after 48–72 hours they may develop biochemical abnormalities, including an increase in SGOT and SGPT levels, mild increases in alkaline phosphatase, an elevated prothrombin time, and hyperbilirubinemia. These patients may then experience fulminant hepatic failure and death within 4 to 10 days.

DIAGNOSIS

The diagnosis of acetaminophen overdosage should be entertained in the appropriate clinical setting, especially if hepatic abnormalities exist without another obvious cause. The diagnosis is confirmed by the plasma concentration of acetaminophen, which also serves as the best predictor of potential for development of liver damage and the need for therapy. Ideally, the plasma level should be obtained at a time between 4 and 24 hours after ingestion. It is then plotted on the nomogram shown in Figure 90–1; levels that fall on or above the treatment line are potentially toxic, and these patients require therapy with the antidote discussed below.

MANAGEMENT

Patients with acetaminophen overdosage should be subjected to forced emesis or gastric lavage to remove unabsorbed drug from the upper gastrointestinal tract. Activated charcoal should not be given, however, because it may absorb the antidote for acetaminophen. If other toxic drugs have been ingested for which charcoal is indicated, it should be instilled, removed by nasogastric tube after 2 hours, and followed by the antidote. Hemodialysis and hemoperfusion may remove acetaminophen from the body but do not alter clinical outcome; they should be used only for the treatment of concurrent overdosage of other drugs.

The commercially available antidote for acetaminophen is *N*-acetylcysteine (NAC, Mucomyst), which prevents the binding of the acylated metabolite of acetaminophen to hepatocytes. It is not known whether NAC substitutes for or helps regenerate glutathione or whether it changes the proportion of acetaminophen that is metabolized by the cytochrome P_{450} system. NAC is effective only in preventing liver damage and is of no benefit if administered 24 or more hours after acetaminophen ingestion.

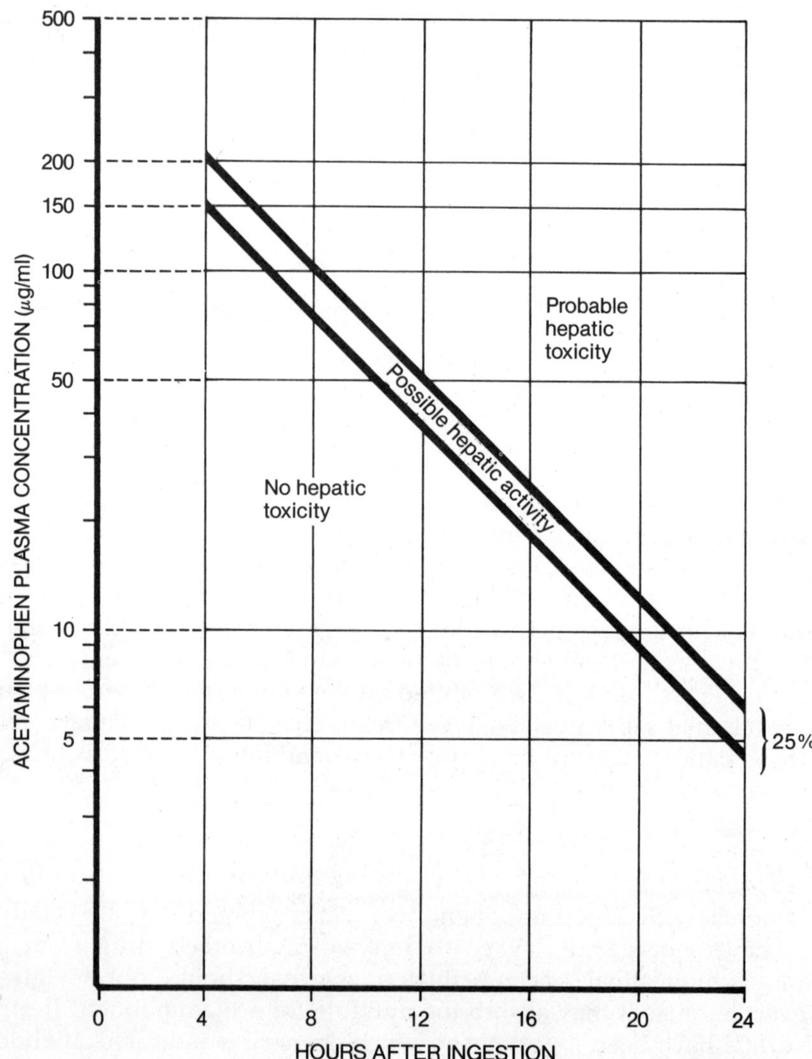

FIGURE 90–1. Nomogram for determining acetaminophen toxicity. See text for explanation. (Modified, with permission, from Rumack BH, Matthew H. Pediatrics 55:871, 1975.)

NAC is available in the United States in 10 percent (100 mg/dl) or 20 percent (200 mg/dl) solutions. It should be given orally in a loading dose of 140 mg/kg followed by 17 maintenance doses of 70 mg/kg each at 4-hour intervals. This regimen should be continued for a total period of 72 hours. NAC may be diluted with water or juice for oral ingestion, or it may be given by nasogastric tube. It may cause nausea and vomiting when given by mouth; intravenous injection has been associated with anaphylactic reactions and cardiovascular collapse.

The treatment of liver failure due to acetaminophen is similar to that of liver failure from other causes and is discussed in Chapter 64.

OUTCOME

As noted earlier, the likelihood of hepatotoxicity and death from acetaminophen may be predicted by plasma levels of the drug. In general, acetaminophen overdosage is one of the most serious overdosages encountered in medical practice.

RECOMMENDED READING

Ameer B, Greenblatt DJ: Acetaminophen. Ann Intern Med 87:202, 1976.
Barker JD, de Carle DJ, Anuras S: Chronic excessive acetaminophen use and liver damage. Ann Intern Med 87:299, 1977.
Black M: Acetaminophen hepatotoxicity. Gastroenterology 78:382, 1980.
Black M, Raucy J: Acetaminophen, alcohol, and cytochrome p-450. Ann Intern Med 104:427, 1986.
Hall AH, Rumack BH: The treatment of acute acetaminophen poisoning. Intensive Care Med 1:29, 1986.
Johnson GK, Tolman KG: Chronic liver disease and acetaminophen. Ann Intern Med 87:302, 1977.
Koch-Weser J: Acetaminophen. N Engl J Med 295:1297, 1976.
Rumack BH, Peterson RC, Koch GG, et al: Acetaminophen overdose: 662 cases with evaluation of oral acetylcysteine treatment. Ann Intern Med 141:380, 1981.
Seefe LB, Cuccherini BA, Zimmerman HJ, et al: Acetaminophen hepatotoxicity in alcoholics. Ann Intern Med 104:399, 1986.

Environmental Disorders

91. Hypothermia

David J. Pierson

David J. Pierson

DEFINITION

Hypothermia is present when a patient's core body temperature is less than 35°C (95°F), as determined by rectal, esophageal, or tympanic membrane measurement. It is further defined both physiologically and clinically as mild (32–35°C; 90–95°F), moderate (30–32°C; 86–89°F), and severe (core temperature less than 30°C or 86°F).

Hypothermia occurs in several distinct clinical settings that have prognostic and therapeutic importance. Accidental hypothermia is seen when otherwise healthy persons are exposed to external factors that overwhelm their ability to maintain normal body temperature as in cold water immersion and other environmental cold exposure. Exhaustion hypothermia can occur in long-distance runners, miners, and certain other workers in whom heat loss outstrips the body's ability to generate heat. Hypothermia also occurs in a variety of disease states. These include sepsis and other overwhelming infections; endocrine/metabolic conditions such as diabetic ketoacidosis, hypoglycemia, and myxedema; severe central nervous system disease (cerebrovascular disorders; head or high spinal cord trauma; anorexia nervosa); hepatic or cardiac failure; and the effects of drugs, typically alcohol, sedative-hypnotic overdose, phenothiazines, and general anesthetics. Loss of the protective function of the skin, as in severe burns and the erythrodermas, also predisposes to hypothermia.

The elderly are particularly vulnerable to subclinical hypothermia because even in the absence of other disease, their thermoregulatory mechanisms are impaired. Studies have found more than 10 percent of elderly individuals living alone to be hypothermic; this disorder can occur in older persons in the summer as well as during cold weather. Controlled deep hypothermia for cardiac or other surgical procedures can also produce the clinical picture discussed in this chapter.

PATHOPHYSIOLOGY

The body's normal responses to cold initially include increased heart rate, dermal vasoconstriction, dilatation of muscle vessels, release of thyroid and adrenocortical hormones, piloerection, and shivering; these decrease heat loss and increase its generation, but they become progressively ineffective with time and continued cooling. Heart rate and blood pressure fall progressively, shivering ceases at aboaut 30°C (86°F), and compensatory mechanisms are lost. Metabolic rate slows progressively to about 50 percent of normal at 28°C. Cerebral blood flow decreases as temperature falls, the pupils are dilated and usually unresponsive at 30°C, and the electroencephalogram (EEG) becomes flat as 20°C is approached.

Other physiologic effects are hematologic (hemoconcentration due to plasma loss from the vascular space; leukopenia and thrombocytopenia from sequestration in the spleen and liver); endocrinologic (hyperglycemia due to decreased pancreatic insulin release and diminished peripheral utilization); and respiratory (impaired ventilatory drive, mucociliary clearance, and cough; leftward shift of the hemoglobin-oxygen saturation curve).

Although many of these changes tend to protect the body from damage induced by cold, the most life-threatening effects of hypothermia are in cardiac conduction and rhythm. Atrial fibrillation commonly occurs as body temperature falls, and as it drops farther, there are extrasystoles and often ventricular tachycardia. Ventricular fibrillation is an immediate hazard at temperatures below 28°C. Dysrhythmias tend to be refractory to all treatment until rewarming to above 30°C is accomplished, making prolonged cardiac resuscitation necessary in many cases.

DIAGNOSIS

Because most clinical thermometers do not register below 34°C, detection and quantitation of hypothermia requires an electronic or other device with an extended range of accuracy. Core rather than pharyngeal or surface temperature must be measured. Physical signs of death and the prognosticators of neurologic reversibility are inapplicable in hypothermia, and patients of any age may recover fully after initially showing no sign of life. A careful search for frostbite, injection sites, and evidence of head injury or other trauma should be made.

Although the presence of underlying sepsis or other infection is a major determinant of prognosis, in a recent study, infected patients could not be distinguished from others by the usual physical signs. Patients with occult infection had decreased systemic vascular resistance and increased cardiac index in comparison with noninfected hypothermic patients, but these measurements require a pulmonary artery catheter, placement and presence of which increases the likelihood of ventricular fibrillation and other dysrhythmias.

MANAGEMENT

General Measures. Although therapy for patients with hypothermia often focuses on rewarming, survival is probably more directly related to adequate general supportive care. Because of the threat of ventricular fibrillation, physical manipulation and transfer of patients between facilities should be avoided if possible, and such procedures as endotracheal intubation and pulmonary arterial catheterization performed with great care. Electrical and chemical cardioversion for ventricular fibrillation are generally unsuccessful at core temperatures below 30°C but may be attempted once; cardiopulmonary resuscitation can effectively support such patients and may be required for a prolonged period while core rewarming proceeds.

Despite higher mortality in the presence of infection, there is no evidence to support routine administration of broad-spectrum antimicrobial drugs to all hypothermic patients. Likewise, corticosteroids are not helpful unless specifically indicated by other conditions. Insulin should be used cautiously despite hyperglycemia, since hypoglycemia can develop precipitously when endogenous insulin release and peripheral utilization increase on rewarming.

Rewarming. Passive rewarming should be adequate in mild hypothermia, particularly that which has developed gradually, as in the elderly. Such patients should be wrapped in blankets and cared for in a warm room. Moderate and severe hypothermia (core temperatures below 32°C) should be treated with active rewarming, although which one of the numerous available techniques should be used is highly controversial. Active surface rewarming, as by immersion in warm water, by radiant heat cradles, or by fluid-circulating heating blankets, was out of favor for a number of years because early studies showed increased mortality with this method, presumably because of "rewarming shock" from cutaneous vasodilation and return of cold blood to the central circulation. More recent work suggests that, although slower than active core rewarming techniques, active external rewarming can be effective and safe if vigorous fluid resuscitation and appropriate hemodynamic monitoring are used.

Severe hypothermia, particularly in the presence of ventricular fibrillation or other severe hemodynamic instability, should probably be treated with active core rewarming techniques if these can be made available. Most readily administered of these, although only modestly effective for rapid rewarming, are inhalation of heated, humidified gas via mask or endotracheal tube (42–46°C, as monitored at the mouth) and heated intravenous fluids. Also relatively easy to administer are irrigation of an intragastric balloon (passage of which, however, may precipitate dysrhythmias) and high colonic irrigation.

Most aggressive, but also most rapidly efficacious, are peritoneal dialysis, hemodialysis, partial cardiopulmonary bypass, and thoracotomy with direct mediastinal irrigation. The last two of these have been successful in some reported cases with cardiovascular collapse, but they are complicated and not immediately available to most clinicians. Peritoneal dialysis, using standard dialysate warmed to 43°C (monitored either intraperitoneally or at the skin), is the least complicated and most readily available invasive method. The dialysate is not retained in the abdomen but is passed in and out rapidly, usually 6–8 times in cases of severe hypothermia. A desired rate of rewarming for all techniques is at least 0.5°C (1.0°F) per hour.

OUTCOME

Survival in hypothermia is primarily determined by the patient's underlying condition. Numerous studies have documented excellent survival in previously healthy individuals with accidental or drug-related hypothermia and mortality rates in excess of 50 percent in patients with underlying chronic disease. Mortality is especially high in patients whose hypothermia is related to sepsis or other serious infection. Neurologic outcome cannot be predicted from initial findings, even after prolonged submersion in cold water or other environmental exposure.

RECOMMENDED READING

Hudson LD, Conn RD: Accidental hypothermia: associated diagnoses and prognosis in a common problem. JAMA 227:37, 1974.

Ledingham I McA, Mone JG: Treatment of accidental hypothermia: a prospective clinical study. Br Med J 280:1102, 1980.

Morris DL, Chambers HF, Morris MG, et al: Hemodynamic characteristics of patients with hypothermia due to occult infection and other causes. Ann Intern Med 102:153, 1985.

Moss J: Accidental severe hypothermia. Surg Gynecol Obstet 162:501, 1986.

Rankin AC, et al: Cardiac arrhythmias during rewarming of patients with accidental hypothermia. Br Med J 289:874, 1984.

Reuler JB: Hypothermia: pathophysiology, clinical settings, and management. Ann Intern Med 89:519, 1978.

Reuler JB, Parker RA: Peritoneal dialysis in the management of hypothermia. JAMA 240:2289, 1978.

Salvosa CB, Payne PR, Wheeler EF: Environmental conditions and body temperatures of elderly women living alone or in local authority homes. Br Med J 4:656, 1971.

Sheehy TW, Navari RM: Hypothermia. Ala J Med Sci 21:374, 1984.

Southwick FS, Dalglish PH Jr: Recovery after prolonged asystolic cardiac arrest in profound hypothermia: a case report and literature review. JAMA 243:1250, 1980.

Welton DE, Mattox KL, Miller RR, et al: Treatment of profound hypothermia. JAMA 240:2291, 1978.

Wong KC: Physiology and pharmacology of hypothermia. West J Med 138:227, 1983.

92. Hyperthermia

David J. Pierson

DEFINITION

Several distinct syndromes involve elevations of body temperature, and it is important to distinguish among them. Fever is a disorder of thermoregulation, in which there is an upward displacement of the set-point with an associated rise in body temperature. Hyperthermia is a condition in which heat gain or heat production exceeds the capacity of the body to dissipate it. The latter occurs in two forms: exertional heat stroke affects previously healthy persons who experience marked elevation in body temperature (typically above 40.6°C [105 °F]) and central nervous system disturbance in the setting of recreational or occupational exercise. Classic or nonexertional heat stroke applies to persons in whom extreme hyperthermia, central nervous system alterations, and anhidrosis occur in the setting of high ambient temperatures. This is the syndrome most likely to be seen in the general hospital and typically occurs in individuals who are elderly, bed bound, or otherwise physically impaired. Heat exhaustion is a less severe form of any of the above, with more modest elevation of core temperature and normal or only mildly disturbed central nervous system function.

Malignant hyperthermia is a pharmacogenetic disorder in which acute hypermetabolic reactions in skeletal muscle are triggered by inhalational anesthetics, skeletal muscle relaxants, or, rarely, other drugs or stresses. Patients are usually children or young adults, and the disorder may follow an autosomal dominant inheritance pattern. Characterized by muscle rigidity and rapidly rising body temperature, malignant hyperthermia is likely to be rapidly fatal unless recognized promptly and treated appropriately.

The neuroleptic malignant syndrome is a separate entity that occurs mainly in patients being treated for psychiatric disorders with major tranquilizers of the phenothiazine and butyrophenone groups (chiefly fluphenazine and haloperidol). It is an idiosyncratic response to the usual doses of these agents and is characterized by akinesia, muscle rigidity, and moderate hyperthermia, developing over a period of 24–72 hours.

PATHOPHYSIOLOGY

Fever, thought to be modulated by the lymphokine interleukin 1 (endogenous pyrogen), may be important in activating the immune response, and so is not necessarily harmful. However, hyperthermia is a pathologic condition adversely affecting numerous body systems. Metabolic rate and tissue oxygen requirements increase progressively as temperature climbs above 37°C. The normal cardiovascular response to elevated temperature is tachycardia, increased cardiac output, and decreased systemic vascular resistance, and this is the pattern seen in exertional hyperthermia. However, the elderly are unable to increase heart rate and cardiac output as effectively and often have paradoxically increased systemic vascular resistance. Circulatory failure due either to peripheral pooling of blood or to hypovolemia is common in elderly individuals exposed to high environmental temperatures. Metabolic acidosis results from inability to meet increased peripheral oxygen demand and is often accompanied by an exaggerated hyperventilatory response. Ingestion of alcohol, phenothiazines, anticholinergics, and other drugs affecting thermoregulation predisposes to both exertional and nonexertional heat stroke. Patients with atherosclerotic cardiovascular disease, diabetes, and chronic alcoholism are especially susceptible to heatstroke during summer heat waves or when otherwise subjected to high environmental temperatures.

Malignant hyperthermia is thought to be due to a sudden rise in intracellular calcium released from sarcoplasmic reticulum in the presence of the triggering agent in a genetically susceptible individual. This leads to intense muscle contraction and rigidity, with a marked increase in heat generation. The pathophysiologic mechanism for the neuroleptic malignant syndrome is unknown. Physical exhaustion, dehydration, concurrent organic brain disease, and use of long-acting depot neuroleptics are all said to predispose to the syndrome.

DIAGNOSIS

Hyperthermia in the setting of exertional or classic heat stroke is usually obvious, although it is important to distinguish hyperthermia from fever; that is, to rule out an infectious cause for elevated temperature. Common symptoms of heat stroke are headache, confusion, and prostration; chills, muscle cramps, nausea, and vomiting are also frequent. Physical examination typically shows a picture of very high core temperature (40.6°C [105°F] or above), circulatory collapse, and impaired mental function, ranging from agitation and delirium to lethargy and coma. Patients with classic heat stroke have hot, dry skin, whereas sweat is commonly present in exertional heat stroke. In the latter, piloerection (gooseflesh) may be seen over the chest and upper arms.

Laboratory findings in both types of heat stroke include hemoconcentration, hypokalemia, hypocalcemia, and hypophosphatemia. Hyperglycemia is common in classic heat stroke, but hypoglycemia may be a feature of the exertional variety. Rhabdomyolysis and hemolysis, common in exertional heat stroke, may rarely occur in the nonexertional variety as well. Disseminated intravascular coagulation, acute renal failure, and hepatic necrosis are also known sequelae. Arterial blood gas values typically show metabolic acidosis and respiratory alkalosis. It should be recalled that the arterial oxygen and carbon dioxide tensions are higher in the hyperthermic patient than when measured at 37°C, by approximately 7 and 4.5 percent per °C, respectively.

In contrast to the situation just described, hypercalcemia and hyperkalemia are characteristic in malignant hyperthermia, along with often extremely high blood levels of creatine kinase. Myoglobinemia and myoglobinuria are common, and acute renal failure is a frequent complication. Consumption coagulopathy, pulmonary edema, and cerebral edema may occur. This condition is often diagnosed in the operating room, heralded by a sudden increase in end-tidal carbon dioxide level in association with blood pressure instability, increased cardiac output, and the appearance of dysrhythmias. Laboratory findings in the neuroleptic malignant syndrome are nonspecific. Creatine kinase levels may be elevated, although not usually so markedly as in malignant hyperthermia.

MANAGEMENT

The treatment of hyperthermia has two components: vigorous general supportive care and monitoring, and specific maneuvers to lower the body temperature as rapidly as possible. Patients with all forms of hyperthermia may require large amounts of fluid resuscitation, and in mild cases, this may be all that is needed, particularly if mental status is normal. More severe cases require active cooling. Traditionally, this has been accomplished by immersion in cold water and ice and by rubbing the neck, axillae, and groin areas with ice. Although cumbersome, these maneuvers are usually rapidly effective. More recently, some clinicians have employed convection and evaporation rather than conduction, by spraying or sponging the patient with tepid water and applying fan-driven air to the skin. This technique lowered core temperature from 106°C or above to below 103°C in ½–1½ hours in one series of patients with classic heat stroke.

Management of malignant hyperthermia requires rapid diagnosis, prompt discontinuation of potential triggering drugs, and administration of dantrolene sodium, which is dramatically effective if given early. The dose is 1–10 mg/kg intravenously, given at a rate of 1 mg/kg/min, until heart rate slows and muscle tone improves, and this can be repeated in 15 minutes before dropping back to 2–10 mg/kg over 4 hours as guided by physical signs. Mannitol and furosemide should be administered in order to maintain high urine output, and dysrhythmias should be treated with procainamide or other agents as necessary.

In the neuroleptic malignant syndrome, all neuroleptic agents should be discontinued and good supportive care given in an intensive care setting. There have been no controlled studies of drug therapy, but dantrolene sodium (1–10 mg/kg intravenously or 50–200 mg orally per day) has been reported effective, as has the dopamine agonist bromocriptine mesylate (2.5–10 mg, orally, 3 times a day). These two agents can be administered concurrently. Recovery parallels elimination of the associated neuroleptic drug from the body.

Whether fever *per se* should be treated remains controversial. Appropriate therapy for the primary disease process is obviously of paramount importance, but once this is done, many clinicians also take measures to lower the patient's temperature. It was previously believed that very high core temperatures, e.g., over 40°C or 106°F, from whatever cause, were in themselves likely to cause brain damage or other complications. Careful reviews of the literature, however, fail to substantiate this.

Temperatures over 39°C (102°F) should definitely be treated in young children with a history of febrile seizures; in patients with fever due to head injury or other central nervous system disease; in psychotic patients with fever and hallucinations; in pregnancy (in which elevated body temperature may be teratogenic); and in individuals with serious cardiovascular disorders such as acute myocardial infarction. In the absence of these factors, whether fever due to infectious diseases is reduced by drugs or by other means apparently has no effect on mortality or morbidity.

Drugs such as aspirin or acetaminophen, which reset the temperature set-point, are preferable to surface cooling for lowering body temperature. Aspirin should not be given to febrile children because of the risk of Reye's syndrome; adults should receive 650 mg every 4 hours until the temperature has returned to normal or symptoms have improved. The dose of acetaminophen is 10–15 mg/kg, 4–5 times daily for children over 2 years of age, and 650 mg 4–5 times daily for adults and children over 13.

OUTCOME

In febrile illness, prognosis is related to the underlying disorder rather than to the magnitude of the temperature elevation. Similarly, in both exertional and classic heat stroke, survival is mainly determined by the patient's underlying state of health. Mortality in classic heat stroke ranges from 10–80 percent in reported series, and is higher in the elderly and in individuals with cardiovascular disease, diabetes, and alcoholism. Prior to widespread recognition of malignant hyperthermia and the use of dantrolene sodium, mortality in this condition was in excess of 50 percent; today it is between 5 and 10 percent, and should approach zero with prompt recognition and management. Mortality in the neuroleptic malignant syndrome is said to be 20–30 percent, often from respiratory failure and aspiration pneumonia. Prompt recognition of this disorder and transfer of patients to intensive care facilities should result in a lowering of this mortality rate as well.

RECOMMENDED READING

Britt BA: Malignant hyperthermia. Can Anaesth Soc J 32:666, 1985.

Exertional heat injury. Med Lett Drugs Ther 27(690):55, 1985.

Graham BS, Lichtenstein MJ, Hinson JM, et al: Nonexertional heatstroke: physiologic management and cooling in 14 patients. Arch Intern Med 146:87, 1986.

Gray JD, Blaschke TF: Fever: to treat or not to treat. Ration Drug Ther 19(12):1, 1985.

Guze BH, Baxter LR: Neuroleptic malignant syndrome. N Engl J Med 313:163, 1985.

Hart GR, et al: Epidemic classical heatstroke: clinical characteristics and course of 28 patients. Medicine 61:189, 1982.

Kilbourne EM, et al: Risk factors for heatstroke: a case-control study. JAMA 247:3332, 1982.

Kolb ME, Horn ML, Martz R: Dantrolene in human malignant hyperthermia. Anesthesiology 56:254, 1982.

Neuroleptic malignant syndrome. (Editorial.) Lancet 1:545, 1984.

Olson KR, et al: Environmental and drug-induced hyperthermia. Pathophysiology, recognition, and management. Emerg Med Clin North Am 2:459, 1984.

Simon HB: Extreme pyrexia. JAMA 236:2419, 1976.

Simon HB: Extreme pyrexia. Hosp Pract 21(5A):123, 127, 1986.

Smego RA, Durack DT: The neuroleptic malignant syndrome. Arch Intern Med 142:1183, 1982.

Sprung CL: Hemodynamic alterations of heatstroke in the elderly. Chest 75:362, 1979.

Temple AR: Review of comparative antipyretic activity in children. Am J Med 75(5A):38, 1983.

93. Near-Drowning

David J. Pierson

David J. Pierson

DEFINITION

Drowning is death by suffocation from submersion in water or other liquid medium. Near-drowning, also called postimmersion syndrome or submersion injury, is the clinical illness that follows initial resuscitation after submersion. Approximately 50,000 cases of near-drowning are seen annually by physicians in the United States, and 7000 persons in this country die of drowning each year.

PATHOPHYSIOLOGY

Near-drowning has two prominent components: pulmonary aspiration of water and other material and hypoxic cerebral injury. The former commonly leads to development of the adult respiratory distress syndrome (ARDS; see Chapter 27), and the latter may be followed by permanent anoxic brain damage.

In 80–90 percent of submersion episodes, water is aspirated into the lungs; in the 10–20 percent in which this does not occur ("dry drowning"), it is presumably prevented by laryngospasm. Fresh water is hypotonic: when aspirated, it is rapidly absorbed from the lungs into the circulation, creating the possibility of hypervolemia, hyponatremia, and acute hemolysis. In contrast, sea water is markedly hypertonic to plasma and, when introduced into the lungs, can trigger a massive shift of fluid from the circulation into the alveolar space, causing pulmonary edema, hypernatremia, hyperchloremia, and hypermagnesemia. Although these pathophysiologic differences between fresh- and salt-water near-drowning have long been appreciated, they are much less clinically important than previously believed and have little impact on management.

Aspiration of either fresh or salt water into the lungs causes diffuse alveolar injury and leads to the clinical picture of ARDS. The severity of pulmonary dysfunction is roughly proportional to the quantity of water aspirated, although the first signs of acute respiratory failure may not develop until several hours following the immersion incident. Bronchospasm is also a prominent feature in many cases. In addition, focal areas

568

of bronchial obstruction from aspirated foreign material or gastric contents may lead to localized areas of pneumonitis or lung abscess.

Metabolic acidosis from tissue hypoxia is common in near-drowning and may be severe. The electrolyte abnormalities described above may occur but are not life-threatening in patients who survive to reach the hospital. Although some hemolysis may also occur, especially in fresh-water near-drowning, it is generally not clinically significant. Disseminated intravascular coagulation is occasionally seen, as is acute renal failure.

Although it is commonly the main determinant of ultimate recovery, cerebral anoxia is difficult to separate clinically from the effects of hypothermia (see Chapter 91) in the initial hours following resuscitation. Because hypothermia lowers the metabolic requirements of the brain, cold-water immersion may be tolerated for longer periods without permanent sequelae than is the case after warm-water near-drowning, especially in children.

Submersion accidents frequently involve head injury or other trauma in addition to near-drowning, and it is important for the clinician to remember these potential reasons for decreased consciousness or for a falling hematocrit.

DIAGNOSIS

The clinical presentation of patients who have experienced near-drowning is highly variable. They may be asymptomatic at initial evaluation or may have cough, dyspnea, or fulminant acute respiratory distress. Neurologically, patients may present with agitation, coma, or recurrent seizures. Dysrhythmias are common, particularly if hypothermia is present. Most patients with near-drowning have fever during the first 24 hours for which no specific explanation may be found; thereafter, temperature elevation often signals the onset of bacterial pneumonia.

Laboratory evaluation shows varying degrees of hypoxemia, usually with respiratory alkalosis, as well as metabolic acidosis, which may be severe. Leukocytosis is common and may exceed 40,000 cells/mm^3. The chest radiograph may initially be normal or may show focal areas of atelectasis, streaky infiltrates, or the diffuse bilateral infiltrates characteristic of ARDS.

MANAGEMENT

Initial supportive therapy should focus on relieving hypoxemia and reversing metabolic acidosis. Positive end-expiratory pressure (PEEP) should be employed if needed to maintain the systemic arterial oxygen tension (PaO$_2$) above 60–65 mm Hg. If the patient is alert and cooperative and does not require mechanical ventilation for other reasons, PEEP may be administered in the form of continuous positive airway pressure (CPAP) by mask. However, most patients with severe near-drowning require endotracheal intubation and mechanical ventilation in addition to PEEP.

The respiratory management of near-drowning is essentially that of ARDS in other settings. Systemic corticosteroids and prophylactic antibiotics are of no benefit and should be reserved for clear, specific indications such as severe bronchospasm or the onset of bacterial pneumonia.

Intracranial hypertension is common in patients with near-drowning, and should be approached in the same way as in other acute diffuse cerebral injuries (see Chapter 77). Whether the aggressive approach to cerebral resuscitation, using barbiturates and other therapy, provides clinical advantages over more conservative approaches remains controversial.

OUTCOME

Survival and eventual neurologic recovery depend upon the severity of respiratory dysfunction and the extent and duration of cerebral hypoxia. Patients who develop full-blown ARDS have the same mortality as that seen in other settings of this syndrome—about 60 percent. However, if the chest radiograph is normal on admission and hypoxemia does not worsen during the initial 24 hours, the outlook for uneventful recovery is good. Progressive pulmonary infiltrates or hypoxemia with onset on the second hospital day or later suggests the development of complicating bacterial pneumonia or sepsis.

Complete neurologic recovery can be expected in those patients who are alert or only moderately obtunded on admission to the intensive care unit, whereas patients who arrive comatose, having required cardiopulmonary resuscitation, are more likely to have sustained permanent neurologic damage; an exception is individuals with cold-water immersion who are markedly hypothermic on admission. In such circumstances, the extent of neurologic recovery cannot be predicted until rewarming and initial stabilization are complete.

RECOMMENDED READING

Knopp RK: Near-drowning. In Rosen P, et al (eds): Emergency Medicine. St. Louis, C. V. Mosby Co., 1983, p. 470.
Martin TG: Near-drowning and cold water immersion. Ann Emerg Med 13:263, 1984.

Modell JH: Biology of drowning. Annu Rev Med 29:1, 1978.

Nussbaum E: Prognostic variables in nearly drowned, comatose children. Am J Dis Child 139:1058, 1985.

Oakes DD, et al: Prognosis and management of victims of near-drowning. J Trauma 22:544, 1982.

Sekar TS, et al: Survival after prolonged submersion in cold water without neurologic sequelae. Arch Intern Med 140:775, 1980.

Spyker DA: Submersion injury: epidemiology, prevention, and management. Pediatr Clin North Am 32:113, 1985.

Wallace JF: Drowning and near-drowning. In Braunwald E, et al (eds): Harrison's Principles of Internal Medicine. 11th edition. Philadelphia, W. B. Saunders Co., 1987, p. 861.

94. Burns

David J. Pierson

David J. Pierson

Definition

Approximately 2 million persons in the United States sustain burn injuries requiring medical attention each year, and 70,000 of these require hospitalization. In recent years, few areas in medicine have seen advances as clinically significant as those that have occurred in burn care. The mortality rate among patients aged 10–30 years with 50 percent total body surface area (TBSA) burns fell from 50 percent in 1964 to about 10 percent in 1984, and similarly impressive gains have been made in rehabilitation and psychosocial outcome among survivors. A major reason for these advances has been the development of specialized centers for burn care, of which there are now 150 in the United States.

Included in the general topic of burns are thermal, chemical, radiation, electrical, and cold injuries, of which only the first will be covered here. Electrical and radiation injuries are discussed in Chapters 99 and 100. Smoke inhalation, an important feature in many patients with thermal burns and a major determinant of morbidity and mortality, is covered in Chapter 95.

Pathophysiology

The physiologic impact of a thermal burn is determined by its depth and how much body surface it involves. First-degree burns may be extremely painful but generally have minimal physiologic impact; only the superficial epidermal layer is devitalized, and healing requires only 4–6 days. Second-degree or partial-thickness burns destroy varying amounts of epidermis and produce blistering, congestion, and coagulation in the subdermal plexus; some skin elements survive, but healing may be prolonged. Third-degree (full-thickness) burns destroy all skin elements, and healing requires skin grafting.

The initial hours following thermal injury are dominated physiologically by massive fluid shifts and resultant cardiovascular impairment, which are proportional in severity to the size of the burn. Increased microvascular permeability and interstitial osmotic pressure lead to massive loss of fluid and protein from the intravascular space, leading to burn shock if fluid resuscitation is not initiated promptly. Diminished renal perfusion from hypovolemia can lead to oliguria and subsequent acute renal failure, which is furthered by massive red blood cell destruction, both immediately and for several days after the burn.

Other hematologic changes include immediate thrombocytopenia and hypofibrinogenemia, which tend to resolve after fluid resuscitation. Gastric and intestinal hypoperfusion and other factors lead to ileus in the majority of patients. A catabolic endocrine pattern occurs, accompanied by increases in metabolic requirements that are markedly greater than those seen in other types of trauma. All aspects of immune function are profoundly affected, roughly in proportion to the size of the burn. Normal temperature regulation is lost; patients with major burns become virtually poikilothermic and are thus prone to rapid heat loss if the ambient temperature is not maintained at 30°C or higher.

DIAGNOSIS

Because fluid resuscitation and prognosis are determined by the depth and size of the burn as well as by body weight, initial estimation of these factors is important. First-degree burns are erythematous and blanch on pressure; they are dry or with small or moderate-sized blisters and are painful. First-degree burns are not considered in calculation of the area of burn. Second-degree burns are pink or mottled red, have bullae or a moist, weeping surface, and are painful. In third-degree burns, the affected skin is white, charred, or translucent; it is hard and dry, with visible thrombosis of superficial vessels, and is without sensation to the touch.

In initial calculation of the TBSA involved, second- and third-degree areas are considered together, since they have the same physiologic impact. The "Rule of Nines" may be used for adult patients: Each upper limb contributes 9 percent; each lower limb, 18 percent; the anterior and posterior aspects of the trunk, each 18 percent; the head and neck, 9 percent; and the perineum and genitalia, 1 percent. This quick method is not appropriate for children, in whom the proportions of body surface area contributed by head and extremities vary with age and size.

Burns may be classified into "moderate" and "major" according to size, depth, and other factors (Table 94–1). Moderate thermal burns can be managed in a general hospital setting, but patients with major thermal burns, inhalation injury, electrical injury, or associated mechanical trauma should be transferred to a specialized burn unit or burn center. Patients whose conditions are medically complicated because of age, coexisting disease, or other factors should also be cared for in a burn unit.

TABLE 94–1. CLINICAL CLASSIFICATION OF BURN INJURIES

MODERATE (can be managed in general hospital)
  Second-degree burns
    Adults: 15–25 percent of body surface area
    Children: 10–20 percent of body surface area
  Third-degree burns
    Adults or children: <10 percent of body surface area
  No involvement of eyes, ears, face, hands, feet, or perineum

MAJOR (should be managed in specialized burn unit or burn center)
  Second-degree burns
    Adults: >25 percent of body surface area
    Children: >20 percent of body surface area
  Third-degree burns
    Adults or children: >10 percent of body surface area
  Inhalation injury
  Electrical injury
  Associated long-bone fractures or other trauma
  Significant underlying medical condition

MANAGEMENT

Initial Care. Removal from the source of injury, assurance of an adequate airway, and establishment of intravenous access are important immediate measures. Because fluid requirements are greatest in the first 8 hours following a burn, intravenous administration of salt-containing fluid should begin as soon as possible in any patient with a burn of greater than 15 percent of TBSA. Tetanus prophylaxis should be administered if the patient has not had this immunization within 12 months.

Fluid Resuscitation. The primary purpose of fluid resuscitation is to maintain vital organ function during the marked and variable volume shifts that occur in the first 48 hours. What fluids to administer and how rapidly to give them are controversial questions, and approaches differ in different centers.

The "gold standard" resuscitation regimen is the Parkland formula: During the first 24 hours, lactated Ringer's solution, 4.0 ml/kg/percent TBSA of burn, is administered, one half of the total being given in the initial 8 hours following injury and one fourth in each subsequent 8 hours. Urine output is kept at 30–70 L/hr. No colloid-containing fluid nor 5 percent glucose is given in the first 24 hours. In the second 24 hours, colloid-containing fluid equivalent to plasma is administered to 20–60 percent of calculated plasma volume plus glucose in water as necessary to maintain a urine output of 30–100 ml/hr.

Some authorities prefer to give less total fluid during the first 24 hours, as in the modified Brooke formula: lactated Ringer's solution, 2.0 ml/kg/percent TBSA of burn in the first 24 hours, followed by 0.3–0.5 ml/kg/percent TBSA of burn of colloid-containing fluid equivalent to plasma, supplemented as necessary with glucose in water to maintain urine output.

Monitoring. Whatever regimen is used, the patient's physiologic response must be monitored carefully and adjustments made as needed. Vital signs and urine output should be monitored at least hourly. Difficult access and the risk of infection make invasive hemodynamic monitoring a larger undertaking in burned patients than in others in the ICU, but most clinicians feel that arterial and pulmonary artery catheters are sufficiently important in management, particularly in the case of serious respiratory dysfunction or underlying cardiovascular disease, to justify their use.

Analgesia and Sedation. Requirements for systemic analgesia and sedation are inversely proportional to burn depth, and patients with extensive third-degree burns require less than might be anticipated. It is important to exclude hypoxemia and hypovolemia as causes for restlessness and agitation, rather than to automatically administer sedation. Repeated small intravenous doses of morphine or other narcotic analgesic should be given rather than subcutaneous and intramuscular injections, especially during the initial period of hemodynamic instability, as the latter may be erratically absorbed with later inadvertent overdosage.

Topical Antibiotics. These have markedly reduced the incidence of burn-wound sepsis, and several types are in wide use. Sodium mafenide (Sulfamylon) requires no dressings but causes pain on application; it may produce metabolic acidosis through inhibition of carbonic anhydrase, and emergence of resistant organisms is frequent. Silver nitrate 0.5 percent requires dressings, may produce electrolyte abnormalities, and can cause methemoglobinemia. Silver sulfadiazine (Silvadene) is not painful on application and requires no dressing, but its use may lead to resistant organisms and allergic reactions. Povidone-iodine (Betadine) is effective but requires a dressing when the cream is used and causes pain on application; it also produces drying of the eschar, which may interfere with healing. Systemic antibiotics should not be given prophylactically but should be reserved for treatment of documented infections and selected according to bacterial susceptibility testing. Burn wound infection is assessed by biopsy of the wound itself; significant infection is defined as a bacterial content of $>10^5$ organisms per gram of tissue. Corticosteroids predispose to infection and have not been shown to improve mortality or morbidity.

Wound Management. Escharotomy to relieve pressure on the peripheral circulation should be considered when cyanosis, impaired capillary refilling, or paresthesias or persistent deep tissue pain occur. More reliable assessment of peripheral perfusion can be obtained by examination of the affected distal palmar arch or posterior tibial artery with an ultrasonic flowmeter. Progressive tachypnea, dyspnea, reduction in vital capacity, and other signs of pulmonary restriction may warrant chest wall escharotomy. Fasciotomy may be necessary, particularly in electrical injury, concomitant long-bone fracture, or deep burns involving muscle.

One important advance in burn care during the last decade has been early excision and closure of the burn wound, instead of the traditional nonoperative regimen. In some centers, sequential excision and grafting of portions of the total burn wound begins 2–4 days after the injury and continues at 4–5 day intervals until the wound is completely closed. This regimen has resulted in significant reductions in hospital stay and infectious complications.

Complications. Multiple organ-system failure in the setting of sepsis syndrome (see Chapter 27) is the leading cause of death in burned patients. The lungs and the burn wound are the usual primary sites. Pneumonia may be either airborne or hematogenous. Nosocomial airborne pneumonia is similar to that seen in other critically ill patients (see Chapter 24). Bloodborne pneumonia tends to occur late in the postburn course and is due to a septic focus elsewhere in the body; common sources are the burn wound, suppurative thrombophlebitis at a current or previous catheter site (which may cause few local signs), an occult visceral perforation, or a soft-tissue abscess. Bacteremia is common in association with wound care procedures and may involve more than one organism. Onset of sepsis syndrome is often heralded by the appearance of new coagulation abnormalities and progressive glucose intolerance.

OUTCOME

Survival after major burns has improved dramatically since the early 1960s, when most patients with burns involving 30 percent of TBSA died. Today the size of burn, expressed as a percent of TBSA, that is fatal to 50 percent of patients (the LA_{50}), is approximately 62 percent for individuals aged 0–40 years, 38 percent for ages 40–65, and 25 percent for age >65 years. Morbidity has also been markedly reduced: In several centers, more than 90 percent of survivors return to occupations as financially remunerative as those they had prior to the burn.

RECOMMENDED READING

Curreri PW, Luterman A: Burns. In Schwartz SI, et al (eds): Principles of Surgery. 4th edition. New York, McGraw-Hill, Inc., 1984, p. 269.
Demling RH: Burns. N Engl J Med 313:1389, 1985.
Demling RH: Infections following burns. In Hoeprich P (ed): Infectious Diseases. Hagerstown, Md. Harper & Row Publishers, Inc., 1984, p. 1348.
Demling RH: Improved survival after massive burns. J Trauma 23:179, 1983.

Engrav LH, et al: Early excision and grafting vs. nonoperative treatment of burns of indeterminant depth: a randomized prospective study. J Trauma 23:1001, 1983.

Gray, DT, et al: Early surgical excision versus conventional therapy in patients with 20 to 40 percent burns: a comparative study. Am J Surg 144:76, 1982.

Herndon DN, et al: Treatment of burns in children. Pediatr Clin North Am 32:1311, 1985.

Luterman A, Dacso CC, Curreri PW: Infections in burn patients. Am J Med 81(1A):45, 1986.

Martyn J: Clinical pharmacology and drug therapy in the burned patient. Anesthesiology 65:67, 1986.

Pruitt BA Jr, Goodwin CW Jr: Burns: including cold, chemical, and electrical injuries. In Sabiston DC Jr (ed): Textbook of Surgery. 13th edition. Philadelphia, W. B. Saunders Co., 1986, p. 214.

Pruitt BA Jr, et al: Current treatment of the extensively burned patient. Surg Annu 15:331, 1983.

95. Smoke Inhalation

David J. Pierson

David J. Pierson

Definition

Inhalation injury is a principal cause of death in fires and is being recognized in burned patients more frequently than in the past. Depending upon population base and location, as many as one third of all patients admitted to specialized burn centers suffer from smoke inhalation injury. As defined here, inhalation injury includes carbon monoxide poisoning, respiratory thermal injury, and chemical injury to the respiratory system from the inhalation of smoke.

Pathophysiology

Carbon monoxide poisoning is the most immediately life-threatening aspect of inhalation injury from fires. By combining preferentially with hemoglobin to produce carboxyhemoglobin (COHb), carbon monoxide displaces oxygen and reduces the systemic arterial oxygen content (CaO_2). It also causes a leftward shift of the oxygen-hemoglobin dissociation curve, further reducing the quantity of oxygen that is released at the tissue level. Carbon monoxide does not affect the systemic arterial oxygen tension (PaO_2), however, so that its presence is not detected by arterial blood gas analysis. Because the peripheral chemoreceptors that mediate hypoxic ventilatory drive are sensitive to PaO_2, not CaO_2, carbon monoxide poisoning does not cause dyspnea or tachypnea until it causes hypoxemia from circulatory dysfunction or lactic acidosis from tissue hypoxia.

Thermal injury affects only those portions of the respiratory tract above the larynx, except in the rare event of steam inhalation. Even with direct exposure to flame, the upper airway absorbs enough thermal energy to prevent the tracheal temperature from rising above 50 °C. Severe upper airway burns may occur, however, and mucosal swelling can rapidly compromise airway patency.

Chemical injury to the lower respiratory tract is a major contributor to morbidity and mortality in fires, and its severity correlates poorly with the presence or severity of cutaneous thermal burns. It is caused by particulate matter and soluble gases generated by the incomplete combustion of wood, plastics, textiles, rubber, and other materials. It is mainly an airway injury, the location of which in the tracheobronchial tree depends upon duration of exposure, particle size, and the solubility of the gases generated; alveolar involvement is unusual in the initial 2–3 days after smoke inhalation.

Burning polyvinyl chloride and other plastics liberate water-soluble gases such as hydrogen chloride, ammonia, and sulfur dioxide, which form strong acids or bases on contact with the moist surfaces of the respiratory tract, producing bronchospasm, mucosal edema, and ulceration. Phosgene from burning plastic also reacts with water to form hydrochloric acid. Lipid-soluble substances such as aldehydes and oxides of nitrogen, which are adsorbed onto carbon particles and carried into the lower airways, damage mucosal cells by denaturing proteins in their cell membranes. Substances inhaled in smoke trigger alveolar macrophages to release potent chemotaxins, which compound the inflammatory response.

Although bronchospasm and mucosal irritation may be immediate, the patient is often only minimally symptomatic during the first day after smoke inhalation, and overt airway edema tends not to be clinically evident for 24 hours or more. By 48–72 hours, pseudomembranes consisting of sloughed tracheobronchial mucosa and inflammatory products may begin to be coughed up, and these can obstruct small and medium-sized airways, producing atelectasis. Bronchopneumonia is a common later sequel.

DIAGNOSIS

The symptoms and signs of carbon monoxide poisoning depend upon the degree to which the patient's hemoglobin becomes replaced by COHb; patients with levels below 10 percent are usually asymptomatic. As COHb increases, however, especially above 20 percent, the patient may have headache, dizziness, confusion, and nausea. Chest pain due to myocardial hypoxia may occur. Semicoma and seizures are common with levels above 40 percent, and death is likely with greater than 60 percent COHb.

Carbon monoxide does not affect PaO_2 or $PaCO_2$ until the level exceeds about 40 percent COHb in most individuals, and cyanosis is absent. Correct diagnosis requires measurement of COHb.

With thermal injury to the upper respiratory tract the principal concern is for airway patency. Inspiratory stridor and progressive mucosal edema of the hypopharynx are indications for urgent endotracheal intubation.

Chemical smoke inhalation injury should be suspected in anyone who was burned in an enclosed space, who has sustained facial burns or singeing of nasal hairs, or who was exposed to smoke during a period of impaired mentation because of alcohol, drugs, or head trauma. More reliably, inhalation injury is likely whenever there is frank inflammation of the oropharyngeal mucosa. Other signs include brassy cough, hoarseness, wheezing, bronchorrhea, and carbon-containing sputum. A patient who is hypoxemic without obvious explanation after a fire, especially if the PaO_2 is less than 300 mm Hg on an inspired oxygen fraction (FIO_2) of 1.0, should be observed for smoke inhalation injury.

More specific confirmation of inhalation injury within the first 24 hours can be obtained by fiberoptic bronchoscopy. Typical bronchoscopic findings include carbonaceous material in the lower airways, bronchorrhea, mucosal edema and inflammation, and the presence of ulcerations, vesicles, or mucosal hemorrhage. Abnormalities on pulmonary function testing (increased airway resistance, diminished peak expiratory flow rate, delayed nitrogen washout) and on radionuclide ventilation scanning have been reported to be early indicators of inhalation injury. These tests may be difficult to obtain in patients with significant burns, however, and their results do not reliably predict the clinical severity of injury.

Findings on the chest radiograph correlate poorly with the clinical picture. The lung fields may remain clear for 48–72 hours despite development of clinical inhalation injury.

MANAGEMENT

Oxygen at $FIO_2 = 1.0$ should be begun immediately whenever carbon monoxide poisoning is suspected. Oxygen displaces carbon monoxide from hemoglobin in direct proportion to its inspired partial pressure. Although a hyperbaric chamber may not be close enough at hand to be practically useful in this setting, oxygen given at 2–2.5 atmospheres greatly increases CaO_2 and rapidly removes COHb. Oxygen at ambient pressure and $FIO_2 = 1.0$ decreases COHb by about 50 percent in 30–40 minutes; empirically, it should be continued for 4 hours before the FIO_2 is reduced, as guided by PaO_2.

Therapy for inhalation injury is supportive, not definitive. Airway protection should be provided if there is any suspicion of upper-airway compromise, although tracheostomy through an area of cutaneous burn is contraindicated. Supplemental oxygen therapy (Chapter 34) should be given, as guided by arterial blood gas measurements; positive end-expiratory pressure (Chapter 36) may also be necessary, either with or without endotracheal intubation and mechanical ventilation. Measures such as incentive spirometry and chest physiotherapy may be helpful in preventing or treating atelectasis.

Bronchospasm should be treated with inhaled bronchodilators, aminophylline, and, if necessary, with systemic corticosteroids. However, steroids should be avoided if possible and should not be administered routinely to patients with smoke inhalation. Similarly, antimicrobial agents should be given to treat documented, specific infections and not used prophylactically.

Outcome

Smoke inhalation injury alone has a mortality rate of 5–10 percent, although this is increased by the presence and severity of underlying illness. Patients under the age of 15 years and those over 40 have a poorer prognosis than those between these ages. The presence of concomitant inhalation injury substantially increases the mortality associated with cutaneous burns. In both burns and inhalation injury, pneumonia and other pulmonary complications are the principal causes of morbidity and mortality. If the patient survives, full recovery of respiratory function is usual. Although the mechanism by which it occurs is uncertain, severe carbon monoxide poisoning can occasionally be followed by long-term neuropsychiatric sequelae.

RECOMMENDED READING

Cahalane M, Demling RH: Early respiratory abnormalities from smoke inhalation. JAMA 251:771, 1984.
Crapo RO: Smoke-inhalation injuries. JAMA 246:1694, 1981.
Curreri PW, Luterman A: Burns. In Schwartz SI, et al (eds): Principles of Surgery. 4th edition. New York, McGraw-Hill, Inc., 1984, p. 269.
Jackson DL, Menges HM: Accidental carbon monoxide poisoning. JAMA 243:772, 1980.
Larkin J, Brahos G, Moylan J: Treatment of carbon monoxide poisoning: Prognostic factors. J Trauma 16:111, 1976.
Levine BA, et al: Prospective trials of dexamethasone and aerosolized gentamycin in the treatment of inhalation injury in the burned patient. J Trauma 18:188, 1978.
Pruitt BA Jr, Goodwin CW Jr: Burns: including cold, chemical, and electrical injuries. In Sabiston DC Jr (ed): Textbook of Surgery. 13th edition. Philadelphia, W. B. Saunders Co., 1986, p. 214.
Robinson NB, et al: Steroid therapy following isolated smoke inhalation injury. J Trauma 22:876, 1982.
Teixidor HS, et al: Smoke inhalation. Radiologic manifestations. Radiology 149:383, 1983.
Winter PM, Miller JN: Carbon monoxide poisoning. JAMA 236:1502, 1976.

96. Decompression Illness and Air Embolism

David J. Pierson

DEFINITION

Dysbarism is a term that covers the complex physical, physiologic, and pharmacologic effects of gas on tissues, resulting either from a change in environmental pressure or from sustained high pressure. This chapter covers two common forms of dysbarism, decompression illness (including decompression sickness and barotrauma, which are encountered in diving), and air embolism, a form of diving barotrauma that also occurs in the hospital setting, frequently as an iatrogenic event.

PATHOPHYSIOLOGY

Both decompression sickness and diving barotrauma are due to the effects of varying environmental pressures on the volume of a gas: volume is inversely proportional to pressure, in accordance with Boyle's law. The most serious effects occur during ascent, either following prolonged deep (saturation) diving or on rising from shallow depths to the surface: Although ascending from 30 m to 20 m (99 ft to 66 ft) increases intrathoracic gas volume by only 33 percent, rising from 10 m (33 ft) to the surface halves the barometric pressure and thus doubles the gas volume. Alveolar rupture can thus occur on ascent after surprisingly shallow dives (reported in as little as one meter of water), especially in the presence of partial airway obstruction or other causes for uneven pulmonary ventilation.

Decompression Sickness. During any dive, extra inert gas (nitrogen or helium, depending upon the depth of the dive and, hence, the breathing mixture used) goes into passive solution in the body. As ambient pressure falls during too-rapid ascent, this inert gas can come out of solution, forming bubbles both in the circulating blood and within tissues. As these bubbles expand, they can block blood vessels and distort or rupture tissues; fibrin and other coagulation elements are also involved, through mechanisms that are incompletely understood. This pathophysiologic sequence is most likely to develop when recommended ascent schedules

582

are violated but also occurs in about one percent of properly conducted saturation dives.

Manifestations of decompression sickness vary in severity from minor to severe and life-threatening. "Type 1 bends" consist of skin mottling and irritation as well as limb pain. "Type 2 bends" include central nervous system involvement, most often affecting the lower cervical, thoracic, or lumbar cord segments, in addition to pulmonary barotrauma and hypovolemic shock, which can occur after excessive diuresis in response to fluid shifts during the weightlessness of diving. Unlike diving barotrauma, which becomes clinically apparent during or immediately after ascent, decompression sickness does not usually appear until some minutes or hours after the dive.

Barotrauma. This consists of direct mechanical damage due to expanding gas. It may affect several air-containing areas of the body, including the middle ear, paranasal sinuses, teeth (involving a pathologic air space in a carious tooth), and, most prominently, the lung. As seen during mechanical ventilation (see Chapter 29), alveolar rupture can become clinically evident in the form of pneumothorax, pneumomediastinum, or subcutaneous emphysema. Air can also enter the pulmonary veins and be embolized systemically (see below).

Air Embolism. Entry of gas bubbles into the pulmonary venous circulation is followed by systemic embolism, most importantly to the brain, where it produces an acute cerebrovascular accident. Air embolism is rare in ventilator-related barotrauma but is a common and dreaded feature of diving barotrauma, perhaps because larger quantities of air enter the circulation as lung volume increases during breath-hold ascent.

A different sequence results from the introduction of air into the systemic venous circulation. This occurs most commonly in the hospital during craniotomy (especially in occipital procedures), when the patient is in the semisitting position, or via central venous catheters. Negative intrathoracic pressure, particularly during inspiration, allows air to be sucked into an opened vein. Venous air embolism can also occur during cardiac bypass and hemodialysis. Small volumes of air generally cause no appreciable effects, but 100 ml or more, if injected rapidly, can be fatal. Because air can enter the venous circulation at up to 100 ml/sec through a 14-gauge needle subjected to a pressure drop of 5 cm H_2O, the potential for serious venous air embolism exists whenever large-bore central venous catheters are used.

Massive venous air embolism obstructs right ventricular forward output, producing sudden cardiovascular collapse. In addition, the mechanical effects of cardiac contraction on the air-blood interface produce a dense froth of air bubbles, which, along with platelets, red blood cells, and fibrin, further impedes pulmonary arterial flow. Increases in dead space and areas of high ventilation in relation to perfusion ($\dot{V}_A/\dot{Q}$) cause the fraction of end-tidal CO_2 ($F_{ET}CO_2$) to fall and arterial PCO_2 to rise. Hypoxemia, which may be severe, results from alveolar hypoventilation, low $\dot{V}A/\dot{Q}$ areas, and diminished cardiac output.

DIAGNOSIS

All three of these disorders produce nonspecific clinical manifestations. Diagnosis in every instance relies on a high index of suspicion and a suggestive clinical setting.

Decompression sickness should be suspected when neurologic changes or musculoskeletal symptoms develop within several hours of diving. Diving barotrauma is evident immediately when the affected individual surfaces after diving. Arterial air embolism produces sudden mental changes or acute neurologic symptoms that may be either focal or generalized. Pneumothorax produces pleuritic chest pain, cough, and dyspnea. In pneumomediastinum, chest pain is the most common symptom and may be either pleuritic or visceral in nature; a characteristic crunching sound may be audible in synchrony with cardiac systole. Subcutaneous emphysema frequently causes no symptoms but is palpable, especially at the base of the neck.

Venous air embolism may cause faintness, dizziness, chest pain, or dyspnea. A "mill-wheel" murmur may be present substernally but is usually transient. Arterial blood gas analysis usually reveals hypoxemia and hypercapnia. During surgery, the initial sign may be a fall in $F_{ET}CO_2$ or detection of air bubbles on cardiac Doppler monitoring. The electrocardiographic signs of air embolism are nonspecific and may include those of cardiac ischemia and acute *cor pulmonale*.

MANAGEMENT

Prevention of dysbarism is a major requirement in all diving, whether for pleasure or for commercial purposes, and decompression tables, indicating the maximum rate of safe ascent, are prominent features of textbooks on diving medicine.

Skin mottling and irritation, the most minor form of decompression sickness, can be treated with oxygen inhalation without further intervention. For all other forms of dysbarism, however, the only effective treatment is recompression, followed by gradual decompression. Decompression sickness involving the central nervous system is a true medical emergency.

If instituted quickly, recompression leads to complete recovery in the majority of cases; since time is crucial, the patient with suspected dysbarism must be transported to a decompression chamber as rapidly as possible. Even when the diagnosis is not made initially, however, or when decompression is otherwise delayed for several hours after onset of symptoms, substantial improvement in neurologic and other symptoms can be achieved. No other treatment can effectively be substituted for recompression.

As soon as the diagnosis of decompression sickness or air embolism is suspected and during transport to the decompression chamber, 100 percent oxygen should be given by mask or by endotracheal tube to facilitate bubble resorption. During decompression, air is briefly substituted for 100 percent oxygen at regular intervals, according to a schedule determined empirically to reduce the risk of oxygen toxicity.

Venous air embolism should be treated by immediately placing the patient's left side down, in the Trendelenburg position, by applying closed-chest compression if necessary, and, if possible, by aspirating the intracardiac air with a Swan-Ganz or other central venous catheter. The patient should be placed on 100 percent oxygen and transported to the nearest hyperbaric chamber as quickly as possible. Air transport is preferable to slower methods, keeping cabin pressure as close to 1 atmosphere as possible.

Diving-related pneumothorax should be treated as in other settings. Patients with pneumothorax who require treatment in a hyperbaric chamber should have a chest tube inserted prior to decompression. Pneumomediastinum and subcutaneous emphysema generally require no treatment other than reassurance.

Emergency information on diving medical problems, including the location of the nearest hyperbaric chamber, can be obtained either from the U.S. Air Force School of Aerospace Medicine (San Antonio, Texas, [512] 536-3281 or 536-3278) or from the U.S. Navy Experimental Diving Unit (Panama City, Florida, [904] 234-4355) on a 24-hour-a-day basis.

OUTCOME

Massive cerebral air embolism causes death within minutes. However, if recompression and gradual decompression are achieved promptly, the majority of patients with all forms of dysbarism sustained during diving will recover completely. Symptoms and signs usually resolve or improve within minutes of recompression. If treatment is delayed, recovery is slower (sometimes requiring many weeks) and is less likely to be complete.

RECOMMENDED READING

Boettger ML: Scuba diving emergencies: pulmonary overpressure accidents and decompression sickness. Ann Emerg Med 12:563, 1983.

Calder IM: Dysbarism: a review. Forensic Sci Int 30:237, 1986.
Denison DM: Disorders associated with diving. In Murray JF, Nadel J (eds): Textbook of Respiratory Medicine. Philadelphia, W. B. Saunders Co., 1988.
Denison DM: Diving medicine. In Weatherall DJ, Ledingham JGG, Warrell DA (eds): Oxford Textbook of Medicine. 2nd edition. New York, Oxford University Press, 1987, p. 6.120.
O'Quin RJ, Lakshminarayan S: Venous air embolism. Arch Intern Med 142:2173, 1982.
Paton W, Elliott DH, Smith EB (eds): Symposium on diving and life at high pressures. Philos Trans R Soc Lond. Series B: Biological Sciences 34(No. 1118):1, 1984.
Peirce EC II: Cerebral gas embolism (arterial) with special reference to iatrogenic accidents. Hyperbaric Oxygen Rev 1:161, 1980.
Strauss RH: State of the art: Diving medicine. Am Rev Respir Dis 119:1001, 1979.

97. Altitude Illness

David J. Pierson

DEFINITION

Two clinically distinct forms of acute high-altitude illness are of interest to clinicians working in critical care: acute mountain sickness (AMS) and high-altitude pulmonary edema (HAPE). The former is common among individuals who travel rapidly to altitudes above 2100–2400 m (7000–8000 ft) and needs to be recognized in order to avoid confusion with more serious conditions. HAPE is less frequent but potentially fatal, making its prompt recognition and treatment a matter of great clinical importance.

PATHOPHYSIOLOGY

Normal Altitude Adaptation. A sequence of physiologic adaptations occurs when healthy individuals ascend from sea level to the relative hypoxia of moderate altitude, several aspects of which are important to an understanding of altitude-related illness. Because of the normal hypoxic ventilatory response (HVR), ventilation increases immediately in order to increase the alveolar and hence the arterial oxygen tension; this increase in ventilation varies in different individuals, and, when substantial, it may be misinterpreted as an abnormal symptom. Within a few hours, diuresis ensues, accompanied by hemoconcentration, effectively increasing blood hemoglobin content. If the individual remains at higher altitude for a period of weeks, red-cell mass gradually increases through increased erythropoiesis.

Acute Mountain Sickness. Although its mechanism is incompletely understood, AMS may be related to maldistribution of body water and inadequate diuresis in response to the relative hypoxia and increased cardiac output that occur at higher altitude. Mild cerebral edema seems to account for many of the symptoms.

The occurrence and severity of AMS depend to some extent upon who the patients are, how high they go and how rapidly they ascend, and how strenuously they exert themselves soon after arrival. It occurs in as many as half of all the healthy trekkers to the base camp of Mt. Everest

587

and in a smaller but significant number of those who travel from the lowlands to the Rockies of Colorado and Utah to ski.

High-Altitude Pulmonary Edema. As with AMS, the pathophysiology of HAPE remains a mystery, although more is understood now than in the past. Some individuals are more susceptible to HAPE than others, especially young persons whose HVR is less brisk than the average, and both rapid ascent and strenuous exertion soon after arrival are predisposing factors. One prominent theory is that HAPE is a form of "overperfusion" pulmonary edema, which results from the combination of hypoxia (accentuated by a poor ventilatory response) and increased pulmonary perfusion brought on by exercise and perhaps abetted by insufficient diuresis. The edema fluid is characteristic of that found in increased vascular permeability but not in acute inflammation.

DIAGNOSIS

Acute Mountain Sickness. The symptoms of AMS may begin a few hours to several days following arrival at altitude and if untreated are usually maximal between days 2–5, although they may last a week or more. Headache, insomnia, and a feeling of "fuzziness in the head" are the most common symptoms, followed in frequency by anorexia, nausea, exertional dyspnea, dizziness, and diarrhea. Lassitude, incoordination, and impairment of judgment may also occur. Tachycardia, cyanosis, and Cheyne-Stokes respiration may be observed.

High-Altitude Pulmonary Edema. The clinical onset of HAPE is usually within 48–96 hours following ascent and often occurs at night. Symptoms begin insidiously and most commonly consist of fatigue, weakness, dyspnea, dry cough, and difficulty sleeping. Headache, nausea, and vomiting may also occur. Symptoms may progress to severe respiratory distress, cough productive of copious pinkish sputum, and shock, and death may follow within hours if evacuation to a lower altitude or oxygen therapy cannot be accomplished. Low-grade fever, tachypnea, tachycardia, cyanosis, inspiratory crackles on chest auscultation, and signs of cerebral edema are frequent findings.

MANAGEMENT

Both AMS and HAPE can be prevented in the majority of individuals, although there are a few persons who appear to be susceptible to repeated attacks of HAPE; for these individuals complete avoidance of altitude is the only sure prevention. The climbers' adage, "Don't go too high too fast," applies, and most authorities recommend a staged ascent, increasing altitude at not more than 300 m/day when above 2500 m. However, many persons on skiing, climbing, or trekking holidays, particularly via air travel, find adhering to such recommendations impractical and difficult.

Acute Mountain Sickness. Acetazolamide (Diamox) is effective in preventing or reducing the symptoms of AMS in most individuals. Treatment (250 mg BID) should start the day before ascent and should be continued for 3 or 4 days. Side effects of this therapy are minor but frequent and include paresthesias of the mouth, fingers, and toes, plus the impartation of an unpleasant taste to carbonated beverages. Other agents such as furosemide (Lasix) have been tried in AMS with less success, although some authors recommend furosemide as well as hyperosmolar agents such as mannitol for cases of frank cerebral edema.

High-Altitude Pulmonary Edema. The primary, life-saving treatment for HAPE is descent to lower altitude. Often an initial descent of only a few hundred meters will result in marked clinical improvement. In those unusual instances in which supplemental oxygen has been available but prompt descent has not been possible, this therapy has been rapidly effective. One study has also shown expiratory positive airway pressure (EPAP) by mask to be effective as a temporizing measure prior to descent.

Because the patient's clinical condition may deteriorate rapidly, early recognition of the symptoms of HAPE in the field is extremely important, and evacuation to lower altitude should be undertaken as soon as the disorder is suspected. Except during actual descent, the patient should be kept at strict bed rest.

Acetazolamide may be effective as preventive treatment in some susceptible individuals, but the clinical evidence for this is less compelling than in AMS. Because patients with HAPE are typically volume-depleted, furosemide and mannitol should not be used.

Patients who have experienced one episode of HAPE are at increased risk for subsequent bouts and should be advised to avoid returning to higher altitude without carefully staging their ascent. They should also avoid strenuous exertion during the first day or two after arrival.

Outcome

Acute mountain sickness is a benign, self-limiting condition that usually subsides in a few days, although headache and other symptoms may persist for weeks in a few individuals. In contrast, HAPE is a potentially fatal disorder with a reported mortality rate as high as 12 percent. Symptoms of HAPE typically improve within a few hours on administration of oxygen or descent to lower altitude, and resolve in 1–3 days. Complete recovery without sequelae can be expected.

RECOMMENDED READING

Crapo JD: Physical, chemical, and aspiration injuries of the lung. In Wyngaarden JB, Smith LH Jr (eds): Cecil Textbook of Medicine. 17th edition. Philadelphia, W. B. Saunders Co., 1985, p. 2287.

Hackett PH, Rennie D, Levine HD: The incidence, importance, and prophylaxis of acute mountain sickness. Lancet 2:1149, 1976.

Heath D, Williams DR: Man at high altitude. 2nd edition. New York, Churchill Livingstone, Inc., 1981, p. 136.

Larson EB, et al: Acute mountain sickness and acetazolamide: clinical efficacy and effect on ventilation. JAMA 248:328, 1982.

Luce JM: Respiratory adaptation and maladaptation to altitude. Phys Sports Med 7:55, 1979.

Mehan RT, Zavala DC: The pathophysiology of acute high-altitude illness. Am J Med 73:395, 1982.

Schoene RB: Pulmonary edema at high altitude: review, pathophysiology, and update. Clin Chest Med 6:491, 1985.

Schoene RB, et al: High altitude pulmonary edema: characteristics of lung lavage fluid. JAMA 256:63, 1986.

Schoene RB, et al: High-altitude pulmonary edema and exercise at 4400 meters on Mt. McKinley: effect of expiratory positive airway pressure. Chest 87:330, 1985.

West JB: Hypoxic man: lessons from extreme altitude. Aviat Space Environ Med 55:1058, 1984.

98. Snakebite

David J. Pierson

David J. Pierson

DEFINITION

45,000 cases of snakebite are reported annually in the United States, of which about 8000 are by venomous species. Of the latter, about 20 percent do not involve actual injection of venom, another 30–35 percent may be classified as minor envenomations, and the remaining 45–50 percent are major, constituting a potential threat to the life of the victim.

Of approximately 120 species of snakes in the United States, 20 are venomous enough to be potentially dangerous to man; these are in two families, the Crotalidae (pit vipers) and the Elapidae (coral snakes). More than 99 percent of bites are by pit vipers, which include the rattlesnake, the copperhead, and the cottonmouth or water moccasin. Most fatal and other major envenomations involve rattlesnake bites, whereas copperhead bites are the least serious, and cottonmouth bites are of intermediate severity.

Although poisonous species can be found in virtually all of the contiguous states, most bites occur in the Southwestern and Southern states, typically between April and October. However, with the current popularity of exotic reptiles, in zoos and in both legal and illegal private collections, snakebites may be encountered in any area of the country at any time, sometimes involving species not native to North America.

PATHOPHYSIOLOGY

Pit Viper Bites. The venoms of crotalid snakes contain mixtures of as many as 25 distinct biologically active components, mostly enzymes. Their effects vary with the species, the quantity of venom injected, and the size, age and state of health of the person bitten. Toxic effects may involve the cardiovascular, hematologic, nervous, and respiratory systems.

A prominent effect of all crotalid venoms is alteration of endothelial permeability, which results in interstitial edema, hemorrhage, and hemolysis. These effects plus the marked local release of histamine, bradykinin, and serotonin lead to local swelling, ecchymosis, and necrosis. Soft-

591

tissue swelling may be dramatic and may contribute to the hypovolemia common in snakebite.

Both coagulant and anticoagulant effects occur by a number of identified mechanisms. These produce an acute hemorrhagic diathesis, which may be manifested by hematuria, melena, hematemesis, epistaxis, or hemoptysis. Prothrombin, partial thromboplastin, and bleeding times are all prolonged.

Most snakebites occur on the hands or feet. Intense, burning pain characteristically begins immediately after envenomation, although in some instances this may be delayed. Advancing edema and ecchymosis usually appear around the puncture site within minutes. Regional lymphadenopathy commonly follows, as can frank necrosis and gangrene of the affected extremity. Muscle fasciculations in the envenomated limb or elsewhere are common, and these may occasionally become generalized and severe.

Systemic symptoms and signs include nausea, vomiting, thirst, diaphoresis, and fever. Numbness and tingling of the tongue, perioral area, scalp, fingertips, and toes are common. Severe envenomation is accompanied by hypotension and prostration; convulsions, acute renal failure, circulatory collapse, and respiratory failure may follow.

Coral Snake Bites. The venom of the coral snake is primarily neurotoxic. Locally, the bite tends to produce only minor discomfort and local swelling, and it may even go unnoticed. Symptoms may not develop for several hours; there may be numbness or tingling in the affected extremity, but the manifestations are characteristically systemic (drowsiness, weakness, nausea, vomiting) and bulbar (tongue fasciculations, dysphagia, paresis of external ocular muscles, respiratory muscle weakness).

DIAGNOSIS

Identification of the Snake. Distinguishing venomous from nonvenomous snakes may be difficult, and it is helpful if the offending reptile can be killed and brought with the patient, so long as this does not delay treatment. The animal's head should be preserved for identification and should be handled with caution: snakes may reflexly inflict venomous bites for up to one hour after death.

Pit vipers have a characteristic deep "pit' on each side of the head, between the eye and the nostril, which functions as an infrared radiation detector for locating warm-blooded prey; nonpoisonous snakes lack this feature. Crotalid snakes also have vertical, slitlike pupils, fangs, and single subcaudal plates, whereas other snakes have round pupils, no fangs, and double subcaudal plates.

Assessment of the Patient. Table 98–1 gives a clinical classification of

TABLE 98–1. PATIENT ASSESSMENT and INITIAL ANTIVENIN ADMINISTRATION IN PIT VIPER ENVENOMATION

DEGREE OF ENVENOMATION	CLINICAL MANIFESTATIONS WITHIN 30–60 MINUTES FOLLOWING BITE	INITIAL LABORATORY ABNORMALITIES	INITIAL ANTIVENIN* DOSE (vials)
None (doubtful)	Pain mild–moderate; swelling in area of bite only; no paresthesias or systemic symptoms	None	None
Minimal	Local pain (may be severe); progressive swelling in area of bite; paresthesias (perioral, scalp, fingers, toes)	None	3–5
Moderate	Severe pain; swelling of entire hand or foot, spreading in involved extremity; paresthesias; muscle fasciculations; cyanosis or ecchymosis in area of bite; nausea, vomiting, or other systemic symptoms	Mild–moderate	6–10
Severe	As above, plus edema or erythema beyond involved extremity; hypotension; shock	Severe	10–20

*Antivenin (Crotalidae) Polyvalent (Wyeth), given in 500 ml intravenous infusion, following manufacturer's instructions in antivenin kit.

pit-viper bites, along with a guide to initial therapy according to the estimated degree of envenomation when the patient is first seen. Even when the snake has been identified as a rattlesnake or other pit viper, envenomation may not have taken place; this is probably the case if the discomfort and swelling are mild and confined to the area of the bite itself. However, in this circumstance, the patient should still be observed for 4–6 hours for the appearance of delayed manifestations.

In order to monitor the venom's effects, and to aid in directing therapy after the initial dose of antivenin, the circumference of the bitten finger, hand, toe, or foot should be measured, along with two more proximal sites (wrist, forearm, and so forth), and these measurements should be repeated every 15 minutes during the first 2–4 hours.

All patients with confirmed venomous snakebite should be monitored in the intensive care unit (ICU). In pit viper bites, especially those involving rattlesnakes, laboratory assessment should include clotting studies (prothrombin time, partial thromboplastin time, platelet count, fibrinogen, fibrin split products), hematocrit or hemoglobin, electrolytes, creatine phosphokinase, indices of renal function, urinalysis, and arterial blood gases. The patient's blood should be typed and crossmatched for possible transfusion. Continuous electrocardiographic monitoring should be instituted if the envenomation is judged moderate or severe.

Patients with coral snake bites should be monitored primarily with serial physical examinations, as laboratory abnormalities are not prominent in this condition.

MANAGEMENT

First Aid. The effectiveness and safety of the traditional triad of tourniquet, incision, and suction have recently been challenged. Most authorities now recommend application of a broad pressure bandage over the bite, extending the wrap firmly over as much of the affected limb as possible, and keeping the patient quiet during transport for definitive therapy. Incision and suction over the wound probably has no effect if begun more than 10–15 minutes after the bite; if used, a single 5 mm incision not more than 2 mm deep should be made parallel with the axis of the bite, and suction should be applied using a rubber cup rather than by mouth to avoid contaminating the wound.

Antivenin. For all but the most minor envenomations, antivenin (antivenom), available in the United States in both polyvalent Crotalidae and Eastern coral snake preparations, is the essential treatment, far overshadowing first aid and other measures in importance. Snakebite is a true medical emergency, and antivenin should be begun as quickly as possible, although it may still be effective if treatment is delayed 24 hours or more. It should be given intravenously. Some clinicians favor local infection of part of one vial into the wound area, but this is of unproven value and should not be done for bites on fingers or toes.

Made with horse serum, antivenin carries a high incidence of associated serum sickness and other adverse effects. Many experienced clinicians routinely perform skin tests for hypersensitivity before proceeding, although in moderate and severe envenomation, antivenin will have to be given anyway, and both false-negative and false-positive results are fairly common. Whether or not skin testing is done, it is advisable to "piggyback" a dilute solution of epinephrine onto the infusion apparatus for use if necessary and to have diphenhydramine (Benadryl) or other antihistamine available in case of acute reaction.

Table 98–1 lists the initial doses of antivenin appropriate for each degree of envenomation, as judged by the patient's clinical state 30–60 minutes after being bitten. For minimal envenomation, the 3–5 units listed will probably be all that are required. In more severe cases, the rate of antivenin administration after the first hour should be determined by the rate of progression or improvement in signs and symptoms; in moderate envenomation, with improvement noted during the first hour, another 5 units during the subsequent 2–4 hours may be sufficient, whereas very severe cases may require 20–40 units or more over the first 4–6 hours.

Bites of the Western (Sonoran) coral snake are relatively minor and do not require specific therapy. In bites of the Eastern coral snake, the earlier strategy of observing the patient for development of systemic manifestations before administering antivenin has proven unduly hazardous. If the diagnosis is clear, 5 vials should be given immediately; although it overtreats some patients, this approach makes irreversible neurologic progression less likely.

Information about availability of antivenins for rare or exotic snake species, names and telephone numbers of regional experts, and other answers to questions about snakebite and its treatment may be obtained from the Oklahoma City Poison Control Center ([405] 275-5454), on a 7-day, 24-hour basis.

Other Therapy. When shock is present, antivenin alone may not restore hemodynamic function, and other treatment for this condition is needed (see Chapter 8). The amount of intravenous fluid given with successive antivenin doses should be appropriate for the patient's state of hydration, electrolyte status, and renal function. Local pain is often intense, and adequate analgesia should be provided along with mild sedation.

All patients should receive tetanus immunization. Antihistamines are appropriate treatment for adverse reactions to antivenin but are not otherwise helpful. Routine administration of corticosteroids or heparin is contraindicated. Antibiotics should be reserved for documented wound infections and not given prophylactically.

Surgical excision of the bite area, fasciotomy, and extensive wound debridement have been used occasionally in the past but are now believed to cause more morbidity than they prevent; surgical procedures should be unnecessary if antivenin treatment is begun promptly. Physical therapy may be necessary to avoid contractures and other complications.

OUTCOME

Prior to the widespread availability of antivenin, mortality from snakebite in the United States was 10–35 percent. It is now well under 1 percent, and both mortality and morbidity should essentially be obviated if therapy can be initiated promptly. In experienced hands, most patients require only 2–3 days' hospitalization.

RECOMMENDED READING

Christopher DG, Rodning CB: Crotalidae envenomation. South Med J 79:159, 1986.
da Silva OA, Lopez M, Godoy P: Intensive care unit treatment of acute renal failure following snake bite. Am J Trop Med Hyg 28:401, 1979.
Jenkins M, Russell FE: Physical therapy for snake venom poisoning. Phys Ther 54:1298, 1974.
Kunkel DB: Bites of venomous reptiles. Emerg Med Clin North Am 2:563, 1984.
Pearn J, et al: First-aid for snake-bite: efficacy of a constrictive bandage with limb immobilization in the management of human envenomation. Med J Aust 2:293, 1981.
Reid HA, Theakston RDG: The management of snake bite. Bull WHO 61:885, 1983.
Russell FE: Snake Venom Poisoning. Philadelphia, J. B. Lippincott Co., 1979.
Russell FE: Snake venom poisoning in the United States. Annu Rev Med 31:247, 1980.
Treatment of snakebite in the USA. Med Lett Drugs Ther 24(619):87, 1982.

99. Electrical Injuries

David J. Pierson

David J. Pierson

DEFINITION

The clinician may encounter three distinct types of electrical injury. Low-voltage injury, as from household current, typically produces sudden death from ventricular fibrillation but may cause no discernible burns or other injuries. High-voltage injury is associated with devastating tissue damage and frequent musculoskeletal injuries, as well as with cardiac arrest and other dysrhythmias. Lightning stroke, only milliseconds in duration but with a current of thousands of amperes and an electrical potential of millions of volts, resembles the other two in some respects but has unique clinical features as well.

PATHOPHYSIOLOGY

Exposure of the body to electric current can cause injury through the direct physiologic effects of electricity (muscle contraction, ventricular fibrillation, or asystole) or through heat. Electric current passing through tissue generates heat according to Joule's law, by which the heat produced (in joules) is the product of the current (in amperes), the resistance of the tissue (in ohms), and the duration of contact (in seconds). Thermal injury can also be produced if an arc is formed to the source of the current, as occurs when physical contact is broken or is only partial and by clothing or other material ignited by the electrical contact.

How severely tissue will be injured by a given exposure to electric current is determined by several factors, including the type of current; alternating current produces tetanic muscle contraction and can "freeze" the victim to the contact source. This usually happens in low-voltage injury, whereas high voltage (>1000 volts) may hurl the patient away from the source.

Different tissues vary in their resistance to the flow of electric current and thus in their propensity for sustaining damage. Bone has the highest resistance, followed by fat, tendon, skin, muscle, blood, and nerve, which is the best conductor of electricity in the body. Calluses increase the skin's surface resistance, whereas moisture markedly reduces it.

596

Other determinants of the occurrence and nature of electrical injury include the pathway taken by the current, which may be unpredictable despite known entry and exit points, the part of the body with which contact is made, the surface area of contact, and the duration of exposure.

Alternating current at 60 hertz is barely perceptible at a current flow of one milliampere (ma). The "let go" current, above which involuntary muscle contraction prevents the victim from releasing the wire or other current source, varies between 8 and 22 ma. 100 ma may induce ventricular fibrillation, and 2 amperes, ventricular standstill; the former is thus more frequent in low-voltage and the latter in high-voltage, electrical injuries.

Immediate and Early Clinical Effects. Sudden death at the scene may result from ventricular fibrillation or asystole; a third possible mechanism in low-voltage accidents in which the victim is "frozen" to the electrical source is suffocation from tetany of the thoracic muscles, although this is speculative. Victims whose dysrhythmias spontaneously reverse or who are resuscitated en route to medical care may experience seizures, paralysis, or alterations of mental status. Hypertension is common, presumably from catecholamine release. Musculoskeletal injuries, including fractures and dislocations, may result either from the force of muscular contraction or from associated falls; spinal cord injury may be present initially or may occur during resuscitative efforts.

Electrical injury produces tissue destruction far exceeding that evident externally. The characteristic pathologic finding is coagulation necrosis of muscle and other tissue. Clinically, this produces profound metabolic acidosis and massive myoglobinuria, frequently leading to acute renal failure. Vascular injury results in widespread thrombosis and hemorrhage.

Late Manifestations. These include incomplete spinal cord transection, ascending motor paralysis, transverse myelitis, and amyotrophic lateral sclerosis, which may not appear for months or even years after the injury. Cataracts are another late sequela.

Clinical Features of Lightning Stroke. Lightning may strike a person directly, usually with high mortality and morbidity, or may strike nearby, with secondary "flash" injury to the individual. In addition, current may spread along the ground and injure one or more persons in the immediate area. If the victim's clothing is wet, the current may "flash over" him or her rather than pass through the body.

Lightning stroke causes death or serious injury in one third of victims, and two thirds of survivors have significant permanent sequelae. Individuals with burns on the head or legs and those with cardiopulmonary arrest at the scene have a worse prognosis than those lacking these features.

Cutaneous burns after lightning stroke have a characteristic "feathery" appearance, which can aid in diagnosis if the lightning itself is not witnessed, and which usually resolve in a few days. Other features distinguishing this from other electrical injuries include a high incidence of tympanic membrane rupture, sensorineural deafness, and ocular defects, which include cataracts, retinal detachment, and optic nerve damage.

Diagnosis

Electrical injury commonly produces cardiorespiratory arrest through either ventricular fibrillation (low-voltage) or asystole (high-voltage or lightning stroke), so that immediate assessment at the scene must focus on cardiorespiratory function. The possibility of coexistent spinal cord injury must be kept in mind during resuscitation and transport.

An entry wound may be present, which is typically depressed and charred, with surrounding edema. There may be one or more exit wounds of various sizes and shapes, along with other burns that may range from first to fourth degree in severity. Tissue damage should be assumed to be more extensive than is initially apparent. Associated skeletal and visceral injuries should be sought.

Initial evaluation should include assessment of fluid and acid-base status and tests for muscle enzymes in blood and for myoglobin in urine. As fluid resuscitation proceeds, urine output should be carefully monitored and involved extremities surgically evaluated for compression syndromes and to assess the need for immediate fasciotomy.

Management

Prolonged initial resuscitative efforts are justified in electrical injury because patients may recover after prolonged cardiac arrest. Electrical injuries clinically resemble crush injuries, and fluid requirements in the initial 24–48 hours may be massive. To this fluid should be added mannitol (25 g initially followed by 12.5 g/hr for 6 hr) if myoglobinuria is present. Initial metabolic acidosis may be profound and may respond poorly to fluid administration.

Two approaches to surgical management exist. The conservative approach relies upon early fasciotomy to decompress affected extremities, followed by reexploration at 48 hours, and then repeated inspections and debridement of devitalized tissues as the wound evolves. Proponents of this approach believe that it permits preservation of initially questionable tissue that turns out to be viable, although to leave devitalized tissue *in situ* may lead to the spread of infection into adjacent, marginally perfused areas. An initially more aggressive approach uses early excision and grafting of the area of injury; advocates of this procedure claim shortened hospitalization, lower mortality, and reduced morbidity from infection.

OUTCOME

Although victims of electrical injury may initially be retrieved from sudden death, tissue destruction and the likelihood of metabolic, infectious, and other early complications tend to make the outlook less optimistic than it might otherwise be. In high-voltage electrical injury, and particularly following lightning stroke, debilitating neurologic and other late sequelae are common, affecting as many as two thirds of survivors. Because many electrical injuries occur on the job, however, and most victims are young, intensive efforts are fully justified.

RECOMMENDED READING

Bartholome CW, Jacoby DW, Ramchand SC: Cutaneous manifestations of lightning injury. Arch Dermatol 111:1466, 1975.
Cooper MA: Electrical and lightning injuries. Emerg Med Clin North Am 2:489, 1984.
Cooper MA: Lightning injuries: prognostic signs for death. Ann Emerg Med 9:134, 1980.
Dixon GF: The evaluation and management of electrical injuries. Crit Care Med 11:384, 1983.
Esses SI, Peters WJ: Electrical burns: Pathophysiology and complications. Can J Surg 24:11, 1981.
Kobernick M: Electrical injuries: Pathophysiology and emergency management. Ann Emerg Med 11:633, 1982.
Rouse RG, Dimick AR: The treatment of electrical injury compared to burn injury: a review of pathophysiology and comparison of patient management protocols. J Trauma 18:43, 1978.
Sances A Jr, et al: Electrical injuries. Surg Gynecol Obstet 149:97, 1979.
Tribble CG, et al: Lightning injuries. Compr Ther 11:32, 1985.
Wright RK, Davis JH: The investigation of electrical deaths: a report of 220 fatalities. J Forensic Sci 25:514, 1980.

100. Radiation Injury

David J. Pierson

INTRODUCTION

Radiation accidents are infrequent, even when radioactive materials are used routinely. However, such accidents may occur not only in nuclear power plants but also in medical centers and research laboratories, in industry, during handling or transport of medical or research radionuclides, or during the disposal of nuclear waste, so that emergency department and intensive care unit (ICU) personnel may encounter patients with acute radiation injury at any time. Such injuries may involve large numbers of patients and may include wounds and other trauma.

Medically important ionizing radiation occurs as accelerated particles (*alpha* and *beta*) and as electromagnetic waves (*gamma* and roentgen or x-rays). Accelerated particles do not penetrate deeply into intact skin and thus cause only surface damage; however, their effects are much more injurious in the presence of open wounds or if they enter the body by inhalation or ingestion. Electromagnetic waves penetrate deeply into the body and cause great damage to radiosensitive tissues.

Technically, radiation injury includes the effects of ultraviolet irradiation and microwaves and also the effects of local radiotherapy for malignancy, but these are not considered here. Likewise, although the effects of radiation injury may occur after years or even generations, this chapter focuses on manifestations only during the first weeks following exposure.

Exposure to radiation is currently measured in grays (Gy), with 1 Gy = 100 rad, or an energy deposition of 1 joule/kg.

PATHOPHYSIOLOGY

Radiation may cause injury through either thermal or ionizing effects, by three basic mechanisms: contamination, in which radioactive dust, solid particles, or liquid becomes physically attached to the victim or to his or her clothing; incorporation, in which radioactive material contaminates an open wound or is inhaled or ingested; and irradiation, in which injury results from the passage of a high flux of electromagnetic waves into or through the victim. The first two of these are medical emergencies,

600

because injury will continue irreversibly as long as the victim is in contact with the radioactive material. Injury in individuals who have been subjected to irradiation has already occurred, and they are not radioactive.

Figure 100–1 depicts the sequence of events that follows acute radiation exposure. Although the actual injury occurs at the time of irradiation, its clinical manifestations appear later and evolve in a characteristic sequence depending upon the radiation dose (Table 100–1).

A prodromal syndrome of anorexia, nausea, and vomiting, of central nervous system origin, has its onset within a few hours of exposure: The larger the dose, the sooner the onset of vomiting. This syndrome resolves spontaneously in 1–2 days and is followed by a quiescent or latent period of up to 2–3 weeks—again, depending upon the dose received.

Exposures to up to 10 Gy (1000 rad) produce a clinical picture of acute radiation sickness that is dominated by damage to the hematopoietic system. Circulating lymphocytes are killed outright and begin to disappear immediately, providing a clinical indicator of the seriousness of the injury. Granulocytes and platelets decline more gradually and reach their nadirs at about 3 weeks. The clinical picture produced is essentially that seen in acute leukemia with pancytopenia, with purpura and hemorrhage, as well as bacterial, viral, and fungal infections, constituting the main threats to life.

A "gastrointestinal syndrome," dominated by diarrhea and fulminating enteritis secondary to loss of small bowel lining, occurs several days after exposure to doses exceeding about 10 Gy (1000 rad). Although survival is theoretically possible with maximal supportive measures and bone marrow transplantation, this syndrome is considered uniformly fatal. When acute exposure exceeds 20–30 Gy (2000–3000 rad), a picture of cardiovascular collapse, encephalopathy, and death ensues within 1–2 days.

Observations of the atomic bomb victims from Hiroshima and Nagasaki in 1945 indicated that the $LD_{50/60}$ (radiation dose fatal within the first 60 days to 50 percent of those exposed) in humans was about 4 Gy (400 rad). With currently available isolation procedures, blood product support, and antibiotics, survival with spontaneous bone marrow regeneration may now occur after doses of up to 6 Gy (600 rad). Experience following the 1986 nuclear power plant disaster at Chernobyl indicates that, with bone marrow transplantation and other maximal support, the $LD_{50/60}$ is now above 6 Gy and is perhaps as high as 10 Gy. Concomitant thermal burns, wounds, and other injuries substantially lower the $LD_{50/60}$, as do preexisting disease and malnutrition.

DIAGNOSIS

Evaluation of the patient with acute radiation injury initially focuses on gauging the severity of exposure because of the pathophysiologic and

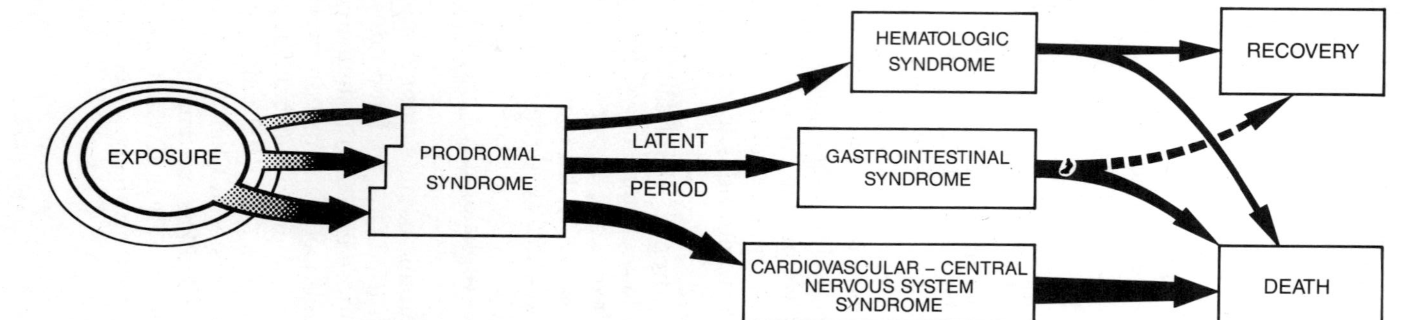

FIGURE 100–1. Natural history of acute radiation injury. Clinical manifestations and their timing are determined by the radiation dose received. See text for further explanation.

TABLE 100–1. MANIFESTATIONS, THERAPY, AND EXPECTED OUTCOME AFTER ACUTE RADIATION EXPOSURE

RADIATION DOSE Gy (Rad)	PRODROMAL VOMITING *Incidence* (Onset)	PREDOMINANT MANIFESTATIONS	THERAPY	EXPECTED OUTCOME
0–1 (0–100)	None	—	Reassurance	Early mortality = 0 Possible late sterility Carcinogenesis, mutagenesis
1–2 (100–200)	25–50 percent (3–6 hr)	Hematologic (lymphopenia)	Observation	Early mortality = 0 Possible late sterility Carcinogenesis, mutagenesis
2–6 (200–600)	75–100 percent (1–2 hr)	*Hematologic* (leukopenia, thrombocytopenia, purpura, hemorrhage, infection)	Erythrocytes Granulocytes Platelets Antibiotics (Bone marrow transplantation)	Mortality = 20–80 percent in first 4–8 weeks—from infection, hemorrhage Possible late effects in survivors
6–10 (600–1000)	100 percent (1 hr)	*Hematologic* (leukopenia, thrombocytopenia, purpura, hemorrhage, infection) Gastrointestinal (diarrhea, enteritis) Epilation	Bone marrow transplantation Erythrocytes Granulocytes Platelets Antibiotics	Mortality = 80–100 percent in first 4–8 weeks—from infection, hemorrhage Likely late effects in survivors
>100 (>1000)	100 percent (½ hr)	*Gastrointestinal* (diarrhea, enteritis) Cardiovascular (shock, circulatory collapse) Central nervous system (acute encephalopathy)	Fluids Electrolytes Symptomatic therapy (?? Bone marrow transplantation)	Mortality = 100 percent in first 2–3 weeks—from enteritis, sepsis

prognostic importance of this factor (see Table 100–1). The radiation dose is estimated using information obtained at the accident site (proximity of patient to source, duration of exposure, inhalation of fumes, dosimetry at the site), from dosimetry of the patient and his clothing on arrival, and from the timing of the onset of vomiting. Physical examination should seek evidence of skin burns, erythema of conjunctiva or other mucous membranes, and associated wounds or other trauma.

Laboratory evaluation on arrival should include a white blood cell count and differential in order to estimate the number of circulating lymphocytes; these counts should be repeated at intervals to assess the rate of lymphocyte disappearance. If the lymphocyte count is >1200 cells/

mm³ 24 hours after the injury, serious bone marrow depression is unlikely; however, if the count is below 500/mm³ in the first 24 hours, the injury is severe. Complete disappearance of lymphocytes from the peripheral blood within 6 hours indicates a fatal exposure. The granulocyte count may be elevated to 10,000/mm³ or more during the first 24–48 hours.

Lymphocyte culture for chromosome analysis may be helpful in assessing the degree of exposure or in confirming the diagnosis of radiation injury if this is uncertain. Blood for cytogenetic studies should be obtained as soon as possible, although the results may be unavailable for several days. When exposure has been such that major bone marrow depression is likely, it is important to obtain consultation early with regard to possible bone marrow transplantation, as blood and bone marrow samples will be needed early if this is to be done.

MANAGEMENT

Management of acute radiation injury consists of removal of the patient from the exposure source (rescue, decontamination, and removal of material ingested or otherwise retained in the body), observation and general supportive care, and specific measures indicated by the clinical onset of leukopenia and thrombocytopenia.

Decontamination should be carried out in the receiving facility according to one of several published protocols (see references) in consultation with a radiation safety officer. Essentially, decontamination consists of removal and isolation of the patient's clothing and gentle but thorough cleansing of all exposed skin with soap and water, retaining and isolating the waste water if possible. Treatment in a specialized radiation treatment facility is indicated if the estimated exposure exceeds 1 Gy (100 rad), if there is residual radioactivity in wounds after initial decontamination, if substantial internal contamination has occurred, or if there is significant complicating illness.

Removal of radioactive substances from the body (decorporation) should commence immediately, as these will continue to injure tissue until removed. Decorporation includes superficial debridement of wounds if contamination persists after irrigation, as indicated by Geiger-Müller meter, and gastric lavage if material has been ingested.

A variety of substances may be administered to bind, precipitate, or otherwise hasten elimination of the radioactive material. These include DTPA (diethylenetriaminepentaacetic acid), the most effective chelating agent for actinide isotopes such as plutonium; DTPA is available only from the U.S. Department of Energy and must be administered promptly. It is given intravenously (0.5–1.0 gm in 250 ml saline, repeated in 1 hour). Other agents for oral administration, depending upon the radiation source, include the following: soluble phosphate (for ^{32}P); magnesium sulfate, epsom salts, or barium sulfate (for radium); aluminum phosphate gel (for strontium); and potassium iodide (to prevent thyroid uptake of ^{131}I, either as 130 mg tablets or several drops of supersaturated solution). Antacids precipitate metal as insoluble salts, and cathartics shorten transit time for any ingested agent.

Patients with radiation injury need specific therapy for associated burns, wounds and other trauma. Appropriate fluid and electrolyte administration is important, as these patients are often dehydrated on initial presentation. Management, once marrow depression is clinically evident, is essentially that of other patients who are pancytopenic, including transfusion, granulocytes, platelets, antibiotics (both prophylactically, when indicated, and for specific infection), hyperalimentation, and careful nursing, using laminar-flow or "life-island" isolation if possible. If bone marrow transplantation is to be considered based on the initial estimate of radiation exposure, this should ideally be undertaken by about 10 days, so that marrow recovery can coincide with the expected nadir of the patient's own cell counts.

OUTCOME

As Table 100–1 indicates, the likelihood of survival in acute radiation injury is mainly a function of the dose of radiation that the patient has received. Concomitant injury or illness worsens the prognosis, as do advanced age and malnutrition. Patients who survive may later develop sterility (sperm count nadir is at 7–8 weeks), cataracts (which may develop 1 or more years after exposure), and persistent T-lymphocyte dysfunction that may last for years.

RECOMMENDED READING

American Medical Association: A guide to the hospital management of injuries arising from exposure to or involving ionizing radiation. Chicago, American Medical Association, 1984.

American National Standards Institute: ANSI guide for hospital emergency departments on handling radiation accident victims. Washington, D.C., American National Standards Institute, ANSI Report N13.28, 1987.

Geiger HJ: The accident at Chernobyl and the medical response. JAMA 256:609, 1986.

Hendee WR: Management of individuals accidentally exposed to radiation or radioactive materials. Semin Nucl Med 16:203, 1986.

Hubner KF, Fry SA (eds): The Medical Basis for Radioactive Accident Preparedness. New York, Elsevier North Holland, 1980.

Leaf A: New perspectives on the medical consequences of nuclear war. N Engl J Med 315:905, 1986.

Leonard RB, Ricks RC: Emergency department radiation protocol. Ann Emerg Med 9:462, 1980.
Phillips TL: Radiation injury. In Wyngaarden JB, Smith LH Jr (eds): Cecil Textbook of Medicine. 17th edition. Philadelphia, W. B. Saunders Co., 1985, p. 2297.
Richter LL, et al: A systems approach to the management of radiation accidents. Ann Emerg Med 9:303, 1980.
Wald N: Diagnosis and therapy of radiation injuries. Bull NY Acad Med 59:1129, 1983.

Index

Page numbers in italics indicate illustrations;
those followed by t indicate tables.